Durgin & Hanan's
PHARMACY PRACTICE FOR TECHNICIANS

Fourth Edition

JANE M. DURGIN, CIJ, RPh, RN, MS, EdD
ZACHARY I. HANAN, RPh, MS, FASHP, FASCP

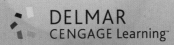

DELMAR
CENGAGE Learning

Australia • Brazil • Japan • Korea • Mexico • Singapore • Spain • United Kingdom • United States

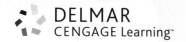
DELMAR
CENGAGE Learning™

Durgin and Hanan's Pharmacy Practice for Technicians

Jane M. Durgin and Zachary I. Hanan

Vice President, Career and Professional Editorial: Dave Garza

Director of Learning Solutions: Matthew Kane

Managing Editor: Marah Bellegarde

Senior Product Manager: Darcy Scelsi

Editorial Assistant: Meaghan O'Brien

Vice President, Career and Professional Marketing: Jennifer McAvey

Marketing Director: Wendy Mapstone

Marketing Manager: Michelle McTighe

Marketing Coordinator: Scott Chrysler

Production Director: Carolyn Miller

Content Project Manager: Kenneth McGrath

Art Director: Jack Pendleton

Technology Project Manager: Mary Colleen Liburdi

For product information and technology assistance, contact us at
Professional & Career Group Customer Support, 1-800-648-7450

For permission to use material from this text or product, submit all requests online at **www.cengage.com/permissions**
Further permissions questions can be emailed to
permissionrequest@cengage.com

Library of Congress Control Number: 2008930282

ISBN-13: 978-1-4283-2032-1

ISBN-10: 1-4283-2032-6

Delmar Cengage Learning
5 Maxwell Drive
Clifton Park, NY 12065-2919
USA

Cengage Learning products are represented in Canada by Nelson Education, Ltd.

For your lifelong learning solutions, visit **delmar.cengage.com**

Visit our corporate website at **www.cengage.com**

Notice to the Reader

Publisher does not warrant or guarantee any of the products described herein or perform any independent analysis in connection with any of the product information contained herein. Publisher does not assume, and expressly disclaims, any obligation to obtain and include information other than that provided to it by the manufacturer. The reader is expressly warned to consider and adopt all safety precautions that might be indicated by the activities described herein and to avoid all potential hazards. By following the instructions contained herein, the reader willingly assumes all risks in connection with such instructions. The publisher makes no representations or warranties of any kind, including but not limited to, the warranties of fitness for particular purpose or merchantability, nor are any such representations implied with respect to the material set forth herein, and the publisher takes no responsibility with respect to such material. The publisher shall not be liable for any special, consequential, or exemplary damages resulting, in whole or part, from the readers' use of, or reliance upon, this material.

Printed in China by China Translation & Printing Services Limited
3 4 5 6 7 12 11 10

Contents

PART I: OVERVIEW OF HEALTH CARE

PART III: PROFESSIONAL ASPECTS OF PHARMACY TECHNOLOGY

PART IV: CLINICAL ASPECTS OF PHARMACY TECHNOLOGY

PART V: ADMINISTRATIVE ASPECTS OF PHARMACY TECHNOLOGY

APPENDIXES

Preface

To meet the needs of technicians in their various training programs, it is the goal and focus of the editors to provide the technician with an understanding of the history of the profession of pharmacy and to bring current professional, clinical, and administrative information and practice trends to the student to increase his or her understanding, knowledge, and competencies of the pharmacy profession.

It is our vision and hope that this textbook will provide the background knowledge, values, attitude, and skills to assist pharmacy technicians in meeting his or her desired goals and professional participation in the practice of pharmacy.

Nearly 40 years ago in 1972, our first Manual for Pharmacy Technicians was published by C. V. Mosby Publishers. It is our distinct honor to continue to contribute to the profession and the advancement of pharmacy technicians.

Jane M. Durgin, CIJ, RPh, RN, MS, EdD
Zachary I. Hanan, RPh, MS, FASHP, FASCP

Reviewers

Glenn D. Appelt, PhD, RPht
Columbia Southern University
Orange Beach, Alabama

Donald Becker
San Jacinto College
Houston, Texas

David P. Elder, RPh
Skagit Valley College
Mt. Vernon, Washington

Michael Ellis
Trinity College
Fairfield, California

Michelle C. McCranie, CPhT, AAS
Ogeechee Technical College
Statesboro, Georgia

Jim Mizner, RPh, MBA
Pharmacy Technician Training Program Coordinator
Applied Career Training
Rosslyn, Virginia

Diana Rangraves, PharmD, RPh
Santa Rosa Junior College
Santa Rosa, California

Traci Tonhofer
Davis Applied Technology College
Kaysville, Utah

Reviewers of Second and Third Editions

Renee Ahrens, PharmD, MBA
Shenandoah University
Winchester, Virginia

Cheri Boggs, BA, CPhT
El Paso Community College
La Mesa, New Mexico

Carolyn Bunker, RPh
Salt Lake City Community College
Salt Lake City, Utah

Sharon Burton-Young, RN
POLY Tech Adult Education
Woodside, Delaware

Jane Doucette, RPh
Salt Lake City Community College
Salt Lake City, Utah

Emery C. Fellows, Jr., CPhT
Pima Medical Institute
Denver, Colorado

Elizabeth Johnson
Houston Community College System
Southeast College
Houston, Texas

Percy M. Johnson
Bidwell Training
Pittsburgh, Pennsylvania

Carol Miller, EdD, CPhT
Miami-Dade Community College
Miami, Florida

Kathy Moscou, BS Pharmacy
North Seattle Community College
Seattle, Washington

Larry Nesmith, BS Ed
Academy of Health Sciences, AMEDD Center & School
Pharmacy Branch, Fort Sam Houston, U.S. Army
San Antonio, Texas

Glen E. Rolfson, RPh
Salt Lake Community College
Salt Lake City, Utah

Peter E. Vondereau, RPh
Cuyahoga Community College
Highland Falls Village, Ohio

Tova R. Wiegand-Green
Ivy Tech State College
Fort Wayne, Indiana

Acknowledgments

We wish to acknowledge and thank our professional colleagues, personal friends, peers, and associates from academia, institutional and community practice, and state and national organizations, who have dedicated their expertise and taken the time to make a personal commitment to participate, and without whom this publication would not have been possible.

Each of our authors has enhanced the content of the fourth edition of our textbook. Their knowledge and experience are evident in their contributions to their respective chapters. Their support of the education and training of pharmacy technicians is very much appreciated.

We also would like to thank our Developmental Editor, Darcy Scelsi, and our Project Manager, Jennifer Bonnar, for all of their coordination, support, and guidance in the development of our textbook. Also, we would like to thank Ken McGrath, Content Project Manager, Meaghan O'Brien, Editorial Assistant, and Jack Pendleton, our Art Director, for all their contributions to the numerous details required for the publication of our textbook.

Lastly, but very importantly, we would like to thank our families, our peers, and our friends for their support and encouragement during the process of the planning, development, composing, and editing of the contents of our fourth edition.

Jane M. Durgin, CIJ, RPh, RN, MS, EdD
Zachary I. Hanan, RPh, MS, FASHP, FASCP

Contributors

Jane Marie Durgin, CIJ, RPh, RN, MS, EdD
Former Professor of Pharmacy
St. John's University
College of Pharmacy and Allied Health Professionals
Jamaica, New York
Chapter 1: A History of Pharmacy

Daniel Walsh, MBA, MHA, FACHE
President and Chief Executive Officer
Winthrop University Hospital
Mineola, New York
Chapter 2: Organizational Structure and Function
   of the Hospital and Pharmacy Department

Brian Malone, RPh, MS
Director of Pharmaceutical Services
Winthrop University Hospital
Mineola, New York
Chapter 2: Organizational Structure and Function
   of the Hospital and Pharmacy Department

Barbara Limburg Mancini, PharmD, BCNSP
President
Home Care Consulting Services
Indian Head Park, Illinois
Chapter 3: Home Health Care

Janet Unger, MPA
Administrator
Chapin Home for the Aging
Jamaica, New York
Chapter 4: Long-Term Care

Dinbandhu Shah, RPh, FASCP
Clinical Director
Shore Pharmaceutical Providers, Inc.
Plainview, New York
Chapter 4: Long-Term Care

Maria Toscano, PharmD
President
Pro Med Care
Mineola, New York
Chapter 4: Long-Term Care

Maria Marzella Sulli, PharmD, CGP
Assistant Clinical Professor
Department of Clinical Pharmacy Practice
St. John's University
College of Pharmacy and Allied Health Professions
Jamaica, New York
Chapter 5: Community Pharmacy

Zachary I. Hanan, RPh, MS, FASHP, FASCP
Former Director of Pharmaceutical Services
Mercy Medical Center
Rockville Centre, New York
President
ZIH Pharmacy Associates, Inc.
Oakdale, New York
Chapter 6: Regulatory Standards in Pharmacy Practice

William N. Kelly, PharmD
Former Professor and Chairman, Department
   of Pharmacy Practice
Mercer University
Atlanta, Georgia
President
William N. Kelly Consulting, Inc.
Oldsmar, Florida
Chapter 7: Drug-Use Control: The Foundation
   of Pharmaceutical Care

Martha L. Mackey, JD
Assistant Professor of Pharmacy Administration
St. John's University
College of Pharmacy and Allied Health Professions
Jamaica, New York
Chapter 8: Ethical Considerations for the Pharmacy
   Technician
Chapter 8: Ethical Considerations for the Pharmacy
   Technician

Debra Feinberg, RPh, JD
Executive Director
New York State Council of Health-System Pharmacists
Albany, New York
Adjunct Professor
Albany College of Pharmacy
Albany, New York
Chapter 9: Pharmacy Associations

Robert Hamilton, RPh, PharmD
Professor, Department of Pharmacy Practice
Director of Continuing Professional Development
Albany College of Pharmacy
Albany, New York
Chapter 10: The Prescription

M. Elyse Wheeler, PhD, MT (ASCP)
Chair, Department of Health Sciences
Albany College of Pharmacy
Albany, New York
Chapter 11: Medical Terminology

P. L. Madan, PhD
Professor of Pharmacy and Administrative Sciences
St. John's University
College of Pharmacy and Allied Health Professions
Jamaica, New York
Chapter 12: Pharmaceutical Dosage Forms

Melinda Reed, RPh, MBA
Instructor, Department of Pharmaceutical Sciences
Albany College of Pharmacy
Albany, New York
Chapter 13: Pharmaceutical Calculations

Lee Anna Obos, RPh
Instructor, Department of Pharmaceutical Sciences
Albany College of Pharmacy
Albany, New York
Chapter 13: Pharmaceutical Calculations

Steve Laddy, RPh
President
MasterPharm Compounding Pharmacy
Richmond Hill, New York
Chapter 14: Extemporaneous Compounding

Thomas Mastanduono, RPh
Vice President
MasterPharm Compounding Pharmacy
Richmond Hill, New York
Chapter 14: Extemporaneous Compounding

Laura Thoma, PharmD
Professor of Pharmaceutical Sciences
Director, Parenteral Medication Laboratory
University of Tennessee
Memphis, Tennessee
Chapter 15: Sterile Preparation Compounding

Sabra Boughton, RN, PhD
Director of Patient Education
University Health Center, Stony Brook
Health Sciences Center, SUNY
Stony Brook, New York
Chapter 16: Administration of Medications

Laura Gianni Augusto, PharmD
Former Director, Drug Information Service
North Shore-Long Island Jewish Health System
Associate Clinical Professor
Assistant Dean for Experiential Pharmacy Education
St. John's University
College of Pharmacy and Allied Health Professions
Jamaica, New York
Chapter 17: Drug Information Centers

Sheldon Lefkowitz, RPh, MS
Director of Pharmacy Services
St. Mary's Medical Center
West Palm Beach, Florida
Chapter 18: Drug Distribution Systems

Jeffrey Spicer, MBA
Faculty
Indian River Community College
Vero Beach, Florida
Chapter 18: Drug Distribution Systems

Linda Kopman, RN, CIC
Infection Control Manager
Franklin Medical Center
Valley Stream, New York
Chapter 19: Infection Control and Prevention
   in the Pharmacy

Robert S. Kidd, MS, PharmD
Associate Professor and Vice Chair
Department of Biopharmaceutical Sciences
Bernard J. Dunn School of Pharmacy
Shenandoah University
Winchester, Virginia
Chapter 20: Introduction to Biopharmaceutics
Chapter 21: The Actions and Uses of Drugs

Regina F. Peacock, PhD
Associate Professor
Department of Biopharmaceutical Sciences
Bernard J. Dunn School of Pharmacy
Shenandoah University
Winchester, Virginia
Chapter 20: Introduction to Biopharmaceutics

L. Michael Marcum, PharmD
Department of Biopharmaceutical Services
Bernard J. Dunn School of Pharmacy
Shenandoah University
Winchester, Virginia
Chapter 21: The Actions and Uses of Drugs

Nicole M. Maisch, PharmD
Associate Clinical Professor
Department of Clinical Pharmacy Practice
St. John's University
College of Pharmacy and Allied Health Professions
Jamaica, New York
Director, Drug Information Service
North Shore-Long Island Jewish Health System
New Hyde Park, New York
Chapter 22: Nonprescription Medications

Dudley G. Moon, PhD
Professor
Basic and Pharmaceutical Sciences
Albany College of Pharmacy
Albany, New York
Chapter 23: Natural Products

Jane Marie Durgin, CIJ, RPh, RN, MS, EdD
Zachary I. Hanan, RPh, MS, FASHP, FASCP
Chapter 24: The Policy and Procedure Manual

Michael Coyne, RPh, MS
Associate Vice President and Director of Pharmacy
Staten Island University Hospital
Staten Island, New York
Chapter 25: Materials Management of Pharmaceuticals

Eric Estes, RPh
Senior Director of Operations
Future Scripts
Philadelphia, Pennsylvania
Chapter 26: The Pharmacy Formulary System

Ilene Estes, RPh, MBA
Former Director of Pharmacy in Long-Term Care
Consultant Pharmacist for Insurance Company
Chapter 26: The Pharmacy Formulary System

Edmund Hayes, RPh, MS, PharmD
Assistant Director of Pharmacy
Department of Pharmaceutical Sciences
University Medical Center, Stony Brook
Health Sciences Center, SUNY
Stony Brook, New York
Chapter 27: Computer Applications in Drug-Use Control

Matthew Grissinger, RPh
Medication Safety Analyst
Institute for Safe Medication Practices
Huntington Valley, Pennsylvania
Chapter 28: Preventing and Managing Medication
    Errors: The Technician's Role

Susan Proulx, PharmD
Vice President, Operations
Institute for Safe Medication Practices
Huntington Valley, Pennsylvania
Chapter 28: Preventing and Managing Medication
    Errors: The Technician's Role

Kenneth R. Cohen, RPh, PhD, PCD
Chief of Clinical Pharmacology and Therapeutics
Brookhaven Memorial Hospital Medical Center
Patchogue, New York
Chapter 29: Reimbursement for Pharmacy Services

Richard J. Lohne, BS, MBA, FACHE, LNHA
Administrator
Rockville Nursing Home
Rockville Centre, New York
Chapter 29: Reimbursement for Pharmacy Services

Lisa S. Lifshin, RPh
Manager, Program Services
Coordinator, Technician Training Programs
Accreditation Services Division
American Society of Health-System Pharmacists
Bethesda, Maryland
Chapter 30: Accreditation of Technician Training
    Programs

Melissa M. Murer Corrigan, RPh
Executive Director/Chief Executive Officer
Pharmacy Technician Certification Board
Washington, DC
Chapter 31: Pharmacy Technician Certification Board

Crystal L. Lipp, PharmD
Associate Director of Stakeholder Relations
Pharmacy Technician Certification Board
Washington, DC
Chapter 31: Pharmacy Technician Certification Board

Introduction

Pharmacy Technicians Are Essential in the Team Effort for Achieving Medication Safety

Five more years have passed since the publication of the third edition of *Pharmacy Practice for Technicians*. We are now nearly a decade into the twenty-first century. So much has changed in advancing the advocacy for the importance of pharmacy technicians in the promotion of a safe medication use process for all avenues of pharmacy. All of the major pharmacy organizations are advocating elevating the role of the pharmacy technician. For example, one of the American Society of Health-System Pharmacists' (ASHP) major priorities in its advocacy agenda is for all pharmacy technicians to have completed standardized accredited education and training, thereby obtaining and maintaining national certification and registration. The Pharmacy Technician Educators Council (PTEC) members have joined together to assist each and every educator to work with their boards of pharmacy when solicited to support mandatory education and recognition for pharmacy technicians.

We have now met the century mark in number of pharmacy technician training programs that have sought ASHP-accreditation. Close to 120 pharmacy technician training programs are now ASHP-accredited, including Walgreens. The larger pharmacy chains are now recognizing the value of diverse, standardized training for their employees and the greater span of functions that they can now provide. Some states now mandate in their regulations that pharmacy technicians must complete an accredited pharmacy technician training program to practice in the state or to be considered state certified (i.e., South Carolina, North Dakota, Nevada). Pharmacy technicians completing accredited programs are even involved in telemedicine practices in North Dakota. I am sure that by the time the next edition of this important training manual is published, we will see a substantial increase of accredited programs serving even greater needs across the county.

More than 250,000 pharmacy technicians have successfully passed the Pharmacy Technician Certification Exam (PTEC). Pharmacy technicians are now testing online to facilitate more accessibility in taking the exam. More states are requiring that pharmacy technicians pass and maintain Pharmacy Technician Certification Board (PTCB) certification.

Another meeting will soon be conducted by the Council on Credentialing in Pharmacy, an organization that works to ensure quality in pharmacy's credentialing programs. The organization's mission includes providing leadership and guidance for these programs in or relevant to pharmacy practice. The group, consisting of fifteen organizations, represents pharmacy in various venues and arenas on a national basis (representatives include the Academy of Managed Care Pharmacy, American Association of Colleges of Pharmacy, the American College of Apothecaries, the American Council of Pharmaceutical Education, the American College of Clinical

Pharmacy, the American Society of Consultant Pharmacists, the Commission for Certification in Geriatric Pharmacy, American Pharmacists Association, PTCB, ASHP, PTEC, Pharmacy Compounding Accreditation Board, National Alliance of State Pharmacy Associations, National Association of Boards of Pharmacy, and the Board of Pharmaceutical Specialties). The meeting serves as a follow-up to one held in 2002 that focused extensively on the importance of education and training for pharmacy technicians.

Some of the same challenges are still evident and growing in providing a safe medication-use system for patients served. The pharmacist shortage is still present. There are an increased number of prescriptions dispensed, not only to our aging population but other populations are now requiring more intensive medication therapies as well. The need for extemporaneously compounded medications for the pediatric and geriatric populations has increased. More automation, technology, and computerization have been developed for use in health care.

What is in the future? It is still difficult to predict. I can tell you one thing—now is the time for pharmacy technicians to grab the best tools they can obtain to enhance their training and education for the ever-changing and advanced pharmacy workplace. Employers are demanding the best employees, new roles are available for pharmacy technicians, and the public is starting to realize that not only pharmacists are involved in providing their medications.

In order to make sure pharmacy technicians are able to undertake future challenges and opportunities, each of them must utilize tools available to make them the best educated in preparation for these new endeavors. The fourth edition of this text represents a major contribution to education and training that will provide a foundation for those who wish to excel as pharmacy technicians. Students using this reference will gain valuable information to advance them in their practices and be integral in the advancement of the role of the pharmacy technician toward 2010 and beyond.

As was once said by the philosopher Rabbi Hillel, "If not now, when?" Good luck in your educational journey in becoming a part of making sure that patients are safe in taking their medications.

Lisa S. Lifshin, RPh
American Society of Health-System Pharmacists
Bethesda, Maryland

How to Use StudyWARE™

The StudyWARE™ software helps you learn terms and concepts in Durgin and Hanan's *Pharmacy Practice for Technicians*. As you study each chapter in the text, be sure to explore the activities in the corresponding chapter in the software. Use StudyWARE™ as your own private tutor to help you learn the material in your Durgin and Hanan's *Pharmacy Practice for Technicians* textbook.

Getting started is easy. Install the software by inserting the CD-ROM into your computer's CD-ROM drive, and follow the on-screen instructions. When you open the software, enter your first and last name so the software can store your quiz results. Then choose a chapter from the menu to take a quiz or explore one of the activities.

Menus

You can access the menus from wherever you are in the program. The menus include quizzes and other activities.

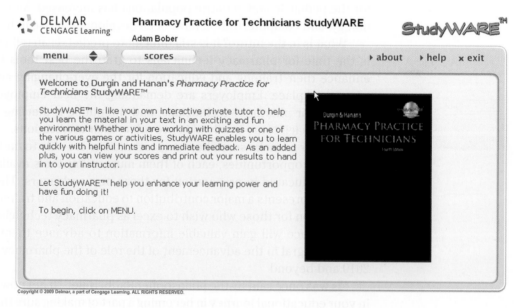

Quizzes. Quizzes include multiple choice, true/false, and matching questions. You can take the quizzes in both practice mode and quiz mode. Use practice mode to improve your mastery of the material. You have multiple tries to get the answers correct. Instant feedback tells you whether you're right or wrong and helps you learn quickly by explaining why an answer was correct or incorrect. Use quiz mode when you are ready to test yourself, and keep a record of your scores. In quiz mode you have one try to get the answers right, but you can take each quiz as many times as you want.

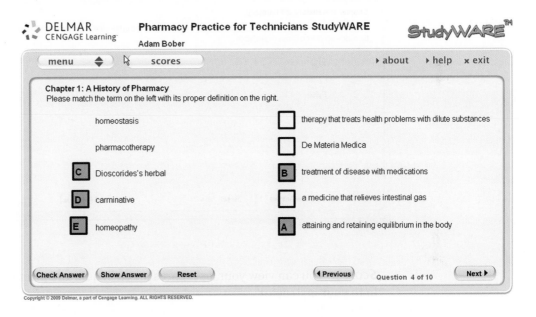

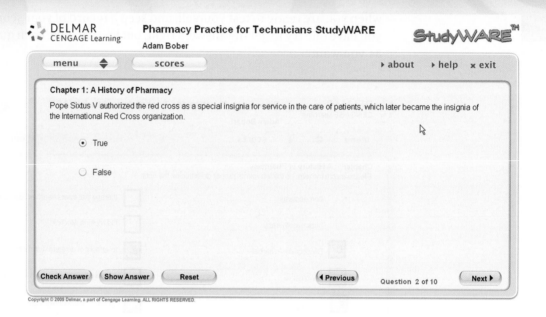

Scores. You can view your last scores for each quiz and print your results to hand in to your instructor.

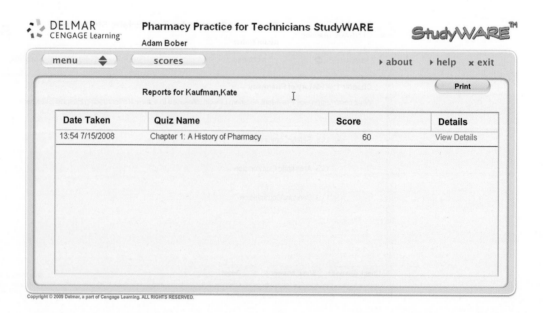

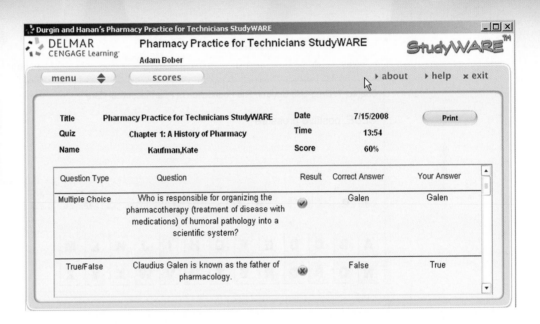

Activities. Activities include hangman, concentration, and the challenge game. Have fun while increasing your knowledge!

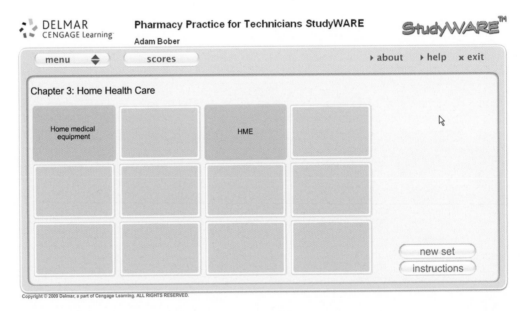

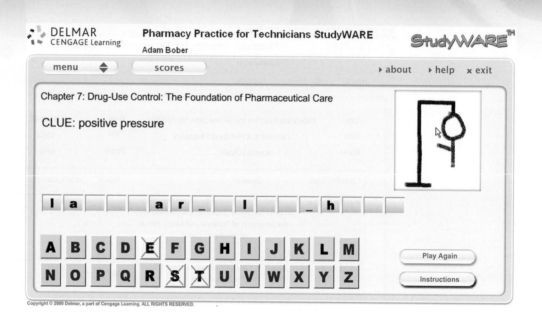

Pharmacy Practice for Technicians StudyWARE

Adam Bober

Chapter 7: Drug-Use Control: The Foundation of Pharmaceutical Care

CLUE: positive pressure

l a _ _ _ a r _ l _ _ _ _ h _ _ _

A B C D E F G H I J K L M
N O P Q R S T U V W X Y Z

Play Again

Instructions

PART

I

Overview of Health Care

A History of Pharmacy

Competencies

Upon completion of this chapter, the reader should be able to

1. Describe the Greek and/or Roman influence on present day health care.

2. Cite the names of pharmacists and/or researchers in the following countries who have contributed to the therapeutic progress of pharmacy in their respective countries: England, France, Germany, Sweden, Canada, and the United States.

3. Describe how research and development of insulin, digoxin, penicillin, and the polio vaccine contributed to the health and well being of Americans.

4. Trace the development of drugs in the United States from colonial days to present.

5. Describe how the history of pharmacy has contributed to increasing knowledge and enhancing an appreciation of the profession of pharmacy.

Key Terms

alkaloid	carminative	malaria
allopathy	deinstitutionalization	monastery
almshouse	dispensatory	Moses Maimonides
antianginal	galenical	pandemic
antiarrhythmic	herb	pharmacognosy
antidote	Hippocrates	pharmacotherapy
antihypertensive	homeopathy	phlegm
asylum	homeostasis	psychiatric
beta blocker	hospice	sanatorium
bile	immunity	Theophrastus
biologicals	immunomodulator	vasodilator

Introduction

Welcome to the world of pharmacy, an honorable profession that has been in existence for more than 5,000 years. This chapter discusses the many drugs used in the old worlds of Mesopotamia (present Persian Gulf area), China, India, Arabia, and Egypt. Many of the drugs mentioned have influenced Eastern medicine for thousands of years.

The Western influence on pharmacy, also known as *materia medica,* was cradled in Greece and Rome, as well as many European countries including Germany, Italy, Switzerland, and Belgium. Many of the drugs brought over from Europe were used by the early colonists in North America.

The history of the field of pharmacology can be pictured as a spiral—it continually evolves and adapts while maintaining and tapping into the roots of previous drug knowledge. While traditional medical research today emphasizes bioengineered drugs and immunomoderators (drugs that activate the immune system for AIDS patients or depress the immune system for human organ recipients), the field of natural remedies has also grown and developed into a billion-dollar business. Almost every pharmacy, whether independent or part of a chain, now contains shelves of herbal, mineral, and nutritional supplements. Still lacking, however, is a system of checks and balances for purity, potency, dosage, and contraindications for these natural remedies. Presently, Germany leads in setting standards for natural remedies. In the world of global communications and international scientific exchange, much of the work done in Germany may soon be shared throughout the world of pharmacy.

Greek Influence

Hippocrates a Greek physician, called the "Father of Medicine."

Some of the earliest examples of healing centers can be found in Greece. A temple dedicated to Aesculapius, the mythical god of medicine, on the island of Cos is one such example. It was here that gods were implored, physicians practiced medicine, and apprentices learned the art of healing. Circa 400 B.C., **Hippocrates**, considered to be the "father of medicine," practiced medicine and pharmacy in ancient Greece in such temples (Figure 1-1). Patients who came to these temples were diagnosed, treated, and cared for until they were able to return home. Treatments included herbal remedies, mineral baths, exercise, fresh sea air, and sunshine. Archaeologists have found admission records and other medical records inscribed in the columns of these temples.

Hippocrates (circ. 460–377 B.C.)

homeostasis a tendency toward stability in the internal body environment; a state of equilibrium.

phlegm viscous mucus secreted orally.

bile a fluid secreted by the liver.

For thousands of years, the writings of Hippocrates occupied a place in medicine corresponding to that of the Bible in the literature and ethics of Western people. Through the use of rational concepts based on objective knowledge, he liberated medicine from the mystic and the demonic.

The concept of **homeostasis**—the attainment and retainment of equilibrium in the body through appropriate drugs and diet—was the traditional benchmark of his numerous practices and writings. Hippocrates theorized that disease resulted from a disturbance of a body fluid (e.g., blood, **phlegm** (viscous mucous secreted orally), and yellow and black **bile** (fluid secreted by the liver), and was thus treated by restoring equilibrium. He believed that health was preserved by caring for the

FIGURE 1-1

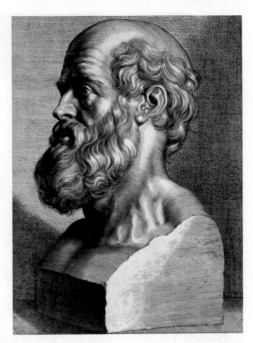

FIGURE 1-1 Hippocrates, the Father of Medicine (Courtesy of the National Library of Medicine).

allopathy a method of treating a disease by administering an agent that has the opposite characteristics of the disease (e.g., antipyretics to reduce fever).

homeopathy assists the body in the treatment or prevention of disease (i.e., giving a minute quantity of a fever-producing substance to reinforce the body's defense system).

Theophrastus a Greek philosopher and botanist who classified plants by pharmaceutical actions.

pharmacognosy the study of therapeutic agents derived from natural sources (e.g., plants).

internal environment (e.g., diet, sleep, exercise) and properly reacting to the external environment (e.g., rain, excess sun, climate changes) to enhance the physical harmony of the body.

More than 200 herbal remedies and a dozen minerals are recommended in the Hippocratic writings. The juice of the poppy, which today we recognize as opium, was among the 200 drugs mentioned. These drugs were available as pills, troches, gargles, eye washes, ointments, and inhalants. In these writings, the word for *drug*—pharmakon—was defined as a purifying remedy; later it was described as a healing remedy. Many of these drug forms are still used today and will be covered in Chapter 12.

Allopathy, a concept employed by the Greeks and in common medical practice in the Western world, treats symptoms and diseases with drugs that restore health by causing the opposite effect. For example, the common cold, seen as cold and damp, was treated with mustard, which is hot and dry. Modern day examples of drugs used in this manner are antacids, antibiotics, and antidiarrheals. This is in contrast to an infrequently used therapy known as **homeopathy**, which treats health problems with very dilute substances that cause the same effect as the symptom (e.g., a person with a fever is treated with minute doses of a fever-producing agent to reinforce the body's defense system).

Theophrastus (circ. 370–287 B.C.)

Theophrastus was a Greek philosopher and botanist who lived circa 300 B.C.. Botany, the study of plants, is closely related to **pharmacognosy**, the science that deals with the medicinal ingredients in living plants. Theophrastus classified plants by their leaves, roots, seeds, and stems (Figure 1-2). His accurate pharmaceutical and pharmacologic observations related to the classification and action of medicinal plants won him the title of "father of botany."

FIGURE 1-2

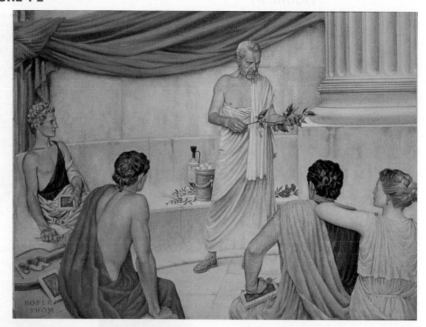

FIGURE 1-2 Theophrastus, the Father of Botany (Printed with permission of the American Pharmacists Association Foundation. Copyright 2007, APhA Foundation).

Pedanios Dioscorides (A.D. 100)

The noted botanist and pharmacologist Dioscorides was the major authority on drugs for sixteen centuries (Figure 1-3). He added to the work of Hippocrates the knowledge he gained while accompanying the Roman armies on their conquests. A major focus of his studies and writings was the use and biological effects

FIGURE 1-3

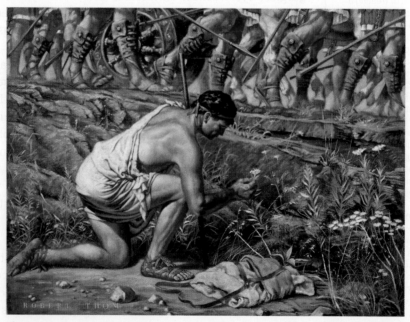

FIGURE 1-3 Dioscorides, noted botanist and pharmacist (Printed with permission of the American Pharmacists Association Foundation. Copyright 2007, APhA Foundation).

of early remedies. For this reason, perhaps he should be called the "father of pharmacology."

Dioscorides's herbal

The information in Dioscorides's herbal, known in Latin as *De Materia Medica*, contained information on more than 600 plants and 90 minerals. Knowledge was collected by Dioscorides from his extensive travels in Africa, Gaul, Persia, Armenia, and Egypt. The remedies of these countries were incorporated into the herbal, which gave plant/mineral descriptions, instructions for growing and preservation, dosage, medicinal uses, and side effects. Considered the most important pharmaceutical guide of antiquity, 35 translations and commentaries had been issued by the year 1540.

Roman Influence

In early Rome (A.D. 200–500), hospitals were often endowed by wealthy citizens who frequently cared for the sick as volunteers. Fabiola, a wealthy Roman woman, donated her palace for the care of the sick and injured and personally cared for their needs. With the fall of the Roman Empire, major changes occurred. The care of the sick became a civil responsibility, and prostitutes and prisoners were assigned health care tasks.

Claudius Galen (A.D. 130–200)

Until 1950, pharmacy students took a course entitled "Galenical Pharmacy." Galen, a Greek-born physician, practiced and taught both pharmacy and medicine in Rome (Figure 1-4). His principles, derived from Hippocrates' theory for the preparation and compounding of medicines, were followed in the Western world for

FIGURE 1-4

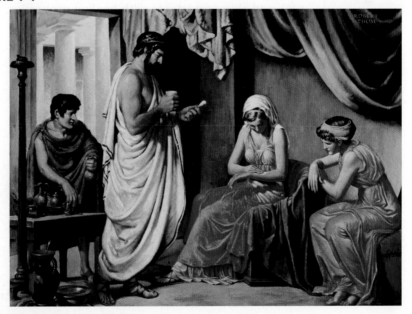

FIGURE 1-4 Galen, a physician, created a scientific system of treating disease with medicine (Printed with permission of the American Pharmacists Association Foundation. Copyright 2007, APhA Foundation).

pharmacotherapy the treatment of disease with medications.

1,500 years. Galen organized the **pharmacotherapy** (treatment of disease with medications) of humoral pathology into a scientific system.

Galen compiled and added to drug information available in Rome in the most famous of his writings, *On the Art of Healing*. This work describes the properties and mixtures of simple remedies and compounded drugs. The treatments describe such **galenicals** (a standard preparation containing one or more organic substances) as tinctures, fluid extracts, syrups, and ointments (see Chapter 12). Galenicals have recently lost popularity due to the present use of synthetic chemicals, antibiotics, and **biologicals**.

galenical a standard preparation containing one or several organic ingredients (e.g., elixir).

Jewish Influence

biologicals medicinal preparations made from living organisms or their products; include serums, vaccines, antigens, and antitoxins.

Moses Maimonides a Hebrew physician, pharmacist, and rabbi (1135–1208); physician to the Sultan Saladin; author of a health book, *Book of Counsels*, and a handbook on poisons.

carminative a medicine that relieves stomach/intestinal gas.

The Jewish influence on health care is demonstrated in biblical records of the Old Testament, as well as by the teachings and works of the famous rabbi and physician **Moses Maimonides** (Figure 1-5). The Prayer of Maimonides for many years continued the pledge of service made by pharmacists as they completed school and began professional practice.

Biblical Records (1200 B.C.)

The Old Testament Book of Sirach (38:4–8) states,

> "The Lord created medicines from the earth and a sensible man will not despise them. Was not water made sweet with a tree in order that His power might be known? And he gave skill to men that He might be glorified in His marvelous works. By them He heals and takes away pain; the pharmacist makes of them a compound. His works will never be finished; and from Him health is upon the face of the earth."

Genesis, the first book of the Bible, mentions myrrh, a remedy used throughout history as an appetite stimulant, **carminative** (a medicine that relieves intestinal gas), and skin protectants with healing properties. Olibanum (frankincense) is a

FIGURE 1-5

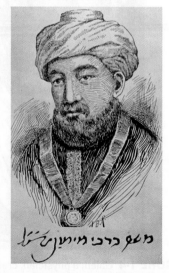

FIGURE 1-5 Moses Maimonides wrote the Prayer of Maimonides, a pledge of service for pharmacists (Courtesy of the National Library of Medicine).

gum resin mentioned in the books of Exodus, Ezra, Jeremiah, Ezekiel, and the Song of Solomon. The Old Testament of the Bible includes the pharmacist's role, professional norms, and many drug examples.

Ancient Hebrews (1200 B.C.)

Several drugs mentioned in the Old Testament are still in use today. Garlic (Numbers 11:5), with a history of thousands of years, is currently being investigated as a means to reduce blood pressure, lower cholesterol, and possibly inhibit the growth of cancer cells. Aloe, mentioned in the New Testament (John 19:39) but available much earlier, is an official ingredient in the compound benzoin tincture. Acacia (Exodus 26:15), used earlier for building purposes, is now commonly used as an emulsifying agent. Other items still in use include coriander, myrrh, almond, and anise. Presently, they are mainly used as foods or flavors.

Moses ben Maimon (Maimonides) (A.D. 1135–1204)

For many decades, pharmacy students were presented with a scroll at graduation containing the Prayer of Maimonides, a Spanish rabbi and scientist. Included are the phrases, "May I be filled with love for my art. Preserve my strength that I may be able to preserve the strength of (others). May there never rise in me the notion that I know enough." Although Maimonides is best known for this document, he also published a glossary of drug terms and a manual of poisons.

Christian Influence

The spread of Christianity brought the teachings of Jesus to the care of the sick and infirm. At the Council of Nicaea in the 4th century A.D., bishops were required to provide a shelter for the care of the sick in each diocese. The Basilius, built by St. Basil the Great in the 4th century, has influenced hospital design to this day. Bishop Landry founded the Hotel Dieu in Paris in A.D. 660. This hospital still cares for the sick from its location on the Seine River in Paris.

Cosmas and Damian (d. A.D. 303)

While the early Greeks had their mythical gods and goddesses of healing (e.g., Aesculapius, Hygeia, and Panacea), the early Christians venerated those saints who significantly contributed to healings. Cosmas was a physician; Damian, his twin brother, practiced pharmacy (Figure 1-6). They were among many who were martyred for their Christian beliefs during Diocletian's persecutions (A.D. 303–313). Over the years, they have been honored as the patron saints of medicine and pharmacy.

monastery a dwelling place for persons under religious vows, who live in ascetic simplicity.

The early Christian **monasteries** (dwellings for persons under religious vows) included an infirmary in their structural design. These infirmaries served the sick monks and persons in the neighborhood who required special care. During periodic plagues, the monks cared for persons with deadly and frightening diseases. Monasteries also contributed to health service by growing, preserving, and preparing herbal medicines and retaining and printing drug information available at the time. These early manuscripts were the medical textbooks of the day.

Monastic Manuscripts (A.D. 500–1200)

The impact of political, intellectual, religious, social, and cultural upheavals of the Middle Ages gave rise to medieval monasteries as centers of learning and science, including medical/pharmaceutical knowledge. Manuscripts from throughout

FIGURE 1-6

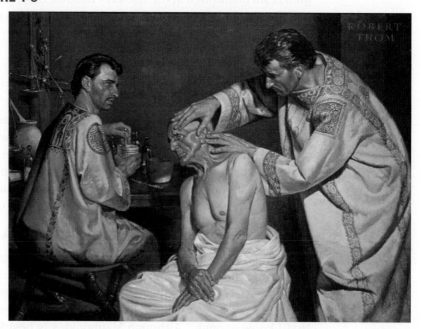

FIGURE 1-6 Damian and Cosmas, the patron saints of medicine and pharmacy (Printed with permission of the American Pharmacists Association Foundation. Copyright 2007, APhA Foundation).

the world were translated or copied in the famous monastic *scriptoria* (libraries). Among the most famous treaties are *De Viribus Herbarum* ("herbs used by people"), composed in a French abbey by Abbott Odo, and *Causae et Curae*, written by the Abbess Hildegard in a monastery in Bingen, Germany. Both manuscripts were completed during the 11th to 12th centuries. In addition to compiling existing knowledge, the monks added to the knowledge through studying the effects of the numerous plants grown in the monastery gardens (Figure 1-7).

FIGURE 1-7

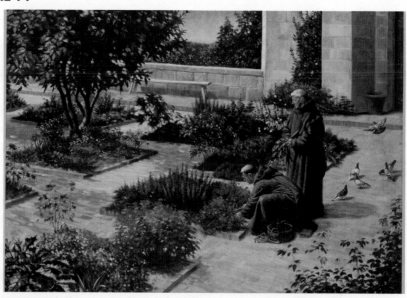

FIGURE 1-7 Herbal remedies and medicines were often grown in the gardens at monasteries (Printed with permission of the American Pharmacists Association Foundation. Copyright 2007, APhA Foundation).

Christian Renaissance Period (A.D. 1300–1550)

At the beginning of the Renaissance, several encouraging events occurred. In 1586, St. Camillus de Lellis founded a religious order, Clerics Regular Servants of the Sick, at the Hospital of St. James in Rome. Through his efforts, the deplorable, filthy conditions in hospitals and miserable treatment by civil servants were scrutinized. St. Camillus took his new community of men and centered their activities in the Hospital of the Holy Spirit, which had been founded in A.D. 717 and was one of the largest hospitals in Europe. The brothers provided personal care for the patients, with special attention to diet. Hospital of the Holy Spirit soon became a major site for the education of lay physicians, with nearly 100 physicians in attendance. The hospital still contains an impressive library of medical literature. Thus, hospitals were beginning to emerge from the Dark Ages. After St. Camillus founded his religious order, Pope Sixtus V authorized the red cross as a special insignia designating the special service provided by the order in the care of patients, many with diseases. To this day, a fourth vow of service, which originated at the time of pestilence, is made by members of this order who wear the red cross on the breast of their habit. The red cross was soon seen on battlefields and ultimately became the insignia of the famous relief organization, the International Red Cross (recently renamed the International Movement of the Red Cross and Red Crescent).

Eastern Influence

The earliest recordings for the use of healing remedies goes back in time to 3000 B.C. These early findings include inscriptions on clay tablets found in Mesopotamia and the *Pen T'sao*, found in China written on bamboo slats, which covered more than 10,000 remedies. Eastern pharmacy and medicine have influenced the health sciences and care and treatment of disease for more than 5,000 years.

Clay Tablets of Mesopotamia (3000–2500 B.C.)

Among thousands of clay tablets unearthed in the present Iraq and Persian Gulf region, more than 800 tablets contained *materia medica* information. These first pharmaceutical texts contained more than 500 remedies from plant, mineral, and other sources. The Code of Hammurabi was also discovered, containing a section on ethical standards for health practitioners.

Pen T'sao (3000 B.C.)

The Chinese document *Pen T'sao*, freely translated as "the botanical basis of pharmacy," describes more than 1,000 plants and 11,000 prescriptions handed down by oral tradition from Shen-Nung, considered the father of Chinese pharmaceutics. The early Chinese texts were inscribed on bamboo slats. They indicated the name of the drug, the dosage, and the symptoms it was used to treat. About 500 B.C., Lao-tsu, a Taoist philosopher, composed an herbal compendium called "Tao te Ching" (The Way).

China (500 B.C.)

Drugs used in early China include ephedra, cassia, rhubarb, camphor, and ginseng. "Yin" drugs were cold and wet, and "yang" drugs were warm and dry. "Red" drugs treated heart conditions, and "yellow" drugs were used to treat liver problems.

FIGURE 1-8

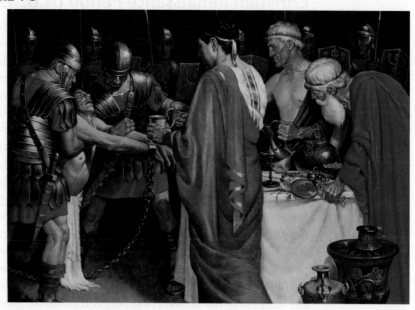

FIGURE 1-8 Mithradates studied prevention of poisoning and possible antidotes (Printed with permission of the American Pharmacists Association Foundation. Copyright 2007, APhA Foundation).

Mithradates VI (d. 63 B.C.)

Early in history, the adverse or poisonous effects of drugs were a matter of concern. Mithradates might be called the "father of toxicology" for his investigation and writings related to the prevention and counteraction of the poisonous effects of drugs through the use of appropriate **antidotes** (a remedy for counteracting a poison) (Figure 1-8).

> **antidote** a remedy for counteracting a poison.

> **psychiatric** relating to the medical treatment of mental disorders.

Arabia and Persia (A.D. 700–800)

In Arab countries, attitudes were humane and compassionate. Asylums for **psychiatric** (mentally ill) patients were built that provided gardens, fountains, pleasant music, and a healthy setting where drugs, baths, and good nutrition were given to the patients.

New dosage forms were introduced as syrups and jams that contained active ingredients such as aloes, senna, nutmeg, clover, camphor, and musk. The *Minhaj* (*Handbook for the Apothecary Shop*) stated that a pharmacist "ought to have deep religious convictions, consideration for others, especially the poor and needy, a sense of responsibility and be careful and God-fearing."

Avicenna (Ibn Sina) (A.D. 980–1037)

Avicenna, also known as Ibn Sina, is called the "Persian Galen" (Figure 1-9). His Arabic writings unified pharmaceutical and medical knowledge known at the time. His teachings were accepted in the West until the 17th century and to this day remain influential in the East.

India (1000 B.C.)

More than 2,000 drugs are mentioned in Charaka's writings, including cinnamon, cardamom, ginger, pepper, aconite, and licorice. These condiments and spices are

FIGURE 1-9

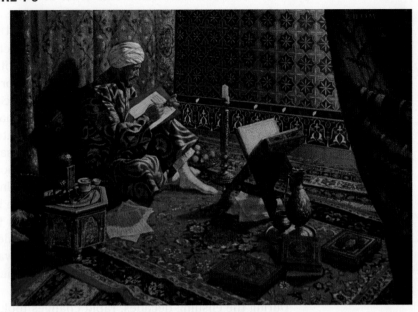

FIGURE 1-9 Avicenna, the "Persian Galen" (Printed with permission of the American Pharmacists Association Foundation. Copyright 2007, APhA Foundation).

in use today. Mercury was used in numerous preparations and is used today as an external antiseptic in Mercurochrome and Merthiolate.

Egyptian Influence

Ebers papyrus (1500 B.C.)

The parchment (papyrus) scroll found in Egypt by George Ebers (1837–1898) is one of 11 medical scrolls that preserve the knowledge of early Egyptian medicine. More than 700 drugs are mentioned, with formulas for more than 800 remedies. According to these scrolls, the pharmacist selected the drugs, prepared them in a magically correct way, and then said a prescribed benediction over them. The use of mortars and pestles, hand mills, sieves, and weighing scales is mentioned in the papyrus.

The great Al-Mansur hospital (A.D. 1285)

The great Al-Mansur Hospital in Cairo, Egypt, is an example of the Arabs' interest and dedication to health care. The hospital had special wards for particular diseases, outpatient clinics, convalescent areas, diet kitchens, and a large medical library. Both men and women were trained to provide care for the sick.

Military Influence

Wars accelerate the need for health care. Military medicine throughout history has provided the stimulus for improvement in infection control, surgical interventions, and trauma management. The Crusaders brought personal and financial support to the hospitals in the areas of conquest between A.D. 1096 and 1291. The Crusaders built hospitals in the Holy Lands. During this period, the Hospitalers of the Order of St. John of God were established to staff the hospitals and care for the wounded on the battlefield. This order continues to maintain health facilities throughout the world.

Hospitals began to take shape in what is now the United States in approximately the same way. It is known that military hospitals functioned during the Revolutionary War in New York (Manhattan), Pennsylvania (Lititz), Massachusetts, and other areas of battle. For the most part, these were temporary field hospitals.

A historic example of a hospital formulary was compiled in Pennsylvania during the Revolutionary War. Known as the "Lititz Pharmacopoeia," it was used in preparing medications for the military hospital located in that town.

During the Civil War in the United States, Louisa May Alcott served as a volunteer and observed the wanton conditions of poor sanitation, the depressing environment, and patient and staff misery at the Union Hospital in Georgetown, Virginia. She describes these conditions in detail in her published book, *Hospital Sketches*. This book influenced President Abraham Lincoln to establish the U.S. Sanitary Commission, which had as its goal a single desire and resolute determination to secure for the men who had enlisted in the war the care that was the duty of the nation to give them. Lincoln also requested the Sisters of Charity to care for the wounded on the battlefields in the Civil War.

During the ensuing decades, rapid changes took place. The wars of the 20th century brought significant changes to hospitals and health care delivery systems. World War I brought about the need to care for patients suffering from major trauma, burns, poison gas, and infections of all kinds. Hospital design reflected these needs in dealing with the masses of the injured, maimed, and sick. Ships designed as floating hospitals (begun during the Civil War) were in great demand to handle large numbers of casualties away from the immediate battlefield. They were also used to transport the sick under treatment to land-based institutions.

World War II saw major advances in trauma surgery, the introduction of systemic sulfonamides, penicillin, and the wide use of blood and plasma for transfusion. The volume of injured increased, and very large hospitals were built to provide the services needed. The Cadet Nurse Corps was developed in the early 1940s to answer the need for large numbers of professionally trained people to nurse the sick. Because of the kinds of injuries, new forms of treatment for war injuries were developed. The professions of occupational therapist and physical therapist came into being. Emotional problems resulting from the war gave new impetus for hospital facilities to deal with war-related psychiatric problems.

One vivid reminder of the Korean conflict was the television series *M*A*S*H*. The weekly series brought us the experience of war through the eyes and emotions of a mobile army surgical hospital staff. It was the close proximity of these mobile operating rooms and support resources that resulted in saving the lives of hundreds, if not thousands, of victims.

Influences of Western Europe (A.D. 500–1200)

herb a leafy plant used as a healing remedy or a flavoring agent.

Medieval physicians prescribed approximately 1,000 natural substances, most of plant origin. **Herbs** (leafy plants used as medicinal or flavoring agents) were the main source of medication. *Materia medica* was derived from the Greeks, Romans, and Arabs. The monasteries in England, Germany, and France preserved this information and added to it the medicinal herbs grown in the monastery gardens. Early explorers of American shores brought back to Europe native remedies such as quinine, found in the bark of South American trees.

During the Middle Ages, medical advancement came close to a standstill. A church edict in 1163 forbade clerics from performing any surgery that caused a loss of blood. At this time, monks were the primary health care practitioners, so surgical procedures were eliminated. Between 1347 and 1350, the Black Plague killed almost one-third of the inhabitants of Europe. Although most people were cared for and/or died in their own homes, many either died on the street or were brought to overcrowded hospitals. Hotel Dieu, one of the finest hospitals in Europe at the time, was reported to dismiss up to 500 bodies a day for burial during the height of the plague.

Throughout the centuries, persons afflicted with mental health problems were often secluded from society in confined custodial care. The poor conditions of care are reflected in the memory of Bethlehem Hospital in London, called Bedlam. (The word continues in the English language to convey the idea of confusion and disorder.) Modern health care requires concern for those afflicted with mental disorders. In Italy, mental hospitals were built in Metz, Uppsala, Bergamo, and Florence, in which patients were treated in a humane way. The town of Gheel in Belgium was outstanding in the care of psychiatric patients, where the focus of town employment and activities was on the care of psychiatric patients who were given residence in the homes of the townspeople. It was in this town that St. Dymphna, the patron saint for mental disorders, was murdered by her deranged father (the king of Ireland), who pursued his daughter in a rage after she had fled his abuse. To this very day, the town of Gheel is given over to the care of the mentally ill with support from the Belgian government.

Swiss Influence

Paracelsus (1493–1541) was born Philippus Aureolus Theophrastus Bombast von Hohenheim. This Swiss alchemist changed his name to indicate his superiority over the great herbalist, Celsus. A product of the Renaissance, Paracelsus revolutionized pharmacy from a botanical science to the beginnings of a chemical orientation in the profession. He replaced the four body fluids identified by Hippocrates (blood, phlegm, yellow bile, and black bile) with three chemical constituents of the body. Paracelsus was the prime mover in bringing pharmacy from a botanical to a chemical science. Sulfur, mercury, and salt were the materials of the body, and drugs were used to overcome excess acid or alkalinity in the body. Alcohols, spirits, acids, and oils were used, as well as mercurials and other minerals.

German Influence

For the first time in the history of Western Europe, pharmacy was declared an independent profession separate from medicine through the official Edict of 1231. Emperor Frederick II of Germany was the author of this edict, known as the Magna Carta of Pharmacy. By it, pharmacies were subject to government inspections; the pharmacist was obliged, under oath, to prepare drugs as prescribed in a reliable and uniform method. This edict influenced the practice of pharmacy across all of Western Europe.

Pharmacopoeias

dispensatory a treatise on the quality and composition of medicine.

Books that contain official drug standards have been known through the ages as recipe books, formularies, **dispensatories**, and pharmacopoeias. The distinction of having the first legal pharmacopoeia goes to the city of Nuremberg, Germany, where the municipal authorities in 1546 made it the official book of drug standards

FIGURE 1-10

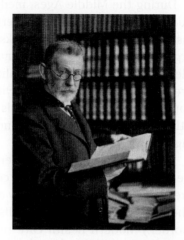

FIGURE 1-10 Paul Ehrlich introduced the concept of chemotherapy (Courtesy of the National Library of Medicine).

for that city. This book, known as *Dispensatorium Pharmacopolarum*, also became official in Augsburg, Cologne, Florence, and Rome.

Frederick Serturner (1783–1841), a pharmacist, won international recognition when he prepared salts of morphine (1804), a drug of universal acclaim in the control of intractable (not easily managed) pain.

Johannes Buchner (1783–1852), a pharmacist and professor of pharmacy in Munich, discovered salicin in willow bark and nicotine in tobacco. These discoveries paved the groundwork for aspirin (acetylsalicylic acid) and nicotinic acid. The latter was synthesized from nicotine in 1867 and is used today as niacin, a member of the vitamin B complex.

Rudolph Brandes isolated hyoscyamine (1819) and, with fellow pharmacist Philipp Geiger (1785–1836), collaborated in research to discover atropine (1835). Atropine, used to this day, is a prototype for antispasmodic drugs.

Although Emil von Behring (1854–1917) was a physician and not a pharmacist, his contribution to pharmacy was a landmark. His work with antitoxins to combat the effects of diphtheria, and later tetanus, initiated serum therapy. Diphtheria antitoxin (1892) created a whole new category of pharmaceuticals.

The concept of chemotherapy was introduced by Paul Ehrlich (1854–1915), who researched 606 chemical combinations until he found an arsenical that would be effective in combating the contemporary **pandemic** (a disease affecting a global population): syphilis. Arsphenamine was patented in 1907 and achieved fame as the "magic bullet" against syphilis. Ehrlich was a German physician and a pioneer in cellular pathology (Figure 1-10). Specific remedies, many of a chemical nature, were targeted at specific microbial and specific human cells. An intensive warfare against infection had begun.

Gerhard Domagk (1895–1964), a German scientist, discovered a sulfa drug, prontosil, to be effective against hemolytic streptococci. The use of this drug became widespread as its effectiveness against a wide range of microorganisms became evident.

pandemic a global epidemic disease.

Swedish Influence

Karl Scheele (1742–1786) was a Swedish pharmacist who made numerous chemical discoveries in the laboratory of his pharmacy shop. Among his discoveries were arsenic (1771), chlorine (1774), glycerin (1783), and numerous organic acids.

English Influence

During the 18th century, many hospitals were built in England to provide treatment for the poor. The Bristol Royal Hospital claims to be the first voluntary hospital in the provinces. One of the most famous hospitals, Guy's Hospital in London, was built in 1740 and provided free care through a ticket admission system.

William Withering (1741–1799), a clinician and a botanist in England, investigated the active ingredient in a folk remedy used to cure dropsy (an accumulation of fluids due to heart impairment). He called attention to digitalis (1741) as the active **alkaloid** (a nitrogenous basic substance found in plants or synthetic substances with structures similar to plant structures) in the foxglove plant. Digoxin, a form of digitalis, is widely used today as a cardiotonic drug.

Edward Jenner (1749–1823), an English physician, vaccinated against smallpox with the cowpox vaccine (1789) (Figure 1-11). This discovery in turn led to the eradication of smallpox in the 20th century.

Ten years later, a new class of anti-infective drugs became available in limited quantities. Penicillin (1942), the first antibiotic to be used in therapy, was available to treat 100 patients. It was first observed as an inhibitor of microbial growth by Alexander Fleming at St. Mary's Hospital in London in 1928. Later, Howard Florey (1898–1968) and his coworkers succeeded in first isolating and then making available this lifesaving antibiotic to treat gram-positive infections.

alkaloid a nitrogenous basic substance found in plants or synthetic substances with structures similar to plant structures (e.g., atropine, caffeine, morphine).

FIGURE 1-11

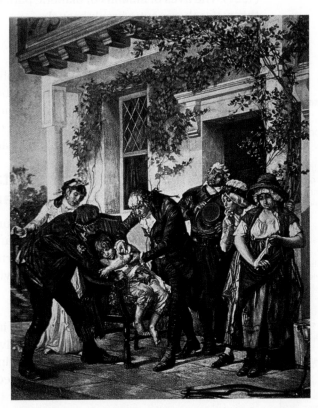

FIGURE 1-11 Edward Jenner discovered the vaccine for smallpox (Courtesy of the National Library of Medicine).

French Influence

Bernard Courtois (1777–1838) discovered iodine (1811) in marine algae. In 1826, the year he graduated from pharmacy school in Montpellier, Antoine Balard discovered bromine in sea water. He later became a faculty member of the same school.

Joseph Caventou (1795–1877), a pharmacist, collaborated with Pierre Pelletier (1788–1842) in the discovery of quinine (1820), which has become a worldwide treatment for **malaria** (an infectious fever-producing disease, transmitted by infected mosquitoes). He made other discoveries as well, including the identification of caffeine (1821).

Pierre Robiquet (1788–1840), a pharmacist who was also a phytochemist, made a number of significant discoveries, including codeine (1832). Codeine, an analgesic weaker than but similar to morphine, is a drug widely used to control pain.

Henri Moissan (1852–1907) obtained free fluorine (1886) by electrolytic methods, thus completing the elements in the halogen family of drugs.

malaria an infectious fever-producing disease, transmitted by infected mosquitoes.

Other Influences

The scientific discoveries in one country are never limited to only applications in that country. Their impact can be felt across the globe.

Canadian Contributions

Another dramatic and lifesaving discovery was made by Frederick Banting (1891–1941) and Charles Best (1899–1978) when they collaborated to discover insulin (1922). The lives of millions of diabetic patients have been saved and enhanced by this major therapeutic breakthrough.

World Health Organization

The World Health Organization (WHO) published the first *International Pharmacopoeia* in Geneva, Switzerland, in 1951. This book was published in English, French, and Spanish and later in German and Japanese. Although not a legal document, it assists in setting internationally acceptable drug standards. Drugs included in any pharmacopoeia are those of proven pharmaceutic and therapeutic value.

almshouse a home for the poor and indigent.

asylum an institution for the relief or care of the destitute or afflicted and especially the insane.

hospice an institution that provides a program of palliative and support services to terminally ill patients and their families in the form of physical, psychological, social, and spiritual care.

sanatorium an institution for the treatment of chronic diseases, such as tuberculosis or nervous disorders.

Developments in the United States Related to Health Care and Drug Therapy

Hospitals have emerged over the years, from **almshouses** for the sick poor, **asylums** for the care and confinement of orphans and the mentally ill, infirmaries for short-term acute care, **hospices** for the terminally ill, and **sanatoriums** for long-term care of tuberculosis patients and the victims of other chronic diseases.

Nonmilitary hospitals

Nonmilitary hospitals came into existence in New Amsterdam, New York; Salem, Massachusetts; and Philadelphia, Pennsylvania. Philadelphia General Hospital was started in 1713 by the Quakers as an almshouse to give relief to the sick, the incurable, the poor, orphans, and abandoned infants.

Benjamin Franklin obtained a grant in 1751 to found the first American hospital, known as the Pennsylvania Hospital. Jonathan Roberts was recruited as the pharmacist and enjoys the reputation of being the first American hospital pharmacist. This institution has had a reputation for excellence from its earliest beginnings. The New York Cornell Medical Center was initially supported by King George III in a charter granted in 1771. The apothecary-in-chief was one of the four administrative officers named in the original charter.

Psychiatric care

In the United States, the physician Benjamin Rush introduced new methods of treatment for psychiatric patients based on moral principles. His concerns and methods were outlined in a treatise on the topic that he published in 1812.

Dr. Rush was a friend of Benjamin Franklin and cared for the mentally ill at Pennsylvania Hospital. The hospital was a forerunner in the care of the mentally disturbed in a general hospital, although at that time, psychiatric patients were housed in the lower level of the hospital and separated from the medical treatment areas.

Custodial care. The 19th century continued the manner of dealing with mental patients by separating them from family and society. At the same time, the term *hospital* was substituted for the term *asylum*. The growth in the number and size of mental hospitals after the turn of the century was tremendous. Custodial care in gigantic facilities became the norm, with half the hospital beds in the United States occupied by mental patients. During the middle of the 20th century, the trend reversed.

Deinstitutionalization. Appropriate use of psychiatric drugs and various psychiatric treatment methods allowed many psychiatric patients to leave custodial care and assume the activities of daily living in society. Under this concept of **deinstitutionalization**, large numbers of persons were discharged to communities and, in some cases, to fend for themselves in the streets. The movement received strong support from civil liberty groups. State governments were only too willing to unburden themselves of the financial responsibilities involved in institutional care. What seemed to be a humane approach only increased the number of homeless in society. Now efforts are being made by professionals to develop small housing facilities for their care. Some now recognize that continued structural support and care are still required.

deinstitutional-ization discharge of persons with a history of long-term mental health care in a hospital back to the community.

Surgical care

Massachusetts General Hospital in Boston was the first hospital to use general anesthesia in surgery. The first operation was performed in 1842, with anesthesia provided by Dr. Crawford Long. Soon chloroform and ether became standard anesthetic agents, which allowed for more frequent, less painful surgery.

Contemporary Medical Practices

"Miracle drugs" are a major part of the medical fabric of the 20th century. Numerous researchers in universities, in pharmaceutical firms, and under government sponsorship have made and continue to make drug discoveries that stave off death and improve the quality of life.

Polio Vaccine

Poliomyelitis was a disease that crippled American President Franklin Roosevelt and killed and crippled many children. Eventually, two vaccines were developed: an

FIGURE 1-12

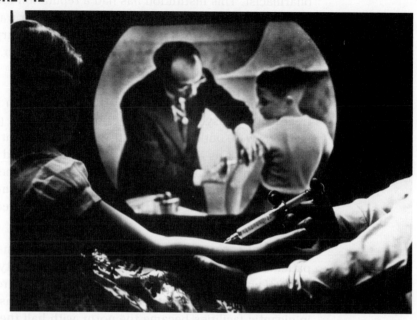

FIGURE 1-12 Jonas Salk discovered the injectable vaccine for polio (Courtesy of the National Library of Medicine).

injectable vaccine (by Jonas Salk, 1955, Figure 1-12) and an oral vaccine (by Albert Sabin, 1961). These vaccines have practically eliminated the disease commonly known as infantile paralysis.

Streptomycin

Selman Waksman (1888–1973) and his colleagues at Rutgers University in New Jersey began an intensive search to find another antibiotic to treat tuberculosis, known as the Great White Plague, which was claiming numerous lives. Streptomycin, discovered in 1944, was the first antibiotic to be effective against tubercle bacillus, the infective agent in tuberculosis.

Whole hospital buildings were changed or eliminated as a result of new treatments. Tuberculosis sanatoriums and poliomyelitis facilities are examples of treatment centers outmoded by new therapy. The famed Willard Parker Hospital of New York was declared obsolete after drug and antibiotic treatments reduced contagion and the need for isolation in hospital buildings. More recently, ambulatory (outpatient) treatment of childhood disease has caused a dramatic reduction in the need for pediatric hospital beds.

Review of Therapeutic Advances Discovered in the 19th and 20th Centuries

The first book of drug standards published in the United States is known as the U.S. Pharmacopoeia (USP) and in 1975 it was combined with another compendium, the National Formulary (NF), to form the USP-NF. Standards in the combined compendia apply to both manufactured and compounded drug preparations and, in addition to being enforceable under federal law, may also be enforceable under state and local laws.

Drug Standards Set by Pharmacopoeias

The first U.S. Pharmacopoeia (USP) was published in Philadelphia in 1820 by the U.S. Pharmacopoeia Convention. This convention, founded on the American principle of representation, had physician representatives from all of the existing states. The goal of the convention was to select the "official" drugs and to set up standards for their identity, purity, and assay methods. By 1850, pharmacists and physicians were members of the convention. The pharmacopoeia is revised every 10 years. The first pharmacist to be chairman of the convention was Charles Rice, superintendent of the General Drug Department at Bellevue Hospital in New York. He laid the foundation for the sixth edition of the USP, published in 1882.

Biologicals

immunity the condition of being resistant to a particular disease (e.g., polio).

Serum therapy was initiated with the discovery of the germ theory by Robert Koch, Edward Jenner's discovery of vaccination to provide **immunity** (the condition of being resistant to a particular disease), and Emil von Behring's discovery of antitoxins to neutralize microbial toxins. The vaccines, toxoids, and antitoxins, which utilize the clear fluid of the blood, were the first biologicals used in serum therapy. The smallpox vaccine was introduced in the early 1900s, followed by vaccines for typhus, whooping cough, measles, mumps, rubella, diphtheria, tetanus, influenza, and polio. In 1987 a genetically engineered hepatitis B vaccine was marketed.

Hormones

Isolation of human hormones began in 1897 with adrenaline, followed by thyroxine (1916), insulin (1922), cortisone, adrenocorticotropin (ACTH), estrone (1929), and testosterone (1935). These substances are important for replacement therapy and other therapeutic needs. Human insulin (Humulin), a product of genetic engineering, was introduced in 1982.

Anti-Infectives

antianginal a drug used to relieve chest pain.

antiarrhythmic an agent that restores normal heart rhythm.

antihypertensive an agent that reduces blood pressure.

beta blocker a drug that selectively blocks beta receptors in the autonomic nervous system.

vasodilator an agent or drug that causes dilation of the blood vessels; increases the caliber of the blood vessels.

immunomodulators agents that adjust the immune system to a desired level.

Anti-infective therapy began with salvarsan (1907) and then prontosil (1935). A major breakthrough occurred with the discovery of penicillin (1928–1940). Other antibiotics soon followed: streptomycin (1944) and chloramphenicol (1947), known as the first broad-spectrum antibiotic.

Synthetics

Synthetic chemicals were rapidly developed, including phenobarbital (1912), Raudixin (1953), Thorazine (1954), lithium (1960), and Valium (1963). **Antianginals** (agents that reduce chest pain), **antiarrhythmics** (agents that restore normal heart rhythms), **antihypertensives** (agents that lower blood pressure), **beta blockers** (agents that block beta receptors in the autonomic nervous system), and **vasodilators** (agents that dilate blood vessels) all improved cardiac and circulatory problems. Drugs were developed to meet problems in the major biologic systems.

Immunomodulators

The most recent category of drugs to be developed is the **immunomodulators** (agents that regulate the immune system). Based on the theory of preserving the integrity of the immune system, immunostimulators are used when there is a deficiency, and immunosuppressants are used to prevent organ transplant rejection and to treat autoimmune diseases. These modulators preserve equilibrium in the second most complicated biologic system, the immune system. (The most complex is the nervous system.)

Drug Development

The use of medicinal substances is a part of every culture. Plants, minerals, and animal parts were the drug components until the early 19th century. Drug therapy was advanced more in the 20th century than all contributions of ages past, and the United States remains the world's leader in production of vaccines, biologicals, and synthetic drugs.

Today the use of natural products, mainly herbal remedies, is a billion-dollar market. Most pharmacies, while carrying the latest remarkable drugs, are now also including a few shelves of natural products. However, due to inconsistencies in strength and purity, discretion and knowledge is needed in their use. Alternative medicines, which are often labeled as food supplements, is a growing industry.

Summary

The author hopes that this introductory chapter focusing on the contributions of many persons in many countries over the centuries to the knowledge and use of drugs will lead to an appreciation of the art and science of pharmacy. Even in a profit-oriented culture, professionals still gain a sense of satisfaction for contributing to the relief of human needs. Pharmacy seeks to prevent illness, especially through biologicals, to treat sickness with appropriate drugs and natural products, and to maintain health through education.

TEST YOUR KNOWLEDGE

Multiple Choice

1. Clay tablets found inscribed with names of plants and minerals used as medicinals were found in present-day
   a. Afghanistan.
   b. Romania.
   c. Iraq.
   d. Egypt.

2. The "botanical basis of pharmacy" was written in
   a. China.
   b. Arabia.
   c. Germany.
   d. Egypt.

3. Hippocrates based his pharmacy practice on the concept of homeostasis, which includes
   a. the principle of restoring and maintaining balance in the body.
   b. the practice of treating symptoms with drugs that have the opposite effect.
   c. the treatment of allergic conditions with antihistamines.
   d. all of the above.

4. The Magna Carta of Pharmacy, which promoted the independence of pharmacy as a profession, was an edict developed and enforced in
   a. the United States.
   b. Great Britain.
   c. Germany.
   d. France.

5. Digoxin, a form of digitalis, is derived from
   a. the poppy plant.
   b. the foxglove plant.
   c. garlic.
   d. frankincense.

Matching

Match the drug to the condition it was used to treat.

1. _____ quinine   a. heart problems
2. _____ arsphenamine   b. malaria
3. _____ streptomycin   c. syphilis
4. _____ digitalis   d. tuberculosis
5. _____ codeine   e. pain control

Match the drugs used in early China with their designated categories.

1. _____ yin drugs   a. colds
2. _____ yang drugs   b. heart conditions
3. _____ red drugs   c. fevers
4. _____ yellow drugs   d. liver conditions

Match the historical figure to what he or she is known for.

1. _____ Hippocrates   a. toxicologist
2. _____ Damian   b. botanist
3. _____ Mithridates   c. patron of pharmacy
4. _____ Theophrastus   d. applied scientific principles to drug therapy

Fill In The Blank

1. Insulin was discovered by _____ and _____.
2. Polio vaccines were developed by _____ and _____.
3. Penicillin was discovered and developed by _____ and _____.
4. The concept of chemotherapy was introduced by _____.
5. _____ discovered the germ theory.

References

Cowen, D. L., & Helfand, W. H. (1990). *Pharmacy: An illustrated history*. New York: Harry N. Abrams, Inc.

Cowie, L. (1986). *Plague and fire*. London: Wayland Publishing.

Donahue, P. (1996). *Nursing, the finest art* (2nd ed.). St. Louis: C. V. Mosby.

Dorland's illustrated medical dictionary (31st ed.). (2007). Philadelphia: W. B. Saunders Company.

Dubos, R. (1988). *Mirage of health*. New York: Harper and Row.

Garrison, F. H. (1960). *History of medicine* (4th ed.). Philadelphia: W. B. Saunders Company.

Ziegler, P. (1997). *The black death*. New York: Penguin Books.

Organizational Structure and Function of the Hospital and Pharmacy Department

Competencies

Upon completion of this chapter, the reader should be able to

1. Explain the primary function of a hospital.
2. List five functions related to patient "processing" activities.
3. Name four treatment services available in a hospital for patient care.
4. Explain the hospital's role in the promotion of health and wellness.
5. Describe the roles of the hospital's governing board.
6. List the functions of the director of a pharmacy department.
7. Identify the major diagnostic and treatment units in the hospital.
8. List major functions of a pharmacy technician in the hospital pharmacy department.

Key Terms

board of directors
board of trustees
credentialing
diagnosis
matrix management
product line management
utilization review

Introduction

> **diagnosis** the determination of the nature of a disease or symptom through physical examination and clinical tests.

Hospitals today are complex networks of health care services. These services focus on **diagnosis** (identification of a medical condition), treatment, prevention, and health maintenance of the community which it serves. This chapter will explore the organizational structure and the functions of a hospital that enable it to maximize optimum therapeutic outcomes for the patients served.

When asked to explain what running a hospital was like, an experienced administrator once described it as running the largest hotel in town, the largest restaurant, the largest laundry, the largest laboratory, the largest employment office, the largest cleaning service, and so forth, all wrapped up into one. This scenario, although somewhat amusing, can be particularly helpful in understanding how patient care is delivered and how a hospital functions on a day-to-day basis.

This chapter explores two concepts: (1) the functions of today's modern hospital, and (2) how the hospital is organized to achieve those functions.

Hospital Functions

The primary functions of any hospital are to provide resources for and assist the physicians in diagnosing and treating their patients. In carrying out these primary functions, various secondary or support functions must also be provided (e.g., record keeping, billing, discharge planning). This simple breakdown of functions is shown in Figure 2-1.

FIGURE 2-1

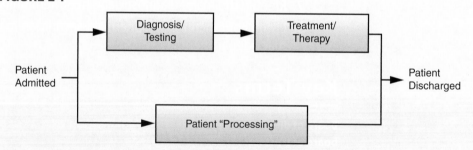

FIGURE 2-1 Simplified diagram of hospital functions.

The "processing" of patients refers to all the functions and paperwork associated with a patient's stay in the hospital. These include the medical records function, utilization review, billing, and discharge planning, to name a few.

The physician orders tests to confirm or identify the patient's diagnosis or medical condition. These tests are carried out in the various departments (e.g., radiology, medical laboratory, cardiopulmonary). Once the diagnosis has been determined, a treatment plan is developed, which may include surgery, physical therapy, respiratory therapy, or drug therapy with medications. Each is carried out by the appropriate clinical service. Some essential departments, such as nursing (patient care services), play an ongoing role in both the diagnosis and treatment functions.

The diagnosis and treatment of a patient is rarely a simple, straightforward process. It is often complicated, involving multiple disciplines within the hospital.

In today's aging society, older patients frequently present themselves at the hospital with multiple diagnoses and conditions, some interrelated to varying degrees, making the diagnosis/treatment functions quite complex. For purposes of understanding the hospital's overall functions, however, it is important to recognize the sequence of diagnosis and treatment and the corresponding patient "processing" as being of primary significance to the structure and function of the hospital.

Health education and wellness promotion are other major functions of hospitals that have gradually developed over the past 10 to 15 years. Hospitals have taken on responsibility not only for helping patients recover good health, but also for helping them maintain good health. To this end, hospitals have sponsored smoking cessation programs, stress reduction classes, weight loss programs, and instruction in how to identify potential health problems, such as self-examination for breast cancer. Community screening efforts for blood pressure, mammography, cholesterol, and glucose levels are representative of similar efforts to uncover those people at risk of becoming ill before their health actually begins to deteriorate (early detection). In addition, hospitals have developed support groups for patients and families with such health problems as diabetes and cancer. Finally, hospitals have begun to play a coordinating role in helping whole groups of patients assess their health care needs and gain access to the appropriate health care providers. Senior citizens are one group of people for whom this service is vital.

If we are to superimpose these additional functions on Figure 2-1, it will now appear as shown in Figure 2-2. Anyone who has ever been in a hospital recognizes that there are a great many other things that go on that have not yet been addressed. Dietary services include counseling patients and preparation and service of meals to patients and employees. Housekeeping keeps the hospital clean and plays an integral role in infection control. Plant engineering maintains the facility and provides the necessary heating, air conditioning, and other utilities. Coordination of all of these activities and others is essential to the successful operation of a hospital (Figure 2-2).

Hospital Organization

Hospital organization and governance have traditionally been characterized by (1) the governing body, (2) the medical staff, and (3) the hospital clinical and administrative staff. All three elements must be effectively integrated for a hospital to successfully support itself.

The governing body is usually called a **board of trustees** or **board of directors**. (In a governmental hospital these are sometimes known as a board of supervisors.) The board is charged with the ultimate responsibility of governing the hospital in the community's best interest. To this end, it is ethically, financially, and legally responsible for everything that goes on in the hospital. The board organizes itself into various committees to perform the detailed activities required to govern the hospital. These committees encompass financial activities, community relations, planning, quality assurance, and personnel, as well as a variety of other areas of responsibility.

The medical staff consists of physicians, psychologists, podiatrists, dentists, physician assistants, and nurse practitioners, each credentialed in their specialty or subspecialty to practice at the hospital. The medical staff is organized into departments such as medicine, surgery, family practice, OB/GYN, and pediatrics, and is further subdivided into subspecialty sections or groups such as cardiology,

board of trustees/ directors the body responsible for governing the hospital in the community's best interest.

FIGURE 2-2

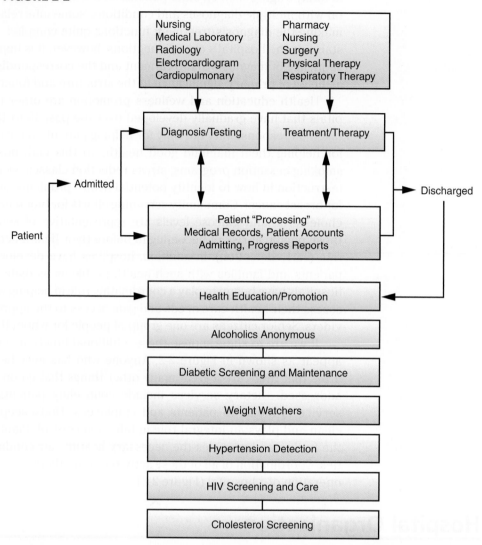

Nursing
Medical Laboratory
Radiology
Electrocardiogram
Cardiopulmonary

Pharmacy
Nursing
Surgery
Physical Therapy
Respiratory Therapy

Diagnosis/Testing

Treatment/Therapy

Admitted

Discharged

Patient

Patient "Processing"
Medical Records, Patient Accounts
Admitting, Progress Reports

Health Education/Promotion

Alcoholics Anonymous

Diabetic Screening and Maintenance

Weight Watchers

Hypertension Detection

HIV Screening and Care

Cholesterol Screening

FIGURE 2-2 Expanded diagram of hospital functions.

orthopedics, and neurology. The president of the medical staff functions as the liaison between the medical staff and the hospital administration.

The clinical departments have a department director or chair who oversees the functioning of the department. Typically, these functions include establishing standards of practice for the department's specialty, providing continuing education for its members, monitoring individual physicians' performance, and providing a forum for the exchange of ideas and new techniques. The medical staff also organizes itself into multidisciplinary committees to perform specific activities for which the medical staff as a whole is responsible. These committee activities include reviewing pharmacy and therapeutics, **credentialing**, quality improvement, and utilization review. For example, the Pharmacy and Therapeutics Committee is responsible for reviewing requests for pharmaceutical agents for inclusion in the hospital pharmacy's formulary. Both the medical staff and the board of trustees also have executive committees to coordinate the work of all other committees. They typically share sponsorship of a joint conference committee made up of representatives from both the board and the medical staff.

credentialing a process in which a formal, organized agency recognizes and documents the competencies and abilities performed by an individual or an organization.

Like the medical staff, the hospital staff is organized around common functions separated into departments or services. Each department or service performs one or more of the following general categories of functions:

- Assist with the diagnosis via testing.
- Help treat the patient via therapy.
- "Process" the patient's paperwork, or monitor the patient's treatment.
- Maintain the physical environment, or support the patient's stay in the hospital.
- Support the functioning and management of the individual departments and hospital as a whole.

Diagnostic testing is typically carried out in departments such as the medical laboratory, radiology, nuclear medicine, and EKG (electrocardiography). Therapy is provided in the departments of pharmacy, physical therapy, speech therapy, and radiation therapy. Some departments, such as nursing, psychiatry, and respiratory therapy, spend significant amounts of time both determining diagnoses and providing treatments.

Other departments perform "processing" functions that assist the patient throughout the stay without directly affecting diagnosis or treatment. Examples of these departments include medical records, admitting, patient accounts (billing), **utilization review**, and social services.

> **utilization review** a committee that determines how use of resources meets criteria and standards.

Another group of departments support the patient's stay either by contributing to the physical environment or by supporting the coordination of services to the patient. Included in this group would be communications, housekeeping, volunteer services, laundry, plant engineering and maintenance, safety and security, and pastoral care. The dietary department, while providing support to the patient through ongoing nutrition, can also play a therapeutic role and a health education role.

Finally, a variety of departments and services are vital to the overall success of a hospital, but patients may never hear of them while around the hospital. These departments support the ongoing operation of the hospital and the individual services and include the departments of materials management, human resources, community relations and fund development, planning, risk management, and accounting and finance. In addition, clerical personnel support the activities of the medical staff.

Each hospital department/service is generally run by an administrative director or a section supervisor. These middle managers report to administrators or vice presidents who in turn report to either the executive vice president or directly to the president. Historically, the departments were grouped according to common operating characteristics into four categories: nursing services, clinical services (testing and treatment departments), support services (support and facilities departments), and financial services (accounting, patient accounts). The organizational chart in Figure 2-3 reflects this historical division of responsibility.

However, hospital organizational structure has changed dramatically over the years and is now tailored specifically to each hospital's activities and the capabilities of its department heads and administrative staff. Although some elements are common to all organizational charts, there is no longer one dominant organizational structure.

> **matrix management** an organizational concept that emphasizes the interrelationship between departments and the common area of decision-making.
>
> **product line management** an organizational concept that emphasizes the end product or category of services being delivered.

Matrix management and **product line management** are only two examples of organizational theory applied to the rapid technological and service delivery evolution that has taken place in health care. Matrix management structurally emphasizes the overlapping areas of responsibility among departments and the common areas of decision making. Product line management organizes the hospital

FIGURE 2-3

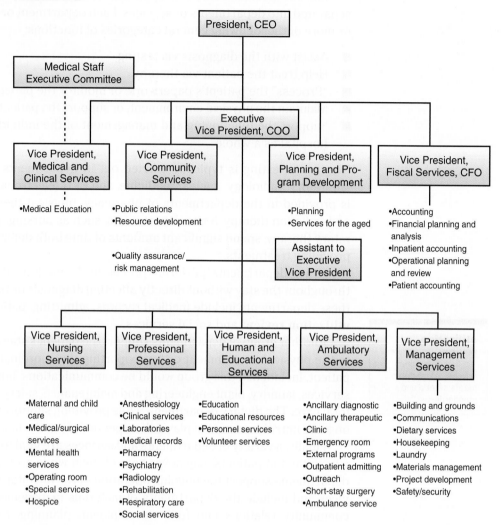

FIGURE 2-3 Hospital organizational chart according to traditional divisions of responsibility.

not along the lines of comparable operating principles, but by the end product or category of service being delivered.

Fully understanding organizational theory is not essential to appreciate how a hospital functions. What is important is appreciating the great variety in the ways hospitals organize themselves and that, in each case, communication and collaboration among departments is vital.

As a way of enhancing communications, the hospital staff, such as the board of trustees and the medical staff, forms committees. Some committees are ongoing, such as safety and quality improvement committees. Many, however, are ad hoc working groups brought together to address a specific problem or concern. Once the desired resolution is achieved, these groups disband or form new committees to address different problems and issues. These ad hoc committees bring various departments together in a problem-solving situation without dramatically altering the organizational structure of the hospital or interfering with the reporting relationships carefully developed over time. As such, they represent a flexible, informal organizational structure that allows the hospital to get its work done.

Hospital Pharmacy Technicians: A Changing Role

Hospital pharmacy technicians perform a broad range of clinical, technical, and clerical tasks necessary to the efficient operation of a hospital pharmacy. They enable the licensed pharmacists to concentrate on professional functions, such as providing medical staff and patients with clinical information and guidance. The principal responsibility of technicians is to prepare, package, and distribute medications prescribed by physicians for hospitalized patients. Medication orders are written by physicians and other licensed practitioners on the patient's medical record. Copies of these orders are sent either manually or electronically from all the patient care units to the pharmacy. After pharmacists review the orders for appropriateness and perform clinical interventions when applicable, the medical order is processed and technicians assist in preparing the medications for dispensing.

The most common method used by technicians for preparing and distributing prescribed medications is known as "unit-dose distribution." Each day, technicians assist in assembling a complete 24-hour supply of medications for every hospital patient. Individual, patient-specific doses of each drug are separately packaged and labeled. All of these unit doses are then placed in the patient's medication cassette either manually or by robotic and automated systems that technicians must be trained to utilize. Many commonly used medications are prepackaged in unit-dose form by drug manufacturers so that technicians need only select the right package. When prepackaged unit doses are not available, supervised technicians must measure or count the prescribed amount from bulk containers and create the packaging with the use of a unit-dose packaging machine. Many hospitals are utilizing bar-coded medications for electronic medication dispensing and patient safety checking. Technicians often assist the pharmacists with this newly added packaging necessity. (Please refer to Chapter 18, "Drug Distribution Systems," for a review of this topic.)

When unit doses are to be administered by the injection route, technicians may assist the pharmacist in the transfer of the medication from vials and ampoules, using aseptic techniques, to the proper dispensing container. In addition, the technician may assist in the preparation of IV admixtures, adding drugs or nutrients (IV additives) to commercially prepared or compounded intravenous solutions. (See Chapter 15, "Sterile Preparation Compounding," for information on this topic.) Pharmaceutical calculations must be accurate and checked by a pharmacist, and extreme care must be taken to ensure sterile conditions and aseptic techniques. (Refer to Chapter 13, "Pharmaceutical Calculations," for information related to this topic.)

Inventory control is another responsibility for some pharmacy technicians. Technicians keep track of medications and other supplies and prepare orders for additional quantities when stock diminishes. They also receive incoming supplies; reconcile invoices against quantities ordered, received, and billed; and put supplies into the appropriate secured storage areas. (Please refer to Chapter 25, "Materials Management of Pharmaceuticals," for information on this topic.)

Additional duties performed by pharmacy technicians may include delivering drugs and pharmaceutical supplies to nursing stations (either manually or by utilizing a hospital-wide pneumatic tube transport system); refilling emergency crash cart medications; maintaining automated dispensing and robotic machines; keeping pharmacy work areas well-stocked, clean, and orderly; and responding to telephone questions or requests from other hospital personnel.

The hospital pharmacy technician's increasing role, responsibilities, and employment requirements may vary not only from hospital to hospital, depending on the pharmacy department's scope of service, but from state to state, as state boards of pharmacy regulations governing the practice of pharmacy are different.

Due to a current nationwide shortage of pharmacists, along with an increasing need for clinical pharmacists on multidisciplinary hospital care teams to ensure good patient outcomes, the need and reliance for well-trained, skilled, and competent technicians will increase. Hence, many states will soon require a formal training program with a competency certification or license examination. Currently, there is a National Pharmacy Technician Certification Board Examination that provides an opportunity for a pharmacy technician to demonstrate that he or she has mastered knowledge and skills across various pharmacy practice settings. (Please see Chapter 31, "Pharmacy Technician Certification Board," for additional information on this topic.)

Structure and Organization of a Pharmacy Department Within a Hospital Organization

In hospitals, nursing homes, or assisted living-type facilities, the role of the pharmacy staff has evolved in response to technological, financial, and other operational influences. The pharmacy director is responsible for the overall operations of the department including staff hiring, scheduling, competency assessment,

FIGURE 2-4

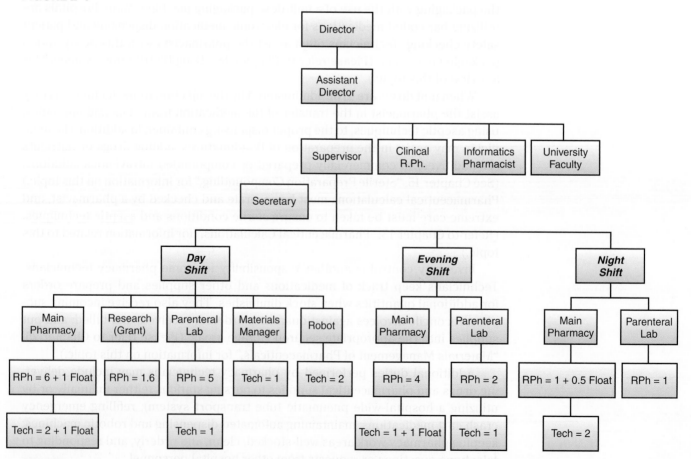

FIGURE 2-4 Hospital pharmacy organizational staffing chart with the pharmacist and technician teams.

budgeting, and regulatory compliance. The director participates on committees and other interdisciplinary activities.

The role of the pharmacist in hospitals today has expanded beyond the preparation of pharmaceutical prescriptions and provision of information on medication administration and interactions. Today pharmacists can obtain advanced training to obtain a Doctor of Pharmacy (PharmD) degree. The PharmD provides enhanced support to the health care team by providing guidance on the type of medications available to treat specific conditions, as well as the most appropriate, and often most cost-effective, route of administration of the drug (Figure 2-4).

Summary

If one conclusion about hospital organizational structure and function can be reached, it is that they will continuously change. New technologies and programs continue to be developed, resulting in changes to the hospital's organizational structure. New roles are continuously being proposed for the nation's hospitals and new organizational structures are being developed to meet the challenges that lie ahead. In short, it is far from clear what hospitals will look like in the future or precisely how they will function. In light of the financial crisis hospitals are currently facing, compounded by the technological revolution we are experiencing, we can be sure that hospitals will remain complex organizations that patients depend upon to adequately provide the required quality care. We can also be sure that proper and appropriate health care will continue to depend on accurate and precise communication of information and, most importantly, on the skill and dedication of those who staff our hospitals.

TEST YOUR KNOWLEDGE

Multiple Choice

1. The primary functions of a hospital are to provide for which of the following:
   a. diagnosis
   b. treatment
   c. both a and b
   d. none of the above

2. Patient "processing" activities include
   a. the admission process.
   b. utilization review.
   c. discharge planning.
   d. all of the above.

3. Most hospitals provide the following treatment modalities:
   a. surgery
   b. hypnosis
   c. acupuncture
   d. massage therapy

4. Wellness programs in hospitals typically include
   a. smoking cessation.
   b. special Olympics.
   c. strength training.
   d. aerobics.

5. The role of the hospital governing board includes responsibility for all the following except
   a. ethical concerns.
   b. hiring supervisory personnel.
   c. legal matters.
   d. financial matters.

Matching

Match the responsible parties with the role they play in the hospital. The answers may be used more than once.

1. _____ maintains physical environment   a. board of trustees
2. _____ establishes medical standards of practice   b. medical staff
3. _____ responsible for overall hospital governance   c. hospital staff
4. _____ provides social services
5. _____ monitors physician's performance

Fill In The Blank

1. In the last century, a major development in hospitals were _____ programs.

2. The governing body of the hospital is called the _____.

3. To enhance communications and efficiencies of the hospital, _____ may be formed.

4. The principal responsibility of _____ is to prepare, package, and distribute medications prescribed by physicians for hospitalized patients.

5. Pharmaceutical _____ must be accurate and checked by a pharmacist, and extreme care must be used to ensure sterile conditions and aseptic techniques.

Home Health Care

Competencies

Upon completion of this chapter, the reader should be able to

1. Describe the evolution and future of the home health care industry, particularly related to the role of the pharmacy in home health care.

2. Explain the scope of services available to a patient requiring home health care.

3. List at least three nontraditional positions a pharmacy technician might have in home health care.

Key Terms

durable medical equipment (DME)
home care
home equipment management services
home health agencies
home health care
home health services
home infusion therapy
home medical equipment (HME)
home medical services
personal care and support services

Introduction

Home health care in the United States is a diverse and rapidly growing segment of health care services. As ambulatory (outpatient) services have largely replaced in-hospital care, home health care has become an increasingly important site of care. Many elderly and infirm Americans, who may experience significant difficulty or hardship in accessing the health care delivery system, may receive a variety of skilled professional services without the need to leave their own home. The Centers for Medicare and Medicaid Services (CMS) estimated in 2004 that more than 7.6 million persons in the United States were receiving home care, by more than 20,000 providers.

As home health care has evolved, the role of the pharmacy in providing services in the home health care setting has grown. As a result of the growth in pharmacological services being provided at home, the need for pharmacological management of these services is growing. The pharmacy technician must understand the services that are provided in the home and the role the pharmacy department plays in providing these services.

The Evolution of Home Health Care

home health care provision of health care services to a patient in his or her place of residence.

home care care given to the patient in their own home.

Home health care, or **home care**, may be defined as the provision of health care services to patients in their place of residence. By this definition, home health care is as old as mankind. The first formal home health care agencies were established during the 1880s. Pharmaceutical services were not a component of these early agencies, which consisted primarily of nurses, therapists, and home health aides. Retail pharmacies provided medications (primarily oral drugs) to patients in their home through home deliveries by the pharmacy or the home health care nurse who picked up the medications for the patient. Pharmacy's role in home health care was then minor and indistinguishable from community pharmacy practice.

The first major boom in the number of home health care agencies occurred in 1965 with the enactment of Medicare. Medicare made home health care services available to the elderly and, beginning in 1973, to certain disabled younger Americans. Between 1967 and 1985, the number of home health agencies grew more than threefold, from 1,753 to 5,983. However, pharmacy's role in home health care had increased very little because medications were not a Medicare-covered benefit.

In 1983 Medicare initiated a method of reimbursement that provided economic incentives for hospitals to discharge patients as early as possible, reducing the length of a patient's stay in the hospital in an effort to reduce health care costs. This dramatically shifted patients from requiring in-hospital care to receiving the provision of care in the home setting.

Home infusion therapy began in the early 1970s and as a result the role of pharmacy in the home care setting began to grow. Several university-based medical centers demonstrated the feasibility of providing nutrition intravenously (IV), or total parenteral nutrition (TPN), in the home for patients unable to eat orally or via feeding tubes. Technological advances in central venous catheters and smaller, more sophisticated infusion pumps made long-term treatment in the home not only possible but sufficiently safe and practical for patients, their caregivers, and providers. Since Medicare was willing to pay for home TPN at about one-third of the inpatient rate, home infusion therapy became the more economical option.

Once the market for home TPN was established, many companies opened pharmacies to provide TPN and other home infusion services, including IV antibiotic therapy and parenteral pain management. Today, many other injectable medications are being administered safely in the home setting.

Health care costs in the United States are a higher percentage of the economy than in any other country. For this reason, employers, the U.S. government, and insurance providers are increasingly looking for ways to manage costs. One predominant way of doing this is by managing the provision of care itself. This concept is called *managed care*. Managed care may direct patients to the most appropriate and most cost-efficient health care setting based on their identified needs. For example, managed care may determine if a patient should be treated at an outpatient clinic, in an inpatient setting, or in the home. An appropriate site of care can reduce costs without reducing (and sometimes increasing) the quality of the care provided. With many pharmacies providing home care, competition has created incentives for many home care providers to contract with managed care networks.

The numbers of patients receiving home care will continue to grow as the population ages. On the basis of satisfaction surveys, most patients prefer home health care to hospital care. One can easily see that delivery of care and services in the home is still a growing market and has not yet reached its peak. Even home infusion therapy, which has seen virtually no breakthroughs in technology and new therapies administered in the home in the past few years, is still experiencing a significant annual growth rate. The growth of pharmacy in home health care will continue into the next century. Many predict it will become the predominant health care setting for the provision of drug therapies and pharmacy practice.

Home Health Care

Home health care encompasses a wide range of services. These services include nursing care and therapies, personal aides to assist with the activities of daily living, delivery and maintenance of medical equipment, and pharmacy services. As these services continue to grow and expand, the pharmacy technician can expect a wider range of professional opportunities. It is therefore helpful to gain a working knowledge of these areas of service in home health care.

Home Health Services

home health services the provision of health care services by a health care professional in the patient's place of residence on a per-visit basis.

The most frequently-provided services falling under the umbrella of home health care are **home health services**, defined as the provision of health care services by a health care professional in the patient's place of residence, usually on a per-visit basis. Home health services consist of a wide variety of health care services. The predominant form of home health services is nursing. Nursing services can be high tech (e.g., infusion therapy) or low tech (e.g., diabetic teaching and monitoring) on an intermittent visit schedule or in 4- to 12-hour shifts. Other services include those of dietitians, medical social workers, physical therapists, occupational therapists, and speech therapists. Some people also include respiratory therapists, dentists, and physicians in this group. Respiratory therapists are usually associated with the home medical equipment industry, rather than with home health agencies. The provision of dental services in the home is relatively new and extremely rare at present.

home medical services physician services in the home.

home health agencies public (governmental) agencies, nonprofit agencies, proprietary agencies, and hospital-based agencies that provide home health services.

Most people prefer to differentiate physician services in the home, referring to them as **home medical services**. Providers of home health services are called **home health agencies**. Home health agencies can be classified as public (governmental) agencies, nonprofit agencies, proprietary agencies, and hospital-based agencies. Most states require home health agencies to be licensed. According to the National Association of Home Care and Hospice, approximately 55 percent of freestanding home health agencies are Medicare-certified. To be Medicare-certified, and thus eligible to take care of and receive payment for Medicare patients, the organization must meet the Medicare Conditions of Participation (a lengthy list of standards and requirements), have a Medicare provider number, and undergo unannounced inspections by CMS staff or approved status-accrediting bodies.

Personal Care and Support Services

personal care and support services the provision of nonprofessional services for patients in their place of residence.

The second most common form of home health care is **personal care and support services**, defined as the provision of nonprofessional services for patients in their place of residence. These services include homemaking, food preparation, personal care, and bathing. The individuals who provide these services are called home health aides, homemakers, or personal care attendants. Most personal care and support services are provided by home health agencies, although some companies (non-Medicare-certified) specialize in this form of care exclusively.

One of the growing areas for personal care and support services is private duty services. Private duty involves the provision of personal care services around-the-clock or for 8 to 18 hours per day, sometimes by a live-in attendant. These services are generally not reimbursed by Medicare or Medicaid and rarely by insurance, so the payment for personal care services is cash payment by the patients and/or their families. Home health or nursing services can also be provided on a private duty basis and it, too, is a growing area. It was estimated in 2003 that 18 percent of all home care services were paid for out-of-pocket.

Home Equipment Management Services

home equipment management services the selection, delivery, set up and maintenance of equipment and the education of the patient in the use of the equipment, all performed in the home or patient's place of residence.

home medical equipment (HME) the equipment used at home (e.g., hospital beds, crutches).

durable medical equipment (DME) includes health-related equipment that is used for long periods of time, is not disposable, and is rented or sold to patients for home care, such as wheelchairs, hospital beds, walkers, canes, and crutches.

The third most prevalent form of home health care is **home equipment management services**, also referred to as **home medical equipment (HME)** services or **durable medical equipment (DME)** services. Home equipment management services can be defined as the selection, delivery, setup, and maintenance of equipment and the education of the patient in the use of the equipment—all performed in the patient's place of residence. Medical equipment includes wheelchairs, canes, walkers, beds, and commodes. It also includes higher-technology items such as oxygen tanks, oxygen concentrators, ventilators, apnea monitors, phototherapy lights, infusion pumps, enteral pumps, and uterine monitors. Many providers include the sale of medical equipment and supplies (such as ostomy supplies) in this home care definition. However, the federal government and the Joint Commission, which accredits such providers, do not include the provision of products without services in their definition of home care. So such sales, without the corresponding services, would not be considered home care.

Home medical equipment providers are not required to be licensed in most states, although the U.S. Food and Drug Administration (FDA) and the Department of Transportation (DOT) require registration for distribution and transportation of oxygen. Numerous pharmacies are involved in the provision of home medical equipment services and sales, which may be included in the definition of home care. Many HME organizations also provide clinical respiratory services, which include the professional services of a registered respiratory therapist for performing in-home assessments, monitoring of vital signs (temperature, blood pressure and pulse rate), oximetry testing (the percent of oxygen saturation in the blood), and/or administrating therapeutic treatments (e.g., nebulized medications). Pharmacies must be involved in providing the respiratory medications (since these are prescription drugs) either as providers or under contract with the HME provider. There are specialty pharmacy practices (e.g., medications by inhalation) that are compounded and delivered by a common carrier.

Home Pharmacy Services

The last major type of home health care is the provision of home pharmacy services. Home pharmacy services do not have a clear and concise definition since there is considerable overlap with retail or community pharmacy practice. However, home care pharmacy generally has the following characteristics:

- All medications are delivered, mailed, or shipped to the patients' home. The patient has never been present in the pharmacy or communicated face-to-face with a pharmacist (except perhaps in the home).
- The patient may be receiving home health (nursing) services and sometimes medical care in his or her home and may be homebound (Figure 3-1).
- The pharmacy is usually responsible for monitoring the patient's medication and clinical response on an ongoing basis. If not the pharmacy, then someone else is responsible (e.g., home health nurse, hospice team, or another pharmacist).

FIGURE 3-1

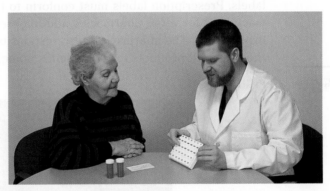

FIGURE 3-1 Home nursing services may include delivery of and assistance with medications provided by a pharmacy.

More than 90 percent of home pharmacy service is home infusion therapy. However, pharmacies specializing in providing services to hospice patients or hospice pharmacies are also categorized as providing home pharmacy services, as are a growing number of specialized mail-order pharmacies. The predominant specialty areas for such mail-order pharmacies include patients with hemophilia, cystic fibrosis, post-transplant and other immune-compromised states, short stature due to growth hormone deficiency, respiratory diseases, multiple sclerosis, and those needing various biotech and injectable products. Pharmacists and pharmacy technicians employed in home care have a significant opportunity to develop special skills and knowledge of these disease states and how to care for these individuals.

Home Infusion Therapy

home infusion therapy intravenous drug therapy provided in a patient's own home.

According to the U.S. Office of Technology Assessment, **home infusion therapy** is described as a medical therapy that involves the prolonged (and usually repeated) injection of pharmaceutical products, most often delivered intravenously, but sometimes delivered via other routes (e.g., subcutaneously, intramuscularly, or epidurally) into patients in their residence. Home infusion therapy is generally thought of as consisting of three services: pharmacy, nursing (home health), and equipment management services.

Pharmacy Services

Pharmacy services generally involve both compounding and dispensing the intravenous solutions into a ready-to-administer form (Figure 3-2). In many ways, this process is similar to the IV room of a hospital pharmacy. Preparation of sterile admixtures for home administration may require special techniques and more stringent environmental controls than a hospital IV admixture room. Unlike in a hospital, where a medication is usually prepared within 24 to 48 hours of administration, home care may involve up to one month between preparation and administration, thus allowing a greater potential for microbial growth. More extensive quality control and end-product testing are also performed on the prepared products for the same reasons. Home infusion pharmacies are required to comply with the United States Pharmacopoeia (USP) Chapter <797> when compounding sterile preparations.

Home care and hospital pharmacy IV admixtures have significantly different labels. Prescription labels must conform to the requirements for the state pharmacy laws for retail pharmacies and may require more detailed administration instructions. The pharmacy is also responsible for the packaging and delivery of the prepared products to the patient's home. Delivery techniques vary from the

FIGURE 3-2

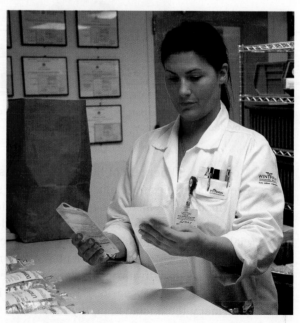

FIGURE 3-2 Pharmacy services for home infusion may involve the compounding of intravenous solutions.

use of one's own delivery vehicles and drivers, to the use of external contracted delivery services—both local and national (e.g., Federal Express), to having the nurse pick up and deliver the medications. Regardless of the delivery method, the pharmacy must always ensure that the product is packaged to control the factors affecting the stability of the product (temperature, light, humidity, etc.) during delivery to the patient's residence.

Although the pharmacist is primarily responsible for the pharmaceutical care and clinical monitoring of the patient, many home infusion pharmacies rely greatly on the pharmacy technician to assist the pharmacist in data collection. For example, the pharmacy technician may be responsible for obtaining copies of laboratory reports, calling patients for their weight, and inventorying supplies to assess compliance with prescribed therapies and administration techniques. The pharmacist monitors the drug therapy through evaluation of information received from the patient's nurse, the patient or family member or caregiver, and the laboratory test results. Frequent and extensive communication regarding the patient may be needed with the physician and nurse, other health care professionals, and the patient or caregiver. The pharmacy maintains not only the normal prescription and dispensing records, but also a clinical record of the patient called a *chart* or *home care record*.

The home infusion pharmacy generally operates under outpatient or retail pharmacy laws, although many state boards of pharmacy have either additional or different regulations for home care pharmacies. The pharmacy is often involved in providing the nursing supplies, catheter care supplies, and the access device for the infusion therapy to patients. These infusion-related supplies and devices are sent with the medications to the patient, for use by the patient or nurse, in the patient's home.

Home Nursing Services

At least initially, most patients receiving home infusion therapy will also be receiving home nursing services. Nurses usually have considerable experience in handling IVs in an acute care setting before they care for home infusion patients. Major responsibilities of the home care nurse include educating the patient and/or family caregiver regarding administration of the infusion and care of the infusion site, performing dressing and infusion site changes, making in-home physical assessments, and monitoring the patient's health status. Nurses will also administer the medications initially, but the eventual goal is to train the patient or a caregiver to perform this task. Periodic visits are then made to monitor the patient's status and response to therapy.

Equipment Management Services

Equipment management services primarily include the selection, delivery, and set-up of an infusion control device (i.e., an infusion pump). They also include the separation of clean (patient-ready) and dirty (returned) equipment, cleaning and disinfecting of equipment between patient use, and routine and preventative maintenance of the equipment, including inspection, testing, and performing maintenance on the equipment. Equipment sent to patients also needs to be tracked at all times in compliance with the Safe Medical Devices Act (SMDA) of 1990. Backup equipment and/or services are needed for equipment malfunctions. In many home infusion pharmacies, pharmacy technicians are responsible for the routine cleaning and volumetric testing of infusion and enteral pumps and the associated documentation.

As in a hospital or clinic setting, not all home infusion patients will need an infusion pump. Gravity administration of the drug using the rate controller or clamp on the administration set or tubing can be safely used at home for some drugs and administration rates. Special infusion pumps and devices have been developed for the special needs of home infusion patients, providing another opportunity for special skills development of pharmacy technicians. Disposable administration devices and small lightweight pumps that do not require an IV pole are commonly used. When drug dilution is not required and the administration time is short, some patients may receive their medication as an IV push (a term used when the active ingredient goes directly into the vein). Pharmacy staff must be able to decide whether an infusion device is required and what device or pump is appropriate for the patient and for the drug being used, and the administration rate and stability of the medication in the system selected.

Types of Home Infusion Providers

Home pharmacy services, as part of home infusion therapy, can usually only be provided by a licensed pharmacy, either alone or as part of a broader health care organization. The exception is physician practices, which can provide these services without a pharmacist or pharmacy out of their office under the auspices of their physician's license. Other types of settings where home infusion services are provided include retail or community pharmacies, institutional or long-term care pharmacies, hospital pharmacies, home health agencies, HME-based providers, infusion therapy specialty providers, and ambulatory infusion centers.

Physician-Based Practices

Physician-based practices are most commonly seen in oncology and infectious disease practices. Usually, physicians run an ambulatory infusion center as part of their office. Patients receive cancer chemotherapy, antibiotics, or any type of infusion while they are in the physician's office. Between physician visits, patients may return to the infusion center to receive their IV medications or have them provided through home care. Even in cases when the patient mainly receives care in the infusion center, at times a nurse may need to assist the patient in the home (e.g., leaking IV access on the weekend). Home care is usually provided by the nurses from the physicians' offices and is usually considered a sideline to their office-based practice. In these physician-based practices, nurses—not pharmacy technicians or pharmacists—are usually responsible for compounding and admixing the IV medications. Sometimes a local pharmacy is contracted to compound and deliver the medications to the physician's office.

Retail or Community Pharmacies

Independent retail or community pharmacies are most likely to provide a variety of services, including HME, ostomy care products, and diabetic care. Infusion therapy is usually a low-volume component. Pharmacists, and sometimes technicians, usually provide home infusion therapy services in addition to retail and other pharmacy duties. Most are "pharmacy-only" providers; however, a few pharmacies hire nurses to help coordinate home infusion therapy services and perhaps provide a limited amount of home health services. Delivery services are provided by nurses or the same delivery mechanism as the retail pharmacy/HME business.

Some are part of a franchise in home infusion or participate in a home infusion network. Many are one-owner operations.

Institutional or Long-Term Care Pharmacies

Institutional or long-term care (LTC) pharmacies primarily provide drug distribution services to numerous nursing homes, independent senior residences, prisons, and other institutional facilities. Although the primary business is oral medications, many also provide IV therapies to long-term care facilities with subacute units (patients needing more skilled care than a nursing home and less than an acute care hospital). Expanding the provision of IV services from the nursing home to the home care environment is very easy. Thus, many LTC pharmacy providers have entered the home care market. However, home infusion therapy is usually a very low percentage of their overall business. These organizations have extensive internal delivery systems (e.g., their own fleet of vans) and usually provide enteral and infusion pumps, though some may also supply other HME. Although these pharmacies may employ a nurse to assist with care coordination and education of the long-term care facility staff, home health services are rarely provided directly by these organizations, which tend to be pharmacy-only operations.

Hospital Pharmacies

Home infusion therapy is often provided by the hospital department of pharmacy in the inpatient IV admixture room or the outpatient pharmacy, utilizing the existing staff. A pharmacist is assigned clinical responsibilities in home care and for interacting with the home health care team. The hospital usually provides a broad array of home health services, although these are operationally in a different department and may not even be on the hospital premises. Infusion pumps are either handled by the biomedical engineering department, the home health services department, materials management, or the pharmacy department, or a combination of these. Delivery services are usually provided by the home care nurses who pick up the medications from the pharmacy. Some hospitals have created a separate home infusion pharmacy independent of the inpatient pharmacy, especially when the volume remains high, which may be located on the campus of the hospital. Some hospitals have created a home infusion division (home health plus pharmacy) that resides off-campus—sometimes as a separate corporate entity. The home infusion division functions like an infusion therapy specialty provider.

Home Health Agencies

Home health agencies have purchased or implemented a pharmacy to supplement their home health services provision. These are usually large home health agencies that provide a wide array of home health services and may have multiple home health offices. The pharmacy may service multiple home health branches and usually looks and operates similar to an infusion therapy specialty provider.

HME-Based Providers

HME providers may also provide home infusion pharmacy services. Usually the primary role of pharmacies is to supply respiratory therapy medications required for the home medical equipment and clinical respiratory needs of their patients. The home infusion pharmacy may operate similarly to a retail pharmacy-based infusion program or an infusion therapy specialty provider.

Infusion Therapy Specialty Providers

The infusion therapy specialty provider specializes only in the provision of home infusion therapy. Generally, this organization provides home health services, although the nurses specialize in home infusion therapy only. Pharmacy occupies a prominent role in this type of organization. Infusion and enteral pumps are usually the only type of medical equipment provided by this company. Maintenance of the infusion and enteral pumps is usually performed by the company's employees, often pharmacy technicians. The infusion therapy specialty providers tend to have their own delivery staff and vans, depending on the size of the organization. This type of provider may service up to 1,000 infusion patients per day. Smaller volume independent providers in this category also exist.

Ambulatory Infusion Centers

Ambulatory infusion centers (AICs) consist of an office, usually in a doctor's office building. Patients are referred here to receive their infusions in a comfortable setting. The office may consist of a series of rooms, each with a relaxing chair, infusion pump, and television. Nurses manage and run the office and administer the medications. AICs are more cost effective than home care for patients whose infusion may take two to six hours. In this setting, the nurse may safely care for multiple patients at the same time. The AICs are generally licensed as pharmacies and have a pharmacist or pharmacy technician present to prepare the IV admixtures for the nurses to administer. The nursing staff may provide limited home care services to patients treated by the center. As discussed, a nurse will need to visit the patient in the home and provide almost all deliveries. Many ambulatory infusion centers are owned by infusion therapy specialty providers and operate in a similar manner. Others are owned by physicians or health care systems.

In all of the preceding cases, the provider can be independent or part of a regional or national chain. Some pharmacies serve patients seen by multiple home health agencies or home medical equipment providers, and service patients in multiple states whose geography is limited only by the areas serviced by overnight delivery services (such as Federal Express). Others are single-site providers serving only their local community.

Preparing and Dispensing Medications for Home Care

The preparation and dispensing of medications in home infusion therapy requires specialized knowledge and skills. Both pharmacists and technicians from other pharmacy practices (e.g., community, hospital, or long-term care) often take at least a year before they are comfortable with the processes and differences of home care practice.

The pharmacist and technician must first be aware of the differences in pharmacy laws and regulations. In most states, home infusion therapy (even if dispensed by the hospital pharmacy) must adhere to retail pharmacy laws and/or special home care regulations, which are different from those of hospital pharmacy practice. For instance, inpatient pharmacists can often accept verbal orders relayed from a hospital nurse. In outpatient pharmacy regulations, most states prohibit the pharmacist from accepting the verbal prescription from anyone but the physician directly (or the physician's employee agent). When the physician gives medication orders or changes to the home care nurse, the pharmacist must call back the physician to verify the orders or receive a written order or fax directly from the physician. Prescription records and labeling requirements are different from those of the inpatient requirements. Second, the pharmacist and technician must be aware of extended stability and beyond-use dates of the products they compound and dispense. In hospital pharmacy, most parenteral medications are used within 24 hours, which is impractical in home care practice. Special packaging may be required for delivery. Products must often be packed in ice chests or Styrofoam-lined boxes for delivery in extremely hot or cold weather. Third, pharmacists and technicians need to be aware of special preparation techniques based on the infusion pump the patient will be using. For instance, the use of a fluid dispensing pump may be needed in preparing drugs in elastomeric devices because of the tremendous pressure needed to fill them. Technicians will need knowledge and training to compound some of the special containers used for ambulatory infusion pumps and other home care-friendly devices. Fourth, home care patients (particularly those with HIV infections) have heightened needs for confidentiality, of which home infusion staff must be aware, and thus show extra sensitivity. For example, delivery staff should never leave supplies with a neighbor or other person unless specifically agreed to in advance by the patient.

Compounding practices *must* adhere to the United States Pharmacopoeia (USP) Chapter <797>. Many state pharmacy laws also have special requirements for IVs prepared for home use. All pharmacists and technicians involved in compounding sterile preparations should become familiar with these regulations. USP <797> gives pharmacy staff the basic guidelines for the compounding environment based on the type of compounding which is to be done. Most pharmacies will only be preparing low- or medium-risk preparations, so they must have a primary engineering device, such as a laminar airflow workbench (LAFW) or biological safety cabinet (BSC), which maintains an ISO Class 5 area (previously called Class 100 environment, since there can be only 100 particles of dust and particulates per cubic foot of air). Training and responsibilities of compounding, policies and procedures, beyond-use dating, quality control, and cleaning and disinfection of the compounding environment are some of the other important contents of USP <797>.

Most importantly, the timing of preparation and dispensing is critical in ensuring that the delivery of a stable, sterile product is coordinated with the needs and dosing regimen of the patient and nurse who may be administering the product. This is considerably more complex and difficult than meeting the service needs of inpatients.

Role of Technicians in Home Infusion Therapy

The role of the technician is more varied and more progressive in home infusion therapy than almost any type of pharmacy. It can be both challenging and provide the opportunity for job changes or advancement. Pharmacy technicians have knowledge and skills that can adapt to other job functions and responsibilities in home infusion pharmacy practice.

The traditional and key role of the technician in home infusion therapy is in the preparation of sterile products under the supervision of a pharmacist. Some states have more stringent requirements for technician supervision by a pharmacist in outpatient and home care settings (e.g., a pharmacist must be physically present within eyesight of the technician at all times) than in a hospital pharmacy. In some expanded health systems, there may be a retail or outpatient pharmacy, institutional pharmacy or hospital pharmacy, and clinic or satellite pharmacies in addition to the home infusion pharmacy, making the technician's role more varied and possibly including duties and responsibilities in these other areas as well. Other roles for pharmacy technicians in home infusion therapy include:

- Equipment management technician.
- Patient service representative.
- Purchasing agent or manager.
- Warehouse supervisor.
- Billing clerk/case manager.
- Home infusion delivery representative.

Equipment Management Technician

Detail-oriented pharmacy technicians accustomed to keeping accurate, thorough documentation of their work are ideally suited to becoming equipment management technicians. As previously described, the location of all infusion pumps must be known at all times. Additionally, since technicians are used to working with the metric system, syringes and measuring devices, they can easily learn to operate the infusion pumps and test their volumetric accuracy.

Patient Service Representative

Pharmacy technicians who enjoy dealing with the people can move into the role of the patient service representative or coordinator (PSR or PSC). This person is responsible for telephoning patients and making sure they have an appropriate inventory of ancillary supplies and medications (Figure 3-3). The PSR is the patient's primary customer service representative and may assist in transmitting

FIGURE 3-3

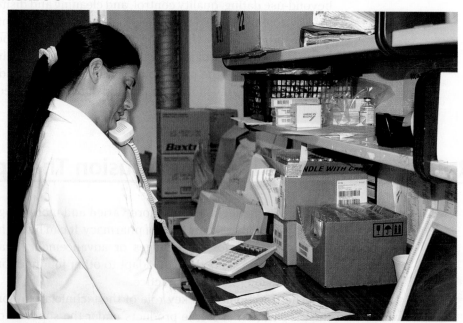

FIGURE 3-3 Technicians serving as patient service representatives should have a professional demeanor and good people skills.

the patient's desires and requests to other staff in the organization. They are very helpful to the professional staff by monitoring compliance with therapy and product usage and often identify patient issues before they can become problematic. Pharmacy technicians in this role learn the use of the ancillary supplies and can help the pharmacy effectively manage supply costs. The PSR may also help coordinate deliveries with the warehouse supervisor/technician. This job is less "hands-on" and is generally more of a desk job.

Purchasing Agent or Manager

Since pharmacy technicians are accustomed to maintaining a sufficient inventory of the prescription drugs and dealing with the drug manufacturers and wholesalers, they may easily move into an expanded role of purchasing all of the ancillary patient supplies and office supplies required by the pharmacy. This employee may also be responsible for negotiating prices and purchasing contracts and handling drug and product recalls.

Warehouse Supervisor/Technician

Pharmacy technicians who enjoy a challenge and are able to multitask may have the opportunity for promotion to the warehouse supervisor/technician position. This person needs to effectively and efficiently schedule patient medication and supplies deliveries to different locations in a timely manner. Each patient's supplies must be accurately picked and packed to assure stability and prevent breakage during delivery. With the purchasing coordinator, an appropriate inventory of ancillary supplies must be maintained. Hazardous materials and wastes must be stored and disposed of according to law and regulation.

Billing Clerk/Case Manager

Pharmacy technicians who have been involved in verifying prescription drug coverage have had an introduction to the reimbursement process. The billing clerk/case manager is responsible for processing patient invoices with insurance companies, Medicare carriers (the organizations responsible for paying the bills for Medicare patients), and/or state Medicaid programs. In addition, this individual may be responsible for verifying a patient's insurance coverage, getting authorization from payers, and negotiating prices with insurance company case managers. This person may also be responsible for the intake process, or obtaining the initial information from the patient and referral source (physician, hospital, insurance company) to admit the patient to service.

Home Infusion Delivery Representative

The delivery representative transports the products to the patient's home and thus must be competent in infusion pump set-up, troubleshooting, and the basics of equipment management; proper storage of the products in the home (i.e., which product must go in the refrigerator); infection control procedures; handling of hazardous materials and wastes; confidentiality; advanced directives and responding in emergency situations; identifying patients who may be abused or at nutritional risk; and so forth. It is important to remember that this individual may be the only employee of the home infusion provider who sees and talks to the patient directly. This individual may have to gather information from the patient or caregiver as well as provide information and care to the patient in addition to routine delivery services.

Summary

Home health care is a new practice territory for many health care professionals who receive their training in a clinical institutional environment. Not every health care provider is ready to take on the challenge of caring for patients in the home. There are many things to consider before taking on such a challenge. The following are some of these considerations:

- A real interest in personal patient care and in adapting to a new practice site.
- Previous experience in the preparation of sterile products.
- Completion of special courses on the care and use of home medical equipment.
- Professional and social ease in the home setting and in dealing with patients and their family members, or with single, homebound patients.
- Ability to be in contact with the pharmacist or home care nurse to communicate routine and unusual occurrences encountered while providing services.
- Ability to collaborate with an entire health care team.

The past few decades have witnessed the remarkable patient care shift from residential institutions to the home. For patients to remain in the home, a team of physicians, nurses, pharmacists, and rehabilitative and physical therapists are involved in maintaining the health and lifestyle of the patient. In every clinical situation, medications are an essential part of the patient's care. The pharmacist and pharmacy technician are important members of the health care team involved in the preparation and monitoring of drugs used in infection control, TPN, pain control, cancer management, and hydration.

Home health care, both the newest and the oldest form of patient care, is a quickly expanding method of patient care. Pharmacists and pharmacy technicians have the challenge and opportunity to enjoy the satisfaction of their professional contributions in home health care.

TEST YOUR KNOWLEDGE

Multiple Choice

1. How many patients were estimated to receive home care in the United States in 2004?
    a. 100,000
    b. 20,000
    c. 1,000,000
    d. 7,600,000

2. Individuals called home health aides are involved in providing which of the following home care services?
    a. home infusion therapy
    b. home medical equipment
    c. home pharmacy services
    d. personal care and support services

3. Home care and hospital pharmacy practice differs in which of the following areas?
   a. different pharmacy laws
   b. packaging products properly for delivery
   c. beyond-use dating
   d. all of the above are different in home care and hospital practices

4. Home infusion therapy providers are licensed in many states as
   a. hospital pharmacies.
   b. long-term care pharmacies.
   c. community or retail pharmacies.
   d. home equipment companies.

5. Home infusion therapy services involve the provision of home pharmacy services with
   a. home health services.
   b. home medical equipment.
   c. personal care and support services.
   d. clinical respiratory services.

6. Which type of equipment is most frequently used in home infusion therapy?
   a. oxygen cylinders
   b. blood glucose monitors
   c. pumps
   d. ventilators and concentrators

7. The types of pharmacies involved in the provision of home infusion therapy include:
   a. retail pharmacies.
   b. hospital pharmacies.
   c. institutional or long-term care pharmacies.
   d. all of the above.

8. The most common form of home infusion therapy is
   a. antibiotics.
   b. TPN.
   c. pain management.
   d. cancer chemotherapy.

Matching

Match the health care provider to the services rendered.

1. _____ monitors vital signs

2. _____ reviews and monitors drug regimens

3. _____ compounds sterile products for intra-venous delivery

4. _____ assists with activities of daily living

a. pharmacy technician

b. home health nurse

c. home health aide

d. pharmacist

Fill In The Blank

1. The provision of health care services to patients in their place of residence is called _____.

2. More than 90 percent of home pharmacy services is _____.

3. _____ is described as a medical therapy that involves the prolonged (and usually repeated) injection of pharmaceutical products, most often delivered intravenously, but sometimes delivered via other routes (e.g., subcutaneously, intramuscularly, or epidurally) into patients in their residence.

4. Pharmacy technicians who are detail oriented and accustomed to keeping accurate detailed documentation of their work are ideally suited to becoming _____.

5. Pharmacy technicians who enjoy a challenge and are able to multitask may have the opportunity for promotion to the _____.

References

American Society of Health-System Pharmacists. *Best practices for hospital & health-system pharmacy: Position and guidance documents of ASHP, 2006–2007.* Bethesda, MD.

American Society of Health-System Pharmacists. ASHP guidelines on quality assurance for pharmacy-prepared sterile products. (2000). *American Journal of Hospital Pharmacy,* 50, 1150–69.

Buchanan, E. C., & Schneider, P. J. (2005). *Compounding sterile preparations* (2nd ed.). American Society of Health-System Pharmacists: Bethesda, MD.

Catania, P. N., & Rosner, M. M. (Eds.). (1994). *Home health care practice* (2nd ed.). Palo Alto, CA: Markets Research.

Conners, R. B., & Winters, R. W. (Eds.). (1995). *Home infusion therapy: Current status and future trends.* Chicago: American Hospital Publishing.

Congress, Office of Technology Assessment. *Home drug infusion therapy under Medicare* (OTA-H-509). Washington, DC.

National Association for Home Care and Hospice. (2004). *Basic statistics about home care.* Washington, DC.

United States Pharmacopeial Convention Chapter 797 Pharmaceutical Compounding-Sterile Preparations. *United States Pharmacopoeia 27th Ed/National Formulary 22 rev.* First supplement. January 1, 2004.

Web Sites

National Association for Home Care (NAHC)   www.nahc.org

Long-Term Care

Competencies

Upon completion of this chapter, the reader should be able to

1. Define long-term care, as well as who receives care and how the care is provided.
2. Identify the three different types of long-term care facilities by sponsorship, and explain the historical significance of each one.
3. Identify the major sources of funding for the long-term care field.
4. Differentiate between a service pharmacist and a consultant pharmacist.
5. Describe the supportive role of the pharmacy profession to the nursing profession.
6. Discuss the role of the pharmacist and pharmacy technician in the delivery of long-term care.

Key Terms

adult day care facility
assisted living facility
automatic stop order
consultant pharmacist
long-term care (LTC)
medication regimen review (MRR)
not-for-profit
nursing home
preferred drug provider (PDP)
proprietary
rehabilitation facility
skilled nursing facility (SNF)

Introduction

long-term care (LTC) health care provided in an organized medical facility for patients requiring chronic or extended treatment.

adult day care facility an institution for adults that provides long-term care, which supplements the care an individual may be receiving at home by providing opportunities for socialization and care while the primary caregiver is at work.

Society has struggled with the obligation to care for those who can no longer care for themselves. Historically, this obligation fell to immediate family members or people of the same religion, tribe, or national background. The very earliest institutions had these religious or fraternal philosophies. Individuals not fortunate enough to be taken in by one of these charitable organizations were forced to live on the streets or to seek admission to institutions created by the governing entity (e.g., the county poorhouse, the almshouse, or the local asylum).

In 1965, Congress passed two laws that would have a profound effect on this historical situation. The Medicare and Medicaid programs changed the way America provided for its frail and elderly population. Under Medicare, the elderly were guaranteed health care and, just as importantly, the children of the elderly were absolved of the legal responsibility of paying for care for their parents. The Medicaid legislation guaranteed payment for those deemed to be indigent. Thus, a new type of medical welfare was created. With these sound sources of income guaranteed, the growth of institutions willing to provide care mushroomed. Just as a generation earlier Social Security had guaranteed a source of income to the elderly and blind, these two pieces of legislation, commonly referred to as Articles 18 and 19, changed the way care was financed and who would ultimately pay the cost.

Long-Term Care

assisted living facility a community-like institution that provides care (such as meal service) for individuals who can no longer remain in their homes, but do not need the level of care provided in nursing homes.

nursing home or skilled nursing facility (SNF) an institution that provides long-term care to individuals needing extensive medical care as well as personal care around the clock.

Long-term care (LTC) is defined as the provision of health and personal care (meeting physical and emotional needs) to individuals over an extended period of time. Long-term care may be required due to traumatic injury, disability, or acute and chronic illness. The need for long-term care may be temporary, spanning a few weeks or months, or ongoing over a period of many years. According to the Administration on Aging, in 2007 about nine million Americans over the age of 65 will need long-term care services. By 2020 that number will increase to 12 million. While most people who need long-term care are age 65 or older, a person can need long-term care services at any age. Forty percent of people currently receiving long-term care are adults 18 to 64 years old.

Long-term care may be provided in a number of settings. The majority of long-term care is provided at home through family members or personal care providers such as home health aides. **Adult day care facilities** provide long-term care that supplements the care an individual may be receiving at home by providing opportunities for socialization and care while the primary caregiver is at work. For individuals who are unable to remain in the home for care but who do not need the level of care provided in nursing homes, there are **assisted living facilities**. These types of facilities provide a community setting for the residents while having basic needs provided such as meal service, assistance with activities of daily living, and emergency support if necessary. **Nursing homes** or **skilled nursing facilities (SNF)** provide long-term care to individuals needing extensive medical care as well as personal care around the clock.

Business Models for Nursing Homes or Skilled Nursing Facilities

proprietary a type of long-term care facility that is owned by one person, a family, a partnership, or a corporation, is run like a corporate business, and makes a profit for its investors.

not-for-profit a type of long-term care facility that does not pay a profit with its extra income, but rather reinvests the revenue back into programs or building improvements for the benefit of the serviced population.

There are three types of business models for LTC nursing facilities: government-sponsored, **proprietary**, and **not-for-profit**. The smallest percentage of LTC facilities are those institutions run by the government at the federal, state, or county level. These may be veterans' homes and hospitals or county-owned homes run for the benefit of their citizens or some other similar grouping. These are the direct descendents of poorhouses and almshouses.

The second type of nursing home is referred to as *proprietary*. This type of long-term care facility is by far the most numerous. These are owned by one person, a family, a partnership, or a corporation. They are run like a corporate business and should make a profit for their investors. The most advanced types of this kind are the large corporations, like Beverly Enterprises, that are traded on the stock market.

The last major type of long-term care facility is referred to as voluntary or not-for-profit. These homes are the direct descendants of those charitable institutions that took care of their own particular followers. The term voluntary refers to the composition of the board of directors, who serve without personal benefit or inurement, but do so from a wish to benefit society in some fashion. The secondary term, not-for-profit, defines what these institutions do with extra income. Instead of paying a profit or dividend to their shareholders like a for-profit institution rightly does, these facilities are obliged to reinvest the excess revenue back into programs or building improvements for the benefit of the serviced population. These facilities are not obligated to pay taxes and have the ability to raise funds for charitable purposes.

Regulation of Long-Term Care Facilities

The various types of facilities providing long-term care have differing levels of regulations, which makes for a complex system of laws, regulations, directives, and governmental oversight activities at the federal, state, and local municipality levels. Sometimes these regulations are similar, sometimes they are not. The Centers for Medicare and Medicaid Services (CMS) has taken an extremely active role in standardizing these rules, regulations, and directives for the entire nation. Still, each state may create a more stringent set of rules, and the facilities must comply with the higher standards. The length and breadth of these rules, regulations, and directives are so extensive that it has been opined that only the nuclear energy field has more rules.

Regulations related to provision of pharmaceutical care range from prescription transcription (i.e., only a licensed nurse may take a telephone order from an off-site physician), to (most recently) a standardized prescription for all doctors. Additionally, storage must be secure and in some cases must be in a double-locked, permanently affixed cabinet with a certain thickness of construction. Controlled drugs must be counted by both off-going and on-coming licensed nursing personnel before keys are transferred. Proper destruction of unused or expired drugs has its own protocol. Recent regulations further dictate how pain-relieving transdermal patches must be handled. The contents and use of the emergency box is also well defined in regulation. Most recently, CMS has issued extensive new regulations concerning gradual dose reductions and tapering of medications and discontinuance of unnecessary medication.

While many of these rules and regulations are written for the macro management of facilities, one example of a very direct rule (with implications every day on every unit on the micromanagement level) is the regulation that the medication nurse has only a one-hour grace period on either side of the stated medication time to successfully complete his or her drug pass. The challenge is to administer all of the drugs that must be given to the entire population that must be medicated, with the proper protocols, within this time span. During annual surveys, the medication nurse is closely watched by state inspectors for possible errors. The error rate cannot exceed 5 percent; otherwise the facility receives an unfavorable citation. This margin of error actually creates a de facto threshold of 95 percent for passing—a very high standard to achieve in any field and typical of the regulations that the long-term care industry struggles to meet.

Funding for Long-Term Care

Funding for long-term care can be divided primarily into three categories: (1) tax dollars through Medicare and Medicaid, (2) private pay, and (3) third-party payors (Figure 4-1). For information related to reimbursement for services see Chapter 29.

Medicare and Medicaid

Medicare Parts A, B, and C account for a large percentage of the dollars spent in health care. Part A usually covers hospital stays and some nursing home time. Part B covers doctor's visits, specialized tests, and supplies. Part C comprises the managed care and/or hospice benefit. Medicare is funded partially by the government through taxes and premiums for individuals and is part of the Social Security benefits package. Medicaid, which is considered the payor of last resort, is an entitlement program paid by federal, state, and local taxes. When all other sources of revenue are exhausted, Medicaid pays for the legitimate costs associated with

FIGURE 4-1

Funding for Long-Term Care

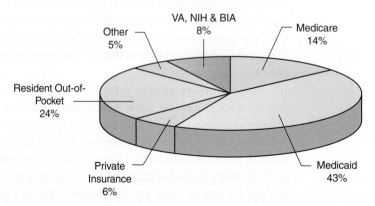

FIGURE 4-1 Funding for long-term care (Source: 2005 Statistical Abstract of the United States, Health and Nutrition. U.S. Census Bureau).

rehabilitation facility an institution that provides services to patients recovering from acute or traumatic events on a short-term basis.

providing care. In skilled nursing facilities, Medicare coverage is limited to up to 100 days, 80 of which have a significant co-pay requirement. To access this benefit, the patient must be considered to be receiving a "skilled service." Most frail elderly do not qualify and thus do not receive these covered days. **Rehabilitation facilities** (which provide services to patients recovering from acute or traumatic events on a short-term basis) are more successful in meeting these Medicare eligibility requirements. Many community elderly still are under the assumption that Medicare will pay for long-term care. Medicare functions better for acute or short-term episodes and not continuing care needs.

Medicare Part D is a new federal government program that began on January 1, 2006. It has created another payor source that is so massive and powerful it may well be years before its full impact is understood. With this legislation, all individuals who qualify for Medicare Part A or Medicare Part B can purchase drug coverage for their needs. Dually eligible patients who have both Medicare and Medicaid are not subject to co-pays. The scope of the coverage differs with the plans. Participation is voluntary, co-pays vary greatly, and as first conceived, gaps exist after certain cost levels are reached and before so-termed "catastrophic coverage" begins.

Historically, it is worthy to note that pharmaceutical costs to the long-term care facility under the previous all-inclusive rate system were often as high or higher than the entire food budget for the facility. This was the impetus for restricted formularies, cost containment initiatives, and pressure on the prescribing doctors to be mindful of costs. This latter was only mildly successful, as most physicians were only somewhat aware of drug costs. Suggestions from both the vendor and consultant pharmacy professionals were often ignored or delayed in the day-to-day business of rendering health care.

preferred drug provider (PDP) a gatekeeper between individual and government payors under Medicare Part D.

Under Medicare D, all patients are assigned to **preferred drug providers (PDPs)**, which act as gatekeepers between the individual and government payors. Each PDP has its own formulary, and there was much initial confusion about what was the best particular PDP for an individual. Additionally, drugs can be removed or added to these formularies, which could then mandate a switch from one PDP to a different one to obtain optimal coverage. If a non-formulary medication or a non-covered medication is ordered, a prior approval for that medication from the PDP is required. A technician, in consultation with a pharmacist, often assists in collecting information from the prescriber required to obtain the prior approval. In its first year of use, nursing home personnel have seen an increase not only in the costs of drugs but in the amount of drugs prescribed.

Private Pay

Individuals who have assets (wealth) to pay for the care they receive until such time that their resources are low enough to be eligible for Medicaid are classified as "private pays." As stated previously, these individuals may qualify for some coverage under Medicare if they are receiving a skilled service. Since the Medicare program is essentially an insurance program, one's level of wealth would not prohibit benefiting from this coverage. However, when the allotted Medicare days are used up, the patient would have to pay with his or her own resources.

Third-Party Payors

This category of non-governmental payors includes insurance companies that have sold long-term care policies, or Health Maintenance Organizations (HMOs) that offer Medicare supplemental/managed care coverage. These managed care companies usually negotiate a price for those patients they are obligated to care for. In many instances these agreements cover all services, so it is important that the rate is sufficient to cover costly items such as prosthesis and pharmaceuticals. These entities watch costs very closely and often dictate what drug can be used by means of a restricted formulary.

Nursing Home Operation

For the most part, the challenge to those who operate nursing homes is the need to balance between rules, regulations, and efficient practice and the great need to recognize these patients as people who need to continue to participate in society and enjoy what life has to offer them. Because government policy and funding have created an impetus to admit skilled-care patients, the population of today's nursing home does not resemble the population of 10 or 20 years ago. Today's facilities operate at much the same level of intensity as a small community hospital. Floor staffing in the modern long-term care facility consists of, most commonly, a charge nurse, possibly a second nurse on busy shifts, and several certified nursing assistants. Physicians, therapists, and consultants will all be at the facility briefly, but the great bulk of the work is carried out by the nursing staff.

A model nursing unit will have 40 to 45 patients, each of whom will receive an average of nine prescriptions daily (with some drugs given several times a day). This brings the minimum total to about 400 doses daily that the charge nurses must administer. The challenge for the pharmacist and the pharmacy technician working with these types of facilities is to communicate the proper information so that the drug achieves the desired effect. Being mindful that long-term care facilities care for residents 24 hours a day, seven days a week, it is likely that many different individuals will perform the same function. The labeling of medications must be clear to avoid misinterpretations by staff members.

Nurses are charged with the responsibility of properly administrating medication to the residents. One popular medication system that is an effective aid for the charge nurse is the unit dose system. In this system, individual pills are packaged in blister packs on a 30-day calendar card so that the nurse can check at any time to verify that the dosage has been given (Figure 4-2).

FIGURE 4-2

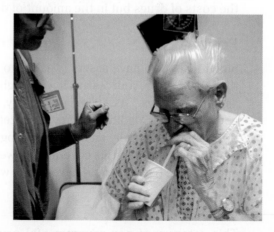

FIGURE 4-2 It is the nursing staff's responsibility to properly and effectively administer medications to patients.

FIGURE 4-3

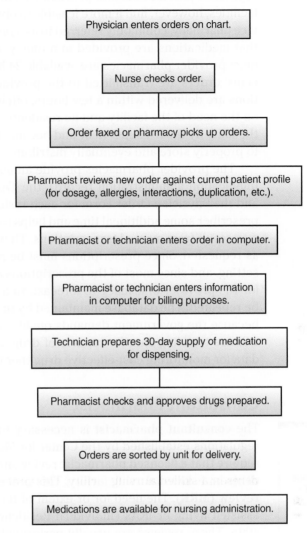

FIGURE 4-3 A medication order entry flow chart.

The medical staff, in coordination with the pharmacy consultant, should develop policies for an **automatic stop order** for particular drugs (e.g., antibiotics and steroids). These drugs and others require that the patient's drug response be reevaluated after specific time intervals (e.g., one week, 10 days, or one month). At that time a medical decision is made to continue the drug, change the dosage, or discontinue the drug. This is a method to assure the proper monitoring of drug usage.

Any procedure or helpful practice that enables the pharmacist or pharmacy technician to assist the nurse in providing a safe medication delivery system is of great value (Figure 4-3). In the future, an automated dispensing machine may be used to blend nursing's need for access with pharmacy's need to control.

Pharmaceutical Personnel in Long-Term Care

Concerning the business aspects of securing prescriptions, there are several types of arrangements by which long-term care facilities obtain the prescriptions for their residents. The larger facilities may have an in-house pharmacy staffed by registered pharmacists and pharmacy technicians. Most small to moderate-sized facilities, however, find it more feasible to obtain medications from a vendor or service pharmacy, commonly referred to as a *provider pharmacy*. In an effort to assure that medications are provided in a timely manner to the long-term care facility, most provider pharmacies are available 24 hours a day, seven days a week. Physicians' orders are transmitted to the provider pharmacy, and the filled prescriptions are delivered within a few hours, often two to three times a day, depending on the need of the facility and its residents. Drugs are then usually distributed to the units by the RN supervisor and become the responsibility of the charge nurse to properly store and eventually distribute.

The provider pharmacies provide an additional service by printing the MAR (medication administration record), the TAR (treatment administration record), and the Physician Order Form for each resident, which saves both the nurse and prescriber some additional time and helps reduce potential medication errors that may result from manual transcriptions. They also produce administrative reports as requested. Since prescriptions must be renewed every 30 days in a long-term setting, and since most of the prescriptions are for chronic ailments, it is possible for the provider pharmacy to forecast, to a large extent, what prescriptions will be repeated. The database maintained by these vendors is increasingly important because the government demands quality assurance activities, while the facility will use trending data for reports of drug usage levels and pharmaceutical cost data for monitoring cost-effective drug therapy.

Consultant Pharmacist

consultant pharmacist responsible for monitoring drug usage and drug therapy of residents in nursing homes.

medication regimen review (MRR) the process established by the Center for Medicare and Medicaid Services requiring that a licensed pharmacist review medication use every month for all residents in a skilled nursing facility.

The **consultant pharmacist** is necessary to the long-term care facility. Federal regulations established by the Center for Medicare and Medicaid Services (CMS) require that a licensed pharmacist review medication use every month for all residents in a skilled nursing facility. This process is called the **medication regimen review (MRR)**. The need for or extent of the MRR in other LTC facilities, such as assisted living or IRAs (Individual Residence Alternatives), varies from state to state. These reviews are usually performed on-site because the pharmacist can use the resident's medical chart. The chart contains information such as laboratory values, physician and nursing notes, and medication administration records. All this information is helpful for identifying a medication problem. The consultant pharmacist reports his or her findings to the medical director, director of nursing, administrator, and the attending physicians (Figure 4-4).

In December 2006, revisions were made to the regulations involving the medication regimen review and the role of the consultant pharmacist. These revisions put greater emphasis on closely evaluating if each medication prescribed is necessary and the consideration of tapering and/or eliminating unnecessary drug consumption. Special attention is given to the use of certain medications known to be a problem in the elderly. In some situations, the consultant pharmacist is now required to perform the MRR more often than once a month.

In addition to the medication regimen reviews, oversight of all pharmacy services is the responsibility of the consultant pharmacist. This careful supervision helps ensure the safe and effective use of medications as well as control of and accountability for the medications throughout the facility. This may include working on policies and procedures, nursing unit inspections, and in-service education to nursing personnel. The consultant pharmacist also works with administration and the medical and nursing staff to help control medication costs, as well as work-

FIGURE 4-4

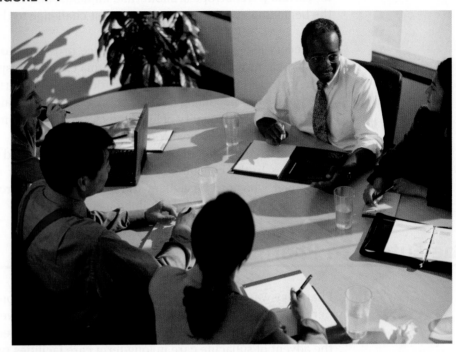

FIGURE 4-4 The consultant pharmacist reports quarterly to the Pharmaceutical Services Committee to provide guidance relating to pharmacy services and unnecessary medications, and to ensure safe administration of medication and education for staff (Courtesy of PhotoDisc).

ing with administration and staff on preparation for annual surveys and the proper disposition of prescription medication. While the actual MRR must be performed by a licensed pharmacist, a technician can be helpful with these other activities.

Emerging Challenges for the Pharmaceutical and Nursing Professional

Several of the growing concerns in the pharmaceutical field include the somewhat different pharmacokinetics of drug absorption, distribution, metabolism, and excretion of drugs in the elderly. Perhaps one of the most pressing is the sheer number of prescriptions that a typical resident needs and the corresponding direct relationship for potential of drug interactions with the increased number of drugs. The changing standard of practice in the treatment of heart disease, for example, currently calls for taking several drugs to control the condition. This is a typical situation in the treatment of many other diseases.

This creates a growing problem for the nurse in a long-term care facility. We are rapidly approaching a point where the number of prescriptions for a patient is so large that it becomes physically difficult, if not impossible, for the elderly resident to ingest. These residents often have difficulty with swallowing or cannot follow instructions. Increasingly, the surveyors are holding nurses to guidelines listed in the package insert of a prescription. This means that for each prescription, eight ounces of water should be ingested; a certain time must elapse between drugs or between drugs and meals; and so forth. It falls to the pharmaceutical professionals to develop other means of delivering the medication. Long-acting injections (used for certain psychotropics, subdermal implants, and transdermal patches) are just the beginning of what is now the greatest challenge to the delivery of good health care.

Recent legislation now allows hospice providers to serve the dying population in long-term care facilities. Before this change, hospice services were mostly home-based. Hospice personnel have developed expertise in pain management. This area is fast becoming not just a concern for the dying, but for all patients who could have a better quality of life if they were able to be more comfortable and less controlled by their medical conditions.

These concerns relating to the number of drugs and patient response present challenges to the consulting and provider pharmacist and medical and nursing personnel, who must be vigilant and work together to provide safe and meaningful drug therapy to the residents in long-term care.

The Future of Pharmacy in Long-Term Care

Pharmacy was probably the first of the caring professions to utilize the computer. Certainly, the logic and structure of the pharmacy is well suited to the strengths of the computer. In the future this natural linkage will become even stronger. With the advent of subacute care in long-term care facilities (with intravenous therapy, as well as a completely new spectrum of high-tech drugs), the need for rational administration and continuous quality improvement will grow. As LTC facilities increase in computer sophistication, information will be rapidly exchanged. Today there are several computer programs that allow physicians to order medications electronically through a computer station or a handheld device. The nurse can review the computer screen and then is able to easily send the vendor pharmacy the computerized reorder, which can then be immediately produced. The savings in time and the lessening of the potential for errors will be great. Quality assurance and risk management functions can also be set up to shadow these prescribing programs.

On the other end of the spectrum, the healthier elderly will gravitate to the assisted living environment—where direct supervision will be less—at a time when their ability to comprehend the drug directions may be diminishing. Hence the challenge will be to package, label, and safeguard the product so that it will be used properly for maximum benefit. A relatively new concept for this market is the color-coded cartridge delivery system. Medication distribution are preloaded into different colored cartridges for different hours of the day. For example, 9 a.m. medications will be in the yellow cartridge, noon meds will be blue, with evening meds being packaged in a different color. This will undoubtedly generate more set-up responsibilities for the pharmacy technician, but will also help the elderly maintain independence and safety while getting all of their needed medications.

Cost containment will increase in importance as a "managed health care model" becomes more popular. Some experts predict that the managed care model will depend more heavily on drug therapy as opposed to more expensive invasive procedures, while others maintain more drugs will become over-the-counter items, a situation that presents a challenge for the dispensing pharmacist to be able to monitor and avoid drug interactions with prescription and nonprescription drugs. Access to databases and "smart cards" that contain entire drug histories for individuals could help in these situations.

Extensive research is being carried out in the use of psychotropic drugs for geriatric (elderly) patients at home. The target goal is to find effective psychotropic drugs with maximum therapeutic benefits and fewer undesirable side effects (e.g., lethargy, apathy, ataxia, and so forth). The pharmacist consultant, in conjunction with the medical staff, needs to maintain up-to-date information to provide effective therapy. The future may well see increased use of combination drugs, longer intervals between doses, implants, pumps, discs, and/or rods. All of these innovations need to be understood, blended for maximum benefit, and tracked for safety. These functions will be within the scope of the pharmacy technicians who understand computers and who stay on the cutting edge of this information explosion.

Summary

Pharmaceutical care provided in long-term care will continue to be a vital service to the care and well being of the growing elderly population. The challenge will be to provide rational drug therapy that is safe, effective, and affordable. The expanding geriatric population will need help, direction, and counseling to maximize good health. The challenge for the pharmaceutical professional is to make information clear and easily understood for a population with increasing deficits.

TEST YOUR KNOWLEDGE

Multiple Choice

1. Legislation that changed the way long-term care was financed was
   a. Medicare.
   b. Medicaid.
   c. Social Security.
   d. both Medicare and Medicaid.

2. The most common type of long-term care facility is
   a. voluntary, not-for-profit.
   b. government-sponsored.
   c. proprietary.
   d. hospice.

3. The most important goal of a long-term care pharmacist is to
   a. fill the prescription per the doctor's order.
   b. write the directions so that no error can be made.
   c. help the nursing personnel properly administer the medication through education and support.
   d. perform all of the above.

4. Drug regimen reviews on each patient are required
   a. upon admission.
   b. upon change of orders.
   c. monthy.
   d. weekly.

5. The consultant pharmacist must report errors and discrepancies to
   a. the medical doctor.
   b. the director of nursing services.
   c. the administrator.
   d. all of the above.

6. Technicians will most probably be responsible for
   a. the packaging of the unit-dose cards.
   b. credit on returned drugs.
   c. administrative computer duties.
   d. all of the above.

7. Managed care companies will probably
   a. use more drug therapy than invasive procedures.
   b. become more aggressive in cost-cutting procedures.
   c. exercise greater control over doctors' prescribing habits.
   d. all of the above.

8. To survive in the future, pharmacists and technicians will have to become comfortable with
   a. quality assurance activities.
   b. continuous monitoring/risk identification.
   c. computerization/information sharing.
   d. all of the above.

9. The governmental body driving the standardization of rules and regulations for long-term care facilities is the
   a. Department of Health and Human Services.
   b. Centers for Disease Control and Prevention.
   c. Center for Medicare and Medicaid Services.
   d. Federal Drug Enforcement Agency.

10. Funding for prescription medications is covered under
    a. Medicare Part A.
    b. Medicare Part B.
    c. Medicare Part C.
    d. Medicare Part D.

Fill In The Blank

1. The provision of health and personal care (meeting physical and emotional needs) to individuals over an extended period of time is called _____.

2. _____ covers doctor visits, specialized tests, and supplies.

3. A gatekeeper between the individual and government payor provided under Medicare Part D is the _____.

4. _____ covers hospital stays and some nursing home time.

5. _____ provide long-term care to individuals needing extensive medical care as well as personal care around the clock.

References

Dean, Nancy L. (April 2007). *An extra dose of safety.* Health Management Technology. Retrieved from www.healthmgttech.com/features/2007_april/0407extra_dose.aspx.

Hagland, Mark. (September 2006). *Right patient, right dose.* Healthcare Informatics. Retrieved from www.healthcare-informatics.com.

The long-term care state operations manual. HcPro Inc., 483.60 Pharmacy Services. www.hcpro.com.

U. S. Census Bureau. (2007). *2005 statistical abstract of the United States, health and nutrition.* Washington, DC.

Web Sites

National Care Planning Council
   www.longtermcarelink.net
National Clearinghouse for Long-Term Care Information
   www.longtermcare.gov
U.S. Department of Health and Human Services Medicare Web Site
   www.medicare.gov

Community Pharmacy

Competencies

Upon completion of this chapter, the reader should be able to

1. Define community pharmacy as a branch of ambulatory care.
2. Discuss the knowledge and skills necessary to practice as a pharmacy technician in the community pharmacy setting.
3. Differentiate between available opportunities within community pharmacy.
4. Outline the process of preparing a prescription for dispensing.

Key Terms

ambulatory care
chain pharmacy
collaborative drug therapy agreement
independent pharmacy
medication therapy management (MTM)

Introduction

This chapter will provide an overview of community pharmacy practice, highlighting the role of the pharmacy technician. The various types of community pharmacy settings will be explored, with an emphasis on the skills and attributes of this popular and rewarding area of practice.

Community Pharmacy Practice

Community pharmacy is a diverse, dynamic, and constantly changing practice environment comprised of several different practice settings and offering many opportunities for the pharmacy practitioner. First and foremost, community pharmacy is a practice environment that requires good people skills and excellent communication, because the pharmacy practitioner deals with patients on a daily basis (Figure 5-1). Pharmacy technicians play a vital role in the community pharmacy, assisting the pharmacist in preparing prescriptions, collecting information from patients, and performing several important functions that will be discussed later in this chapter.

Pharmacists have been at the top of the Gallup poll of most trusted professionals every year, and many people use their community pharmacist as their sole source of health care information. Most people visit their community pharmacy more often than any other health care setting and look to their community pharmacist for information, advice, and counseling. In the community pharmacy, practitioners can recommend a cough and cold remedy in one minute and then help a transplant patient decipher his complex medication regimen in the next minute. Basically, in the community pharmacy, practitioners have to be ready for anything,

FIGURE 5-1

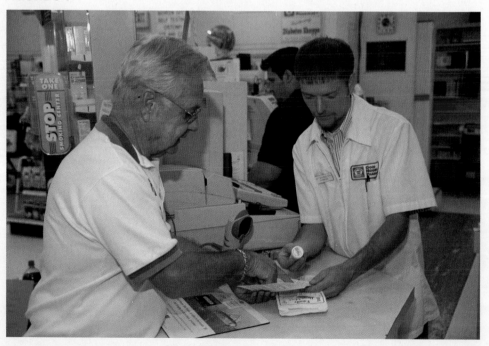

FIGURE 5-1 Working in a community pharmacy requires good interpersonal skills.

and every day offers new and exciting opportunities to assist people in improving their health care and quality of life.

Community pharmacy is a branch of ambulatory care practice. **Ambulatory care** simply means that the patients being treated are not hospitalized or institutionalized, or that they walk in and out in the same day. Other ambulatory care settings include physicians' offices, clinics, and emergency rooms. Another term for ambulatory care is the "outpatient setting." When patients are in the hospital or reside in a long-term care facility, they are referred to as *inpatients* because they are living, usually temporarily, in the facility. When they are residing at home, they are referred to as *outpatients*. Community pharmacy is recognized as an outpatient or ambulatory care setting.

The number of prescriptions being filled has increased dramatically over the last few years and is only expected to keep rising. One of the reasons the number of prescriptions is rising is the aging of the population. People are living longer and are healthier than ever before. As people age, their requirements for medications increase, and more prescriptions are needed. In addition to the aging of the population, advances in medicine are allowing physicians to treat patients without putting them in the hospital, adding to the numbers of prescriptions processed in the outpatient or community pharmacy setting. More and more medications are available each year, the more prescriptions that will be generated. These factors, along with an increased access to insurance programs, add up to more prescriptions requiring processing in community pharmacies.

Because of the rapid growth in the number of prescriptions each year, the community pharmacy environment needs to be open to changing and adapting to meeting increased needs. One change we are consistently witnessing is the growing role of technology in processing prescriptions. Virtually all community pharmacies utilize computers to varying degrees in the prescription-filling process (Figure 5-2).

FIGURE 5-2

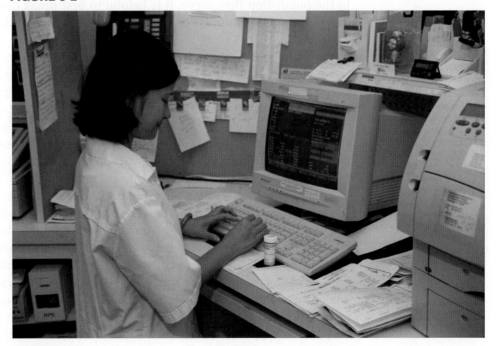

FIGURE 5-2 A solid foundation of computer skills is also necessary to work in the community pharmacy.

Besides keeping a computerized patient profile, computers in the pharmacy can be used to screen phone calls and accept refill orders, scan prescriptions to prevent errors, and, in some cases, count the units of medication, fill the container, and label the vial. Computers are also used to alert the pharmacist to drug interactions and transmit insurance information to a patient's insurance company. Many pharmacies utilize e-prescribing technology, where a prescription can be generated at the prescriber's office and electronically transmitted directly into the processing computer at the local pharmacy, eliminating the need to enter information off a paper prescription. In the future we may not even be surprised to see various types of medication-dispensing kiosks where consumers can pick up an attached phone and have a video conference with a pharmacist in some remote location off the premises. With prescription volume increasing and the shortage of pharmacists worsening, this may become more common than we would like to think.

In addition to increasing technology, another expanding area in community pharmacy is the role of pharmacy technicians. Pharmacists are expanding their role as patient-care providers and incorporating more patient-care activities into their daily practice. With the increasing complexity of drug regimens, pharmacists need to be spending more time with the patients, counseling and educating them on their disease states and medication therapy. This proves to be a difficult task with the increasing volume of prescriptions being handled, so technicians in this area are vital to patient care. By performing many of the technical functions in support of the pharmacist, pharmacy technicians are enabling patients to spend more time with the pharmacist, receiving care and information that can help them get the most benefit from their therapy.

Types of Community Pharmacies

independent pharmacy a retail pharmacy owned and operated by an individual pharmacist or group of individuals as compared to chain drug stores.

chain pharmacy a retail pharmacy owned by a corporation that consists of many stores in a particular region or nationally.

There are different types of community pharmacies, offering varying services to the population they serve. It is helpful to first break down the pharmacies by definition and then discuss the different services each of the types of pharmacies can provide.

Independent pharmacies consist of one to four stores owned and operated by an individual pharmacist or group of individuals. They are not part of a large corporation. They vary greatly in size, volume of prescriptions, and services. A benefit of working for an independent pharmacy would be that there is usually direct access to the owner or main decision maker, so suggestions can go right to the top. Also, independent pharmacies are sometimes more likely to specialize in one area of pharmacy, such as surgical supplies or home infusion therapy. These types of services are discussed later in the chapter.

Chain pharmacies also vary in size, volume, and services and can be differentiated from one another based on the setting in which they are housed. Chain drugstores are the most common, and although these stores sell mostly traditional drugstore merchandise, many of them carry a large variety of products. Chain drugstores can be regional, where they only operate stores in one geographic area, or national, with stores spread out all over the country. Examples of national chain drugstores include CVS and Rite-Aid. In addition to chain drugstores, chain pharmacies can be located in supermarkets, and again, be regional or national in scope. Other types of stores that sometimes house chain pharmacies are mass merchandisers like Target, Costco, and Kmart. So even within chain pharmacy, the settings vary greatly and the practices can be quite different from place to place.

Community Pharmacy Services

The services that different types of community pharmacies provide are as diverse as the stores that house them. Customary pharmacy services include prescription processing and basic over-the-counter and general merchandise provision. But the services do not have to end there. Many community pharmacies base the services they provide on the population they serve and the demand in the area in which they are located.

Surgical Supply/Durable Medical Equipment

Some community pharmacies provide surgical supplies to patients in their community. This would include durable medical equipment such as knee braces, neck collars, hospital beds, canes, walkers, commodes, and other products. A pharmacy specializing in durable medical equipment will have a pharmacist and specially-trained staff to assist patients in choosing the best products, fitting patients for products like braces and orthotic supplies, and obtaining proper reimbursement from insurance providers for these services.

Long-Term Care

Community pharmacies can also provide medications to long-term care facilities in addition to providing prescription processing services to the community. Some long-term care facilities, like nursing homes, have their own pharmacies in the building, but many, because of their size or budget, may not. In these cases the facilities use pharmacies that generally prepare the orders on a daily basis for the inpatients and deliver the medications to the facility. This type of setting combines inpatient and outpatient services into one environment.

Home Infusion

Similar to long-term care provision, some pharmacies provide home care organizations with parenteral medications. These products are prepared in the community pharmacy and then delivered or shipped to the patient's home, where a skilled nurse will administer the medication. Home infusion services are discussed in detail in Chapter 3 of this textbook.

Specialty Compounding Services

Many community and/or compounding pharmacies across the country specialize in compounding pharmaceutical products that are not readily available in a particular dosage form or in the dose necessary for the patient. Compounded pharmaceutical products can take the form of oral suspensions or solutions, intravenous admixtures, capsules, topical preparations, or even the unusual, like lollipops. Compounding services are an important part of many community pharmacy services. They are especially useful in special patient populations such as children and veterinary practices. Many times children will suffer from illnesses that can be treated only with adult medications. In these cases, the medications may only be available as a tablet or capsule or only in a dosage that would far exceed what would be recommended for a child. The medication needs to be diluted into a child-appropriate dose and possibly into a dosage form that can be taken by a child who cannot swallow tablets or capsules. In these situations, the pharmacist would prepare a solution or suspension by grinding the available tablets into a powder,

FIGURE 5-3

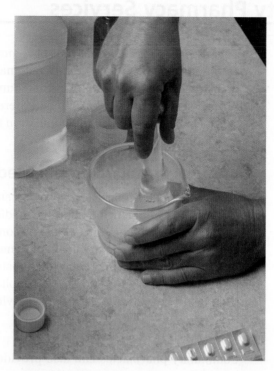

FIGURE 5-3 Some community pharmacies specialize in compounding services for special populations such as pediatrics or veterinary practices.

adding an appropriate amount of water or other diluent, and then flavoring the preparation to make it palatable (Figure 5-3). This is just one example of how pharmacists use compounding services to improve the care offered to patients.

Veterinary practices also use compounding services on a routine basis. Many veterinarians use human medications to treat their animals. The doses or dosage forms they need are not commercially available. They will then go to a community pharmacy that specializes in compounding veterinary products and use their services to get what they need.

The pharmacy technician offers many types of services to the compounding pharmacist. A technician may be involved in almost any step in the process, from gathering the necessary ingredients to be incorporated, to mixing the products together under the supervision of the pharmacist. Some of the skills necessary to participate in compounding services are meticulous attention to detail, knowing how to properly using equipment necessary to weigh and measure wet and dry ingredients, and knowledge of the metric and apothecary system for weights and measures. Extemporaneous compounding is covered in detail in Chapter 14.

Mail-Order Pharmacies

Mail-order pharmacies can be divided into two categories: those affiliated with large pharmacy benefits management (PBM) companies and smaller, independent operations. PBMs are used by employers, or the insurers of employers, to manage and handle pharmacy claims.

Mail-order pharmacies accept new prescriptions from patients through the mail, dispense the prescriptions, and send them back through the mail to the patients. Refills for medication are requested by telephone, e-mail, or a postcard. Sometimes the mail-order pharmacy is located in a state other than the state where the patient lives. The lack of one-on-one contact with a pharmacist and the delay in receiving medication are the main reasons people do not use mail-order pharmacies. Examples of mail-order pharmacies are those associated with AARP, Express Scripts, Medco, AdvancePCS, and PharmaCare Direct.

Internet Pharmacy

Recently some Internet or cyber-pharmacies have emerged. The first question about these is usually "Are they legal?" They are if they are licensed in the state where they are located and in the states where they are doing business. These pharmacies function much like mail-order pharmacies, but with a few exceptions. Some Internet pharmacies are establishing personal contact between pharmacists and patients via e-mail. They are also using patient profiles, offering over-the-counter (OTC) sales, and providing a wide choice of delivery options including mail, express delivery, or pick up at an affiliated retail pharmacy. Examples of Internet pharmacy services are www.drugstore.com, www.planetrx.com, and www.soma.com.

Outpatient Pharmacies in Hospitals

Some larger hospitals have outpatient pharmacies within the hospital, usually close to the entrance, the clinics, or emergency room. These pharmacies dispense medication to their ambulatory patients. They also fill prescriptions written by doctors on the hospital staff and dispense the first filling of a new prescription for a patient being discharged from the hospital and prescriptions for employees of the hospital.

Prescription Processing

The primary activity involved in community pharmacy practice is processing prescriptions and delivering them to a patient or caregiver with provision of appropriate medication information. While several types of community pharmacy settings offering an array of services exist, this basic function remains consistent across all types. The process begins when a prescription is presented, either by phone, fax, e-prescribing technology including e-mail, or in person. The prescription is then entered into the computer and cross-checked with the patients' existing profile. If this is the first time the patient is visiting the pharmacy, additional information needs to be collected from the patient and entered into the record. Once the prescription is entered into the computer, it usually goes on to be processed and filled. If the prescription requires making a clinical decision or some type of pharmacist intervention, the pharmacist needs to be alerted so he or she can resolve the problem (Figure 5-4). Once the prescription is deemed adequate to process, the medication is retrieved from the inventory, and then the appropriate number of dosing units is counted or measured, placed in a container, and labeled. At this point, the pharmacist will perform one final check to ensure no errors have been made. The prescription is then delivered to the patient or caregiver or put in a location of the pharmacy designated for prescriptions waiting to be picked up. A pharmacy technician can participate in virtually every step of this process. However, when a clinical decision needs to be made, such as how to handle an inappropriate dose or drug interaction, the pharmacist is the only person who should ever make those decisions.

FIGURE 5-4

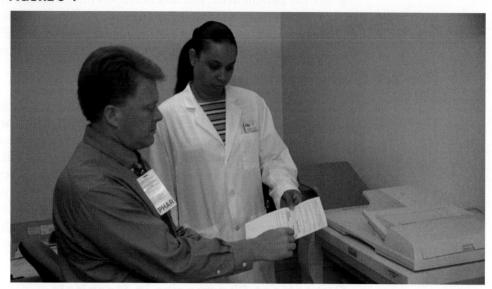

FIGURE 5-4 If the pharmacy technician has a question about a prescription, the pharmacist must be consulted for confirmation before proceeding to dispense.

The Pharmacy Technician in the Community Pharmacy

Because of the process just outlined, which comprises most of a community pharmacy technician's time, there are certain qualifications people should possess if they are considering a position as a pharmacy technician in this setting. As previously mentioned, communication and interpersonal skills are a necessity, and potential technicians should pay extraordinary attention to detail because of the nature of their responsibility. Community pharmacies can sometimes be busy, stressful places; and an ability to properly handle these types of situations is crucial. The ability to stay focused among different types of distractions is also necessary. Working in a community pharmacy processing prescriptions also requires knowledge of prescription medications—most importantly, their brand and generic names—as well as computer literacy and an understanding of pharmacy billing and third-party (insurance) reimbursement. Many of these skills can be learned through on-the-job training, but formalized training and technician certification programs are making for higher-quality personnel.

The pharmacy technician's role in the community pharmacy includes:

■ Greeting each patient in a respectful, professional manner—a friendly personality is a great attribute. The pharmacy technician is usually the first person the patient encounters at the pharmacy and represents the entire department. As the saying goes, "First impressions are everything."

■ Collecting information from the patient to ensure the prescription is processed efficiently and accurately. This includes information such as the patient's name and address, date of birth, individual health information, and insurance information.

■ Assisting in the technical aspects of prescription preparation. This includes typing information into the computerized database, retrieving medications from stock, counting dosage units, labeling prescription vials, returning

FIGURE 5-5

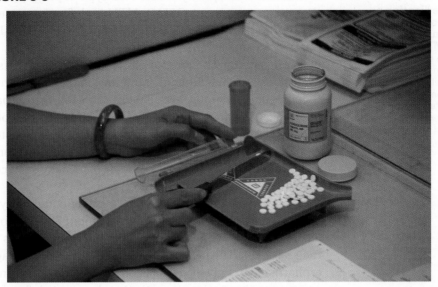

FIGURE 5-5 One aspect of preparing a prescription may be to count the pills to be dispensed.

items to stock, and keeping the pharmacy department orderly and organized (Figure 5-5).

■ Submitting electronic claims to insurance providers, and addressing all issues related to the claims.

■ Alerting the pharmacist when clinical intervention is necessary.

■ Complying with the various federal and state laws governing the practice of pharmacy. The pharmacy technician should be familiar with all the laws that govern practice and aid the pharmacist in complying with those laws.

Patient Care

With the expansion of the pharmacy profession to incorporate more patient-care activities into practice, many community pharmacies are offering direct patient-care services such as medication therapy management, screenings for conditions such as osteoporosis, diabetes, and high blood pressure, and immunizations. All pharmacists in the community setting provide clinical services to some degree because any prescription being processed in the pharmacy requires some patient-oriented activity. However, some pharmacies are expanding the types of clinical services they provide and are offering various patient education programs, disease-state management services, and medication administration services.

The increasing complexity of many medication therapy regimens requires patients to be well educated about their illnesses and the medications being used to treat them. Pharmacists are an excellent source of this information, and many pharmacies offer services to assist patients in managing their illnesses through patient education. The patient education services offered in community pharmacies usually focus on common disease states such as diabetes, asthma, hyperlipidemia, smoking cessation, and hypertension. The pharmacy may offer special counseling sessions with the pharmacist where patients are taught about their illness, the medications that manage it, and some lifestyle changes they can make

medication therapy management (MTM) pharmacists are reimbursed for non-drug services such as drug therapy management for diabetes, anticoagulation, anemia, hypertension, and renal failure.

to increase their quality of life. This type of program is referred to as **medication therapy management (MTM)**. MTM is defined as a service or group of services that optimize therapeutic outcomes for an individual patient. The patients and pharmacist meet either on a one-on-one basis or as a group and discuss their disease, monitor their progress, and in many disease management programs, even perform clinical monitoring and make treatment decisions. The results of their regular meetings are usually reported to the patient's physician, and the pharmacist is part of that patient's treatment team. Some clinical monitoring that takes place in community pharmacies includes cholesterol testing, blood sugar or diabetes testing, and blood pressure screening and monitoring. These types of services go along with the expansion of pharmacy services to more patient-focused activities.

Another area of involvement for many community pharmacists is immunizations. Almost all of the states in the United States allow pharmacists to administer immunizations, and many community pharmacies have made that a focus of their services. Through a collaborative drug therapy agreement with a physician, a pharmacist is given permission to administer an immunization, such as a flu or pneumonia vaccine, to patients who meet defined criteria spelled out in the agreement. A **collaborative drug therapy agreement** allows a physician to designate certain responsibilities to a pharmacist. It is a voluntary written agreement between a pharmacist and prescriber that permits expanded authority for the pharmacist, such as the ability to initiate or modify drug therapy or order and perform laboratory tests. The agreements are not limited to the practice of immunizations; we see them being incorporated into programs for diabetes, cholesterol, and anticoagulant therapy.

collaborative drug therapy agreement an agreement between a physician and a pharmacist that allows the pharmacist expanded prescription authorization regarding managing drug therapy.

Since clinical services are directly related to patient care, the pharmacy technician should express that same dedication to caring for patients by offering a courteous, respectful, caring, professional attitude. Frequently, it is the pharmacy technician who has the initial contact with the patient and holds the responsibility for generating patient confidence and comfort in the ensuing interaction. A poor greeting and discourteous attitude may create a less-than-favorable situation for the patient, pharmacist, and staff. A pharmacy technician should be committed to providing patient care, which goes beyond the customer service found in retail outlets. Persons presenting to pharmacy for assistance or to have a prescription filled are considered patients, which means the relationship goes beyond that of a purveyor and customer. The rewards of such patient interactions and the opportunity to develop relationships with patients is one of the most gratifying aspects of becoming a pharmacy technician.

Summary

In summary, community pharmacy is a diverse, fast-paced environment that requires good interpersonal skills and attention to detail. Pharmacy technicians are an increasingly important part of the expansion of pharmacist services to include more patient-focused activities such as medication therapy management. The role of pharmacy technicians will increase in the future as the volume of prescriptions increases. Community pharmacy can be a tremendously rewarding area of pharmacy practice, because practitioners get the opportunity to impact peoples' health and care for patients on a daily basis.

TEST YOUR KNOWLEDGE

Multiple Choice

1. Community pharmacy practice is an example of
   a. long-term care.
   b. acute care.
   c. ambulatory care.
   d. nuclear pharmacy.

2. In recent years, the number of prescriptions processed in the community pharmacy setting has
   a. steadily increased.
   b. steadily decreased.
   c. remained the same.
   d. varied.

3. The pharmacy technician can perform all of the following tasks in the community pharmacy *except*
   a. counting the correct number of medication units to be dispensed.
   b. labeling the medication container.
   c. receiving the written prescription to be processed from the patient.
   d. counsel the patient on the appropriate use of the medication and side effects.

4. Community pharmacies vary in their delivery of services and may provide which of the following?
   a. prescription compounding
   b. durable medical equipment
   c. medication therapy management
   d. all of the above

5. A single pharmacy owned and operated by an individual or group of individuals is an example of a/an
   a. independent pharmacy.
   b. chain pharmacy.
   c. regional pharmacy.
   d. long-term care pharmacy.

6. Which of the following is an ambulatory care setting?
   a. nursing home
   b. community pharmacy
   c. rehabilitation center
   d. intensive care unit

7. Pharmacy technicians are experiencing an increase in roles in community pharmacy due to
   a. pharmacists expanding their roles as patient-care providers.
   b. decreases in technology used in the pharmacy.
   c. people living healthier and longer lives.
   d. increasing needs to compound medications.

8. The primary activity involved in community pharmacy practice is
   a. preparing medications for inpatients.
   b. processing prescriptions.
   c. managing drug regimens.
   d. delivering medications to patients.

9. The pharmacy technician's role includes which of the following?
   a. counseling patients
   b. making recommendations for over-the-counter products
   c. collecting information from patients
   d. developing drug regimens for patients

10. Types of direct patient-care services being offered in the community pharmacy include
    a. medication therapy management.
    b. collaborative drug therapy agreements.
    c. drug reviews.
    d. all of the above.

Fill In The Blank

1. Care provided to patients who walk in and out in the same day is called _____ care.

2. The primary reason for the rising number of prescriptions is _____.

3. A pharmacy owned and operated by a pharmacist or group of pharmacists is called a/an _____ pharmacy.

4. A pharmacy that is a part of a large business and sells retail items as well as pharmaceuticals is called a/an _____ pharmacy.

5. One of the primary qualifications for working in a community pharmacy is good _____ skills.

References

American Pharmacists Association. (2003). White paper on pharmacy technicians: Needed changes can no longer wait. *Journal of the American Pharmacists Association*, 43(1): 93–107.

Hagel, H. P., & Rovers J. P. (Eds.). (2002). *Managing the patient-centered pharmacy*. Washington, DC: American Pharmacists Association.

Tindall, W. N., Beardsley, R. S., & Kimberlin, C. L. (Eds.). (2007). *Communication skills in pharmacy practice* (5th ed.). Philadelphia: Lippincott Williams & Wilkins.

Web Sites

National Community Pharmacists Association   www.ncpanet.org

PART

II

The Profession of Pharmacy

CHAPTER

6

Regulatory Standards in Pharmacy Practice

Competencies

Upon completion of this chapter, the reader should be able to

1. Describe the difference between statutes, rules and regulations, and quasi-legal standards.
2. Identify several federal regulatory agencies.
3. Explain the reason for rules, regulations, and practice standards in health institutions.
4. State the need for the Food, Drug, and Cosmetic Act.
5. Discuss the Investigational Drug Approval Process.
6. List several requirements of the Controlled Substance Act (CSA).
7. Recognize drugs that fall under regulation of the Controlled Substance Act.
8. Explain the need for Material Safety Data Sheets (MSDS).
9. Cite appropriate categories of drugs requiring patient package inserts.
10. State several basic components of the patients' bill of rights.

Key Terms

Bureau of Alcohol, Tobacco and Firearms (ATF)

Controlled Substances Act (CSA)

covered entities

Drug Enforcement Administration (DEA)

Durham-Humphrey Amendment

Federal Food, Drug, and Cosmetic Act (FDCA)

Federal Hazardous Substances Act

federal statutes

Food and Drug Administration (FDA)

Food and Drug Administration Modernization Act of 1997 (FDAMA)

Food, Drug, and Cosmetic Act of 1938

Hazard Communication Standard (HCS)

Health Insurance Portability and Accountability Act (HIPAA)

Joint Commission

Kefauver-Harris Amendment

medication administration record (MAR)

Occupational and Safety Act of 1970

Omnibus Budget Reconciliation Act (OBRA)

orphan drugs

patient package insert (PPI)

patients' bill of rights

Poison Prevention Packaging Act

prospective drug review

protected health information (PHI)

Pure Food and Drug Act of 1906

quasi-legal standards

rules and regulations

Schedule I

Schedule II

Schedule III

Schedule IV

Schedule V

state board of pharmacy

Introduction

Rules and regulations are necessary to ensure the orderly and safe functioning of society while protecting and respecting individual prerogatives. No individual or enterprise is without regulation.

Regulations in health care provide for assurance of the safety and welfare of health care recipients, provide for the provision of minimum standards of a health care service, and provide standards by which to judge reasonable and prudent practice in a court of law. Additionally, the implementation of new regulations has, overall, a very positive impact on the elevation and expansion of health care services and responsibilities.

Health care institutions are complex entities providing services to every segment of our society. Because of the complexity of health care, every profession in a health care institution is subject to regulation in some form. The profession of pharmacy—with its direct relationship to public health, safety, and welfare—is, as such, under the watchful eye of regulatory agencies.

One objective of this chapter is to give the pharmacy technician an understanding of some federal and state regulatory agencies and the laws, rules, and practice standards affecting pharmacy practice. The other objective is to provide an appreciation of the relationship of these regulatory standards to the specific activities of the pharmacist and the pharmacy technician in the practice of pharmacy.

Statutes, Rules, Regulations, and Quasi-Legal Standards

Federal statutes enacted by a legislative body (Congress at the federal level or the legislature at the state level) outline the conduct of persons or organizations subject to the law. They also enable regulatory agencies to regulate a field pursuant to the mandate of the legislative body. Examples of federal agencies and their respective regulatory statutes are the Food and Drug Administration, which administers the Food, Drug, and Cosmetic Act (FDCA), and the Drug Enforcement Administration, which administers the federal Comprehensive Drug Abuse and Prevention Control Act, more commonly known as the Controlled Substances Act (CSA). These agencies and statues will be discussed in more detail later in the chapter.

Rules and regulations are administrative enactments that are implemented by government agencies at the local, state, and federal levels and meet the intent of statutory policies and procedures. For example, regulatory agencies such as the **Food and Drug Administration (FDA)** and the **Drug Enforcement Administration (DEA)** can implement rules and regulations to enforce the Federal Food, Drug, and Cosmetic Act and the Controlled Substances Act, respectively. State boards of pharmacy issue detailed regulations to carry out the policies and procedures of the state pharmacy acts.

Quasi means "similar to." **Quasi-legal standards** are established by semi-governmental or private organizations, such as professional pharmacy organizations. These standards are recognized by the federal government and many state governments. They have been sanctioned through statutes and regulations. The American Society of Health-System Pharmacists (ASHP) has developed an extensive series of practice standards covering numerous aspects of institutional pharmacy practice. Practice standards provide a basis for evaluation, review, and goal-setting for hospital pharmacy directors and their staffs. In a court of law, the practice standards define accepted professional practice and assume quasi-legal status. The system of law in the United States relating to the practice of medicine, pharmacy, and other health professions is based on "reasonable and prudent" practice. Practice standards define reasonable and prudent practice. A practitioner who fails to meet these standards may be found negligent by the courts.

Federal Versus State Drug Control Laws

Federal laws and regulations vary from those of particular states; therefore, practicing pharmacists and technicians must learn certain basic rules in order to know where they stand in complying with the law. These rules can be summarized as follows:

1. Pharmacists are equally responsible for compliance with both federal and state laws and respective regulations governing their pharmacy practice.
2. If the federal law or regulation is more stringent than the comparable state law or regulation, or vice versa, the more stringent law or regulation must be followed. In many cases, the state law or regulation is more stringent than its federal counterpart.

State Regulatory Agencies

Every state will have its own unique structure for the regulation of the education, licensing, and discipline of the profession of pharmacy. It should be recognized that laws may change from state to state, as different boards of pharmacy will have different roles and responsibilities for both the pharmacist and pharmacy technician that may vary significantly.

State Boards of Pharmacy

state board of pharmacy body established to ensure that the public is well served professionally by pharmacists.

In most states, responsibilities of the **state board of pharmacy** are to ensure that the public is well served professionally by pharmacists, and the drugs distributed and dispensed within each state meet standards for purity and potency and are properly labeled. Other responsibilities include but are not limited to the following:

- Licensing and registering pharmacies.
- Dealing with complaints of professional misconduct.
- Carrying out disciplinary proceedings.
- Developing regulations relating to filling and refilling prescriptions.
- Substituting generic and therapeutic drugs.
- Labeling.
- Performing inspections.
- Defining poisons and mandating records to be maintained upon retail sale.

Federal Laws Regulating Drug Control and Pharmacy

A number of federal laws and subsequent amendments to these laws have been enacted over many years, with a goal to protect the public health.

Federal Food, Drug, and Cosmetic Act (FDCA)

Federal Food, Drug, and Cosmetic Act (FDCA) federal law through which the Food and Drug Administration promulgates its rules and regulations.

The **Federal Food, Drug, and Cosmetic Act (FDCA)** is the federal law (statute) through which the Food and Drug Administration enforces its rules and regulations. Up until 1906, there were few safeguards on the distribution of foods and drugs, cosmetics, and medical devices. Products were often contaminated, were not consistent in strength, and were poorly labeled. Since 1906, several important amendments have shaped the current FDCA regulations.

Pure Food and Drug Act of 1906

Pure Food and Drug Act of 1906 this law was passed by Congress because of concern about the risks to public health and safety associated with unsanitary and poorly labeled foods and drugs

The **Pure Food and Drug Act of 1906** was passed by Congress because of concerns about the risks to public health and safety associated with unsanitary and poorly labeled foods and drugs. The law prohibited the adulteration and misbranding of foods in interstate commerce.

Food, Drug, and Cosmetic Act of 1938

Food, Drug, and Cosmetic Act of 1938 the federal statute through which the FDA promulgates its rules and regulations.

A major push for the enactment of the **Food, Drug, and Cosmetic Act of 1938** was the sulfanilamide elixir tragedy of 1937, which caused 107 deaths. Sulfanilamide was one of the first of the miracle anti-infective sulfa drugs marketed, but a manufacturer mistakenly used diethylene glycol (automobile antifreeze) as an agent in its preparation of sulfanilamide elixir. The new law required that no new drug could be marketed until proven safe for use when used according to directions on the label. The new law applied to cosmetics and devices as well.

Drug products marketed prior to 1938 were exempted or "grandfathered" from the law and did not have to be labeled or proven safe under the law. For example, digoxin, nitroglycerin, and phenobarbital were drugs on the market prior to 1938 and are grandfathered from this law.

Durham-Humphrey Amendment of 1951

Durham-Humphrey Amendment established two classes of drugs, over-the-counter and prescription, and mandated that labels of prescription drugs include the legend *"Caution: Federal law prohibits dispensing without a prescription."*

A number of drug products covered by the 1938 FDCA were not safe to use without medical supervision. The **Durham-Humphrey Amendment** (also referred to as the Prescription Drug Amendment) was enacted in 1951 to solve this problem. The amendment established two classes of drugs—prescription and over-the-counter drugs—and provided that the labels of prescription drugs did not have to list "adequate directions for use," but were required to include the legend *"Caution: Federal law prohibits dispensing without a prescription"* on the manufacturer's label. When dispensed by a pharmacist, "adequate directions for use" was satisfied by the pharmacist placing directions by the prescriber on the label of the dispensed product. These drugs became known as prescription or *legend drugs*.

Drugs that did not require medical supervision for their use had to have adequate directions for use on their label and were referred to as *over-the-counter* or *nonprescription drugs*.

Kefauver-Harris Amendment of 1962

Kefauver-Harris Amendment an amendment to the Federal Food and Cosmetic Act that required all new drugs marketed in the United States to be shown to be not only safe, but also effective.

The **Kefauver-Harris Amendment** was adopted as a result of a popular sedative, thalidomide, that was being marketed in Europe but was not approved by the FDA for the U.S. market. In 1961 it was confirmed that thalidomide had caused serious birth defects in thousands of infants in Europe. The Kefauver-Harris Amendment to the FDCA (also known as the Drug Efficacy Amendment) required that all new drugs marketed in the United States had to be proven both safe and effective. This efficacy requirement was made retroactive to all drugs approved between 1938 and 1962.

This amendment also provided for the following areas:

■ The oversight of prescription drug advertising by the FDA.
■ The establishment of Good Manufacturing Practices (GMP) requirements.
■ Informed consent of patients for clinical drug investigations.
■ Implementation of reporting of adverse drug reactions.

Medical Device Amendment of 1976

Congress amended the FDCA in 1976 to provide for more extensive regulation regarding the safety and efficacy of medical devices. The Medical Device Amendment requires classification of devices according to their function.

Orphan Drug Act of 1983

orphan drugs
drugs used for diseases and conditions considered rare in the United States, for which adequate drugs have not yet been developed and do not generate incentives for drug manufacturers to research and develop treatments.

Orphan drugs are those used to treat relatively rare diseases. A *rare disease* is one that affects less than 200,000 persons in the United States or one that affects more than 200,000 persons, but for which there is no reasonable expectation that the cost of developing the drug and making it available will be recovered from the sales of the drug. The law provides various tax and licensing incentives to drug manufacturers to develop and market orphan drugs for the diagnosis, treatment, or prevention of rare diseases or conditions.

Food and Drug Administration Modernization Act of 1997

Food and Drug Administration Modernization Act of 1997 (FDAMA) legislation that streamlined regulatory procedures and encouraged manufacturers to conduct research for new uses of drugs and perform pediatric studies of drugs.

The **Food and Drug Administration Modernization Act of 1997 (FDAMA)** was passed as it was felt that the FDCA had produced a too-burdensome regulatory system for drug approval. This legislation includes:

■ Streamlining regulatory procedures to ensure the expedited availability of safe and effective drugs and devices.
■ Encouraging manufacturers to conduct research for new uses of drugs and to submit supplemental New Drug Applications (NDAs) for these uses.
■ Encouraging drug manufacturers to perform pediatric studies of drugs.

The Controlled Substances Act

Controlled Substances Act
federal law regulating the manufacture, distribution, and sale of drugs that have the potential for abuse.

The **Controlled Substances Act (CSA)** of 1970 is the major federal law regulating the manufacture, distribution, and sale (dispensing/administration) of certain drugs or substances that are subject to or have a potential for abuse or physical or psychological dependence. These drugs or substances are designated as "controlled substances." The law provides a "closed" system for legitimate handlers of these drugs, which should help reduce the widespread diversion of these drugs into the illicit market.

The Drug Enforcement Administration (DEA) is the federal law enforcement agency charged with the responsibility for combating controlled substance abuse. The DEA was established July 1, 1973. It resulted from the merger of the Bureau of Narcotics and Dangerous Drugs, the Office for Drug Abuse Law Enforcement, and other drug enforcement agencies. The DEA was established to more effectively combat narcotic and dangerous drug diversion and abuse through enforcement and prevention.

Controlled substances are classified into five schedules (Table 6-1):

Schedule I a controlled substance with no currently approved medical use, with a high potential for abuse.

Schedule II drugs with high potential for abuse, with severe psychological and/or physical dependence liability.

Schedule III a controlled substance whose abuse may lead to moderate or low physical dependence or high psychological dependence.

- **Schedule I:** The controlled substances in Schedule I include drugs with a high abuse potential that have no currently approved medical use in the United States.

- **Schedule II:** The controlled substances in Schedule II include drugs having a high abuse potential with severe psychological or physical dependence liability. Some drugs included in Schedule II are also found in other schedules when combined with other drugs. The dispensing of Schedule II controlled substances requires affixing an orange label with the caution statement *"Controlled substance, dangerous unless used as directed."* Additionally, this federal transfer warning statement is required: *"Caution: Federal law prohibits the transfer of this drug to any person other than the patient for whom it was prescribed."*

- **Schedule III:** The controlled substances in Schedule III include drugs that have an abuse potential less than those in Schedule I and Schedule II. Abuse of these drugs may lead to moderate or low physical or high psychological dependence. Any compound, mixture, or preparation containing amobarbital, secobarbital, or pentobarbital, combined with one or more other active ingredients, is listed as a Schedule III drug, as the drug's abuse potential is not great enough to warrant a Schedule II classification. It should be noted that anabolic steroids are classified in Schedule III by the federal government, but New York State (and perhaps other states) classifies them in Schedule II.

Schedule IV a controlled substance with less abuse potential and limited risk of physical and psychological dependence.

Schedule V contains preparations with limited quantities of certain narcotic drugs.

- **Schedule IV:** The controlled substances in Schedule IV include drugs having an abuse potential less than those listed in Schedule III and have limited physical or psychological dependence as compared to drugs in Schedule III.

- **Schedule V:** The controlled substances in Schedule V include drugs having an abuse potential less than those listed in Schedule IV, and abuse of these drugs may lead to limited physical dependence or psychological dependence as compared to drugs in Schedule IV. Drugs in Schedule V consist mainly of preparations containing limited quantities of certain narcotic drugs (codeine), generally for antitussive indications and others for anti-diarrheal indications.

Each commercial container of a controlled substance is required to have on its label a symbol designating the schedule to which it belongs. The symbols for controlled substances are C-I, C-II, C-III, C-IV, and C-V. Alternatively, the symbol may be a C with the schedule designation inside it.

Maintenance of controlled substances

Hospitals and other health care facilities authorized to purchase, possess, and use controlled substances must keep a number of records both within the pharmacy and at the individual nursing units to ensure appropriate use and control of the controlled substances. These records and reports include the following:

- An order signed by a person authorized to prescribe, specifying the controlled substance medication for a specifically indicated person.

- A separate record at the main point of supply for controlled substances. This shows the type and strength indicating the dates and amounts of such drugs received and dispensed.

- A record of authorized requisitions for such drugs for distribution to the nursing units. Such records must indicate the signature of the dispensing pharma-

TABLE 6-1   Examples of Controlled Substances by Drug Schedule

SCHEDULE I	SCHEDULE II	SCHEDULE III	SCHEDULE IV	SCHEDULE V
heroin	alfentanyl	acetaminophen with codeine (Tylenol with codeine)	alprazolam (Xanax)	
marijuana	amobarbital	anabolic steroids (Testoderm, Winstrol)	butorphanol (Stadol)	Actifed with codeine
LSD	amphetamines	butabarital (Fiorinal)	chloral hydrate (Noctec)	Dimetane DC
peyote	cocaine	dronabinol (Marinol)	chlordiazepoxide (Librium)	Phenergan with codeine
mescaline	fentanyl (Sublimaze, Duragesic)	nalorphine (Nalline)	clonazepam (Clonopin)	Robitussin A-C
hallucinogenic substances	hydromorphone (Dilaudid)	thiopental (Pentothal)	diethylpropion (Tenuate)	Diphenoxylate with atropine (Lomotil)
	levorphanol (Levo-Dromoran)		eszopicione (Lunesta)	
	meperidine (Demerol)		flurazepam (Dalmane)	
	methadone		midazolam (Versed)	
	methylphenidate (Ritalin, Concerta)		oxazepam (Serax)	
	morphine (MS Contin)		pemoline (Cylert)	
	methamphetamine (Desoxyn)		pentazocine (Talwin)	
	oxycodone (OxyContin, Pecodan, Percocet)		phenobarbital	
	pentobarbital (Nembutal)		propoxyphene (Darvon, Darvocet)	
	phenmetrazine (Preludin)		sibutramine (Meridia)	
	secobarbital (Seconal)		temazepam (Restoril)	
	sufentanyl (Sufenta)		triazolam (Halcion)	
	tincture of opium			

cist and receipt at the nursing unit by the signature of a person authorized to receive controlled substances.

■ With each substock (amount on a nursing unit) of controlled substances, a documentation record must be furnished. The administration sheet lists the type of controlled substance, dose, and number of doses furnished to the nursing unit.

The sheet also indicates the

■ Name of the patient.
■ Name of the prescribing physician or practitioner.
■ Date and hour of administration.
■ Quantity of administration.
■ Balance on hand after each administration.
■ Signature of the administering nurse.
■ Upon administration of the controlled substance, an entry must be made in the patient's **medication administration record (MAR)**. The entry includes

medication administration record (MAR) a record maintained by the nursing staff containing information about the patient's medication and its frequency of administration.

the name of the administering nurse and the date and hour of administration. Partially-used doses of controlled substances must have wastage documented by the administering nurse and another nurse as a witness. Additionally, at the end of each shift or at the end of the day for controlled drug activities, two nurses must count the controlled substances for that substock and sign their name, verifying that the counts are correct.

It should be noted that for those institutions that have their pharmacy inventories and/or nursing substocks of controlled medications in automated dispensing machines, the same requirements for recordkeeping as noted above must be met by the automated system.

Registration

The Controlled Substances Act exerts its control by way of federal registration of all persons (except the ultimate user or patient) in the legitimate chain of purchase to distribution or dispensing of controlled drugs (Figure 6-1). Every person or firm who manufactures, distributes, conducts instructional activities with, conducts chemical analysis with, conducts research with, exports, imports, prescribes, administers, or dispenses controlled substances or who proposes to engage in the same must register with the federal Drug Enforcement Administration (DEA) of the U.S. Department of Justice. Registration for dispensers is effective for three years. This registration must be displayed prominently in the pharmacy.

Ordering controlled substances

Under the Controlled Substances Act, a federal triplicate order form (DEA-222) is necessary for the ordering of controlled substances in Schedules I and II and is required for transfer of Schedule I and II products from one pharmacy to another and for returns to the wholesaler or manufacturer (Figure 6-2).

DEA forms may be requisitioned on DEA Form 222a or by contacting any Division Office or the Registration Unit of the DEA. No charge is made for order forms. Each order form must be signed and dated by a person authorized to sign an application for registration. Copy 1 (brown) and Copy 2 (green) go to the supplier, and Copy 3 is retained by the purchaser.

Lost or stolen order forms, drug theft or loss

Both federal and state laws have requirements for drug security and regulations for reporting lost or stolen order forms and controlled drug theft and/or loss. Controlled drug theft or loss must be immediately reported to the DEA Diversion Field Office (using DEA Form 106), and a controlled drug theft should also immediately be reported to the local police (Figure 6-3).

Inventory requirements

The Controlled Substances Act requires each registrant to make a complete and accurate record every two years of all stocks of controlled substances on hand. The biennial inventory date of May 1 may be changed by the registrant to fit the regular general physical inventory date, so long as the date is no more than six months from the biennial date that would otherwise apply. The inventory must be maintained at the location appearing on the registration certificate for at least two years.

Most hospital pharmacy departments take a physical inventory of their controlled drugs much more frequently than required by federal law. Some

FIGURE 6-1

Form-224	**APPLICATION FOR REGISTRATION** Under the Controlled Substances Act	APPROVED OMB NO 1117-0014 FORM DEA-224 (10-06) Previous editions are obsolete

INSTRUCTIONS — Save time - apply on-line at *www.deadiversion.usdoj.gov*
1. To apply by mail complete this application. Keep a copy for your records.
2. Print clearly, using black or blue ink, or use a typewriter.
3. Mail this form to the address provided in Section 7 or use enclosed envelope.
4. Include the correct payment amount. FEE IS NON-REFUNDABLE.
5. If you have any questions call 800-882-9539 prior to submitting your application.

IMPORTANT: DO NOT SEND THIS APPLICATION **AND** APPLY ON-LINE.

DEA OFFICIAL USE :

Do you have other DEA registration numbers?   ☐ NO   ☐ YES

MAIL-TO ADDRESS — Please print mailing address changes to the right of the address in this box.

FEE FOR THREE (3) YEARS IS $551 **FEE IS NON-REFUNDABLE**

SECTION 1   APPLICANT IDENTIFICATION   ☐ Individual Registration   ☐ Business Registration

Name 1   (Last Name of individual -OR- Business or Facility Name)

Name 2   (First Name and Middle Name of individual - OR- Continuation of business name)

Street Address Line 1 (if applying for fee exemption, this must be address of the fee exempt institution)

Address Line 2

City   State   Zip Code

Business Phone Number   Point of Contact

Business Fax Number   Email Address

DEBT COLLECTION INFORMATION — Mandatory pursuant to Debt Collection Improvements Act

Social Security Number (*if registration is for individual*)

Provide SSN or TIN. See additional information note #3 on page 4.

Tax Identification Number (*if registration is for business*)

FOR Practitioner or MLP ONLY: Professional Degree : *select from list only*   Professional School :   Year of Graduation :

National Provider Identification: Date of Birth (*MM-DD-YYYY*):

SECTION 2 BUSINESS ACTIVITY — Check one business activity box only
☐ Central Fill Pharmacy
☐ Retail Pharmacy
☐ Nursing Home
☐ Automated Dispensing System
☐ Practitioner (DDS, DMD, DO, DPM, DVM, MD or PHD)
☐ Practitioner Military (DDS, DMD, DO, DPM, DVM, MD or PHD)
☐ Mid-level Practitioner (MLP) (DOM, HMD, MP, ND, NP, OD, PA, or RPH)
☐ Euthanasia Technician
☐ Ambulance Service
☐ Animal Shelter
☐ Hospital/Clinic
☐ Teaching Institution

FOR Automated Dispensing System (ADS) ONLY: DEA Registration # of Retail Pharmacy for this ADS

An ADS is automatically fee-exempt. Skip Section 6 and Section 7 on page 2. You must attach a notorized affidavit.

SECTION 3 DRUG SCHEDULES — Check all that apply
☐ Schedule II Narcotic   ☐ Schedule III Narcotic   ☐ Schedule IV
☐ Schedule II Non-Narcotic   ☐ Schedule III Non-Narcotic   ☐ Schedule V

☐ Check this box if you require official order forms - for purchase or transfer of schedule 2 narcotic and/or schedule 2 non-narcotic controlled substances.

NEW - Page 1

FIGURE 6-1 DEA application for registration.

FIGURE 6-1 (Continued)

SECTION 4

STATE LICENSE(S)

Be sure to include both state license numbers if applicable

You MUST be currently authorized to prescribe, distribute, dispense, conduct research, or otherwise handle the controlled substances in the schedules for which you are applying under the laws of the **state** or jurisdiction in which you are operating or propose to operate.

State
License Number
(required)

Expiration
Date
(required)   /   /
MM - DD - YYYY

What state was this license issued in? _____

State Controlled Substance
License Number
(if required)

Expiration
Date   /   /
MM - DD - YYYY

What state was this license issued in? _____

SECTION 5

LIABILITY

IMPORTANT

All questions in this section must be answered.

1. Has the applicant ever been **convicted of a crime** in connection with controlled substance(s) under state or federal law, or is any such action pending?   YES ☐   NO ☐

   Date(s) of incident MM-DD-YYYY: ☐☐ - ☐☐ - ☐☐☐☐

2. Has the applicant ever surrendered (for cause) or had a **federal** controlled substance registration revoked, suspended, restricted, or denied, or is any such action pending?   YES ☐   NO ☐

   Date(s) of incident MM-DD-YYYY: ☐☐ - ☐☐ - ☐☐☐☐

3. Has the applicant ever surrendered (for cause) or had a **state** professional license or controlled substance registration revoked, suspended, denied, restricted, or placed on probation, or is any such action pending?   YES ☐   NO ☐

   Date(s) of incident MM-DD-YYYY: ☐☐ - ☐☐ - ☐☐☐☐

4. If the applicant is a **corporation** (other than a corporation whose stock is owned and traded by the public), association, partnership, or pharmacy, has any officer, partner, stockholder, or proprietor been **convicted of a crime** in connection with controlled substance(s) under state or federal law, or ever surrendered, for cause, or had a **federal** controlled substance registration revoked, suspended, restricted, denied, or ever had a **state** professional license or controlled substance registration revoked, suspended, denied, restricted or placed on probation, or is any such action pending?   YES ☐   NO ☐

   Date(s) of incident MM-DD-YYYY: ☐☐ - ☐☐ - ☐☐☐☐   *Note: If question 4 does not apply to you, be sure to mark 'NO'. It will slow down processing of your application if you leave it blank.*

EXPLANATION OF "YES" ANSWERS

Applicants who have answered "YES" to any of the four questions above **must provide a statement to explain each "YES" answer.**

Use this space or attach a separate sheet and return with application

Liability question # _____   Location(s) of incident: _____

Nature of incident:

Disposition of incident:

SECTION 6   **EXEMPTION FROM APPLICATION FEE**

☐ Check this box if the applicant is a federal, state, or local government official or institution. Does not apply to contractor-operated institutions.

Business or Facility Name of Fee Exempt Institution. **Be sure to enter the address of this exempt institution in Section 1.**

The undersigned hereby certifies that the applicant named hereon is a federal, state or local government official or institution, and is exempt from payment of the application fee.

FEE EXEMPT CERTIFIER

Provide the name and phone number of the certifying official

Signature of certifying official (**other than applicant**)

Date

Print or type name and title of certifying official

Telephone No. (required for verification)

SECTION 7

METHOD OF PAYMENT

Check one form of payment only

☐ Check   Make check payable to: **Drug Enforcement Administration**   See page 4 of instructions for important information.

☐ American Express   ☐ Discover   ☐ Master Card   ☐ Visa

Credit Card Number

Expiration Date ☐☐ - ☐☐

Sign if paying by credit card

Signature of Card Holder

Printed Name of Card Holder

Mail this form with payment to:

U.S. Department of Justice
Drug Enforcement Administration
P.O. Box 28083
Washington, DC 20038-8083

FEE IS NON-REFUNDABLE

SECTION 8

APPLICANT'S SIGNATURE

Sign in ink

I certify that the foregoing information furnished on this application is true and correct.

Signature of applicant (sign in ink)

Date

Print or type name and title of applicant

WARNING: Section 843(a)(4)(A) of Title 21, United States Code states that any person who knowingly or intentionally furnishes false or fraudulent information in the application is subject to imprisonment for not more than four years, a fine of not more than $30,000, or both.

NEW - Page 2

FIGURE 6-2

| | | | | | | | | | | | | | | | | | | | | | | | | | | | | | | |

BLANK DEA FORM-222
U.S. OFFICIAL ORDER FORM—SCHEDULES I & II

See Reverse of PURCHASER'S Copy for Instructions	No order form may be issued for Schedules I and II substances unless a completed application form has been received, (21 CFR 1305.04).	OMB APPROVAL NO. 1117-0010

TO: *(Name of Supplier)* | STREET ADDRESS

CITY and STATE | DATE | **TO BE FILLED IN BY SUPPLIER** SUPPLIERS DEA REGISTRATION No.

LINE No.	No. of Packages	Size of Packages	Name of Item	National Drug Code	Packages Shipped	Date Shipped
	TO BE FILLED IN BY PURCHASER					
1						
2						
3						
4						
5						
6						
7						
8						
9						
10						

NO. OF LINES COMPLETED | SIGNATURE OF PURCHASER OR HIS ATTORNEY OR AGENT

Date Issued | DEA Registration No. | Name and Address of Registrant

Schedules 2, 2N, 3, 3N, 4, 5

Registered as a PHARMACY | No. of this Order Form

DEA Form-222 | **U.S. OFFICIAL ORDER FORMS—SCHEDULES I & II** DRUG ENFORCEMENT ADMINISTRATION SUPPLIER'S COPY 1

FIGURE 6-2 DEA order form.

departments take manual controlled drug inventories on a daily basis to ensure appropriate accountability and reconciliation. Many departments of pharmacy have automated dispensing cabinets specifically for controlled substances, where an ongoing perpetual inventory is maintained for each controlled drug transaction.

Please refer to Chapter 18, "Drug Distribution Systems," for a comprehensive review of automated dispensing technology and the role and responsibilities of the pharmacy technician.

FIGURE 6-3

REPORT OF THEFT OR LOSS OF CONTROLLED SUBSTANCES

Federal Regulations require registrants to submit a detailed report of any theft or loss of Controlled Substances to the Drug Enforcement Administration.

Complete the front and back of this form in triplicate. Forward the original and duplicate copies to the nearest DEA Office. Retain the triplicate copy for your records. Some states may also require a copy of this report.

OMB APPROVAL No. 1117-0001

1. Name and Address of Registrant (include ZIP Code)
ZIP CODE
2. Phone No. (Include Area Code)

3. DEA Registration Number — 2 ltr. prefix — 7 digit suffix
4. Date of Theft or Loss
5. Principal Business of Registrant (Check one)
1 Pharmacy 2 Practitioner 3 Manufacturer 4 Hospital/Clinic 5 Distributor 6 Methadone Program 7 Other (Specify)

6. County in which Registrant is located
7. Was Theft reported to Police? Yes No
8. Name and Telephone Number of Police Department (Include Area Code)

9. Number of Thefts or Losses Registrant has experienced in the past 24 months
10. Type of Theft or Loss (Check one and complete items below as appropriate)
1 Night break-in 2 Armed robbery 3 Employee pilferage 4 Customer theft 5 Other (Explain) 6 Lost in transit (Complete Item 14)

11. If Armed Robbery, was anyone:
Killed? No Yes (How many) ___
Injured? No Yes (How many) ___
12. Purchase value to registrant of Controlled Substances taken? $
13. Were any pharmaceuticals or merchandise taken? No Yes (Est. Value) $

14. IF LOST IN TRANSIT, COMPLETE THE FOLLOWING:
A. Name of Common Carrier
B. Name of Consignee
C. Consignee's DEA Registration Number
D. Was the carton received by the customer? Yes No
E. If received, did it appear to be tampered with? Yes No
F. Have you experienced losses in transit from this same carrier in the past? No Yes (How Many) ___

15. What identifying marks, symbols, or price codes were on the labels of these containers that would assist in identifying the products?

16. If Official Controlled Substance Order Forms (DEA-222) were stolen, give numbers.

17. What security measures have been taken to prevent future thefts or losses?

PRIVACY ACT INFORMATION

AUTHORITY: Section 301 of the Controlled Substances Act of 1970 (PL 91-513).
PURPOSE: Report theft or loss of Controlled Substances.
ROUTINE USES: The Controlled Substances Act authorizes the production of special reports required for statistical and analytical purposes. Disclosures of information from this system are made to the following categories of users for the purposes stated:
A. Other Federal law enforcement and regulatory agencies for law enforcement and regulatory purposes.
B. State and local law enforcement and regulatory agencies for law enforcement and regulatory purposes.
EFFECT: Failure to report theft or loss of controlled substances may result in penalties under Section 402 and 403 of the Controlled Substances Act.

In accordance with the Paperwork Reduction Act of 1995, no person is required to respond to a collection of information unless it displays a ly valid OMB control number. The valid OMB control number for this collection of information is 1117-0001. Public reporting burden for this collection of information is estimated to average 30 minutes per response, including the time for reviewing instructions, searching existing data sources, gathering and maintaining the data needed, and completing and reviewing the collection of information.

FORM DEA - 106 (11-00) Previous editions obsolete
CONTINUE ON REVERSE

FIGURE 6-3 DEA form: report of theft or loss.

FIGURE 6-3 (Continued)

FORM DEA-106 (Nov. 2000) Pg. 2   **LIST OF CONTROLLED SUBSTANCES LOST**

Trade Name of Substance or Preparation	Name of Controlled Substance in Preparation	Dosage Strength and Form	Quantity
Examples: Desoxyn	Methamphetamine Hydrochloride	5 mg Tablets	3 x 100
Demerol	Meperidine Hydrochloride	50 mg/ml Vial	5 x 30 ml
Robitussin A-C	Codeine Phosphate	2 mg/cc Liquid	12 Pints
1.			
2.			
3.			
4.			
5.			
6.			
7.			
8.			
9.			
10.			
11.			
12.			
13.			
14.			
15.			
16.			
17.			
18.			
19.			
20.			
21.			
22.			
23.			
24.			
25.			
26.			
27.			
28.			
29.			
30.			
31.			
32.			
33.			
34.			
35.			
36.			
37.			
38.			
39.			
40.			
41.			
42.			
43.			
44.			
45.			
46.			
47.			
48.			
49.			
50.			

I certify that the foregoing information is correct to the best of my knowledge and belief.

_____   _____   _____
Signature   Title   Date

Destruction of controlled substances

To dispose of any excess or undesired stocks of controlled substances, a pharmacy is required to contact the state Bureau of Controlled Substances and/or the Drug Enforcement Agency (DEA) office for disposal instructions and to request the necessary form(s) from each (DEA Form 41).

Issuing prescriptions and dispensing controlled substances

A prescription for a controlled substance may be issued only by an individual practitioner authorized to prescribe controlled substances in the state in which he/she is licensed to practice. An employee of the individual practitioner (a nurse, secretary) may communicate a prescription issued by a practitioner to a pharmacist. Only a pharmacist, or a pharmacy intern under the supervision of a pharmacist, may fill a prescription for a controlled substance. Whether a pharmacy technician may engage in the dispensing of a controlled substance under the supervision of a licensed pharmacist depends on state law.

Controlled drug prescriptions must be dated on the day when written and must include:

■ The name and address of the patient.
■ The drug name, strength, and dosage form.
■ The quantity prescribed.
■ Directions for use.
■ The name and address and registration number of the prescriber.

The prescription must have the name of the prescriber stamped, typed, or hand-printed on it, as well as the signature of the physician.

The responsibility for the proper prescribing and dispensing of controlled substances rests with both the prescriber and the pharmacist who fills the prescription. A prescription ordered by a person knowingly prescribing a controlled substance that is not within the usual course of his/her legitimate practice is not deemed a legal prescription. Individuals prescribing such a prescription and a pharmacist knowingly filling it are in violation of the CSA.

Emergency situations

An emergency situation is an exception to the requirement that a pharmacist dispense a Schedule II drug only pursuant to a written prescription. A pharmacist may dispense a Schedule II drug on oral authorization of the prescriber under the following emergency circumstances:

■ The quantity prescribed is limited only to the amount necessary to treat the patient for the emergency.
■ The prescription must be immediately reduced to writing by the pharmacist.
■ The prescriber must deliver to the dispensing pharmacist within seven days a written prescription for the emergency quantity prescribed. The prescription must have written on its face *"Authorization for Emergency Dispensing."* On receipt, the pharmacist must attach this prescription to the oral emergency prescription. Failure of the prescriber to deliver the written prescription within the seven-day period requires the pharmacist to notify the DEA. Failure of the pharmacist to do so voids the prescription.

Recordkeeping requirements

Controlled substances records (e.g., inventory, records of receipt, records of disposition, records of theft or loss, prescriptions, and so forth) must be kept for at least two years at the place of registration. Specific states may require maintaining controlled drug records for more than the federal requirements of two years. For example, New York State's requirement is five years.

Federal Hazardous Substances Act

The **Federal Hazardous Substances Act** was enacted in 1960. This act requires that certain hazardous household products ("hazardous substances") bear cautionary labeling to alert consumers to the potential hazards that those products present and to inform them of the measures they need to protect themselves from those hazards. The Consumer Product Safety Commission (CPSC) enforces this act. The CPSC was created to protect the public "against unreasonable risks of injuries associated with consumer products." The CPSC is an independent agency that does not report to, nor is it part of, any other department or agency in the federal government.

Poison Prevention Packaging Act

The **Poison Prevention Packaging Act** of 1970 is an amendment to the Federal Hazardous Substances Act. It regulates certain substances defined as household substances. It requires that these substances be packaged for consumer use in "special packaging" that will make it significantly difficult for children under the age of five to open, but not difficult for adults to open. The "special packaging" is often referred to as *child-resistant containers*.

Drugs dispensed on prescription or on a medical practitioner's order are exempt from the special packaging requirement if the prescribing doctor specifies a noncomplying container in the prescription or if the patient or customer receiving the drug requests a noncomplying container. Another exemption is made for over-the-counter items for elderly or handicapped persons. But for the exemption to apply, such noncomplying packaging must contain the printed statement, *"This package for households without young children"*.

The following is a list of substances that are currently required to be sold or dispensed to consumers in the special child-resistant containers:

- Aspirin-containing preparations.
- Controlled substances.
- Prescription only (legend) drugs, unless the patient or guardian requests a non-child-resistant container and signs a release to this effect.

Exempt from the special packaging requirement for legend drugs are sublingual nitroglycerin preparations and sublingual and chewable isosorbide dinitrate (Isordil) preparations, as these drugs are prescribed for cardiac patients who must be able to quickly get at their medication.

Occupational and Safety Act

The **Occupational and Safety Act of 1970** was passed to assure every working man and woman in the nation safe and healthy working conditions. Under the Occupational and Safety Act, the Occupational Safety and Health Administration (OSHA) was created to decrease hazards in the workplace, to maintain a reporting system for monitoring job-related injuries and illnesses, and to develop mandatory job safety and health standards. OSHA is authorized to conduct workplace inspections to determine whether employers are complying with standards issued by the agency for safe and healthful workplaces. Workplace inspections are performed by OSHA compliance safety and health officers.

Hazardous drugs and chemicals

On May 23, 1988, an OSHA regulation became effective requiring that employees know about the hazards of all chemicals to which they are exposed. The **Hazard Communication Standard (HCS)** is based on the simple concept that employees have both a need and a right to know the hazards and identities of the chemicals to which they are exposed when working. They also need to know what protective measures are available to prevent adverse affects.

The purpose of this standard is to ensure that the hazards of all chemicals are evaluated and that information concerning these hazards is transmitted to affected employees. This transmission of information is to be accomplished by a comprehensive hazard communication program that includes container labeling and other forms of warning, material safety data sheets, and employee training.

Written hazard communication program

Employers must develop and implement a written hazard communications program that includes a list of the hazardous chemicals known to be present by obtaining the appropriate material safety data sheets (MSDS) for all toxic/hazardous substances in every department.

MSDS must be provided by the manufacturer, importer, or distributor for each hazardous chemical used in a workplace. The MSDS must be in English and must contain the following information:

- Chemical and common names.
- If a mixture, chemical and common names of ingredients.
- Physical and chemical characteristics, such as flash point and vapor pressure.
- Physical hazards, including potential for fire, explosion, and reactivity.
- Health hazards, including signs and symptoms of exposure.
- Routes of entry into the body.
- Precautions for safe handling and use, including hygienic practices and protective measures during repair or maintenance.
- Procedures for cleanup of spills and leaks.
- Emergency and first aid procedures.
- Date of preparation of MSDS or date of latest revision.
- Name, address, and telephone number of manufacturer, importer, or distributor.

The employer must maintain copies of the required MSDS for each hazardous chemical in the workplace and ensure that they are readily accessible to employees during each work shift. Alternatively, the employer may subscribe to a service that will fax an MSDS upon request of the employee by calling a toll-free telephone number.

Air contaminants

Employees are to be protected from air contaminants and chemicals that could cause injury or illness with regard to potential carcinogenic agents. OSHA published *Guidelines for Handling Cytotoxic (Antineoplastic) Drugs* as a meaningful tool for pharmacy employers and employees handling chemotherapy drugs. The publication provides information regarding personal protective equipment, monitoring, and training.

Flammable and combustible liquids

Appropriate storage (e.g., vault, cabinet) must be provided for pharmaceuticals such as alcohol, acetone, and flexible collodion.

Portable fire extinguisher

A sufficient number of portable fire extinguishers of the appropriate type, depending on the hazards in the department, must be available and immediately accessible.

Storage of hazardous chemicals

Bulk storage and receiving areas, such as the pharmacy storeroom, must have unobstructed aisles, shelving must be secured to prevent accidental falling, and the area must be kept clean and dry.

Omnibus Budget Reconciliation Act of 1990

> **Omnibus Budget Reconciliation Act (OBRA)** mandated three provisions that affect the profession of pharmacy, including the provision that drug manufacturers are required to provide their lowest prices to Medicaid patients, and the provision that pharmacists are to provide drug use review and patient counseling.

In adopting the federal **Omnibus Budget Reconciliation Act (OBRA)** of 1990, Congress recognized the escalating pressure to expand social programs—particularly those that impact active older citizens—and that the pharmacist could play a key role in improving the effectiveness of drug therapy and reducing the overall costs.

OBRA 90 mandated three main provisions affecting the profession of pharmacy, including the provision that drug manufacturers are required to provide their lowest prices to Medicaid patients, the provision that drug-use review and patient counseling are now mandated.

OBRA 90 requires states to implement regulations consistent with the objectives of the federal law prior to January 1, 1993. Although the original federal regulations mandate such programs for Medicaid patients only, virtually every state has implemented the new regulations for all patients to ensure all patients a high level of professional service.

Pharmacists are now required to maintain individual patient medication profiles that must contain—in addition to patient demographic information such as name, address, telephone number, gender, and date of birth—information including known allergies and drug reactions, chronic diseases, a comprehensive list of medications and medical devices and other appropriate information necessary for counseling about the use of prescription and over-the-counter drugs. Utilizing this patient medication profile, pharmacists are expected to conduct a **prospective drug review** before dispensing or delivering a prescription to a patient, or the patient's caregiver, which would include screening for the following:

> **prospective drug review** a review of the patient's medication profile by a pharmacist to screen for any drug problems prior to the drug being dispensed.

- Therapeutic duplication.
- Drug-drug interactions, including serious interactions with any over-the-counter drugs.
- Incorrect drug dosage or duration of treatment.
- Drug-allergy interactions.
- Clinical abuse or misuse.

After a prospective drug review, regulations require that counseling be provided to each patient and must include all "matters which in the pharmacist's professional judgment, the pharmacist deems significant," including the following:

- The name and description of the medication.
- The dosage form, dosage, route of administration, and duration of drug therapy.
- Special directions and precautions for preparation, administration, and use by the patient.
- Common severe side effects or adverse effects or interactions that may be encountered, including their avoidance and action required if they occur.
- Techniques for self-monitoring drug therapy.
- Proper storage.

- Prescription refill information.
- Action to be taken in the event of a missed dose.

For mail-order pharmacies, counseling and patient profile information may be conveyed by toll-free, long-distance telephone and is usually patient-initiated. Although any qualified employee of a pharmacy, such as a technician, may initiate the offer to have the pharmacist counsel a patient, only a pharmacist or a pharmacy intern can provide the actual counseling. The objective of counseling the patient or the patient's caregiver is to improve patient medication compliance, to avoid medication misadventures, and to improve drug therapy outcomes.

Today, with the degree of Doctor of Pharmacy being conferred on all pharmacy graduates, pharmacists should view these requirements as an opportunity to utilize their education and training in their professional role as drug therapy experts. The public has a need for a readily available professional who will assist them in improving their health care outcomes, and the pharmacist is the most logical professional to meet these needs.

Health Insurance Portability and Accountability Act of 1996

Health Insurance Portability and Accountability Act (HIPAA) an important law that requires the adoption of security and privacy standards in order to protect personal health care information.

In 1996 Congress passed the **Health Insurance Portability and Accountability Act (HIPAA)**. Within the law there are two titles: Title I and Title II. Title I, known as *Insurance Reform*, protects health insurance coverage for workers and their families when they change or lose their jobs. Title II, known as *Administrative Simplification*, is the act that will fundamentally change the way health care facilities handle patient information. It aims to improve the efficiency and effectiveness of the American health care system by adopting national standards for electronic health care transactions. The law also requires the adoption of security and privacy standards in order to protect personal health care information.

Overview of Title II

The Department of Health and Human Services (HHS) estimates that currently there are about 400 formats for electronic health claims being used in the United States. This lack of standardization minimizes efficiency of the health care system and makes it difficult and expensive to develop and maintain software. HIPAA requires every provider who does business electronically to use standardized health care transactions, code sets, and identifiers. Standardization creates a common language that encourages development of an information system using electronic data interchange (EDI). Chain and community pharmacies may use NDC code numbers for the transfer of information relating to drugs and pharmaceuticals. EDI allows entities within the health care system to exchange medical billing and to process transactions in a fast and cost-effective manner. HHS estimates that these standards will provide a net savings to the health care industry of $29.9 billion over 10 years.

protected health information (PHI) includes any individually identifiable health information, with the exclusion of employment records.

Health information privacy

Prior to HIPAA, personal health information could be distributed for reasons having nothing to do with a patient's medical treatment or health care reimbursement. Consequently, HIPAA provisions were made to mandate the adoption of federal privacy protections to protect and guard against the misuse of individually identifiable health information. **Protected health information (PHI)** includes any individually identifiable health information transmitted or maintained in any form, with the exclusion of employment records.

Definitions

HIPAA regulations apply to **covered entities**, which include:

1. A *health plan* that provides or pays the cost of medical care (e.g., group health plan, HMO, Part A or Part B of Medicare, the Medicaid Program).
2. A *health care clearinghouse* that facilitates processing of health information from another entity (e.g., billing service).
3. A *health care provider* of medical or health services (e.g., preventative, diagnostic, or therapeutic services; the sale or dispensing of a drug, device or equipment).
4. A *business associate* who, on behalf of a covered entity, performs or assists in a function or activity involving the use or disclosure of individually identifiable health information.

> **covered entities**
> entities which HIPAA regulations apply to; namely, health plans that provide or pay the costs of medical care, health care clearing-houses that facilitate the processing of health information from another entity, and health care providers of medical or health services.

Preexisting pharmacy privacy requirements

American Pharmaceutical Association Code of Ethics for Pharmacists—Principle 2

A pharmacist is dedicated to protecting the dignity of the patient. With a caring attitude and compassionate spirit, a pharmacist focuses on seeing the patient in a private and confidential manner.

American Association of Pharmacy Technicians Code of Ethics for Pharmacy Technicians—Principle VI

A pharmacy technician respects and supports the patient's individuality, dignity, and confidentiality.

New York State Regulations on Unprofessional Conduct—Regents Rules 29.1(b)(8)

Unprofessional conduct shall include revealing of personally identifiable facts, data, or information obtained in a professional capacity without the prior consent of the patient or client, except as authorized or required by law.

Regulatory Standards for Marketed Drugs

The necessary labeling of medications, for both professional and/or patient information, in the form of package inserts is required for the safe and appropriate prescribing and use of medication.

Prescription Drug Labeling

Prescription drugs are labeled for the health care professional, not the patient. The following information is required on the commercial label:

- Name and address of the manufacturer, packer, or distributor.
- Name of the drug (brand and/or generic) as applicable.
- Ingredients and quantity.
- Name of inactive ingredients.
- Quantity in terms of weight or volume (e.g., 1 pint).

- Quantity of the container (e.g., 100 capsules).
- Statement of usual dose or reference to the package insert.
- Symbol *"Rx Only"* and/or the legend *"Caution: Federal law prohibits dispensing without prescription.*
- If not for oral use, the route of administration.
- Lot or control number.
- Expiration date.
- Statement directed to the pharmacist (where applicable) specifying the type of container to be used in dispensing the drug (e.g., "dispense in tight, light-resistant container").

Unit-Dose Labeling and Packaging

Unit-dose packaging is applicable when a single dosage unit of a drug is packaged and labeled for administration to patients in hospitals, long-term care facilities, and other institutions that use unit-dose systems. This type of packaging is convenient in that it reduces medication errors and diversion and permits the return and crediting of unused, sealed doses. Because of the size of the unit-dose package, the FDA has regulations requiring the label on the unit-dose package to include the following:

- Generic and brand name of the drug, where applicable.
- Quantity of active ingredient in each unit dose package.
- Expiration date.
- Lot number.
- Name of the manufacturer, repackager or distributor.
- Other appropriate information as required (e.g., bar code).

Package Insert

The package insert accompanies the drug product and contains the medical information needed for safe and effective use of the drug by health care professionals. The following information must be contained under the section headings and in the order listed:

- Generic and proprietary name.
- Clinical pharmacology.
- Indications and usage.
- Contraindications.
- Warnings.
- Precautions.
- Adverse reactions.
- Drug abuse and dependence.
- Overdosage.
- Dosage and administration.
- How supplied.
- Date of the most recent revision of the labeling.

patient package insert (PPI) an informational leaflet written for the lay public describing the benefits and risks of medications.

Patient Package Inserts

FDA regulations require the distribution of **patient package inserts (PPIs)** to educate the patient about the proper use and potential dangers inherent in the use of specific prescription medications. The PPI is an informational leaflet written for the lay public describing the benefits and risks of the medication. PPIs must be provided to patients receiving prescriptions for products such as Accutane, as well as those receiving estrogen or progesterone-containing products.

The requirements of the regulation are met if the PPI is provided to the patient before administration of the first dose of the drug and every 30 days thereafter as long as therapy continues. These rules apply to all physicians, community pharmacists, and hospital pharmacists who dispense these drugs. Hospitals and provider pharmacies that provide medications to patients in long-term care facilities are also responsible for providing PPIs to patients (and/or their families or caregivers) receiving these medications.

National Drug Code Number

A National Drug Code (NDC) number is required on all over-the-counter and prescription drug labels. The NDC number assigned to new drugs has 11 digits. The first five digits identify the manufacturer or distributor, and the last six digits identify the drug name, package size, and type of drug. The FDA assigns the number for identification purposes, for facilitating the processing of third-party prescription drug claims, and for distributing products between manufacturers, wholesalers and pharmacies. The FDA requires that all drug labeling include the NDC as a linear bar code to allow health care professionals to scan the bar code to assure that the right drug, dosage, and route of administration is dispensed and administered to the patient.

Bar Codes

Bar coding of pharmaceuticals (prescription drugs, biologicals, and nonprescription drugs) has been mandated by the FDA to help reduce medication errors in hospitals.

A bar code consists of a combination of bars and spaces with varying widths that allow encoding of pertinent information concerning a drug product. A scanner is utilized to read the bar code.

Switch of Prescription Drugs to Over-the-Counter Drugs

The FDA has an over-the-counter drug review process, which is a mechanism for those drugs that have been recommended to switch from prescription to OTC status. If this switch is approved, the FDA publishes an OTC drug monograph for this drug.

In some instances the FDA may approve a switch in OTC status based on a manufacturer's supplemental application to its NDA. This can sometimes be confusing to pharmacists, as approval for one manufacturer's supplemental NDA application does not automatically apply to other manufacturers of the same product. Thus, a product from one manufacturer may be a prescription, and an identical product from another manufacturer is an OTC. Pharmacists and technicians must abide by the label and not sell a legend drug without a prescription, even though the competitor's drug may be OTC.

Orange Book

Every state has enacted generic substitution laws allowing a pharmacist to substitute a generically equivalent drug for the prescribed drug. Pharmacists are responsible for ensuring that the substituted generic drug product is bioequivalent to the prescribed product. To assist pharmacists and technicians in identifying bio-equivalent generic medications, the FDA published *Approved Drug Products with Therapeutic Equivalence Evaluations*. This book is often referred to as *The Orange Book* because of its orange cover. *The Orange Book* can be accessed at the FDA's Web site: www.fda.gov/cder/ob. *The Orange Book* lists thousands of marketed mul-tisource drugs approved by the FDA as safe and effective.

The FDA uses a two-letter coding system for drug products with therapeutic equivalence evaluations.

Drug products with the first letter *A* are considered bioequivalent and are therefore therapeutically equivalent to the brand name product. Drug products with the first letter *B* are not considered to be therapeutically equivalent for vari-ous reasons.

The second letter of the code more specifically describes the different dosage forms of the product. For example:

AA—bioequivalent drug products in conventional dosage forms.
AN—bioequivalent solutions and powders for aerosolization.
AT—bioequivalent topical products.

Investigational Drugs and the New Drug Approval Process

Drugs marketed in this country for either human or animal use must receive the approval of the Food and Drug Administration (FDA). This approval is sought by submission of a New Drug Application (NDA). FDA regulations in effect since 1962 state that to receive approval, the drug must be shown to be both safe and efficacious for the use intended. Since evidence supporting its safety and efficacy must be included sometime prior to this approval, the drug must have been actu-ally used by physicians for the conditions named in the application. It is during this period of preapproval use that a drug is considered to be investigational. An applicant must submit evidence that the drug is safe and effective, and this evi-dence must be obtained through animal and clinical (human) studies. However, it is not permissible to ship a new drug in interstate commerce unless the drug has an approved NDA. Individuals or pharmaceutical companies desiring to ship or receive drugs that are not covered by an approved NDA may obtain an exemption from the FDA for the pursuit of clinical investigations. To receive this exemption, the manufacturer must apply for a Notice of Claimed Exemption, or IND applica-tion, commonly referred to as an *investigational new drug (IND)* exemption. The purpose of the approval process for an IND is to protect the safety of the humans who will participate in the clinical trials.

Preclinical Studies

Administration of biologically active substances to humans carries unavoidable risk, and this risk can be identified through adequate preclinical research. This research uses animals and establishes the drug's biological and toxicological characteristics. These preclinical studies are conducted to determine how the drug is absorbed, distributed, metabolized, and eliminated. This information pro-vides the basis for establishing suitable human dosage regimens.

Phase I Clinical Studies

Phase I clinical studies represent the first time a new drug is introduced into human beings. Emphasis is now placed on describing the safety of the new agent by defining the pharmacokinetic (absorption, distribution, metabolism, and excretion), toxicological, and pharmacological parameters associated with its use in humans. A minimal number of patients are utilized for Phase I clinical trials. Phase I studies with a control group of patients (those receiving a placebo) are usually performed double-blind, with neither the investigator nor the patient aware of which drug—active versus placebo—is being administered.

Phase II Clinical Studies

Phase II clinical studies are a continuation and expansion of those activities initiated during Phase I trials. The relative degree of safety for human use is determined in Phase I studies. In Phase II studies the emphasis is toward establishing the activity of the new drug in patients being treated. Protocols are developed that include the goals and objectives of the research, the dosing used, and the parameters assessed.

Upon completion of Phase II studies, evidence of safety and efficacy must be established before proceeding further. Unfavorable outcomes in Phase II studies may lead to the abandonment of further research, while favorable results may lead to further clinical trials, and Phase III studies are initiated.

Phase III Clinical Studies

The decision to initiate Phase III clinical trials is based on a review and analysis of the study results in the preclinical, Phase I, and Phase II studies. Phase III studies provide for proof of efficacy and establish the acceptable use(s) of the drug. Phase III study protocols are often conducted in a number of hospitals concurrently, as many hundreds of patients may need to be evaluated before meaningful results can be obtained.

Approval for marketing can be sought only upon completion of all of the aforementioned research. To obtain marketing approval, a completed New Drug Application (NDA) must be sent to the FDA for review and approval.

Informed Consent

For all three IND clinical phases, the FDCA requires the investigators to obtain an informed consent of the patient or the patient's representative for the administration of an experimental drug. The informed consent outlines the potential risks, possible benefits, and alternative course(s) of treatment.

Institutional Review Board

The institutional review board (IRB) is a multidisciplinary board or committee designated by an institution to objectively review and approve biomedical research involving human subjects in accordance with FDA regulations. The purpose of the IRB, among others, is to ensure that the risks to the patients are minimized and that a written informed consent will be obtained from each patient.

Handling of Investigational Drugs

The procedures for handling investigational drugs are an important part of hospital drug distribution systems. These procedures will naturally reflect the extent to which an institution is involved with research, the resources available, and the particular needs of the hospital. For most community hospitals, the main activities related to investigational drugs will most likely involve the receipt, storage, dispensing, recordkeeping, and control of investigational drugs. In a large teaching hospital, investigational drug use may result in numerous services and responsibilities requiring full-time personnel.

The basic responsibilities of a hospital pharmacy handling investigational drugs are as follows:

- *Distribution and control of investigational drugs*, including drug procurement, storage, inventory management, packaging, labeling, distribution, and disposition of unused drugs.
- *Clinical services*, including pharmacy and nursing staff in-service education and training, perhaps patient education, and the monitoring and reporting of adverse drug reactions.
- *Research activities*, which may involve participating in the preparation or review of research proposals and protocols, assisting in data collection and analysis, and serving on the institutional review board (IRB).
- *Clinical study management*, which might involve working on study reports to the research sponsor.

Use of Marketed Products for Unapproved Uses

Physicians may use a marketed drug for an indication or in a manner not in the approved product labeling. In doing so, the physician must have acceptable evidence such as published articles in recognized medical journals, or accepted use in the medical community that justifies its intended use. Use of drugs in this fashion is not subject to FDA regulation, nor is it subject to review unless required by institutional policy for review by the institutional review board or the pharmacy and therapeutics committee.

Reporting of Adverse Drug Reactions

One definition of an adverse drug reaction is "any unexpected, or unwanted change in a patient's condition that a physician suspects may be due to a drug, that occurs at doses normally used in humans, and that requires treatment, indicates decrease or cessation of therapy with the drug, or suggests that future therapy with the drug carries an unusual risk in the patient."

Most hospitals have a policy that all suspected adverse reactions to drugs will be brought to the attention of the physician, investigated, documented in the patient's chart, and that severe adverse reactions will be reported to the FDA, and the additional requirements of each respective state for reporting severe reactions to the department of health or other agency within the state will be followed.

Upon suspecting that an adverse drug reaction has occurred, the nurse should follow hospital procedure.

1. Alert the prescribing physician that an adverse drug reaction may have occurred, and initiate appropriate treatment, if necessary.
2. Record the suspected adverse drug reaction on the patient's chart.

3. Using the hospital's procedures established for reporting an adverse drug reaction, notify the pharmacy of the suspected reaction.

The pharmacy will document and review the drug reaction and, where appropriate, pertinent data will be supplied to the Food and Drug Administration. The FDA maintains a voluntary program that allows health care professionals to report adverse drug reaction directly to them. An official reporting form entitled MedWatch (Form FDA 3500) is shown in Figure 6-4. This form can be obtained from the FDA by calling 800-FDA-1088 or by writing MedWatch, 5600 Fishers Lane, Rockville, MD 20852-9787. Reports may be telephoned to the same number or faxed to 800-FDA-0718. Reports may also be entered online at the FDA's Web site, www.fda .gov/medwatch/index.html.

Drug Quality Reporting System (DQRS)

In addition to the adverse drug reaction program, the FDA maintains a voluntary program through which health care practitioners can report drug quality problems. The FDA encourages pharmacists to report any concerns with a drug product, including poor or improper labeling, the lack of efficacy of an injectable product, particulate matter, abnormal color or taste, and so forth. The FDA receives DQRS reports through the MedWatch program.

Drug Recalls

All drug recalls are voluntary, either manufacturer-initiated or FDA-requested, and the result of reports from the manufacturer or health professionals.

The FDA medical staff determines the health hazard potential of a product (e.g., subpotent labeling errors, adverse drug reactions) and assigns a drug recall classification as follows:

1. *Class I*—There is a reasonable probability that the use or exposure to a product will cause severe adverse health consequences or death.
2. *Class II*—The use of or exposure to a product may cause temporary or medically reversible adverse health consequences.
3. *Class III*—The use of or exposure to a product is not likely to cause adverse health consequences.

The manufacturer is responsible for notifying sellers of the recall, and sellers are responsible for contacting consumers if necessary. The FDA requires that written notices for Class I, Class II, and some Class III recalls be sent by first-class mail with the envelope and letterhead conspicuously marked "URGENT: DRUG RECALL."

A pharmacist and/or technician should immediately retrieve all lot numbers of the recalled medication, supplies, and devices from the facility, and place them in a secure, separate area, following the manufacturer's recommendation to destroy or return the recalled drugs. A notation on the recall notice should be made noting the date, amount (if any) of the recalled drugs, and their disposition. It should be noted that dispensing a recalled product may violate the FDCA, because the drug is likely adulterated or misbranded.

A post-recall audit is done by the FDA to verify that manufacturers, wholesalers, pharmacists, or customers have received notification about the recall and have taken appropriate action.

FIGURE 6-4

U.S. Department of Health and Human Services

Form Approved: OMB No. 0910-0291, Expires: 10/31/08
See OMB statement on reverse.

MEDWATCH

The FDA Safety Information and
Adverse Event Reporting Program

For VOLUNTARY reporting of
adverse events, product problems and
product use errors

Page ____ of ____

FDA USE ONLY

Triage unit
sequence #

PLEASE TYPE OR USE BLACK INK

A. PATIENT INFORMATION

1. Patient Identifier	2. Age at Time of Event, or Date of Birth:	3. Sex	4. Weight
In confidence		☐ Female ☐ Male	____ lb or ____ kg

B. ADVERSE EVENT, PRODUCT PROBLEM OR ERROR

Check all that apply:

1. ☐ Adverse Event   ☐ Product Problem (e.g., defects/malfunctions)
☐ Product Use Error   ☐ Problem with Different Manufacturer of Same Medicine

2. Outcomes Attributed to Adverse Event
(Check all that apply)

☐ Death: _____
        (mm/dd/yyyy)
☐ Life-threatening
☐ Hospitalization - initial or prolonged
☐ Required Intervention to Prevent Permanent Impairment/Damage (Devices)

☐ Disability or Permanent Damage
☐ Congenital Anomaly/Birth Defect
☐ Other Serious (Important Medical Events)

3. Date of Event (mm/dd/yyyy)	4. Date of this Report (mm/dd/yyyy)

5. Describe Event, Problem or Product Use Error

6. Relevant Tests/Laboratory Data, Including Dates

7. Other Relevant History, Including Preexisting Medical Conditions (e.g., allergies, race, pregnancy, smoking and alcohol use, liver/kidney problems, etc.)

C. PRODUCT AVAILABILITY

Product Available for Evaluation? (Do not send product to FDA)

☐ Yes   ☐ No   ☐ Returned to Manufacturer on: _____
                          (mm/dd/yyyy)

D. SUSPECT PRODUCT(S)

1. Name, Strength, Manufacturer (from product label)

#1

#2

2.	Dose or Amount	Frequency	Route
#1			
#2			

3. Dates of Use (If unknown, give duration) from/to (or best estimate)	5. Event Abated After Use Stopped or Dose Reduced?
#1	#1 ☐ Yes ☐ No ☐ Doesn't Apply
#2	#2 ☐ Yes ☐ No ☐ Doesn't Apply

4. Diagnosis or Reason for Use (Indication)

#1

#2

8. Event Reappeared After Reintroduction?

#1 ☐ Yes ☐ No ☐ Doesn't Apply

6. Lot #	7. Expiration Date
#1	#1
#2	#2

#2 ☐ Yes ☐ No ☐ Doesn't Apply

9. NDC # or Unique ID

E. SUSPECT MEDICAL DEVICE

1. Brand Name

2. Common Device Name

3. Manufacturer Name, City and State

4. Model #	Lot #	5. Operator of Device
Catalog #	Expiration Date (mm/dd/yyyy)	☐ Health Professional ☐ Lay User/Patient
Serial #	Other #	☐ Other:

6. If Implanted, Give Date (mm/dd/yyyy)	7. If Explanted, Give Date (mm/dd/yyyy)

8. Is this a Single-use Device that was Reprocessed and Reused on a Patient?
☐ Yes   ☐ No

9. If Yes to Item No. 8, Enter Name and Address of Reprocessor

F. OTHER (CONCOMITANT) MEDICAL PRODUCTS

Product names and therapy dates (exclude treatment of event)

G. REPORTER (See confidentiality section on back)

1. Name and Address

Phone #	E-mail

2. Health Professional?	3. Occupation	4. Also Reported to:
☐ Yes ☐ No		☐ Manufacturer
5. If you do NOT want your identity disclosed to the manufacturer, place an "X" in this box: ☐		☐ User Facility ☐ Distributor/Importer

FORM FDA 3500 (10/05)   Submission of a report does not constitute an admission that medical personnel or the product caused or contributed to the event.

FIGURE 6-4 MedWatch form for voluntary reporting by health professionals of adverse events and product problems.

FIGURE 6-4 (Continued)

ADVICE ABOUT VOLUNTARY REPORTING

Detailed instructions available at: http://www.fda.gov/medwatch/report/consumer/instruct.htm

Report adverse events, product problems or product use errors with:

- Medications *(drugs or biologics)*
- Medical devices *(including in-vitro diagnostics)*
- Combination products *(medication & medical devices)*
- Human cells, tissues, and cellular and tissue-based products
- Special nutritional products *(dietary supplements, medical foods, infant formulas)*
- Cosmetics

Report product problems - quality, performance or safety concerns such as:

- Suspected counterfeit product
- Suspected contamination
- Questionable stability
- Defective components
- Poor packaging or labeling
- Therapeutic failures (product didn't work)

Report SERIOUS adverse events. An event is serious when the patient outcome is:

- Death
- Life-threatening
- Hospitalization - initial or prolonged
- Disability or permanent damage
- Congenital anomaly/birth defect
- Required intervention to prevent permanent impairment or damage
- Other serious (important medical events)

Report even if:

- You're not certain the product caused the event
- You don't have all the details

How to report:

- Just fill in the sections that apply to your report
- Use section D for all products except medical devices
- Attach additional pages if needed
- Use a separate form for each patient
- Report either to FDA or the manufacturer *(or both)*

Other methods of reporting:

- 1-800-FDA-0178 -- To FAX report
- 1-800-FDA-1088 -- To report by phone
- www.fda.gov/medwatch/report.htm -- To report online

If your report involves a serious adverse event with a device and it occurred in a facility outside a doctor's office, that facility may be legally required to report to FDA and/or the manufacturer. Please notify the person in that facility who would handle such reporting.

If your report involves a serious adverse event with a vaccine call 1-800-822-7967 to report.

Confidentiality: The patient's identity is held in strict confidence by FDA and protected to the fullest extent of the law. FDA will not disclose the reporter's identity in response to a request from the public, pursuant to the Freedom of Information Act. The reporter's identity, including the identity of a self-reporter, may be shared with the manufacturer unless requested otherwise.

-Fold Here-

-Fold Here-

The public reporting burden for this collection of information has been estimated to average 36 minutes per response, including the time for reviewing instructions, searching existing data sources, gathering and maintaining the data needed, and completing and reviewing the collection of information. Send comments regarding this burden estimate or any other aspect of this collection of information, including suggestions for reducing this burden to:

Department of Health and Human Services
Food and Drug Administration - MedWatch
10903 New Hampshire Avenue
Building 22, Mail Stop 4447
Silver Spring, MD 20993-0002

Please DO NOT
RETURN this form
to this address.

OMB statement:
"An agency may not conduct or sponsor, and a person is not required to respond to, a collection of information unless it displays a currently valid OMB control number."

U.S. DEPARTMENT OF HEALTH AND HUMAN SERVICES
Food and Drug Administration

FORM FDA 3500 (10/05) (Back) **Please Use Address Provided Below -- Fold in Thirds, Tape and Mail**

DEPARTMENT OF
HEALTH & HUMAN SERVICES

Public Health Service
Food and Drug Administration
Rockville, MD 20857

Official Business
Penalty for Private Use $300

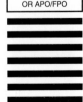

NO POSTAGE
NECESSARY
IF MAILED
IN THE
UNITED STATES
OR APO/FPO

BUSINESS REPLY MAIL

FIRST CLASS MAIL   PERMIT NO. 946   ROCKVILLE MD

MEDWATCH

The FDA Safety Information and Adverse Event Reporting Program
Food and Drug Administration
5600 Fishers Lane
Rockville, MD 20852-9787

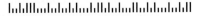

Repackaging of Drugs

Repackaging of drugs in a pharmacy requires the use of a repackaging record. A repackaging record must be maintained, including the name, strength, lot number, quantity, name of the manufacturer and distributor, the date of repacking, the number of packages prepared, the number of dosage units in each package, the signature of the person performing the repackaging operation, the signature of the pharmacist supervising the repackaging, and other identifying marks added by the pharmacy for internal recordkeeping purposes. In the event of a drug recall, the repackaging record is a source of information referred to in an effort to determine if the recalled drug has been repackaged.

Expiration Dating for Repackaged Drugs

Calculation of the expiration date for a repackaged drug may vary as per state board regulations. In New York State drugs repackaged for in-house use must have an expiration date of 12 months or 50 percent of the time remaining of the manufacturer's expiration date—whichever is less—from the date of repackaging. The USP Pharmacists' Pharmacopoeia states the expiration date shall be one year from the date the drug is packaged or the expiration date (of the original container), whichever is earlier.

Product Tampering

The FDA promulgated regulations in 1982 requiring that certain OTC drugs and devices be manufactured in tamper-resistant packaging. A tamper-resistant package is defined as "one having an indicator or barrier to entry which, if breached or missing, can reasonably be expected to provide visible evidence to consumers that tampering has occurred."

The United States Pharmacopoeia and the National Formulary

In 1906 with the passage of the Food and Drug Act and in 1938 with the passage of the Food, Drug, and Cosmetic Act, the United States Pharmacopoeia (USP) became the official compendia of drug standards in the United States. Each chapter of the USP is assigned a number, which appears in brackets along with the chapter name. Chapters 1 to 999 are requirements, as well as official monographs and standards of USP, whereas Chapters 1000 to 1999 are informational.

Chapter 797 of the USP, entitled "Pharmaceutical Compounding: Sterile Preparations" was published on January 1, 2004. The guidelines laid out in this chapter are enforceable by federal and state regulatory agencies. The chapter details the procedures and requirements with which pharmacists, technicians, and other health professionals must comply when they compound sterile preparations. This chapter establishes practice standards that are applicable to all practice settings where sterile preparations are compounded (e.g., hospitals, community pharmacies, home infusion services, ambulatory care services, physician offices, nursing homes, etc.). (Please refer to Chapter 15, "Sterile Preparation Compounding," for a comprehensive review of this topic and the role and responsibilities of the pharmacy technician.)

Medicare

The Medicare program was enacted in 1965 to help provide for federal health insurance for those older than 65 years of age and for certain disabled individuals, regardless of age. The law has two components:

- *Part A* provides hospitalization insurance without any charge to eligible beneficiaries.
- *Part B* covers outpatient diagnostic services such as X-rays and laboratory tests.

On December 8, 2003, the Medicare Prescription Drug Improvement and Modernization Act, also known as Medicare Part D, was signed into law. In 2006 this law added a voluntary prescription drug benefit to Medicare. Beneficiaries will pay an average of a $35 monthly premium, plus $250 deductible, and a 25 percent co-payment up to $2,250. Coverage then stops for drug costs between $2,251 and $5,100. This is known as the "doughnut hole." After $5,100 in drug expenditures, the plan will pay the greater of either $2 for a generic, $5 for a brand name drug, or a 5 percent co-payment.

The law also provides coverage for disease management programs, termed *medication therapy management (MTM)* programs. Pharmacists may receive fees for providing MTM services to patients with chronic diseases who take multiple drugs.

Long-Term Care Facility Regulation

A long-term care facility (LTCF) is a facility that is planned, staffed, and equipped to accommodate individuals who do not require hospital care but who are in need of medical, nursing, and related health and social services. Nursing homes that accept federal funds, including Medicare and Medicaid, are required to comply with federal regulations issued by the Centers for Medicare and Medicaid Services (CMS), formerly called the Health Care Financing Administration (HCFA). Each nursing home is surveyed annually to determine compliance with the federal regulations. These surveys are enforced through appropriate state agencies, with the majority of the states vesting regulatory power in the state department of health. (Please refer to Chapter 4, "Long-Term Care," for a comprehensive review of this topic and the role and responsibilities of the pharmacy technician.)

Tax-Free Alcohol

The federal government's philosophy with respect to the use of tax-free ethyl alcohol is that the alcohol will be used only for specific purposes:

- It will not be used for beverage purposes.
- It is not for resale.
- It is used in accordance with uses stated on the alcohol permit.

Bureau of Alcohol, Tobacco, and Firearms (ATF) a department of the U.S. Treasury, which establishes regulatory standards for procuring, storing, dispensing, and use of tax-free alcohol for specific clinical uses.

If not used according to stated purposes, a tax will be levied for its procurement and subsequent use. In pursuit of this goal, the **Bureau of Alcohol, Tobacco, and Firearms (ATF)** is responsible for controlling tax-free alcohol, which has a number of mandated specific federal forms users of tax-free alcohol must complete.

Pharmacies may purchase 95 percent ethanol, with applicable taxes, for routine compounding of pharmaceutical preparations or filling prescriptions by using Form ATF-11. Institutions with a need for greater volumes of alcohol may purchase tax-free alcohol, which is much lower in cost, as the tax on regular alcohol purchases is quite high. Hospital pharmacies can purchase tax-free alcohol by using Form ATF-1447. Pharmacies purchasing alcohol for use as a beverage must obtain a retail liquor dealer's stamp.

There must be adequate and secure fire-resistant storage facilities available for the prevention of unauthorized access to tax-free alcohol. These facilities must be large enough to hold the maximum quantity of tax-free alcohol that will be on hand at any one time as allowed by the respective institution's tax-free alcohol permit. A bond is required for persons who withdraw more than 1,500 proof gallons of tax-free alcohol per year.

Accurate detailed records of all receipts, shipments, loss, usage, destruction, and withdrawal and use of tax-free alcohol must be kept for easy access by ATF officers. Records must be kept on file for three years after the date of transaction. All records must be kept at the permit premises. A physical inventory must be made of the tax-free alcohol on a semiannual basis. If a loss is incurred, a claim for allowances must be filed with the ATF regional director.

The Joint Commission

Joint Commission not-for-profit organization whose standards are set to ensure effective quality services (e.g., optimal standards for the operation of hospitals).

The **Joint Commission** was formed in 1951 as a not-for-profit, private, nongovernmental organization by the American College of Physicians, American College of Surgeons, American Hospital Association, American Medical Association, and later, the American Dental Association, for the purpose of improving the quality of health care provided to the public. The Joint Commission has changed its mission to not only address the quality of patient care, but also patient safety.

The Joint Commission establishes optimal standards for health care providers and then evaluates organizations for compliance to these standards through an on-site inspection called a *survey*. If the organization is in substantial compliance with these standards, the Commission awards a certificate of accreditation. To maintain accreditation, the organization is expected to correct any identified deficiencies and be in continuous compliance with the standards of the Joint Commission. The organization could be surveyed at any time on an unannounced basis, but must be resurveyed at least once every three years.

The Joint Commission currently sets standards and accredits the following types of health care providers: hospitals, home health care agencies, home infusion providers and home care pharmacies, long-term care pharmacies, ambulatory infusion centers, home medical equipment and home oxygen providers, ambulatory clinics, ambulatory surgicenters and office-based surgery practices, community health centers, college and prison health care centers, nursing homes and subacute facilities, assisted living facilities, clinical laboratories, behavioral health organizations, and alcohol and chemical dependency centers, among others.

Accreditation

Accreditation is a voluntary process, and the organization pays to be surveyed and accredited by the Joint Commission. Currently, more than 80 percent of hospitals are accredited by the Joint Commission, with a significant percentage in other health care areas. So why do health care organizations seek accreditation? Accreditation signifies achievement of a higher level of quality and safety in providing patient care. This brings prestige to the organization, attracting both staff and physicians, and provides a source of pride within the community. Lastly, the Joint Commission has been granted "deemed status" for participation in Medicare. That means that providers accredited by the Joint Commission are "deemed" to meet the Medicare Conditions of Participation and can receive Medicare funding without having separate annual Medicare surveys by state inspectors. Thus, while voluntary in nature, loss of accreditation can mean not only a loss of prestige, but also a loss of significant Medicare and private insurance funding. That is why many hospitals place such importance on preparation for Joint Commission surveys and in adhering to the standards.

The Joint Commission Standards

All standards are published in a Comprehensive Accreditation Manual for each of the major accreditation programs (e.g., hospitals, home care, behavioral health, ambulatory, networks, long-term care), which are provided on a complimentary basis to each organization that has applied for accreditation. Most standards related to pharmacy practice fall within the "Medication Use" section of the "Care of the Patient" chapter. However, other chapters often contain standards pertinent to the pharmacy. For example, the requirement for patient education on medications can be found in the education chapter.

Quality Improvement

The Joint Commission is a strong proponent of the principles of continuous quality improvement. This theory requires collection of data to measure, assess, and ultimately improve all processes within the organization. The Joint Commission calls this *performance improvement* or *PI*. PI forms the cornerstone of all standards. As a result, the performance improvement coordinator of most hospitals is the key person responsible for coordinating the hospital's accreditation preparation efforts.

Survey Process

While there are a number of components to the Joint Commission survey, a pharmacy technician will most likely be involved with visits to patient care settings and tours of the pharmacy. During a typical inpatient hospital unit visit, the surveyor tours the unit to review its overall operation—including appropriate storage of medications—and meets and interviews key unit staff, including physicians, nurses, pharmacists, social workers, dietitians, and possibly even pharmacy technicians. If technicians are interviewed as part of a survey, they need to be able to explain what they do and how they do it, to be knowledgeable about the pharmacy's policies and procedures, and about other hospital policies and procedures that describe their responsibilities both within the pharmacy and/or in their functions in patient care areas.

FIGURE 6-5

Patients' Bill of Rights

As a patient in a hospital in New York State, you have the right, consistent with law, to:

(1) Understand and use these rights. If for any reason you do not understand or you need help, the hospital MUST provide assistance, including an interpreter.

(2) Receive treatment without discrimination as to race, color, religion, sex, national origin, disability, sexual orientation or source of payment.

(3) Receive considerate and respectful care in a clean and safe environment free of unnecessary restraints.

(4) Receive emergency care if you need it.

(5) Be informed of the name and position of the doctor who will be in charge of your care in the hospital.

(6) Know the names, positions and functions of any hospital staff involved in your care and refuse their treatment, examination or observation.

(7) A no smoking room.

(8) Receive complete information about your diagnosis, treatment and prognosis.

(9) Receive all the information that you need to give informed consent for any proposed procedure or treatment. This information shall include the possible risks and benefits of the procedure or treatment.

(10) Receive all the information you need to give informed consent for an order not to resuscitate. You also have the right to designate an individual to give this consent for you if you are too ill to do so. If you would like additional information, please ask for a copy of the pamphlet "Do Not Resuscitate Orders — A Guide for Patients and Families."

(11) Refuse treatment and be told what effect this may have on your health.

(12) Refuse to take part in research. In deciding whether or not to participate, you have the right to a full explanation.

(13) Privacy while in the hospital and confidentiality of all information and records regarding your care.

(14) Participate in all decisions about your treatment and discharge from the hospital. The hospital must provide you with a written discharge plan and written description of how you can appeal your discharge.

(15) Review your medical record without charge. Obtain a copy of your medical record for which the hospital can charge a reasonable fee. You cannot be denied a copy solely because you cannot afford to pay.

(16) Receive an itemized bill and explanation of all charges.

(17) Complain without fear of reprisals about the care and services you are receiving and to have the hospital respond to you and if you request it, a written response. If you are not satisfied with the hospital's response, you can complain to the New York State Health Department. The hospital must provide you with the State Health Department telephone number.

(18) Authorize those family members and other adults who will be given priority to visit consistent with your ability to receive visitors.

(19) Make known your wishes in regard to anatomical gifts. You may document your wishes in your health care proxy or on a donor card, available from the hospital.

Public Health Law(PHL)2803 (1)(g)Patient's Rights, 10NYCRR, 405.7,405.7(a)(1),405.7(c)

FIGURE 6-5 Patients' bill of rights.

Survey Results

While the actual final accreditation report of the organization is confidential, the Joint Commission does publicly post a performance report that includes, among other things, the accreditation decision. The final recommendations of the survey team allow the organization to improve its quality and safety of patient care in a positive, non-punitive environment. For more information about the Joint Commission and the accreditation process, refer to their Web site at www.jointcommission.org.

Patients' Bill of Rights

patients' bill of rights a declaration ensuring that all patients, inpatients, outpatients, and emergency service patients are afforded their rights in a health care institution.

Many states have established a **patients' bill of rights** for hospital and health care institutions. This bill of rights ensures that all patients—inpatients, outpatients, and emergency service patients—are afforded their rights. The hospital's responsibility for assuring patients' rights includes both providing patients with a copy of these rights and providing assistance to patients to understand and exercise their rights.

For the purposes of illustration, Figure 6-5 is an example of the New York State Hospital Patient's Bill of Rights. It is incumbent upon all health care workers to be familiar with the bill of rights and to ensure compliance with it.

Summary

Numerous statutes, rules, regulations, and quasi-legal standards of practice regulate the pharmacy profession. These requirements have been established to protect the patient and to ensure safe and effective drug therapy. Pharmacists and technicians should be familiar with and ensure compliance with these standards in their daily activities and responsibilities. Additionally, both the American Pharmacists Association and the American Association of Pharmacy Technicians have published a Code of Ethics for Pharmacists and Technicians respectively, which outline principles designed to guide professionals in their relationships with patients, other health professionals, and society. Both codes are outlined in Chapter 8, "Ethical Considerations for the Pharmacy Technician."

Legal Citation Format

Legal terminology, format, and symbols in legal reading materials are summarized as follows so that the references noted in this chapter are meaningful and applicable:

- Statutes are arranged into titles and divided into sections. For example, the Food, Drug, and Cosmetic Act begins at 21 U.S. Code § 321 (Title 21 of the U.S. Code, Section 321). The symbol § means *section*. The mark §§ means *sections*.
- Regulations are proposed by federal administrative agencies in a daily publication known as the *Federal Register*. Citations in the *Federal Register* use volume numbers and page numbers, and dates in parentheses. For example, 65 Fed. Reg. 82, 462 (2000).
- Once regulations have been finalized and adopted by the agency, they appear in the Code of Federal Regulations (CFR). The citations in the CFR refer to title number and section. For example, 21 CFR § 120.200.

TEST YOUR KNOWLEDGE

Multiple Choice

1. A patient package insert is required to be given to all patients who are taking
   a. steroids.
   b. analgesics.
   c. estrogenic drugs.
   d. all of the above.

2. Which of the following is considered a controlled substance?
   a. Demerol
   b. morphine
   c. Valium
   d. all of the above

3. Regulations affecting pharmacy practice encompass
   a. federal and state statutes.
   b. state rules and regulations.
   c. CSA regulations.
   d. all of the above.

4. Which of the following is *not* an approved use of tax-free alcohol?
   a. use in educational organizations for scientific purposes
   b. use in hospitals for medical purposes
   c. laboratory use for scientific research
   d. beverage purposes

5. Which of the following is *not* a responsibility of the Food, Drug, and Cosmetic Act (FDCA)?
   a. protection of public health
   b. Consumer Product Safety Commission
   c. collection of adverse drug reaction reports
   d. over-the-counter drugs' labeling requirements for safe consumer use

6. Controlled substances are required by federal law to have appropriate safeguards with their use. Which of the following is *not* an issue?
   a. inventory requirements
   b. dispensing records and reports
   c. administration records
   d. patient consent

7. Which of the following is *not* a reason to report adverse drug reactions to the FDA?
   a. public information
   b. possible revision of prescribing information
   c. possible drug recall
   d. possible warning statement

8. A Class I recall does *not* include
   a. voluntary manufacturer initiation.
   b. possibility of severe health consequences.
   c. FDA initiation.
   d. assignment of the drug recall classification by the FDA.

9. The intent of the Occupational Safety and Health Administration (OSHA) is
   a. to monitor job-related injuries.
   b. to develop job safety and health standards.
   c. to ensure a safe and healthy workplace.
   d. all of the above.

10. Pharmacy practice standards, guidelines, and statements
   a. define reasonable and prudent practices.
   b. establish minimum standards for the profession.
   c. improve the delivery of pharmaceutical care.
   d. establish pharmacist positions.

Matching

Match the legislation with what it enforces.

1. _____ Durham-Humphrey Amendment

2. _____ Orphan Drug Act

3. _____ Controlled Substances Act

4. _____ Poison Prevention Packaging Act

5. _____ Hazard Communication Standard

6. _____ Health Insurance Portability and Accountability Act

a. Regulates the manufacture, sale, and distribution of drugs that have a high abuse potential

b. Creates incentives for manufacturers to research and develop drugs to treat rare diseases and disorders

c. Establishes guidelines to protect patient privacy

d. Establishes requirements for child-resistant containers

e. Establishes prescription versus over-the-counter drugs

f. Establishes the rights of employees to know the dangers of substances used in the workplace

Fill In The Blank

1. _____ and _____ are administrative enactments implemented by government agencies that meet the intent of statutory policies.

2. The _____ prohibits the adulteration and misbranding of foods in interstate commerce.

3. The _____ requires that all new drugs be proven safe and effective.

4. Schedule _____ drugs have no approved medical use in the United States.

5. The FDA requires distribution of _____ to educate patients about the proper use of and potential hazards of drugs.

References

Abbod, R. (2005). *Pharmacy practice and the law* (4th ed.). Sudbury, MA: Jones and Bartlett Publishers.

American Society of Health-System Pharmacists. (2007-2008). *Best practices for health system pharmacy.* Bethesda, MD.

Facts and Comparisons. (2006). *Pharmacy law digest* (40th ed.). St. Louis, MO.

Joint Commission. (2007). *Comprehensive accreditation manual for hospitals.* Oakbrook Terrace, IL.

Pharmaceutical Compounding-Sterile Preparations, Chapter 797 (2005). *The USP pharmacists' pharmacopoeia* (1st ed.). United States Pharmacopeial Convention: Rockville, MD.

Reiss, B., & Hall, G. (2006). *Guide to federal pharmacy law* (5th ed.). Delmar, NY: Apothecary Press.

University of the State of New York, the New York State Education Department, and the New York State Board of Pharmacy. (2007). *Pharmacy guide to practice.* Albany, NY.

Some Relevant Federal Statutes and Regulations

Statutes

Alcohol Tax Law
Controlled Substances Act of 1970
Federal Food, Drug, and Cosmetic Act
Hazardous Substances Act
Health Insurance Portability and Accountability Act
Occupation and Safety Act
Poison Prevention Packaging Act of 1970
Social Security Amendments of 1965 (Medicare and Medicaid)
U.S. Statutes at Large, 1670

Regulations

Consumer Product Safety Commission (Poison Prevention Packaging Act). 16 CFR §§ 1700–1704.
Drug Enforcement Administration
Food and Drug Administration
Health Care Financing Administration (Medicaid)
Internal Revenue Service (Alcohol Tax Law)
Social Security Administration (Medicare)

Drug-Use Control: The Foundation of Pharmaceutical Care

Competencies

Upon completion of this chapter, the reader should be able to

1. State the mission of pharmacy practice.
2. Explain the foundational elements of pharmaceutical care.
3. Briefly describe the elements in the drug use process, once the drug is approved for distribution.
4. Explain how important control is in the drug use process.
5. Explain the role of pharmacists in the drug use process.
6. Discuss the role of technicians in the drug use process.
7. Discuss trends in the drug use process and how these trends may affect the roles of the pharmacist and pharmacy technician.

Key Terms

adverse drug reaction (ADR)
alternative medicine
drug manufacturer
drug order
drug use process
drug wholesaler
formulary
group purchasing
IV admixtures
Kardex
laminar flow hood
medication-related problem (MRP)
non-adherence
pharmaceutical care
retailer
side effects
unit dose

Introduction

drug use process an organized, complex, and controlled system of manufacturing, purchasing, distributing, storing, prescribing, preparing, dispensing, administering, using, controlling, and monitoring a drug's effects and outcomes to ensure that drugs are used safely and effectively.

Once a drug is approved for use in the United States, a defined process is used to distribute the drug product and make it available for use. This organized, complex, and controlled procedure is called the **drug use process**. Pharmacists and pharmacy technicians are intimately involved in the drug use process, and they are responsible for controlling parts of the process so the drugs are used safely and effectively and not diverted into the wrong hands.

This chapter describes how drugs make their way to the patient after being made by the manufacturer. It will begin with a review of drug distribution, the self-use of medication, the prescribing, dispensing, and administrating of prescription medication, and what it means to provide quality drug therapy. The primary focus is on control of the drug use process and how pharmacists and pharmacy technicians exert that control.

The Drug Use Process

Once a drug is approved for distribution, the drug use process encompasses manufacturing, purchasing, distributing, storing, prescribing, preparing, dispensing, administering, using, controlling, and monitoring drugs and their effects and outcomes (Figure 7-1). In short, the drug use process consists of the steps and procedures used to get a drug to its eventual destination safely, securely, and effectively.

Pharmacy technicians spend most of their time in the ordering, storing, preparing, dispensing, and controlling parts of this process. However, it is important for them to understand the entire drug use process and do what they can to add proper control as needed.

Manufacturing the Drug

The drug use process begins with the pharmaceutical company or manufacturer who develops and creates drugs. It is the responsibility of the manufacturer to prepare drugs that are safe and effective for use. Drug research, development, and creation is heavily regulated.

Drug Distribution

drug manufacturer the company responsible for developing, producing, and distributing pharmaceutical products.

drug wholesaler the company responsible for delivering medication, medical devices, appliances, etc. to pharmacies and retailers.

retailer the company responsible for delivering products to patients.

The United States has the most complex and most efficient drug distribution system in the world. Automation, such as bar coding, computerized inventories, and information systems, keep the products flowing. As drugs flow through the distribution system, they increase in value.

Drug manufacturers, wholesalers, and retailers are the major firms responsible for the supply and distribution of medication in the United States. **Drug manufacturers** develop and produce the pharmaceutical products. **Drug wholesalers** deliver medication, medical devices and appliances, health and beauty aids, and other products to pharmacies and, with the exception of prescription drugs, to other retailers. **Retailers** (like community pharmacies) provide these products to the patient.

FIGURE 7-1

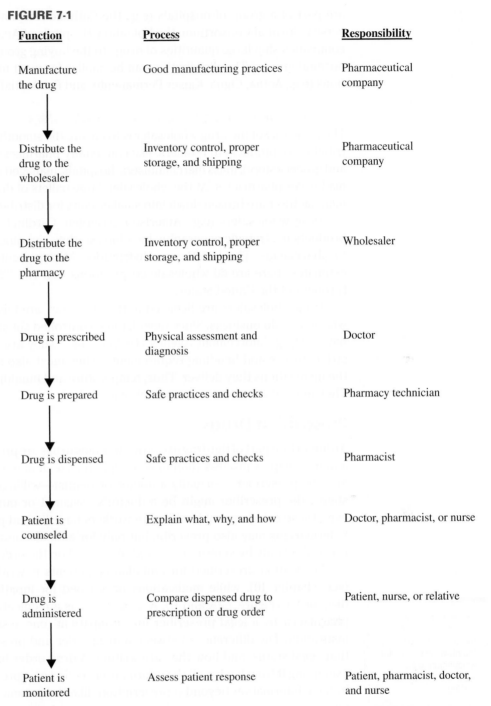

Function	Process	Responsibility
Manufacture the drug	Good manufacturing practices	Pharmaceutical company
Distribute the drug to the wholesaler	Inventory control, proper storage, and shipping	Pharmaceutical company
Distribute the drug to the pharmacy	Inventory control, proper storage, and shipping	Wholesaler
Drug is prescribed	Physical assessment and diagnosis	Doctor
Drug is prepared	Safe practices and checks	Pharmacy technician
Drug is dispensed	Safe practices and checks	Pharmacist
Patient is counseled	Explain what, why, and how	Doctor, pharmacist, or nurse
Drug is administered	Compare dispensed drug to prescription or drug order	Patient, nurse, or relative
Patient is monitored	Assess patient response	Patient, pharmacist, doctor, and nurse

FIGURE 7-1 An overview of the drug use process.

Distribution of drugs from pharmaceutical manufacturers

group purchasing an arrangement where pharmaceutical companies ship large quantities of drugs to the warehouses of hospital buying groups.

Most of the pharmaceutical products made by manufacturers go directly to drug wholesalers and to other major distribution centers. Pharmaceutical companies also deliver their products to distribution centers set up by chain pharmacies (e.g., CVS, Rite Aid, Walgreens), mass merchandisers (e.g., Kmart, Wal-Mart), and grocery store chains that have pharmacies (e.g., Kroger, Publix, Albertsons).

Although some hospitals can buy directly from the manufacturer, most buy their medication through an arrangement called **group purchasing**. Most hospitals are part of a group of hospitals (e.g., the Catholic Hospital Association, the University Hospital Consortium, the Voluntary Hospitals of America). Pharmaceutical companies ship large quantities of drugs to the buying group warehouses of these hospital groups. The distribution can be similar for most managed care organizations (e.g., Aetna, Cigna, Kaiser Permanente, and Prudential).

Distribution of drugs from drug wholesalers

The basic role of the drug wholesaler is to ensure the smooth, safe, and efficient distribution of products to retailers, like community pharmacies (independent, chain, and grocery store), mass merchandisers, hospitals, managed care organizations, and mail-order pharmacies. At the wholesaler, large pallets of drugs delivered from the manufacturer are broken down into smaller units for distribution to pharmacies.

Drug wholesalers (e.g., AmerisourceBergen, Cardinal, and McKesson) store products in strategic geographic locations so they can quickly send the products to pharmacies. The Healthcare Distribution Management Association (HDMA) estimates there are 60 wholesale corporations that run 225 distribution centers throughout the United States.

Drug wholesalers are licensed in the state they are located and in the states where they do business. Since most handle controlled substances, they must also have a Drug Enforcement Agency (DEA) license. They are required to adhere to strict storage and handling requirements. They must also ensure the integrity of the medications they deliver. Thus, temperature and humidity must be controlled. They must also protect against theft of a product.

Prescribing Drugs

An important part of the drug use process is how drugs are prescribed. This involves a more complex process than most people realize. It starts with a patient's need and the prescriber's—usually a doctor or dentist—willingness to help. In some states, the prescriber might be a doctor's assistant or nurse practitioner; however, these categories of health care workers have limited prescribing privileges. Veterinarians may also prescribe but only for animals, and certain drugs can be prescribed only by veterinarians and dispensed on the order of a veterinarian.

Medication prescribed for ambulatory patients is written on a prescription (see Chapter 10), while medications prescribed for inpatients are written in a drug order (Figure 7-2A and B). A **drug order** is a medication order written to a pharmacist by a legal prescriber for an inpatient (one assigned to a bed) of an institution. The differences between a drug order and prescription are in definition, legal status, and how they are written. A drug order has legal requirements exempting it from having all the information needed on a prescription, but it needs to have information beyond a prescription, like the patient's location (e.g., room number).

When prescribing drugs in an organized health care setting, the doctor normally must prescribe those drugs found in the organization's formulary. A **formulary** is a listing of drugs of choice as determined by relative drug product safety, efficacy, and effectiveness, and information about each drug approved by the medical staff of that organization for use within the organization.

Drug samples

Sometimes patients may receive a sample of the medication. Sometimes they will receive a sample of the medication *and* a prescription for the medication. These drug samples are small quantities of the drugs supplied to the doctor, usually

drug order a course of medication therapy ordered by the physician or dental practitioner in an organized health care setting.

formulary a listing of drugs of choice as determined by safety, efficacy, effectiveness, and cost, and approved by the medical staff for use within an institution.

FIGURE 7-2

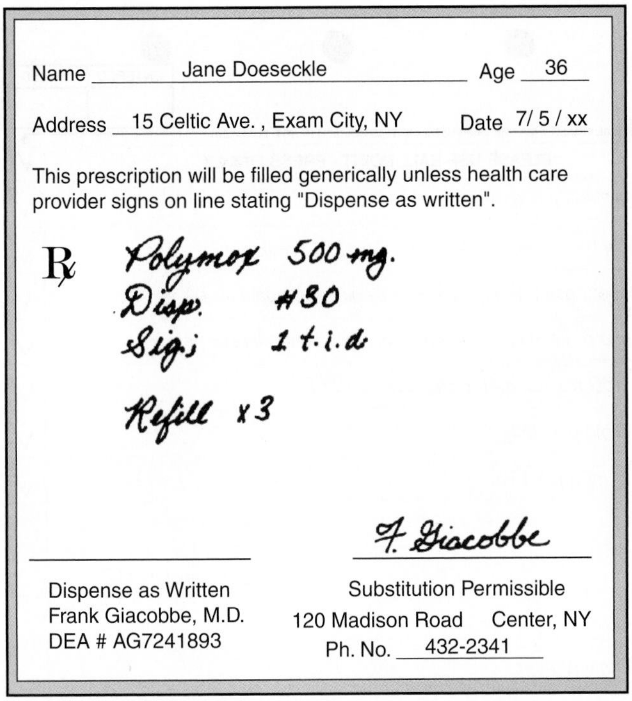

Name _____ Jane Doeseckle _____ Age __36__

Address __15 Celtic Ave. , Exam City, NY__ Date _7/ 5 / xx_

This prescription will be filled generically unless health care provider signs on line stating "Dispense as written".

℞ *Polymox 500 mg.*
   Disp.   #30
   Sig;   1 t.i.d

   Refill x3

                              F. Giacobbe
_____   _____
Dispense as Written   Substitution Permissible
Frank Giacobbe, M.D.   120 Madison Road   Center, NY
DEA # AG7241893   Ph. No. __432-2341__

FIGURE 7-2 A. Prescription.

by sales representatives of drug companies. The idea behind samples is for the patient to try the medication to see if it works and is tolerated before having the prescription "filled" (slang for *dispensed*) at a pharmacy.

Pharmacists and some regulators, like state boards of pharmacy, health departments, and the Joint Commission, frown on samples. This is because of lack of control over samples and, even though they are dated, they sometimes go out of date before they are given to patients. In addition, some doctors feel they may become biased toward a certain drug or start using the most expensive drugs if they are provided samples. Therefore, some doctors refuse to use them.

Preparing and Dispensing the Drug

The dispensing of medication is an organized process. Most patients have never been behind a prescription counter to see what takes place. It is much more than "count and pour" (the medication) and "lick and stick" (the label).

The community pharmacy

Following are the recommended steps in dispensing a prescription in a community pharmacy setting:

1. Accept the prescription and establish the pharmacist-patient relationship.
2. Review the prescription and patient information.
3. Review the patient's medication profile.
4. Review the insurance coverage and bill appropriately.
5. Retrieve the drug or ingredients from storage.
6. Prepare or compound (put together) the medication.
7. Label the container.
8. Perform a final check and dispense the medication.
9. Counsel the patients about their medication.

FIGURE 7-2

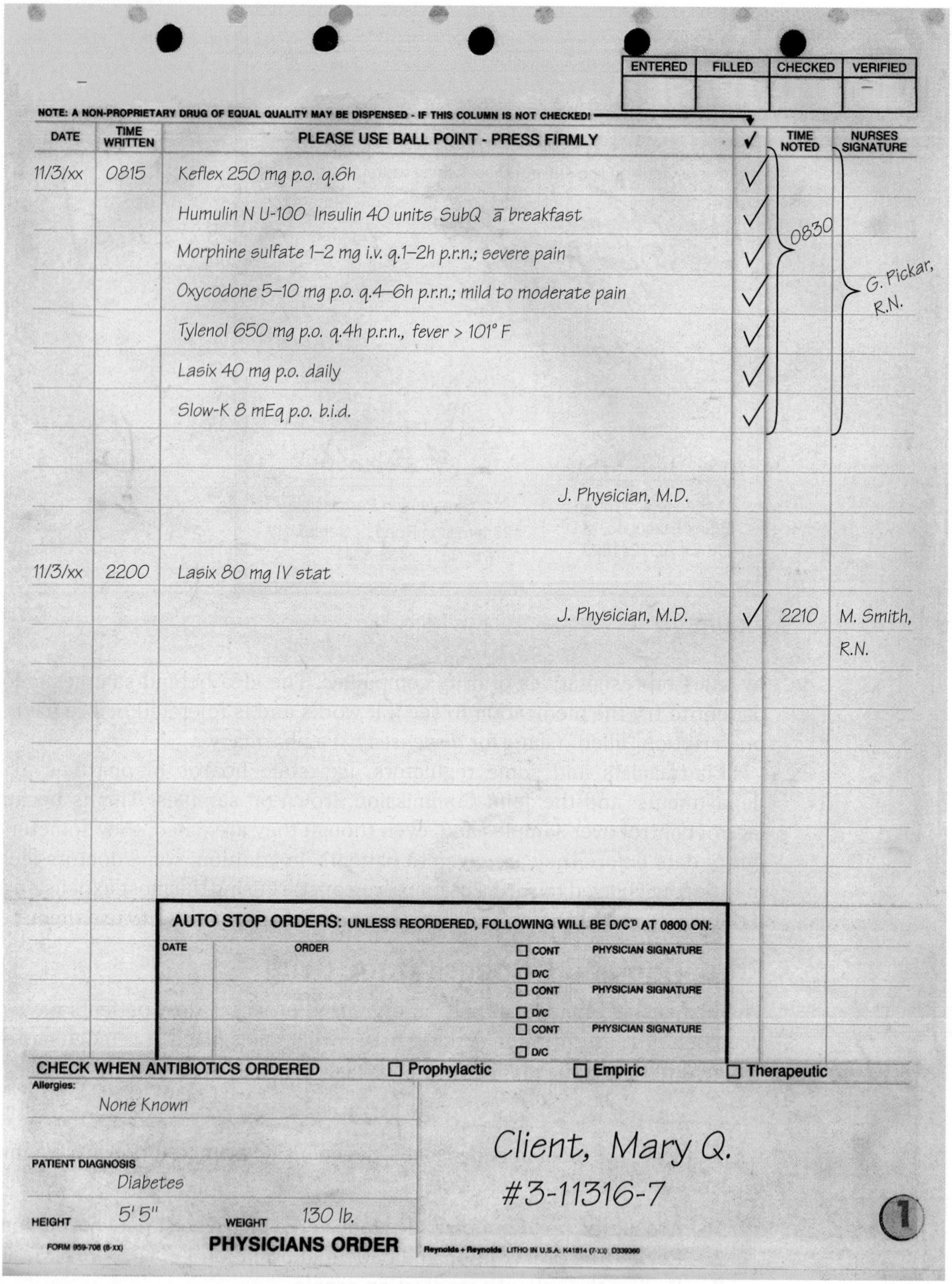

		ENTERED	FILLED	CHECKED	VERIFIED

NOTE: A NON-PROPRIETARY DRUG OF EQUAL QUALITY MAY BE DISPENSED - IF THIS COLUMN IS NOT CHECKED!

DATE	TIME WRITTEN	PLEASE USE BALL POINT - PRESS FIRMLY	✓	TIME NOTED	NURSES SIGNATURE
11/3/xx	0815	Keflex 250 mg p.o. q.6h	✓		
		Humulin N U-100 Insulin 40 units SubQ ā breakfast	✓	0830	
		Morphine sulfate 1–2 mg i.v. q.1–2h p.r.n.; severe pain	✓		
		Oxycodone 5–10 mg p.o. q.4–6h p.r.n.; mild to moderate pain	✓		G. Pickar, R.N.
		Tylenol 650 mg p.o. q.4h p.r.n., fever > 101° F	✓		
		Lasix 40 mg p.o. daily	✓		
		Slow-K 8 mEq p.o. b.i.d.	✓		
		J. Physician, M.D.			
11/3/xx	2200	Lasix 80 mg IV stat			
		J. Physician, M.D.	✓	2210	M. Smith, R.N.

AUTO STOP ORDERS: UNLESS REORDERED, FOLLOWING WILL BE D/CᴰAT 0800 ON:

DATE	ORDER		
		☐ CONT	PHYSICIAN SIGNATURE
		☐ D/C	
		☐ CONT	PHYSICIAN SIGNATURE
		☐ D/C	
		☐ CONT	PHYSICIAN SIGNATURE
		☐ D/C	

CHECK WHEN ANTIBIOTICS ORDERED   ☐ Prophylactic   ☐ Empiric   ☐ Therapeutic

Allergies:
None Known

PATIENT DIAGNOSIS
Diabetes

HEIGHT 5' 5"   WEIGHT 130 lb.

FORM 959-708 (8-XX)   **PHYSICIANS ORDER**   Reynolds + Reynolds LITHO IN U.S.A. K41814 (7-XX) D339360

Client, Mary Q.
#3-11316-7

①

FIGURE 7-2 B. Drug order.

For safety reasons, pharmacy technicians should not be performing duties that encompass clinical judgment or are required by law to be performed by pharmacists. Duties four through seven in the list above clearly can be performed by pharmacy technicians.

The institutional pharmacy

Although some organized health care settings, like hospitals, have outpatient pharmacies that dispense medication on the order of a prescription for their ambulatory patients, most of the medication dispensed is for inpatients. There are three primary systems for dispensing drugs in hospitals and other organized health care settings: floor stock, unit dose, and centralized IV admixtures.

Floor stock. Medication can be stored on the patient care units in the form of a floor stock system; however, this is not recommended (Figure 7-3). If this is done, medication should be limited. The caution on storing medication in this manner is due to safety. Floor stock offers more opportunity for error because there is no check and balance system to avoid mistakes. The nurse can go to floor stock where the medication is stored—usually on a shelf or in a drawer—take out what is needed, and provide it directly to the patient.

FIGURE 7-3

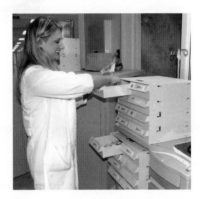

FIGURE 7-3 Floor stock system.

The most common drugs in floor stock are narcotics (which are always under lock and key with strict counting requirements), various intravenous solutions (IVs), and emergency drugs (usually in a kit). Some patient care units, like the emergency room (ER), intensive care units (ICUs), the operating room (OR), and recovery room (RR), have more floor stock than others.

Unit dose. Drugs may also be prepared and dispensed as a unit dose. A **unit dose** is a dose dispensed from the pharmacy that is ready to be given to the patient, which means that no further dosage preparation, calculation, or manipulation is required. Unit-dose systems are safer because there is less opportunity for error, and there is a built-in check and balance system.

In the unit-dose system of medication distribution, there are two medication drawers for each patient. One drawer is in the pharmacy being filled, while the other is on the patient care unit being used by the nurse to give medication to that patient (Figure 7-4). Each drawer is usually divided into two sections: one for regularly scheduled medication and the other for PRN (as needed) medication. The pharmacy allocates enough medication for the patient for the next shift (7 a.m. to 3 p.m., 3 p.m. to 11 p.m., or 11 p.m. to 7 a.m.) or the next 24-hour period. At the end of the shift or 24-hour period, the drawers are exchanged.

The built-in check and balance system in the unit-dose system is based on three sets of medication records: the doctor's orders in the patient's record, the patient's pharmacy profile, and the nursing Kardex.

unit dose a single-use package of a drug. In a unit-dose distribution system, a single dose of each medication is dispensed prior to the time of administration.

FIGURE 7-4

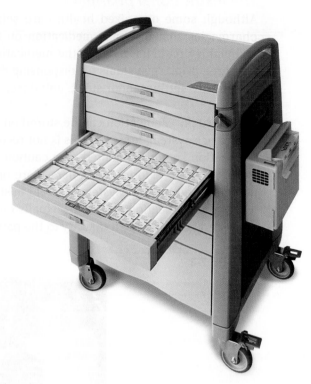

FIGURE 7-4 Unit-dose system (Courtesy of Artromick International, Inc.).

The pharmacy receives a copy of the patient's medication orders. Ideally, pharmacy technicians, rather than pharmacists, enter the medication orders into the patient's profile, which is part of the pharmacy computer system. If the hospital has a total information system, the orders flow directly from the doctor's electronic orders into an electronic version of the patient's pharmacy profile in the computer system. On the patient care unit the unit clerk transcribes (copies) the medication orders into the nursing **Kardex** (a card for each patient in a folder). The nurse must check and initial these transcriptions. The nurse uses the Kardex as a reminder of what, when, and to whom to administer medication. In an automated system, the nurse receives a printed list showing what to administer, to whom, and at what time.

There are three sets of medication records for each patient: the doctor's order, the pharmacy patient profile, and the nursing Kardex. They should be identical. The best procedure for checking a patient's unit-dose drawer is for the pharmacist to check the contents of the drawer against the nursing Kardex, rather than the pharmacy patient profile from which the drawer was filled. If the drawer is not correct, one of three things happened: (1) the drawer was filled improperly, (2) there was a computer entry error made in the pharmacy, or (3) there was a transcription error made between the doctor's order and the nursing Kardex. Which error occurred? The answer can be found by checking the doctor's order in the patient's record.

IV admixtures. The third drug distribution system is for IV (intravenous) admixtures. **IV admixtures** are IV solutions to which medication is added. Such medication is administered to patients intravenously (into their vein) and must be sterile (i.e., free of anything that can cause infection, including germs such as bacteria,

> **Kardex** a card for each patient in a folder noting his or her pharmacy profile and medication orders.

> **IV admixture** an intravenous solution to which medications are added.

FIGURE 7-5

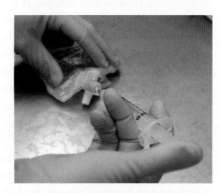

FIGURE 7-5 The pharmacy technician must take care to prepare IV admixtures in a sterile environment.

> **laminar flow hood** a sterile work area with positive pressure air flow that filters the air.

viruses, and fungi). The technique of adding medication to IV solutions should be done carefully and under ideal aseptic conditions (Figure 7-5). For years, nurses prepared the IV solution on the patient care unit, a place full of germs. If this is still allowed in the hospital, there must be a policy on how nurses should do this.

American Society of Health-System Pharmacists (ASHP) and Joint Commission standards now recommend that IV admixtures be prepared in the pharmacy using aseptic (germ free) techniques and a laminar flow hood. A **laminar flow hood** is a sterile work area with positive pressure air flow that filters the air. Pharmacists and pharmacy technicians are trained to prepare IV admixtures properly and should be recertified on how to do this. Once the IV admixtures are prepared, preferably by a pharmacy technician rather than a pharmacist, they should be checked by a pharmacist. When an IV additive solution is contaminated during preparation, the bacteria grow quickly with time and temperature. Therefore, IV additive solutions should be prepared just before they are needed and refrigerated between the time they are prepared and the time they are used. Delivery of IV admixtures to the patient care units is usually done by a courier or a pneumatic tube system.

Drug preparation and dispensation can be done from a large central pharmacy or from a central pharmacy and smaller, decentralized satellite pharmacies. Decentralized pharmacies are located in strategic locations in the hospital and serve several patient care units. Central pharmacies are more efficient, as they need less inventory and personnel. The advantages of decentralized, satellite pharmacies are faster service, more service, and more opportunity for staff pharmacists to deliver pharmaceutical care on the floors.

Patient Counseling

The doctor, pharmacist, or nurse is responsible for communicating to the patient about treatment regimens. The patient should be made aware of what drug treatments are being prescribed, why they are being prescribed, and how they work. The patient should be encouraged to ask questions about the drug treatments and care being prescribed. It is the patient's right to be informed of therapeutic treatments and to consent to those treatments.

Medication Administration

Patients usually receive medication one of three ways: (1) self-administration, (2) administration from a friend or relative, or (3) administration from a nurse. Self-administration is the way most medication is taken. It may also be the most dangerous. Unless the doctor, nurse, or pharmacist counsels the patient on taking the medication, the chances of the patient taking it correctly decrease. The patient should understand the name of the medication, what it is for, and what to expect from it. Most importantly, the patient needs to understand how to take the medication correctly. Does taking one tablet three times a day mean three times during the waking hours, or spread out over every eight hours? Does it need to be taken with water, or can it be taken with fruit juice or milk? Can patients stop taking the medication when they feel better, or do they need to take it until it is all gone? If they miss a dose, should they take twice as much next time? How should the medication be stored? What about side effects?

Medication managed by a friend or relative may be needed when the patient is sick and at home. This method of medication administration may be safer than self-administration. Most people are more careful when being responsible for others. They also tend to ask more questions and are afraid to do anything wrong. Friends and relatives also are better at giving the medication on a schedule or reminding the patient when the medication is due.

Nurse-administered medication is the most accurate method of administering medications. Nurses know medication and how to give it, and if they do not, they have been trained to find out how. Nurses pride themselves on this important role. They also have developed ways to administer the medication to the most ornery patient or the youngest child.

No matter who gives the medication, it is easy to make an error like forgetting to give it, giving the wrong drug, giving too much or too little, or giving it at the wrong time. This is unfortunate since so much effort went into making an appointment, seeing the doctor, getting a diagnosis and a prescription, and getting the prescription filled. Not taking the medication properly can result in an extended illness, going back to the doctor, having an adverse reaction, or possibly having to go to the emergency room or hospital. All of this results in more time and expense.

Compliance with taking the medication as prescribed

Some people never get their prescription filled or, if it is called in to the pharmacist, never pick it up. How big is this problem? One study looking at this problem in community pharmacies found that about 2 percent of people never picked up their prescription. This translates into 40 million prescriptions not picked up and $1 billion in lost sales. Reasons cited for this problem were recovery (39 percent), having a similar drug at home (35 percent), did not feel they needed it (34 percent), and did not like taking medication. Preliminary evidence suggests that when a doctor prescribes electronically and sends the prescription to a community pharmacy, up to 20 percent of prescriptions are not picked up by the patient.

The problem of unclaimed prescriptions is also a problem for outpatient pharmacies in hospitals. One proposed solution to this problem is to call the patient as a reminder that the medication is ready for pickup.

Even if a person has a prescription filled, it does not mean he or she will take it as prescribed. Either forgetting or purposely not taking medication as prescribed is called **non-adherence**. Non-adherence is a big problem. There are various means of discovery rates of medication compliance such as urine tests, serum tests, pill counts, patient interviews, and record reviews. As reported in literature, rates of non-adherence with prescribed therapy vary greatly. The variance is explained by different patient populations, the category of drugs, how often the medication is prescribed each day, and by differences in study design. Medication compliance rates vary significantly for several disease states.

non-adherence
forgetting or purposefully not taking medications as prescribed.

The underlying problems associated with medication non-adherence are patient actions (decisions and behaviors). Patients decide whether to take a medication and how often. Reasons for patients not taking their medication or not taking it as prescribed include cost, feeling better, side effects, not realizing the importance, and forgetting.

The cost of medication non-adherence is high in lives lost, time lost, and added care needed. An estimated 125,000 Americans die each year simply because they fail to take their medication as prescribed. Equally disturbing are the unnecessary hundreds of thousands of extra hospital admissions because of medication non-adherence. In one study, 36 of 89 medication-related admissions were related to medication noncompliance. Of these, 54 percent were because of intentional non-adherence.

Another study examined the records of seven patients not taking their medication as prescribed. More than $14,000 was spent on outpatient visits, hospital days, and emergency room visits over one year as a direct result of medication non-adherence.

There is also the cost of time, such as having to stay home or leave work or school to seek medical attention. The estimated cost is a loss of 20 million workdays a year or about $1.5 billion in lost earnings. The annual economic cost of medication non-adherence in the United States is estimated to be more than $100 billion.

Many groups of people, like doctors, nurses, pharmacists, AARP, the Task Force for Compliance, and the National Council on Patient Information and Education (NCPIE) have been working on the problem of medication non-adherence. Much has been learned and more still needs to be done. Each patient not taking medication as prescribed has a different reason or set of reasons for not being in compliance. Thus, the solution for gaining patient compliance will differ from one patient to the next.

Pharmacy technicians should learn methods to discover if there has been non-adherence and alert the pharmacist of this problem. Once it has been determined there is a non-adherence problem, the pharmacist should try to find out why. The most common issues are cost, other needs, fear of the medication not working or causing adverse effects, or forgetfulness.

The most effective way to improve medication adherence is by understanding why the patient is not taking the medication as prescribed and then using a combination of methods specifically designed to address the patient's reasons for not being compliant. Doing this is not only in the patient's best interest, but also in the pharmacist's best interest both clinically and economically.

Monitoring the Patient

The pharmacy profession has decided the mission of pharmacy practice is to help patients make the best use of their medication. To do this, pharmacists need to get out from behind their counters and out of the hospital pharmacy and be in direct contact with patients. In other words, pharmacists need to be more concerned about patients than about drug products. This idea is called *pharmaceutical care.* The definition of **pharmaceutical care** has evolved over the last 20 years. The most current definition is "a practice in which the practitioner takes responsibility for a patient's drug-related needs and is held accountable for this commitment."

There continues to be controversy about the name *pharmaceutical care.* Some pharmacists—mostly community pharmacists—feel the word *pharmaceutical* should be replaced with the words *pharmacy* or *pharmacist* (i.e., pharmacy care

pharmaceutical care the direct, responsible provision of medication-related care for the purpose of achieving definite outcomes that improve a patient's quality of life.

or pharmacist care). The rationale is the word *pharmaceutical* is too closely associated with drug products, and by calling it pharmaceutical care, anyone can provide it. The expression *pharmacy* or *pharmacist care* avoids these problems. However, most professional pharmacy organizations and schools of pharmacy are still using the original term *pharmaceutical care*.

The elements of pharmaceutical care

Regardless of the terminology or definition used, six general principles or elements of care are encompassed.

1. *Responsible provision of care.* The pharmacist should accept responsibility for the patient.
2. *Direct provision of care.* This means the pharmacist must be in direct contact with patients. He or she must see and talk with patients.
3. *Caring.* This virtue, a key characteristic among nurses and doctors, has been the most understated virtue of pharmacy. It is the centerpiece of pharmaceutical care.
4. *Achieving positive outcomes.* Several positive clinical outcomes can occur because of taking medication: cure of disease, elimination or decline of a patient's symptoms, arresting or slowing of a disease process, or preventing a disease or a symptom.

    There are also negative outcomes from taking medication: the medication fails to work as expected; there are nagging side effects; or adverse drug reactions cause moderate patient morbidity (illness), a life-threatening or permanent disability, or death.

    Besides clinical outcomes there are also economic (cost) and humanistic outcomes (functional status, quality of life, and patient satisfaction). Under pharmaceutical care, it is the pharmacists' responsibility to do everything possible to achieve positive patient outcomes and avoid the negative effects of taking medication.
5. *Improving the patient's quality of life.* Everyone has a certain, measurable quality of life. Under the pharmaceutical care model of delivering care, the pharmacist must, with the patient and the doctor, set reasonable treatment goals for each drug prescribed that will improve the patient's functioning and health-related quality of life.
6. *Resolution of medication-related problems.* The task of pharmaceutical care is to resolve medication-related problems. **Medication-related problems (MRPs)** are undesirable events a patient experiences that involve (or are suspected of involving) drug therapy and that actually (or potentially) interfere with a desired patient outcome.

medication-related problems (MRPs) Undesirable events a patient experiences involving drug therapy that interfere with a desired patient outcome.

Pharmaceutical care involves identifying potential and actual MRPs, resolving actual MRPs, and preventing potential MRPs. There are eight MRPs.

1. *Needed drug therapy.* The patient has a medical condition that requires introducing new or additional drug therapy.
2. *Unnecessary drug therapy.* The patient is taking drug therapy that is unnecessary given his or her present condition.
3. *Use of wrong drug.* The patient has a medical condition for which the wrong drug is being taken.
4. *Dosage is too low.* The patient has a medical condition for which too little of the correct drug is being taken.

5. *Dosage is too high.* The patient has a medical condition for which too much of the correct drug is being taken.
6. *An adverse drug reaction.* The patient has a medical condition because of an adverse drug reaction or event.
7. *Not receiving the drug.* The patient has a medical condition for which the patient needs, but is not receiving, the drug.
8. *Drug interaction.* The patient has a medical condition and there is a drug-drug, drug-food, or drug-laboratory test interaction.

Quality Drug Therapy

There is much more to being a pharmacist than making sure the patient receives the drug prescribed and taking actions to ensure the drug is taken as prescribed. Today, pharmacists are trained to help each patient receive quality drug therapy. *Quality drug therapy* is safe, effective, timely, and cost-effective drug therapy delivered with care.

Pharmacists used to fill prescriptions written by doctors and were not allowed to question whether the drug prescribed was the best drug for the patient. This has changed for various reasons. First, the drugs are getting more complex, more potent, and more abundant. Second, doctors cannot know everything about every drug. Third, the clinical education of the pharmacist has expanded. And fourth, the scope of practice and legal duty of the pharmacist to help and protect the patient has expanded.

A doctor prescribes a drug based on what he or she knows and considers best. A pharmacist may see the patient differently, may know information the doctor does not know about the drug, or knows about other drugs that may benefit the patient. Thus, if the pharmacist thinks the patient may benefit from changing the prescribed drug—its dose, route of administration, or dosage form, or changing to another drug—he or she is obligated to call the doctor and discuss it.

Pharmacy technicians should look for problems in prescriptions and drug orders and bring them to the attention of the pharmacist. This helps the pharmacist and helps protect the patient from harm.

Medication Safety and Drug Misadventures

Although medication can be wonderful—helping to cure an illness or helping a patient feel better—it also has the potential for harm. Harm resulting from medication is called a *drug misadventure*.

Side Effects

side effects
known effects of a drug experienced by most people taking the drug; these are usually minor.

All drugs have side effects. **Side effects** are known, usually minor, annoying effects of the drug experienced by most people taking the drug. An example is the drowsiness associated with some antihistamine drugs used for treating hay fever symptoms. Since side effects are expected, minor events, they are not a drug misadventure per se.

Adverse Drug Reactions

Some drugs can cause more dangerous conditions called *adverse drug reactions.* **Adverse drug reactions (ADRs)** are unwanted, more serious, harmful effects of the drug that are not experienced by every patient taking the drug. Here is example of an ADR:

> Sally is a 34-year-old mother of an 8-year-old and a 5-year-old. She is under stress, both at home and at her law firm, and there is no end in sight. Her stress causes her to be irritable and unable to sleep. After seeing her doctor, she is told to exercise more and use stress reduction exercises daily. Sally tries these suggestions, but is just too busy to follow them consistently. Sally's friend Sue has had similar problems, so Sue gives Sally a few tranquilizers to try. The drug helps, so Sally pressures her doctor to prescribe a tranquilizer—five milligrams three times a day. As the days get more stressful, Sally starts taking the drug three times during the day and once at bedtime. Sometimes during the day she gets drowsy, and sometimes she forgets if she has taken the drug. Driving home one day, she almost falls asleep at the wheel. She wakes up just in time to keep from hitting a car in front of her. When she goes to get a refill of her prescription, the pharmacist tells her that she should still have a week's worth of the drug left, but she has only two tablets.

Allergic Drug Reactions

Patients allergic to a drug or an ingredient in the medication, even a color dye, can experience drug reactions that can vary from a minor annoyance to a life threat. It is critical that every pharmacy, patient profile, and computer system contain information on each patient's allergies. Here is an example of an allergic drug reaction:

> A 45-year-old man with low back pain collapsed 15 minutes after an intramuscular injection of diclofenac (generic name). Twenty minutes after successful revival, he went into a coma and never recovered. Before receiving the drug, the patient was asked, "Are you allergic to diclofenac?" The patient said no; however, it was later discovered the patient had a previous reaction to the drug but only knew the drug by its trade name.

Drug-Drug Interactions

Some drugs interact with other drugs, or interact with food or drinks the patient is taking. One drug can make another drug inactive or overactive. The outcome of a drug interaction can range from a minor inconvenience to death. Pharmacists must be vigilant about detecting and stopping these interactions from occurring. Here is an example of a drug-drug interaction:

> A 47-year-old man was prescribed chlordiazepoxide and haloperidol as part of a supervised alcohol detoxification program. He also received 650 milligrams of acetaminophen twice a day for two days. On the third day the patient experienced disorientation, hallucinations, low blood pressure, jaundice, and a tender liver. He progressively worsened and died on his 28th day in the hospital. His doctor suspected a drug interaction between the acetaminophen and alcohol.

---

adverse drug reaction (ADR) any unexpected, obvious change in a patient's condition that the physician suspects may be due to a drug.

Medication Errors

Medication errors rarely occur when considering the millions of prescriptions and doses of medication patients receive yearly. The incidence is a fraction of a percent. However, this is meaningless if the error occurs to you or someone you love. Therefore, the public has zero tolerance for medication errors. That means pharmacists and pharmacy technicians have to be accurate all the time; there is no room for errors. Here is an example of a medication error:

> Mike McClave mixed two spoonfuls of prescription medicine he picked up at a pharmacy for his 8-year-old daughter with some clear soda and gave it to her to relieve a raspy, sore throat. The next morning his daughter never woke up. She had received oral morphine, rather than an anesthetic for her sore throat.

Pharmacists have built-in check-and-balance systems—a safety net—for detecting medication errors before they harm patients. However, medication errors occasionally occur within the drug use process. These errors are usually the result of a medication system failure rather than the failure of one person.

Medication Use in the United States

According to a national survey, over half (51 percent) of American adults take two or more medications each day. In addition, almost half of Americans (46 percent) take at least one prescription medication each day, whereas more than a quarter (28 percent) takes multiple prescription medications daily.

The rates of prescription medication use are highest among older Americans. Seventy-nine percent of those age 65 or older reported taking one prescription medication each day, compared with respondents aged 55 to 64 (63 percent), aged 45 to 54 (52 percent), and aged 44 years or younger (28 percent). Americans aged 65 or older that take prescription medications take an average of four each day.

Among respondents who reported the use of a prescription medication within the past week, the majority (61 percent) showed the medication was for a long-term health condition. Twenty-four percent said they were treating a recurring health problem, whereas 10 percent showed they are treating a short-term, acute health condition.

Besides increased over-the-counter (OTC) sales in the United States, the use of **alternative medicine** (e.g., herbal supplements, megavitamins, and other non-traditional remedies) is increasing dramatically. Overall, four out of 10 Americans are trying alternative health treatments. In an ASHP survey, more than one-third (39 percent) of respondents reported taking an average of four herbal supplements and vitamins in the past week. Forty percent reported taking an average of two herbal supplements or vitamins each day.

alternative medicine herbal supplements, megavitamins, and other non-traditional remedies.

Along with more medications being taken, there has been a shift of where patients are buying their medication. Although every community pharmacy is filling more prescriptions, the two fastest growing pharmacies are mail-order and grocery store pharmacies, and the slowest growing are independent community pharmacies. In fact, there is some concern that the independent corner drugstore may not be able to survive much longer.

Self-Care and the Role of Over-the-Counter Medication

Pharmacists and pharmacy technicians must understand illness and the patient's reaction to it. Seldom do people go to a doctor when they get sick, at least not right away. Most people see how they are feeling and how the illness progresses. Some deny they are ill. Some seek the advice of family or friends. Still others take control and seek out as much information as they can about their problem.

Self-Care

It is helpful when people take a more active role in their health care. Documentation of increased interest in self-care is witnessed by the many self-help books, TV programs, newspaper articles, and talk shows covering these topics. Determining what spawned this self-care revolution is difficult. However, one reason is obvious: consumers are increasingly self-medicating with nonprescription drugs. The Nonprescription Drug Manufacturers Association has surveyed many consumers to learn about their attitudes regarding this practice:

■ Almost seven out of 10 consumers prefer to fight symptoms without taking medication, if possible.

■ Among consumers, 85 percent believe it is important to have access to nonprescription medication.

■ About nine out of 10 consumers realize they should take medication only when necessary.

■ Of consumers who ended the use of their nonprescription medication, 90 percent did so because their medical problems or symptoms resolved.

■ Even though a medication may be available without a prescription, almost 95 percent of consumers agreed that care should be taken when using it.

■ Nearly 93 percent of consumers report that they read instructions before taking a nonprescription medication for the first time.

Over-the-Counter (OTC) Medication

Some ill patients, and those who experience a health problem, will find their way to a pharmacy to browse the over-the-counter (OTC) aisle for a cure. Many will try reading the labels of various OTC medications to see if the medication will cure what ails them. Pharmacy technicians should watch for this and alert the pharmacist when they see a patient in the OTC area needing help.

Fortunately, there is a system of self-medication in the United States, and OTC medications are found everywhere—drugstores, convenience stores, supermarkets, and mass merchandisers. If it were not for this allowance, we would need many more doctors and health care facilities. A recent survey on patient satisfaction with pharmacy services found that patients' highest awareness of OTCs was for cold cures, vitamins, and dental products, and that satisfaction was high with these products.

Control of the Drug Use Process

The drug use process is extensive and complex. It is also designed with many checks and balances to keep patients from experiencing a preventable drug misadventure. At the center of this control is the pharmacist and pharmacy technician. Laws, rules and regulations, accreditation policies, and pharmacy traditions have given the pharmacist this important responsibility. Although pharmacists have accepted this responsibility and they are up to the task, they cannot do it alone. They need the help of pharmacy technicians, other health professionals, and patients who will take responsibility for their own health.

Pharmacy technicians are used extensively in the drug use process (drug purchasing, receiving, storage, inventory control, recordkeeping, and preparation). Although pharmacy technicians are involved extensively in processing prescriptions and drug orders, it is important that they think about what they are doing and not get caught up in being fast. Finding anything out of the ordinary is cause for concern and for taking a "safety time-out" to explore if something is wrong. This also holds true when working alongside pharmacists, all of whom occasionally make errors. It is the technician's job to discreetly but forcefully point out that the pharmacist may be making an error. Patient safety should be everyone's number one concern.

Current Issues in the Drug Use Process

Issues that will have direct impact on the drug use process encompass the "aging of America" and the respective current and projected increase in the numbers of prescriptions that will be generated, along with the continual development and availability of new pharmaceuticals. This, along with the current shortage of pharmacists, will directly affect pharmacists' activities and expand the role of technicians in their collaborative efforts to meet the demands of providing safe and effective drug therapy to their patients.

The Rising Number of Prescriptions and Limited Number of Pharmacists

Due to increased demand and better drugs, the number of prescriptions filled each year is rising at an unprecedented rate. The large "baby boom" generation will soon be reaching age 65, and these individuals will need more medication as they get older. At the same time, the pharmacy profession is being stretched. A shortage of pharmacists is becoming clear because of expanded roles for pharmacists and an increased use of medication.

The profession's response has been to start more schools of pharmacy. However, from all accounts, this may not be enough. To meet the demands and to preserve or expand the pharmacist's clinical role, pharmacy will need to better use pharmacy technicians, reorganize pharmacies to be more efficient, and increase the use of pharmacy automation and information technology.

Pharmacy Automation

Pharmacy departments are slowly moving to maximize the automation available for charting, packaging, labeling, and dispensing medications. The cost of current equipment is high, and the skills needed must be learned. This is an area where pharmacy technicians can excel. The pharmacist's time can be better utilized in patient care if the technicians can ensure an efficient drug distribution system.

Summary

The drug use process is complex and involves manufacture, distribution, pre-scribing, preparation, storing, dispensing, administering, monitoring, and review of drugs and their use. The process is controlled, and at the center of this control are various checks and balances, regulations, and the pharmacists and pharmacy technicians. Even with control, the system is not perfect and thus needs constant attention and improvement.

> **Note:** Much of what has been written by the author in this chapter has been reprinted with permission from *Pharmacy: What It Is and How it Works*, copyright 2002, 2007, CRC Press, Boca Raton, FL.

TEST YOUR KNOWLEDGE

Multiple Choice

1. The societal purpose of pharmacy practice is to
   a. dispense medication.
   b. provide drug information.
   c. help people make the best use of their medication.
   d. prepare drugs.

2. The drug use process is
   a. when people abuse drugs.
   b. methods used to prepare drugs.
   c. steps involved in getting drugs to their final destination.
   d. how drugs are managed.

3. What is drug-use control?
   a. Any method used to reduce the improper use of a drug
   b. Federal drug enforcement regulations
   c. A method to accurately measure who uses drugs
   d. FDA manufacturing rules

4. Why is control needed in the drug use process?
   a. To protect patients from harm
   b. To satisfy FDA requirements
   c. To keep drugs from being illegally diverted
   d. Both a and c

5. Which of the following is not a drug-use control method?
   a. Formulary
   b. Laws, rules, and regulations
   c. Policies and procedures
   d. All of the above

6. Which of the following is not considered a medication misadventure?
   a. Errors
   b. Adverse reactions
   c. Side effects
   d. Drug interactions

7. What primary duty do pharmacists perform for society?
   a. Prepare medication for patients
   b. Help patients use their medication safely
   c. Supply drugs
   d. Price the prescription accurately

8. Pharmacy technicians will legally perform their duties as long as they
   a. check everything they do in the pharmacy.
   b. read all labels at least three times before dispensing the drug.
   c. have all labels and products checked by the pharmacist.
   d. are certified.

9. A major change transforming pharmacy into a true clinical profession is
   a. the use of automation.
   b. the use of more pharmacy technicians.
   c. pharmaceutical care.
   d. all of the above.

10. How will the changes in Question 9 affect pharmacy technicians?
    a. They will be more involved in running automation.
    b. They will be doing higher level functions.
    c. They may need more education.
    d. All of the above.

Matching

Match the function in drug-use control with the party responsible for that function. Answers may be used more than once; some may have more than one correct answer.

1. _____ manufacture the drug
2. _____ distribute the drug to the wholesaler
3. _____ distribute the drug to the pharmacy
4. _____ prescribe the drug
5. _____ prepare the drug
6. _____ dispense the drug
7. _____ counsel the patient
8. _____ administer the drug
9. _____ monitor the patient

a. wholesaler
b. patient or family
c. doctor
d. pharmacy technician
e. pharmaceutical company
f. doctor
g. pharmacist

Fill In The Blank

1. Drug _____ develop and produce pharmaceutical products.

2. Drug _____ deliver medication, medical appliances, and other products to pharmacies.

3. A listing of drugs of choice is called a _____.

4. A sterile work area with positive pressure air flow that filters the air is called a _____.

5. An unwanted, serious, side effect of a drug is a/an _____.

References

Alkhawajah, A. M., Eifawal, M., & Mahmoud, S. F. (1993). Fatal anaphylactic reaction to diclofenac. *Forensic Science International*, 60, 107–110.

Anonymous. (1999). *1999 retail pharmacy digest: Measuring customer satisfaction.* Raritan, NJ: Ortho Biotech.

Anonymous. (1996). No-show customers cost community pharmacies $1 billion annually. *American Journal of Health-System Pharmacy*, 53, 1236, 1239–1240.

Avorn, J. (2004). *Powerful medicines: The benefits, risks, and costs of prescription drugs.* New York: Alfred A. Knopf.

Bentley, J. P., Wilkin, N. E., & McCaffrey, D. J. (1999). Examining compliance from the patient's perspective. *Drug Top*, 143(14): 58–67.

Berg, J. S., Dischler, J., Wagner, D. J., et al. (1993). Medication compliance: Health-care problem. *Ann Pharmacother*, 27, S5–S19, S21–S22.

Brodie, D. C. (1967). Drug-use control: Keystone to pharmaceutical service. *Drug Intell*, 1, 63–65.

Chandrasekaran, R. (1994). Prescription error claims dad's angel. *The Washington Post*. October 31, Page A11.

Col, N., Fanale, J. E., & Kronholm, P. (1990). The role of medication noncompliance and adverse drug reactions in hospitalizations of the elderly. *Arch Intern Med*, 150, 841–845.

Dolder, C., Lacro, J., Dolder, N., & Gregory, P. (2003). Pharmacists' use of and attitudes and beliefs about alternative medications. *American Journal of Health-System Pharmacy*, 60, 1352–1357.

Hamilton, W. R., & Hopkins, U. K. (1997). Survey of unclaimed prescriptions in a community pharmacy. *Journal of the American Pharmacists Association*, NS37, 341–345.

Handbook of non-prescription drugs. (2000). American Pharmaceutical Association. Washington, DC.

Healthcare Distribution Management Association. *Healthcare product distribution: A primer.* Accessed Aug. 5, 2005, at www.healthcaredistribution.org.

Japsen, B. (2001, January 26). Saying yes to free drug samples raises concern. *Atlanta Journal*, January 26.

Kelly, W. N. (1999). Drug use control: The foundation of pharmaceutical care. *Pharmacy practice for technicians* (2nd ed.). Albany, NY: Delmar.

Kelly, W. N. (2006). *Prescribed medication and the public health: Laying the foundation for risk reduction.* Binghamton, NY: Haworth Press.

Kier, K. L., & Pathak, D. S. (1991). Drug-usage evaluation: Traditional versus outcome-based approaches. *Topics in Hospital Pharmacy Management*, 11, 9–15.

Kirking, M. H., Zaleon, C. R., & Kirking, D. (1995). Unclaimed prescriptions at a university hospital's ambulatory care pharmacy. *American Journal of Health-System Pharmacy*, 52, 490–495.

Leppik, I. E. (1990). How to get patients with epilepsy to take their medication: The problem of noncompliance. *Postgraduate Medicine*, 88, 253–256.

Lesser, P. B., et al. (1986). Lethal enhancement of therapeutic doses of acetaminophen by alcohol. *Dig Dis Sci*, 31, 103–105.

Martin, E. W. (1971). The prescription. In *Dispensing of medication* (7th ed.). Easton, PA: Mack Pub. Co.

McQueen, C. E., Shields, K. M., & Generali, J. A. (2003). Motivations for dietary supplement use. *American Journal of Health-System Pharmacy*, 60, 655.

National Council on Patient Information and Education. (2002). *Attitudes and beliefs about the use of over-the-counter medicines: A dose of reality*. Bethesda, MD.

National Council on Patient Information and Education. (1995). *Prescription medicine compliance: A review of the baseline of knowledge*. Washington, DC.

Robbins, J. (1987). Forgetful patient: High cost of improper medication compliance. *U.S. Pharmacist*, 12, 40–44.

Rucker, T. D. (1987). Prescribed medications: System control or therapeutic roulette? In *Control Aspects of Biomedical Engineering*. International Federation of Automatic Control, Oxford, UK.

Salek, M. S., & Sclar, D. A. (1992). *Medication compliance: The pharmacist's pivotal role*. Kalamazoo, MI: Upjohn.

Self-medication in the '90s: Practices and perceptions. (1992). Nonprescription Drug Manufacturers Association: Washington, DC.

Sloan, N. E., Peroutka, J. A., Morgan, D. E., et al. (1994). Influencing prescribing practices and associated outcomes utilizing the drug use evaluation process. *Topics in Hospital Pharmacy Management*, 14, 1–12.

The Task Force for Compliance. (revised April 1994). *Noncompliance with medications*. Baltimore, MD.

Web Sites

AARP   www.aarp.org

Health Care Distribution Management Association
   www.healthcaredistribution.org

National Council on Patient Information and Education   www.talkaboutrx.org

Ethical Considerations for the Pharmacy Technician

Competencies

Upon completion of this chapter, the reader should be able to

1. List the six ethical principles available to resolve an ethical dilemma.
2. Discuss the major concepts presented in the *Code of Ethics for Pharmacy Technicians*.
3. Identify, prospectively, practice situations where ethical dilemmas may occur.
4. Detect and explain the presence of an ethical dilemma in pharmacy practice and present alternative responses.

Key Terms

autonomy
beneficence
ethics
nonmaleficence
pharmacy technician

Introduction

This chapter focuses on ethical challenges faced by practitioners, pharmacists, and pharmacy technicians in our changing health care environment with the adoption of the pharmaceutical care standard. It provides guidance on how to approach an ethical dilemma, presents six ethical principles that may be applied to face these dilemmas, and describes the nature and importance of ethical codes of behavior. Technicians are reminded of the responsibilities and risks imposed on them both by state governments and the pharmacists they assist. Practical considerations are raised in the areas of drug distribution and patient communication, and the tools provided should assist pharmacy technicians in making sound ethical evaluations. Final ethical choices regarding drug therapy reside with the pharmacist.

The Changing Health Care Environment

American society and our health care system are evolving in unexpected, challenging, and sometimes disturbing ways. Diversity and mobility are the norms of existence, not the exception. Scientific and medical discoveries and advances present a health care environment that can produce unprecedented results, but at ever-increasing costs. Federal and state government and third-party payors dominate our health care delivery system and frequently decide what treatment is given or how to distribute lessening resources, shifting decision making from the traditional physician-patient environment to a corporate model. Globalization, computerization, and Internet use provide patients a broader reach and outlook, yet disconnect them and their activities from the local neighborhood that formed the basis of their personal and professional interactions. While individuals and society are more dependent on business, financial, and religious institutions for their well being, recent scandals present disturbing ethical concerns about organizational leadership and make us question whether the trust we have placed in these institutions and their leaders is misguided and unwarranted.

Pharmacy practice is not immune to change. Practitioners are challenged to keep current with numerous drug therapy advances while facing an informed and more assertive patient population that seeks active participation in its treatment. Pharmaceutical manufacturers produce new classes of drugs and new delivery systems that benefit patients. However, some are merely "me too" drugs that just provide more expensive, not better, care. Some drug companies offer financial incentives to doctors, pharmacists, and allied health professionals to prescribe or recommend particular drugs or to switch patients from one medication to another., whether or not this activity is in the best interest of the patient or falls within the context of "pharmaceutical care."

Pharmaceutical Care

Providing a patient with quality pharmaceutical care is now the basic standard for pharmacy practice. *Pharmaceutical care*, as defined by Hepler and Strand, is "the direct, responsible provision of medication-related care for the purpose of achieving definite outcomes that improve a patient's quality of life." Pharmacy education has adopted pharmaceutical care as its endpoint and developed PharmD (Doctor of Pharmacy) curricula to implement its adoption. Pharmaceutical practitioners are under pressure to maximize use of their resources to meet this standard and recognize the need for trained assistants to lessen the pharmacist's burden in drug distribution. Pharmacy technicians are vital partners in the delivery of pharmaceutical care to the patient population.

The Role of the Pharmacy Technician

pharmacy technician a person skilled in various pharmacy service activities not requiring the professional judgment of the pharmacist; has received formal or informal skill training to participate in numerous pharmacy activities in concert with and under the supervision of a registered pharmacist.

According to the ASHP's "White Paper on Pharmacy Technicians," a **pharmacy technician** is "an individual working in a pharmacy, who, under the supervision of a licensed pharmacist, assists in pharmacy activities that do not require the professional judgment of the pharmacist." They are employed in a variety of settings: hospitals, community pharmacies, mail-order pharmacies, long-term care facilities, and home health care, and they assist pharmacists to manage drug distribution and paperwork and enable the pharmacist to concentrate on providing direct patient care. Pharmacists depend on the technician's expertise to facilitate expansion of their professional scope of practice, and technicians are central to maintaining pharmacy's professional stability and growth by performing duties that do not require the professional skills and judgment of a licensed pharmacist. Pharmacy technicians must therefore share the pharmacist's ethical commitment to safe medication use.

Technician training can be based on a structured educational program or provided on the job. Activities may include collecting and organizing information to assist pharmacists in patient care, and developing and managing medication distribution and control systems. On a state-by-state basis, limitations are placed on technician responsibility and authority by the level of recognition they receive (registration, certification, or licensure) and whether or not they have their own scope of practice. Some states currently register, certify, license, or enroll pharmacy technicians. In the other states, health care personnel are performing the activities of the technician but may not receive specific recognition or regulation by a licensing agency. Most states play a direct role in regulating pharmacy technician practice and in determining scope of practice. Communication with the prescriber, including refill authorization, preparation of the label as well as the medication, entering the prescription into the computer system or patient information into the profile, and medication preparation, including compounding and reconstituting of oral liquids, are all activities the state may delegate to the technician.

There are other technician issues decided on a state-by-state basis: the level and type of training, continuing education requirements, and whether or not they can review the work of other technicians. Health care personnel acting as pharmacy technicians in states that do not certify, register, or license and do not have the title, legally derive their power to act from the pharmacist and the pharmacist's scope of practice. Thus, their limitations on practice and ethical considerations must flow directly from the pharmacist they assist.

Those pharmacy technicians recognized separately by a state must still coordinate their activities and ethical conduct with pharmacists, though they are separately responsible for their behavior legally and morally.

Codes of Professional Behavior

Self-discipline and self-regulation are essential components of professional behavior. Ethical codes set standards and responsibilities among members of a group and govern interactions with other organizations, patients, clients, colleagues, and society. Codes declare the collective conscience of a group and the norms of professional behavior they value. They usually focus on dealing honestly with patients, suppliers, and competitors, respecting individual autonomy, recognizing the right to make informed decisions, maintaining confidentiality, and promoting just and effective use of resources. The first medical code was the *Hippocratic Oath*, which dates back to the fifth century B.C.

The aftermath of World War II and its unethical excesses encouraged the World Medical Association to adopt the *Geneva Convention of Medical Ethics*, followed by the *Nuremberg Code*, suggesting guidelines for human experimentation and the need for voluntary consent of a patient. Later, the World Medical Association adopted the *Declaration of Helsinki*, emphasizing the importance of informed consent and full disclosure to the patient.

Health care professional groups and organizations acknowledge the need to declare to the public the values they deem important and by which they wish to be judged. Albert Jonsen, author of *Clinical Ethics*, believes that professionalism should focus on honesty, integrity, respect for patients, a commitment to patients' welfare, a compassionate regard for patients, and dedication to maintaining competency in knowledge and technical skills. Professional organizations recognize that codes make explicit the primary goals and values of the group, and individuals who join make a moral commitment to uphold the values and obligations expressed. The codes may also focus on inspirational ideals, serve as a statement of organizational principles, and provide rules to govern behavior. When these codes are created and ratified by the membership of a professional organization or the profession itself, they have more societal impact than if they are imposed by the leadership of the organization with little or no member input or acceptance.

The Code of Ethics for Pharmacy Technicians

The *Code of Ethics for Pharmacy Technicians* was drafted by the American Association of Pharmacy Technicians in 1996 to deal with the particular duties and responsibilities of technicians. The code has most relevance for technicians who are members of the organization, but also has persuasive impact on all pharmacy technicians, regardless of professional affiliation or work environment. The principles expressed in the technician's code include assisting pharmacists in providing the best care for patients based on the moral guidelines expressed in the pharmacist's code; supporting honesty and integrity; maintaining competence, knowledge, and expertise; respecting patient confidentiality; avoiding activities that bring discredit to the profession; and meeting standards required by law.

Those pharmacy technicians not separately licensed, registered, or certified serve as agents of a pharmacist, and therefore are bound by the principles of the American Pharmaceutical Association's *Code of Ethics for Pharmacists* because their professional activities derive from the pharmacist's responsibilities.

The Pharmacist's Code of Ethics

The pharmacist's code has evolved over the years and reflects behavioral guidelines for pharmacy practice as it exists today. Its principles are designed to guide pharmacists in their relationships with patients, health professionals, and society, including helping patients achieve optimum benefit from medications while maintaining their trust, being caring, compassionate and discreet, respecting a patient's autonomy and dignity, acting with honesty and integrity, maintaining professional competence, respecting the beliefs and values of colleagues, and allocating health resources in a fair and just manner. A copy of the code is shown in Figure 8-1. Pharmacists also have an oath, similar to the *Hippocratic Oath*, which is taken voluntarily by many practitioners and declares values that parallel those expressed in the *Code of Ethics*. See the section on the Prayer of Maimonides (Chapter 1, p. 9).

Ethical Decision Making

Organizations and professional associations cannot carry out their policies as a group, but instead rely on individual members to implement the standards they have adopted. Identifying an ethical question or facing an ethical dilemma is done by an individual, and the actions taken are primarily based on individual moral assumptions or beliefs.

ethics the study of precepts or principles used to assist us in making the correct choice when faced with alternative possibilities in a moral situation.

Ethics is the study of precepts or principles used to assist us in making the correct choice when faced with alternative possibilities for action in a moral situation. Lowenthal and Meth, authors of "The Continuous Review of Courses: A System for Maintaining Curricular Effectiveness," believe the practice of ethics is a "process that resolves dilemmas and judges the appropriateness of one's behavior in situations where a protocol cannot be applied." Practitioners are encouraged to do the right thing, as if all issues are clearly delineated, focusing on right versus wrong or good versus evil. We rarely face such clear-cut situations. In reality, we encounter ethical dilemmas and are challenged to come up with an acceptable response. An ethical dilemma is a difficult moral problem involving two or more mutually exclusive and morally equal courses of action. We are often asked to choose between the better of two imperfectly acceptable alternatives, or the lesser of two objectionable ones.

The methods we use to determine the correctness of our actions are imprecise, and when placed within a health care setting, have a complexity and impact beyond our personal concerns. How, then, do you handle conflict, make the choices you must, and live with the consequences, as health care practitioners and as individuals? Amy Haddad and her fellow authors suggest that "we utilize ethical judgment skills and apply ethical principles based on our personal and professional value system and the needs of our society and the patient." It is hoped we will be able to recognize when a dilemma exists, define the elements of the dilemma, develop alternative solutions, act on the appropriate solution, and evaluate the outcome.

Ethical Principles

Ethicists do not agree on the number of distinct ethical principles used to solve dilemmas. A consensus recognizes the following six: honesty, promise-keeping, nonmaleficence, beneficence, autonomy, and justice.

FIGURE 8-1

American Pharmaceutical Association
Code of Ethics for Pharmacists (1994)

Preamble. Pharmacists are health professionals who assist individuals in making the best use of medications. This Code, prepared and supported by pharmacists, is intended to state publicly the principles that form the fundamental basis of the roles and responsibilities of pharmacists. These principles, based on moral obligations and virtues, are established to guide pharmacists in relationships with patients, health professionals, and society.

I. A pharmacist respects the covenantal relationship between the patient and pharmacist.

Considering the patient-pharmacist relationship as a covenant means that a pharmacist has moral obligations in response to the gift of trust received from society. In return for this gift, a pharmacist promises to help individuals achieve optimum benefit from their medications, to be committed to their welfare, and to maintain their trust.

II. A pharmacist promotes the good of every patient in a caring, compassionate, and confidential manner.

A pharmacist places concern for the well-being of the patient at the center of professional practice. In doing so, a pharmacist considers needs stated by the patient as well as those defined by health science. A pharmacist is dedicated to protecting the dignity of the patient. With a caring attitude and a compassionate spirit, a pharmacist focuses on serving the patient in a private and confidential manner.

III. A pharmacist respects the autonomy and dignity of each patient.

A pharmacist promotes the right of self-determination and recognizes individual self-worth by encouraging patients to participate in decisions about their health. A pharmacist communicates with patients in terms that are understandable. In all cases, a pharmacist respects personal and cultural differences among patients.

IV. A pharmacist acts with honesty and integrity in professional relationships.

A pharmacist has a duty to tell the truth and to act with conviction of conscience. A pharmacist avoids discriminatory practices, behavior or work conditions that impair professional judgment, and actions that compromise dedication to the best interests of patients.

V. A pharmacist maintains professional competence.

A pharmacist has a duty to maintain knowledge and abilities as new medications, devices, and technologies become available and as health information advances.

VI. A pharmacist respects the values and abilities of colleagues and other health professionals.

When appropriate, a pharmacist asks for the consultation of colleagues or other health professionals or refers the patient. A pharmacist acknowledges that colleagues and other health professionals may differ in the beliefs and values they apply to the care of the patient.

VII. A pharmacist serves individual, community, and societal needs.

The primary obligation of a pharmacist is to individual patients. However, the obligations of a pharmacist may at times extend beyond the individual to the community and society. In these situations, the pharmacist recognizes the responsibilities that accompany these obligations and acts accordingly.

VIII. A pharmacist seeks justice in the distribution of health resources.

When health resources are allocated, a pharmacist is fair and equitable, balancing the needs of patients and society.

Source: American Pharmaceutical Association website

FIGURE 8-1 Code of Ethics for Pharmacists (adopted by the membership of the American Pharmacists Association, then the American Pharmaceutical Association, October 27, 1994).

The principle of honesty deals with our obligation to tell the truth in our dealings with others. However, are we bound to do this totally, in every situation, or are there circumstances when it is in no one's best interest to "tell the truth, the whole truth, and nothing but the truth"?

Also, moral people have an obligation to keep the promises they make. However, sometimes even with the best of intentions, we may make promises we are unable to fulfill because circumstances change or the ability to comply is no longer within our control. Does promise-keeping require us to blindly continue with a promise, no matter what the cost to ourselves or others?

Under the principle of **nonmaleficence**, we are obliged to "do no harm" to others, but many people will grudgingly engage in behavior that harms one person, particularly a stranger, if it defends or protects others, particularly family members or friends.

Beneficence requires that we act in a positive way in our dealings with others; that we "do good." It also mandates preventing harm to others if it is in our power.

Autonomy supports the concept that people have the right to live their lives as they see fit. Exercise of autonomy is limited where the rights of one person come in conflict with the rights of another. How do you draw this line?

Justice or equality recognizes the belief that all people should receive respect and that benefits conferred on one individual should be available to all. However, it does not require that all people be treated exactly alike all the time.

Recognizing the presence of these principles in a challenging moral situation may simplify the handling of the situation. However, the use of these principles to solve ethical dilemmas is complicated when the situation presents two or more of them in conflict. You must determine what principle is dominant in your value system, or what will do the most good, or do the least harm, and act accordingly. You have a moral imperative to follow your conscience, regardless of the consequences.

nonmaleficence the principle that pharmacists are obliged to "do no harm" to others in the practice of health care and/or pharmacy.

beneficence the practice of doing good; a kindly action.

autonomy an independent action.

The Decision-Making Process

When an ethical issue arises in a practice setting, try to understand all the implications of your actions before you act. Following these simple steps may help lessen negative impacts that arise from the decisions you make:

- Look at the ethical issue in the broadest context. Who is involved? Who will it affect? What are your options?
- Decide if you are just faced with an ethical question or are dealing with an ethical dilemma, which may have negative consequences regardless of the actions you take.
- If you are facing a dilemma, determine the alternative responses you may make to the situation.
- Look at the risks involved for each response for patients, yourself, your organization or employer, your profession, and society.
- Assess the benefits derived to each group for each alternative.
- Identify the ethical principles present in the situation; see if any are in conflict and determine which principle is most important.
- Make your behavioral decision based on knowledge and evidence, not emotion.
- Afterward, evaluate the consequences of your actions and determine if you would repeat the choice you made.

■ Realize there will always be unintended consequences to your actions. Just because you make the "right" decision does not mean you will not have to deal with personal, professional, and legal fallout.

Practical Application

Situations that may be a source of ethical conflict for pharmacists and pharmacy technicians fall into two general categories: those related to the drug distribution system, and those involving communication with patients, their families, and other health professionals. How would you handle the situations below?

Drug Distribution Issues

■ What would you do when you feel a prescription presented by a patient seems not only inappropriate based on the information you possess, but potentially harmful? Would you be less concerned if the prescription, while inappropriate, was neither harmful nor beneficial?

■ How would you handle a patient who asks for a few pills to tide them over until they get a new prescription? Does it matter how long the patient has been your customer or that the drug involved is habit-forming?

■ Would you dispense a controlled medication to a patient you suspect has a substance abuse problem?

■ When is it necessary to confront or report a colleague you believe is diverting drugs?

■ If you were approached by a medical retailer to participate in a patient "switch" to their generic drug in return for financial compensation, how would you respond?

■ Should you do something if a prescribed drug is not approved for use with the patient's disease?

■ Is it important to make sure patient information gathered in the dispensing function is made available to others only on a "need to know" basis?

■ If you are asked to prepare a medication that contradicts your personal beliefs, ethically or religiously, would you refuse?

These are some of the drug distribution scenarios that pharmacists and pharmacy technicians may have to face and work through.

Communication Issues

Communication scenarios can also present ethical challenges. Patient involvement and consent to treatment is one of the most basic tenets of modern health care. The patient should know what medications he or she is taking, what the side effects may be, what the prognosis is, and what alternative treatments or medications are available.

Everyone agrees patients must provide health professionals with "informed consent." The characteristics of informed consent include shared decision making between the patient and his or her provider, based on mutual respect and good communication. Good communication requires adequate disclosure of the nature of an intervention, its risks, and its benefits. Ethical questions arise as to how much information is enough, how much is too much, where to draw the line, and who should be making these determinations.

Respecting the patient's privacy and maintaining confidentiality are other ethical minefields for pharmacists and pharmacy technicians. It is essential that the patient trust health care providers to ensure the patient will continue treatment. This is particularly true when patients are vulnerable because of their age (e.g., the elderly, a minor child) or their disease state (e.g., AIDS, mental illness, sexually transmitted disease). Intentional or unintentional disclosure of information may have a negative impact on patients, their employment status, their finances, or their personal relationships. However, health professionals also have responsibilities to protect the society they serve. How do you distinguish between these competing health needs? Does your answer differ based on the nature of the disease the patient possesses? Can you contemplate a set of circumstances where you would feel it necessary to keep health information on a child secret from a parent, or information on a husband from a wife?

There are also ethical dilemmas that cross both categories:

■ If a prescriber asks you to incorrectly label a prescription because he or she does not want the patient to know the nature of the medication, or that the patient is receiving a placebo, how would you respond?

■ When a patient asks what a drug is used for, would you assume that the prescriber has not communicated with the patient on the medication and tell the patient everything you know without contacting the prescriber?

■ What is your responsibility to your patients and your profession when it becomes clear that a colleague is no longer functioning well or acting in a competent manner? Would you tell someone? Would you report your colleague anonymously?

■ If a medication mistake was made with a patient and you discovered it after the patient had left, how far would you go to rectify the situation? Would you admit the mistake up front, and if you did, to whom would you admit the mistake?

We are sure you can easily supply more examples of practice situations where ethical questions are raised and ethical dilemmas faced. You will notice that we did not supply the answers. That is your job. We have given you some suggestions on the principles to consider and the ways to approach a dilemma. But in the end, it is your value system that will determine your response.

Risk/Benefit Response

Let us remind you that any decision brings with it the risk of being judged wrong and having to face the consequences of your actions. Accepting responsibility for your decisions is central to acting professionally. Do not be surprised or caught off guard by one of the examples we have raised. Assess your value system and ask yourself what you would do before being faced with the situation. Be prepared.

The extent to which a pharmacy technician may directly experience these situations is dependent on the scope of practice recognized in the state and the relationship the technician has with the pharmacist he or she assists. If you have made ethical mistakes in the past, it is important to analyze retrospectively what you did and why you did it so you do not repeat the behavior.

As the pharmacist becomes more and more involved in providing pharmaceutical care to patients in all practice settings and the need for medications continues to expand, the role of the pharmacy technician will expand and the nature of ethical dilemmas they face will change. Be ready to meet the challenge.

Summary

Because of the changing nature of the health care environment and the emergence of pharmaceutical care as the standard for pharmacy practice, pharmacy technicians and pharmacists are facing ethical challenges not previously anticipated. This chapter provides the information and the tools to deal with ethical dilemmas that may arise in both the drug distribution and patient care arenas. The six ethical principles and the two codes of ethics present a starting point for your quest to seek solutions to these dilemmas, to minimize risk to your patients and yourself, and to provide the public the benefits of pharmaceutical care.

TEST YOUR KNOWLEDGE

Multiple Choice

1. Pharmaceutical care
   a. focuses on medication outcomes that improve the quality of a patient's life.
   b. is of no concern to a pharmacy technician.
   c. is only a pharmacy practice issue, not a pharmaceutical education issue.
   d. has yet to be accepted as a standard of pharmacy practice.

2. Pharmacy technicians
   a. are licensed by all states.
   b. all have the same scope of practice.
   c. are meant to assist pharmacists in their practice.
   d. do not have ethical obligations to the patient population.

3. The earliest known example of an ethical code in medicine was
   a. *The Nuremberg Code.*
   b. *The Hippocratic Oath.*
   c. *The Declaration of Helsinki.*
   d. *The Geneva Convention of Medical Ethics.*

4. The *Code of Ethics for Pharmacy Technicians*
   a. has direct application to the activities of all pharmacy assistants.
   b. has direct application to the activities of all pharmacy technicians.
   c. has direct application to the activities of all pharmacists.
   d. has direct application to the activities of members of the American Association of Pharmacy Technicians.

5. Which of the following statements is false?
   a. Ethical principles help us make choices between moral alternatives.
   b. Ethical dilemmas always present clear-cut choices between right and wrong.
   c. Our ethical choices sometimes force us to select the lesser of two evils.
   d. Personal and professional values have a place in the ethical decision making process.

6. The principle of beneficence means
   a. you can do harm.
   b. you should do good.
   c. you should treat everyone equally.
   d. you should let people do what they want.

7. The ethical decision-making process
   a. can be a complex, time-consuming activity.
   b. takes no time or thought.
   c. never has any unintended consequences.
   d. is free of risk.

8. Ethical conflicts in the drug distribution system may include
   a. intentional disclosure of patient information in violation of patient confi-dentiality.
   b. dispensing a controlled substance to a patient you believe has a drug abuse problem.
   c. not getting "informed consent."
   d. releasing patient information under a public health initiative.

9. Ethical conflicts in the patient communication area may include
   a. finding a colleague who may be diverting drugs.
   b. being asked to prepare a medication whose purpose conflicts with your religious beliefs.
   c. being asked by a husband about his wife's medication and its purpose.
   d. being asked by a patient to supply a few pills to tide them over.

10. Facing ethical dilemmas
    a. will bring about the same result in every person.
    b. will always make you pleased with the results of your decisions.
    c. will never subject you to professional or legal consequences.
    d. will always be a personal and professional challenge.

Matching

Match the ethical principle with its description.

1. _____ honesty
2. _____ promise-keeping
3. _____ nonmaleficence
4. _____ beneficence
5. _____ autonomy
6. _____ justice

   a. doing good
   b. all people receive the same benefits
   c. be truthful in dealing with others
   d. do no harm
   e. doing what you say you are going to do
   f. having the right to do what you see fit

Fill In The Blank

1. The direct, responsible provision of medication-related care for the purpose of achieving definite outcomes that improve a patient's quality of life is the definition of _____.

2. A _____ is "an individual working in a pharmacy, who, under the supervision of a licensed pharmacist, assists in pharmacy activities that do not require the professional judgment of the pharmacist."

3. Self-discipline and self-regulation are essential components of _____.

4. _____ is the study of precepts or principles used to assist us in making the correct choice when faced with alternative possibilities for action in a moral situation.

5. There are two primary sources presenting ethical conflict in the pharmacy setting: _____ and _____.

References

American Society of Health-System Pharmacists. (1996). White paper on pharmacy technicians. *American Journal of Health-System Pharmacy*, 53, 1991–1994.

Haddad, A. M., Kaatz, B., McCart, G., McCarthy, R. L., Pink, L. A., & Richardson, J. (1993). Report of the ethics course content committee: Curricular guidelines for pharmacy education. *American Journal of Pharmacy Education*, 57, 34S–43S.

Hepler, C. D., & Strand, L. M. (1990). Opportunities and responsibilities in pharmaceutical care. *American Journal of Health-System Pharmacy*, 47, 533–543.

Jonsen, A. R. (2006). *Clinical ethics*. New York: McGraw-Hill.

Lowenthal, W., & Meth, H. (1993). The continuous review of courses: A system for maintaining curricular effectiveness. *American Journal of Pharmacy Education*. 57, 134–139.

National Association of Boards of Pharmacy. (2001). Status of pharmacy technicians. In *Survey of Pharmacy Law*. Park Ridge, IL.

Strandberg, K. (2007). *Essentials of law and ethics for pharmacy technicians*. Boca Raton: CRC Press.

Web Sites

American Pharmacists Association   www.aphanet.org

Pharmacy Associations

Competencies

Upon completion of this chapter, the reader should be able to

1. Identify pharmacy associations in the United States and internationally.
2. Describe the two major issues that resulted in the formation of national pharmacy associations.
3. Explain the history behind the formation of the first college of pharmacy in the United States.
4. Discuss the early problems associated with the issue of drug safety and efficacy in the United States.
5. Match the acronyms to the full names of the various pharmacy associations.

Key Terms

Academy of Managed Care Pharmacy (AMCP)
American Association of Colleges of Pharmacy (AACP)
American Association of Pharmacy Technicians (AAPT)
American College of Apothecaries (ACA)
American College of Clinical Pharmacy (ACCP)
American Council for Pharmaceutical Education (ACPE)
American Pharmaceutical Association (APhA)
American Pharmacists Association
American Society of Consultant Pharmacists (ASCP)
American Society of Health-System Pharmacists (ASHP)
National Association of Boards of Pharmacy (NABP)
National Association of Chain Drug Stores (NACDS)
National Community Pharmacists Association (NCPA)
National Pharmacy Technician Association (NPTA)
Pharmacy Technician Certification Board (PTCB)
Pharmacy Technician Educators Council (PTEC)
reciprocity

Introduction

Professional associations are comprised of like professionals who meet for a common goal or purpose. Professional associations serve a vital role in shaping the future of that profession. Through a united voice, the professional association provides its members with an opportunity to develop and regulate professional policy and procedure. Associations are instrumental in establishing best practices for the profession. There are many diverse pharmacy associations, each representing the interests of different practitioners. Most national associations (and numerous state and local associations) were formed to further the professional objectives of their members. Pharmacy and pharmacy technician associations, their web addresses, and their professional publications are listed in Table 9-1.

The goals of this chapter are to familiarize the reader with pharmacy associations and to demonstrate the important role they play in the practice of pharmacy in the United States.

Historical Developments

Two major issues stimulated the formation of the first local and national pharmacy association in the United States:

1. The development of educational standards for pharmacy practice; and
2. The concern about the safety and efficacy of drug products available in the United States.

Education

The first national pharmacy association in the United States, the American Pharmaceutical Association (APhA), was responsible for the formation of the first college of pharmacy, Philadelphia College of Pharmacy, formed in 1821. This educational institution was developed due to the association recognizing the need to standardize educational requirements for pharmacists. As a result of educational standardization, schools of pharmacy have been established throughout the United States and internationally. There are currently more than 125 schools of pharmacy in the United States, with new schools on the horizon. All schools of pharmacy in the United States and many schools outside of the United States are accredited through the Accreditation Council for Pharmaceutical Education (ACPE). Pharmacy education does not end upon graduation from a school of pharmacy. All pharmacists licensed in the United States are required to obtain continuing pharmaceutical education for license maintenance and professional development.

Safety and Efficacy of Drug Products

The integrity of drug products was first recognized by the federal government in 1906 when the Pure Food and Drug Law was implemented. This law was a start at regulation; however, it did very little to improve the integrity of the drug products on the market. In 1938 a tragedy in Europe caused the Food and Drug Administration to implement the Food, Drug, and Cosmetic Act, requiring that all drugs be

TABLE 9-1   Pharmacy and Pharmacy Technician Associations

A directory of pharmaceutical and health-related societies around the world can be found at www.pharmweb.net.

U.S. Pharmacy and Pharmacy Technician Associations

AMCP	Academy of Managed Care Pharmacy	www.amcp.org
ACPE	Accreditation Council for Pharmacy Education	www.acpe-accredit.org
AACP	American Association of Colleges of Pharmacy	www.aacp.org
AAPS	American Association of Pharmaceutical Scientists	www.aapspharmaceutica.com
AAPT	American Association of Pharmacy Technicians	www.pharmacytechnician.com
ACA	American College of Apothecaries	www.americancollege ofapothecaries.com
ACCP	American College of Clinical Pharmacology	www.accp1.org
ACCP	American College of Clinical Pharmacy	www.accp.com
AIHP	American Institute of the History of Pharmacy	www.pharmacy.wisc.edu/aihp
APhA	American Pharmacists Association	www.pharmacist.com
ASAP	American Society for Automation in Pharmacy	www.asapnet.org
ASCPT	American Society for Clinical Pharmacology and Therapeutics	www.ascpt.org
ASCP	American Society of Consultant Pharmacists	www.ascp.com
ASHP	American Society of Health-System Pharmacists	www.ashp.org
ASP	American Society of Pharmacognosy	www.phcog.org
BPS	Board of Pharmaceutical Specialties	www.bpsweb.org
CCGP	Commission for Certification in Geriatric Pharmacy	www.ccgp.org
CRS	Controlled Release Society	www.controlledreleasesociety.org
DEA	Drug Enforcement Administration	www.usdoj.gov/dea/index.htm
DIA	Drug Information Association	www.diahome.org
FDA	Food and Drug Administration	www.fda.gov
HDMA	Healthcare Distribution Management Association	www.healthcaredistribution.org
HIMSS	Healthcare Information and Management Systems Society	www.himss.org
ICPT	Institute for the Certification of Pharmacy Technicians	www.nationaltechexam.org
ISMP	Institute for Safe Medication Practices	www.ismp.org
ICR	Institute of Clinical Research	www.instituteofclinicalresearch.org
IVT	Institute of Validation Technology	www.ivthome.com
	The Joint Commission	www.jointcommission.org
NABP	National Association of Boards of Pharmacy	www.nabp.net
NACDS	National Association of Chain Drug Stores	www.nacds.org
NADDI	National Association of Drug Diversion Investigators	www.naddi.org
NCPA	National Community Pharmacists Association	www.ncpanet.org
NISPC	National Institute for Standards in Pharmacist Credentialing	www.nispcnet.org
NPhA	National Pharmacists Association	www.npha.com
NPTA	National Pharmacy Technician Association	www.pharmacytechnician.org
PCMA	Pharmaceutical Care Management Association	www.pcmanet.org
PERI	Pharmaceutical Education and Research Institute	www.peri.org
PhRMA	Pharmaceutical Research and Manufacturers of America	www.phrma.org
PCAB®	Pharmacy Compounding Accreditation Board	www.pcab.info
PTCB	Pharmacy Technician Certification Board	www.ptcb.org
PTEC	Pharmacy Technician Educators Council	www.rxptec.org
PQRI	Product Quality Research Institute	www.pqri.org
USP	U.S. Pharmacopeia	www.usp.org

(continued)

TABLE 9-1 Pharmacy and Pharmacy Technician Associations (continued)

Foreign Pharmacy and Pharmacy Technician Associations		
ACP	Alberta College of Pharmacists	www.pharmacists.ab.ca
AFP	Association of Finnish Pharmacies	www.apteekkariliitto.fi
APTUK	Association of Pharmacy Technicians, UK	www.aptuk.org
AAHP	Austrian Association of Hospital Pharmacists	www.aahp.at
	Austrian Federal Board of Pharmacy	www.apotheker.or.at
OPhG	Austrian Pharmaceutical Society	www.oephg.at
BIRA	British Institute of Regulatory Affairs	medizin.li/profiles/company_br/br_00033480.htm
CACDS	Canadian Association of Chain Drug Stores	www.cacds.com
CAPT	Canadian Association of Pharmacy Technicians	www.capt.ca
CAPT Alberta	Canadian Association of Pharmacy Technicians Alberta	www.captalberta.org
CAPT Vancouver	Canadian Association of Pharmacy Technicians Vancouver	www.captvancouver.ca
CPhA	Canadian Pharmacists Association	www.pharmacists.ca
CSPS	Canadian Society for Pharmaceutical Sciences	www.cspscanada.org
EFPIA	European Federation of Pharmaceutical Industries and Associations	www.efpia.org
ESCP	European Society of Clinical Pharmacy	www.escpweb.org/site/cms
SFPT	French Society of Pharmacology	www.pharmacol-fr.org
IACP	International Academy of Compounding Pharmacists	www.iacprx.org
IFPMA	International Federation of Pharmaceutical Manufacturers and Associations	www.ifpma.org
IFPW	International Federation of Pharmaceutical Wholesalers	www.ifpw.com
INRUD	International Network for the Rational Use of Drugs	www.inrud.org
FIP	International Pharmaceutical Federation	www.fip.org
IPSF	International Pharmaceutical Students' Federation	www.ipsf.org
ISPE	International Society for Pharmacoepidemiology	www.pharmacoepi.org
ISPhC	International Society of Pharmaceutical Compounding	www.isphc.com
NPA	National Pharmacy Association	www.npa.co.uk
NDMAC	Nonprescription Drug Manufacturers Association of Canada	www.ndmac.ca
OCP	Ontario College of Pharmacists	www.ocpinfo.com
PSA	Pharmaceutical Society of Australia	www.psa.org.au
PFLI	Pharmacists for Life International	www.pfli.org
WHO	World Health Organization	www.who.int
International Pharmaceutical Web Sites		
ABPI	Association of the British Pharmaceutical Industry	www.abpi.org.uk
EPSA	European Pharmaceutical Students' Association	www.epsa-online.org
RPSGB	Royal Pharmaceutical Society of Great Britain	www.rpsgb.org.uk
RSC	Royal Society of Chemistry	www.rsc.org
SBS	Society for Biomolecular Sciences	www.sbsonline.org

State Associations: The major national pharmacy associations have state affiliates listed on their Web sites. For state association listings, check out the sites for the ASHP, APhA, and ASCP.

proven safe prior to marketing. In 1962 another tragedy in Europe caused the Food and Drug Administration to take action. All drugs needed to be safe and effective for the use for which they were intended. The Food and Drug Administration has the authority to seize or enjoin misbranded or adulterated drugs from being introduced into inter- or intrastate commerce.

National Associations of Pharmacists and Pharmacy Technicians

American Pharmaceutical Association (APhA), now the **American Pharmacists Association** founded in 1852, this is the largest association in pharmacy with more than 60,000 members.

The first national association of United States pharmacists was the **American Pharmaceutical Association (APhA)**, which is now known as the **American Pharmacists Association**. Formed in Philadelphia in 1852, the APhA has grown into the largest of the national associations in pharmacy, with approximately 60,000 members. The original objectives of the association have not changed since its inception. These objectives include:

- Quality, improvement of and regulation of the drug supply.
- Inter- and intra-professional relations.
- Improvement of the scientific knowledge base of the profession.
- Dissemination of new knowledge through publication.
- Identification of educational standards for practice of the profession.
- Restriction of drug-dispensing functions.
- Creation of ethical standards of practice.

The APhA supports voluntary certification of technicians by the pharmacy profession but opposes licensure, registration, or certification by state law or regulation.

In addition to being the first national professional pharmacy association, the APhA is also considered to be the "parent" of many other pharmacy associations, such as the American Society of Health-System Pharmacists (ASHP), the National Community Pharmacists Association (NCPA), the American College of Apothecaries (ACA), the American Association of Colleges of Pharmacy (AACP), and the American Association of Pharmaceutical Scientists. These associations were all initiated by special interest groups originally a part of the APhA.

The APhA is organized into three academies: the Academy of Pharmacy Practice and Management (APhA-APPM), the Academy of Pharmaceutical Scientists (APhA-APRS), and the Academy of Student Pharmacists (APhA-ASP). The APhA also has a research foundation and a Political Action Committee (PAC). The APhA co-founded the Pharmacy Technician Certification Board (PTCB) with ASHP, the Illinois Council of Health-System Pharmacists, and the Michigan Pharmacists Association. The PTCB offers certification and recertification exams for pharmacy technicians several times each year. Information on certification exam contents and processes are available on the PTCB Web site, www.ptcb.org. As of 2006, PTCB certified more than 250,000 pharmacy technicians.

The APhA formed a task force on specialties in pharmacy in 1973 to address the issue of pharmacy specialization. The Board of Pharmaceutical Specialties (BPS) was then formed, with four primary responsibilities:

1. Identifying and recognizing critical specialty practice areas.
2. Setting standards for certification and recertification of pharmacy specialists.

3. Objectively evaluating professionals seeking certification and recertification.
4. Serving as a resource for information, and as the agency coordinating the process.

The **American Society of Health-System Pharmacists (ASHP)** was founded at the 1942 meeting of the APhA, and from its founding until 1972, membership in the parent organization (APhA) was required for membership in ASHP. The American Society of Health-System Pharmacists is a 30,000-member national professional association that represents pharmacists who practice in hospitals, health maintenance organizations, long-term care facilities, home care, and other components of the health care system. ASHP has had a long history of focusing on medication-error prevention and promoting pharmacists as the professionals that assist people in making the best use of their medications. ASHP currently focuses its programs and resources on practice domains, including acute care; ambulatory care; clinical specialists and scientists; home, ambulatory and chronic care; inpatient care; pharmacy practice managers; pharmacy informatics and technology; and technicians. ASHP has taken strong positions regarding the education of pharmacists and technicians and has accrediting standards for pharmacy residencies designed for pharmacy graduates, and for pharmacy technician training programs.

Since continuing education or continuing professional development is a requirement for the pharmacy profession, it is very important for associations to provide educational programming for its members. Both the APhA and ASHP have been leaders in providing relevant educational programming for pharmacists. The APhA now provides a framework for specialty certification of pharmacists in areas such as diabetes, immunization, medication therapy management, hypertension, and anticoagulation. The APhA and ASHP each host two annual meetings that provide leadership skills, as well as educational programming for pharmacists and pharmacy technicians. These meetings also provide a forum for industry and practicing pharmacists, pharmacy students, and pharmacy technicians to network.

The **National Community Pharmacists Association (NCPA)**, formerly the National Association of Retail Druggists (NARD), developed from the parent APhA's Section on Commercial Interests as an independent association in 1898. The NCPA has strongly represented the interests of the independent pharmacy owner since its inception and has championed the independent practice alternative to students of pharmacy. In 1991, the NCPA created the National Home Infusion Association (NHIA). A special focus of the NCPA has been the training and certification of pharmacists in various areas of "pharmacist care" through the National Institute for Pharmacist Care Outcomes (NIPCO), including diabetes, osteoporosis, respiratory disease, hypertension, hyperlipidemia, arthritis and pain management, infectious disease, nutrition, and weight management. The NCPA Management Institute was established in 1989 to provide independent pharmacists with management information, as well as the training and support necessary for successfully running their pharmacies. The NCPA has a reputation for being a vigorous defender of the independent owner's rights and has been very influential in lobbying in the United States. The NCPA lobbied for more than a decade for legislation to make armed robbery a federal offense. The NCPA was the first to recognize the importance of a Political Action Committee, thereby establishing a Political Action Committee (PAC) in pharmacy with the slogan "Get into politics or get out of pharmacy." Political Action Committees serve a vital role in supporting the legislative efforts of the association through personal monetary contributions to the committee.

American College of Apothecaries (ACA) a small, selective association of community-based practitioners whose membership is granted only if the pharmacy and practitioners comply with specified pharmacy professional standards.

American Association of Pharmacy Technicians (AAPT) membership is open to pharmacy technicians with access to educational services and availability at an annual meeting.

The **American Society of Consultant Pharmacists (ASCP)** is an association of pharmacists providing drug therapy management services and medication distribution to older adults and patients with chronic illness, focusing on advancing the practice of consultant and senior care pharmacy. The ASCP provides health care practitioners with a particular interest in the geriatric and chronically ill patient with education and resources to improve their practice skills. Health professionals other than pharmacists are eligible to become members of the ASCP.

The **Academy of Managed Care Pharmacy (AMCP)** is a professional association of pharmacists and associates who serve patients in the managed health care system environment. The goals of the AMCP, ASHP, and APhA often overlap, and multiple memberships in these associations are not uncommon.

The **American College of Clinical Pharmacy (ACCP)** consists primarily of PharmD clinical practitioners and faculty members. Its stated mission is to facilitate the creation, transmission, and application of new knowledge in the science of pharmacotherapy.

The **American College of Apothecaries (ACA)** is a small, selective association of community-based practitioners. Membership is granted only if the practitioners and their pharmacy comply with certain standards of professional service and appearance. Dual membership in the APhA is required.

Pharmacy Technician Associations

National Pharmacy Technician Association (NPTA) the world's largest professional organization for pharmacy technicians in practice sites including community practice, hospitals, home care, long-term care, nuclear sites, military sites, prison facilities, as well as management, education and drug sales.

Pharmacy Technician Certification Board (PTCB) established in 1995 to provide a voluntary mechanism for a national certification program for pharmacy technicians.

The **American Association of Pharmacy Technicians (AAPT)** was the first pharmacy technician association, formed in 1979. The mission statement of the AAPT is to provide leadership and to represent the interests of its members to the public as well as health care organizations; to promote the safe, efficacious, and cost-effective dispensing, distribution, and use of medications; to provide continuing education programs and service to help technicians update their skills and keep pace with changes in pharmacy services; and to promote pharmacy technicians as an integral part of the patient care team.

The **National Pharmacy Technician Association (NPTA)** is the world's largest professional organization established specifically for pharmacy technicians. The association is dedicated to advancing the value of pharmacy technicians and the vital roles they play in pharmaceutical care. Technician practice settings include retail, independent, hospital, mail-order, home care, long-term care, nuclear, military, correctional facility, formal education training, management, and sales settings. Both associations hold annual meetings during the summer months and provide their members with access to educational services. In addition to the AAPT and NPTA, the APhA and ASHP offer technician membership.

The **Pharmacy Technician Certification Board (PTCB)** was established in January 1995 through the efforts of the APhA, ASHP, the Illinois Council of Health-System Pharmacists (ICHP), and the Michigan Pharmacists Association (MPA). It provides a voluntary mechanism for a national certification program for pharmacy technicians.

The PTCB offers the certification examination several times each year in a computer-based testing format. Computer-based testing is beneficial to the technician candidate by providing results within a few weeks of the testing and creating more flexibility for exam scheduling. To be eligible to take the examination, the candidate must have a high school diploma or General Equivalency Diploma (GED).

For 2007, the application fee for the exam is $129. The PTCB requires recertification every two years and 20 hours of continuing education within that two-year time period. Technicians play a major role in the practice of pharmacy, and they are a valuable and essential component to the care of the patients that pharmacists treat every day.

The **Pharmacy Technician Educators Council's (PTEC)** mission is to assist the profession of pharmacy in preparing high-quality, well-trained technical personnel through education and practical training. In addition, the council's goal is to promote the profession of pharmacy through professional activities and dissemination of information and knowledge to members, pharmacy organizations, and other specialists and professions. The PTEC usually meets jointly with the American Association of Colleges of Pharmacy (AACP) at the AACP annual meeting. Members of the PTEC include faculty members of formal technician training programs, most often associated with community colleges.

Other Related Associations

Many other national associations in pharmacy represent special segments of the profession. These are presented here with a brief description of their membership and mission.

The **National Association of Chain Drug Stores (NACDS)** is an association of corporations, generally represented by their chief executive officers, many of whom are not pharmacists. The title is misleading, because the NACDS represents a variety of businesses, not only chain or multi-outlet pharmacies. Chain membership is contingent on the chain having four or more retail pharmacies open to the public. Grocery chains, department stores, and various discount outlets with pharmacies belong to the NACDS. The strength of this organization lies in its size and large financial capabilities. Chains are the largest employer of practicing pharmacists. The NACDS is composed of more than 200 retail chain pharmacy companies, employing more than 112,000 pharmacists. Chain community pharmacies consist of of approximately 20,700 traditional chain drug stores, 9,400 supermarket pharmacies, and nearly 6,400 mass merchant pharmacies. The NACDS membership base operates more than 36,000 retail community pharmacies with annual sales totaling nearly $650 billion—including $193 billion in sales for prescription drugs, over-the-counter (OTC) medications, and health and beauty aids. Chain-operated community retail pharmacies fill more than 70 percent of the 3.2 billion prescriptions dispensed annually in the United States.

The **American Association of Colleges of Pharmacy (AACP)**, founded in 1900, is the national association representing the interests of pharmacy education and educators. The AACP comprises all 105 U.S. colleges and schools of pharmacy, including more than 4,300 faculty, 48,500 students enrolled in professional programs, and 3,600 individuals pursuing graduate study. The AACP is committed to excellence in pharmacy education.

The AACP adopted a policy for supportive personnel (pharmacy technicians), which states that the training of such personnel be based on sound educational principles. The AACP also recommended that its member schools offer their assistance for the development of those objectives.

The **American Council for Pharmaceutical Education (ACPE)** is the national, independent accrediting agency for professional degree programs in pharmacy and for providers of continuing education programs in pharmacy. Formed in

---

Pharmacy Technician Educators Council (PTEC) mission of the council is to assist the profession of pharmacy to prepare high-quality, well-trained technical personnel through education and practical training programs.

National Association of Chain Drug Stores (NACDS) an association of corporations represented by Chief Executive Officers, many of whom are not pharmacists, and includes chains, grocery, department stores and discount outlets.

American Association of Colleges of Pharmacy (AACP) an organization of pharmacy colleges primarily concerned with education issues, such as curricula and teaching methodology.

American Council for Pharmaceutical Education (ACPE) the accrediting body for colleges of pharmacy, by which high educational standards are established and monitored.

1932 through the efforts of the APhA, AACP, the National Association of Boards of Pharmacy (NABP), and the American Council on Education (ACE), the ACPE has proposed and published the standards that schools must meet to obtain and maintain accreditation. Providers of continuing pharmacy education must meet certain criteria, involving budget, governance, faculty quality and quantity, admission standards, physical facilities, library, curricula, and achievement when accrediting education programs. Accreditation is voluntary, but inasmuch as all states require graduation from an accredited school of pharmacy as a prerequisite of licensure, an unaccredited program could not survive. Accreditation is also needed to qualify for various state and federal financial aid programs.

National Association of Boards of Pharmacy (NABP) formed in 1904 to assist member boards in developing pharmacy standards to protect the public health.

reciprocity mutual exchange or interchange between two parties.

The **National Association of Boards of Pharmacy (NABP)** is the independent, international, and impartial association that assists its member boards and jurisdictions in developing, implementing, and enforcing uniform standards for the purpose of protecting the public health. Since its inception in 1904, the NABP has worked to standardize the requirements for pharmacist licensure while maintaining the posture of individual states' rights. Transfer of licensure among most states, or **reciprocity**, has been facilitated through the NABP. The NABP makes available the North American Pharmacist Licensure Exam (NAPLEX®), the Multi-State Pharmacy Jurisprudence Exam (MPJE®), and the Foreign Pharmacy Graduate Equivalency Exam (FPGEE®) to assist state pharmacy boards in their evaluation of candidates for pharmacy licensure.

Association Publications

One of the first actions of a professional association is the publication of a journal for the dissemination of scientific and professional information for the membership and the profession. The founders of the Philadelphia College of Pharmacy were responsible for the publication of the first American pharmacy journal, the *Journal of the Philadelphia College of Pharmacy*, in 1825. In 1835 the title was changed to the *American Journal of Pharmacy* and is now recognized as the *Journal of the American Pharmacists Association* (JAPhA). Today, the APhA also publishes *Pharmacy Today*, *Pharmacy Student*, *APhA DrugInfoLine*, and *JPharmSci*. Many national associations of pharmacy have continued and expanded on this action, publishing their own journals and newsletters (Table 9-2). In addition, several associations—most notably the APhA and ASHP—have produced publications providing pharmacists and other health professionals with needed drug information.

TABLE 9-2   Organizational Publications

AACP	*American Journal of Pharmaceutical Education (AJPE)*
AAPS	*AAPS; Pharmaceutical Research; AAPS PharmSciTech*
AMCP	*Journal of Managed Care Pharmacy*
APhA	*Journal of the American Pharmacists Association (JAPhA)*
ASCP	*The Consultant Pharmacist; Supplements to the Consultant Pharmacist; ASCP Update; Clinical Consult*
ASHP	*American Journal of Health-System Pharmacy (AJHP)*
CRS	*Journal of Controlled Release (JCR)*
ISMP	*ISMP Medication Safety Alerts® Newsletter*
NACDS	*NACDS Foundation Chain Pharmacy Industry Profile; The Practice Memo*
NCPA	*America's Pharmacist*
NPTA	*Today's Technician™*

Summary

There are numerous professional associations that meet the specialty needs of their membership. Associations represent members practicing in community, chain, hospital, consulting, and clinical pharmacy practices. Colleges of pharmacy, accrediting agencies, state boards of pharmacy, wholesalers, and more comprise additional specialty membership groups in pharmacy practice. Many of these associations offer membership to pharmacy technicians, as do several specialty pharmacy technician associations.

The various associations in pharmacy link together all pharmacy personnel and provide a system for networking and a mechanism to establish best practices for the profession. As a result, all pharmacists have the opportunity to enter the mainstream of the constantly evolving growth and development of the profession of pharmacy.

TEST YOUR KNOWLEDGE

Multiple Choice

1. Professional associations provide their members with which of the following?
   a. Common interest
   b. Best practices in the profession
   c. United front on legislative issues
   d. All of the above

2. Of the following issues, which two stimulated the formation of the first national pharmacy association?
   i. Laws restricting the practice of pharmacists
   ii. Educational standards for the practice of pharmacy
   iii. Safety and efficacy concerns about drug products
   iv. Boycotts of pharmacies
   a. i and ii
   b. i and iii
   c. ii and iii
   d. ii and iv

3. In what state was the first pharmacy formed?
   a. New York
   b. Texas
   c. California
   d. Pennsylvania

4. What organization is responsible for accrediting colleges of pharmacy?
   a. APhA
   b. ACPE
   c. ASHP
   d. ASCP

5. What entity is responsible for the oversight of food and drug products in the United States?
   a. DEA
   b. ACPE
   c. FDA
   d. PTCB

6. The Pharmacy Technician Certification Board is responsible for which of the following?
   a. Accredited technician programs
   b. Registration of technicians for all states in the United States
   c. Certifying technicians who successfully pass an examination
   d. All of the above

Matching

Match the organization to its primary membership base.

1.	_____ ASHP	a.	open to all pharmacists
2.	_____ NCPA	b.	independent community retail pharmacists
3.	_____ AACP	c.	hospital pharmacists
4.	_____ APhA	d.	pharmacy educators
5.	_____ PTEC	e.	pharmacy technicians

References

Flanagan, M. E. (1995). Voluntary technician certification program reflects changes in practice. *American Pharmacy*, NS35 (5), 18–23.

Murer, M. M. (1996). Technician certification leads to recognition, better patient care. *Journal of the American Pharmaceutical Association*, NS36, 514–520.

Smith, J. E. (1995). The national voluntary certification of pharmacy technicians. *American Journal of Health-System Pharmacy*, 52, 2026–2029.

Web Sites

Academy of Managed Care Pharmacy (AMCP)
    www.amcp.org
American Association of Colleges of Pharmacy (AACP)
    www.aacp.org
American Association of Pharmacy Technicians (AAPT)
    www.pharmacytechnician.com
American College of Apothecaries (ACA)
    www.americancollegeofapothecaries.com
American College of Clinical Pharmacy (ACCP)
    www.accp.com
American Pharmacists Association (APhA)
    www.pharmacist.com

American Society of Consultant Pharmacists (ASCP)
   www.ascp.com
American Society of Health-System Pharmacists (ASHP)
   www.ashp.org
National Association of Boards of Pharmacy (NABP)
   www.nabp.net
National Community Pharmacists Association (NCPA)
   www.ncpanet.org
Pharmacy Technician Certification Board (PTCB)
   www.ptcb.org

PART

III

Professional Aspects of Pharmacy Technology

The Prescription

Competencies

Upon completion of this chapter, the reader should be able to

1. Identify the various parts of a prescription.
2. Describe methods for transmitting prescriptions to pharmacies.
3. Explain the differences between transmitting prescriptions or drug orders to pharmacies in community settings and institutional settings.
4. Identify roles for the pharmacy technician in handling and interpreting prescriptions.

Key Terms

collaborative drug therapy management (CDTM)
dispense as written (DAW)
inscription
medication order
prescription
script
sig
signa
signatura
subscription
superscription
therapeutic substitution

Introduction

Pharmacists are an important part of the health care team, which is made up of physicians, nurses, and many other health care professionals. Unlike many of these health care workers, the pharmacist works in a separate location. For this team to function, there must be a method of communication between its members. The *prescription* is the method of communication. While prescriptions are typically written, they may also be verbal or electronic. Whatever the format, it is essential that the pharmacy technician understand the prescription.

The Prescription

prescription
permission, granted orally or in writing, from a physician for a patient to receive a certain medication on an outpatient basis that will help relieve or eliminate the patient's problem.

script an abbreviated form of prescription.

The **prescription**, or **script** as it is also known, instructs a pharmacist to dispense—select, count, place in an appropriate container, and label—a specific drug in a specific dose and dosage form for a specific patient. While most prescriptions are for prescription (or legend) drugs, prescriptions may also be written for over-the-counter (OTC) medications.

The prescription is written on a prescription blank that is usually preprinted with frequently-used information, such as the prescriber's name, phone number, and Drug Enforcement Administration (DEA) number, as well as the prescriber's address. The prescription blank will also have prompts for important information such as the patient's name, address, date of birth, number of refills, and the date the prescription was written.

In New York State an official prescription exists. It is issued by the state with numerous safeguards built in to reduce the chance of fraudulent use of the prescriptions to obtain medications illegally. While it is only required for use in New York State, it can serve as a fairly typical example of a prescription (Figure 10-1).

Parts of the Prescription

Each state specifies the necessary components of a prescription. Typically, the following items are required on every prescription (the numbers identify the corresponding information in Figure 10-1):

1. *Name, address, and date of birth of the patient.* It is obviously important to identify the patient accurately. While the name may be sufficient to identify the patient, the patient's address and date of birth (DOB) may be necessary in some situations; for instance, with patients who have common names (e.g., Mary Smith) or if two members of a family share the same or very similar names (e.g., Mike and Mickey). The DOB is also important as it helps the pharmacist determine the appropriateness of drug choice, dose, and dosage form for younger patients. The prescriber may not always provide the address or date of birth. The pharmacist can add this information from the patient profile. The prescriber must, however, provide the patient's name; this the pharmacist cannot add. If the technician is in the position of receiving the prescription from the patient, it should always be reviewed for the address and date of birth. If the information is missing or illegible, it is appropriate for the technician to ask if other prescriptions are on file that can be used to add this data. In some pharmacies, it may be part of the technician's responsibilities to add the address, date of birth, or correct spelling of the patient's name. If the pharmacist does not

FIGURE 10-1

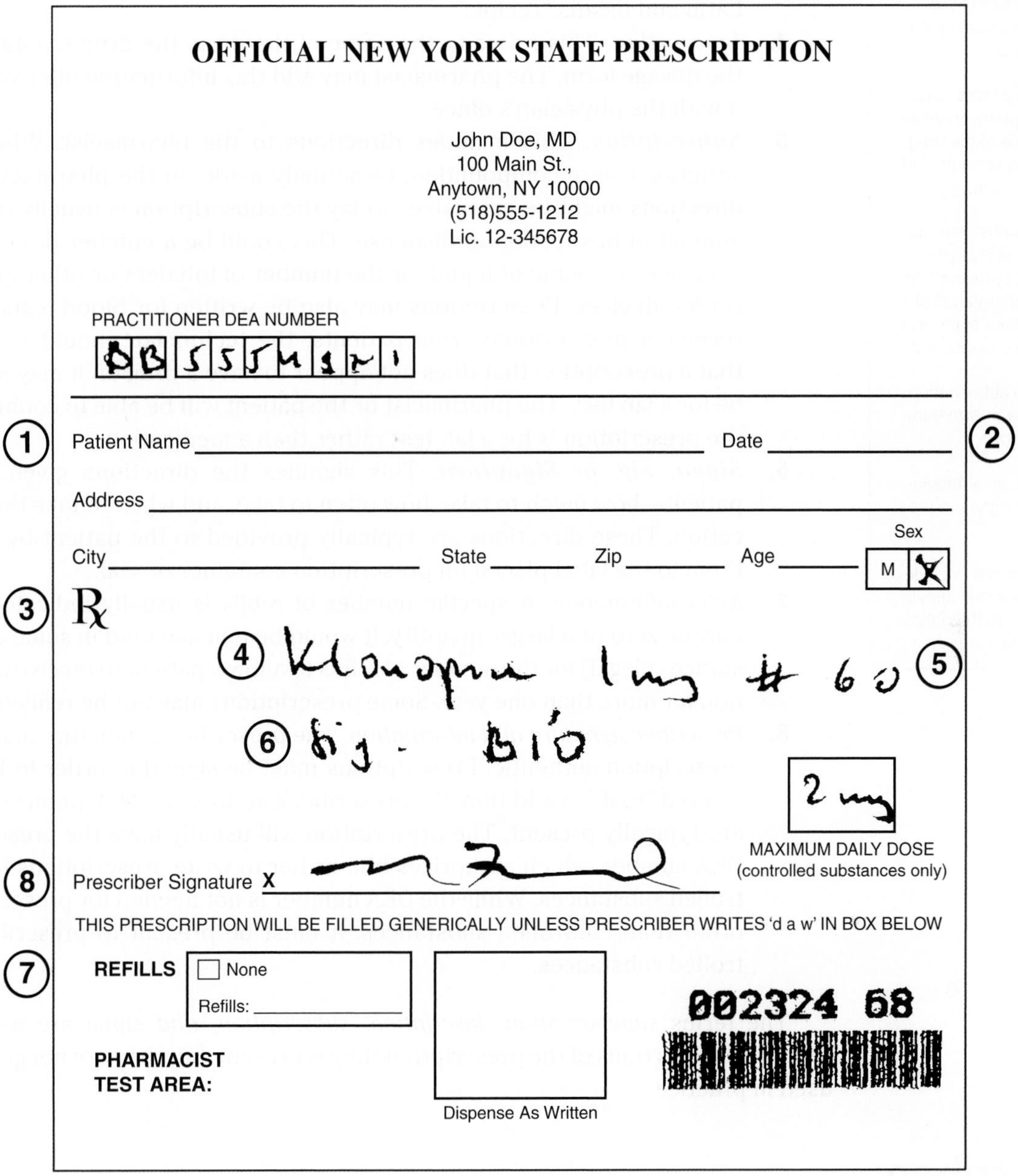

OFFICIAL NEW YORK STATE PRESCRIPTION

John Doe, MD
100 Main St.,
Anytown, NY 10000
(518)555-1212
Lic. 12-345678

PRACTITIONER DEA NUMBER

① Patient Name _____ Date _____ ②

Address _____

③ City _____ State _____ Zip _____ Age _____ Sex M ☒

R̶x̶

④ Klonopin 1mg # 60 ⑤

⑥ sig - bid

2 mg

MAXIMUM DAILY DOSE
(controlled substances only)

⑧ Prescriber Signature X ~~~~~~~~

THIS PRESCRIPTION WILL BE FILLED GENERICALLY UNLESS PRESCRIBER WRITES 'd a w' IN BOX BELOW

⑦ REFILLS ☐ None

Refills: _____

PHARMACIST
TEST AREA:

Dispense As Written

002324 68

FIGURE 10-1 Prescription.

explain his or her expectations to the pharmacy technician, the technician should clarify the expectations in this regard.

2. *Date script was issued.* The date that the prescription was written is important. Prescriptions are typically written for a specific purpose, as part of a specific treatment plan, and should usually be presented to the pharmacy shortly after the prescription was written. Sometimes during an annual visit with their physician, patients will receive a prescription for a medication they are currently receiving. These prescriptions may not be filled for a few months as patients wait for their current prescription refills to run out. If the prescriber failed to date the prescription, the pharmacist may add the date unless the prescription is for a controlled substance. If the prescription is for a controlled substance, the pharmacist must verify the date with the prescriber.

superscription
the Rx symbol on the prescription.

inscription on a prescription, contains the name of the drug, the drug strength and dosage form.

subscription an indication on a prescriber's prescription to the pharmacist of the amount of medication to be dispensed.

sig an abbreviation for *signa* or *signatura* (see below).

signa an abbreviation for signature (see below).

signatura includes directions that should be given to the patient and so labeled.

3. *Superscription.* This is the *Rx* symbol on the prescription. It derives from Latin and means "recipe."

4. *Inscription.* This refers to the name of the drug, the drug strength, and the dosage form. The pharmacist may add this information after verifying it with the physician's office.

5. *Subscription.* This includes directions to the pharmacist. When prescriptions were compounded, or actually made, in the pharmacy, these directions might be extensive. Today the subscription is usually only the amount of medication to dispense. This could be a number of tablets or capsules, a volume of liquid, or the number of inhalers or other administration devices. Prescriptions may also be written for blood tests. When receiving prescriptions from patients, the technician should recognize that a prescription that does not appear to have a drug on it may actually be for a lab test. The pharmacist or the patient will be able to confirm that the prescription is for a lab test rather than a medication.

6. *Signa, Sig, or Signatura.* This signifies the directions given to the patient—how much to take, how often to take, and when to take the medication. These directions are typically provided to the patient by adding them to the label placed on prescription container or vial.

7. *Refill information.* A specific number of refills is usually indicated. This may be zero or a larger quantity. It would be unusual (and in some circumstances illegal) for the number of refills to allow a patient to receive medication for more than one year. Some prescriptions may not be refilled at all.

8. *Prescriber signature and information.* The prescriber's signature makes the prescription authentic. Prescriptions must be signed in order to be considered "real." In addition, the prescriber's address and telephone number are typically present. The prescription will usually have the prescriber's DEA number, which authorizes him or her to write prescriptions for controlled substances. While the DEA number is not needed for prescriptions other than controlled substances, it must be present to prescribe controlled substances.

The terms *superscription, inscription, subscription, and* signa are useful to describe the portions of the prescription they represent, but they are not generally used in practice.

Prescribers

collaborative drug therapy management (CDTM) an agreement between a physician and a pharmacist that allows the pharmacist expanded prescription authorization regarding managing drug therapy.

Licensed prescribers are most often physicians (MD, doctor of medicine, or DO, doctor of osteopathy), but they may also be dentists, podiatrists, physician's assistants (PAs), nurse practitioners (NPs), optometrists, and pharmacists. While each of these non-physician groups may have the right to prescribe, ethical or legal limits are often imposed on their ability to prescribe. For example, dentists should only be prescribing for dental concerns; PAs and NPs may only prescribe when they have a specific relationship with a physician. Similarly, some states permit pharmacists to prescribe through a process known as **collaborative drug therapy management (CDTM)**, in which the pharmacist has a formal arrangement with specific physicians that allow the pharmacist to prescribe certain drugs for specified conditions under a written agreement between the physician and pharmacist that only applies to that physician's patients. Obviously, the nature of these agreements between non-physician prescribers and physicians is determined by each state's laws, and considerable variation is present from state to state.

Methods of Receiving a Prescription

When a licensed prescriber determines that a patient requires drug therapy, he or she typically communicates that information to a pharmacist by using a written prescription. The prescription is often given to the patient by the physician, and the patient presents the prescription to the pharmacist. While all of the above is provided in reference to a written prescription, prescriptions may also be given to the pharmacist orally, typically over the telephone. An oral prescription must have all of the information that a written prescription contains. The pharmacist is required to immediately transcribe, or write, the oral prescription.

Prescriptions may also be transferred electronically to pharmacies. Perhaps the most common method of doing this is using a facsimile or fax machine, but other methods are continuously being developed. Because of security concerns, e-mail is generally not considered an acceptable method of transferring prescriptions; however, computerized physician order entry (CPOE) is being developed and advocated as a method of reducing medication errors. CPOE is not currently in widespread use, but is more common in hospital settings than community settings. State law may require that a hard copy of electronically-transmitted prescriptions be produced and maintained just as regular written prescriptions would be filed.

Medication Orders

When patients are in institutional settings, such as hospitals or nursing homes, they still require medications, but they obviously do not take prescriptions to the pharmacy to obtain their medications. In these situations, directions to give patients medications are called **medication orders** rather than prescriptions. Medication orders are written on order sheets. A sample order sheet is shown in Figure 10-2.

medication order orders for all medications and intravenous solutions written on an order sheet (or via computerized physician order entry) on a hospital-wide computer system.

While several differences between prescriptions and medication orders exist, some of the more important differences are that multiple drugs may be written on the same order sheet, and many things other than drugs may be ordered on an order sheet. Thus, it is important for the technician to review order sheets carefully to identify all of the medications ordered, realizing that all of the drug orders may not be next to one another.

The requirements for medication orders are usually specified by the hospital or nursing home, but are somewhat similar to those described previously for prescriptions. Some differences include that a patient is usually identified by a room number instead of an address; a quantity to dispense is not needed; and refills are not required. However, instead of a number of refills or a quantity to dispense, most institutions have automatic *stop order policies.* These policies specify that medications will be stopped after so many days and must be reordered if they are to be continued. Stop order policies will also permit prescribers to order therapy for a specific number of days or doses, which may exceed the number stated in the stop order policy.

FIGURE 10-2

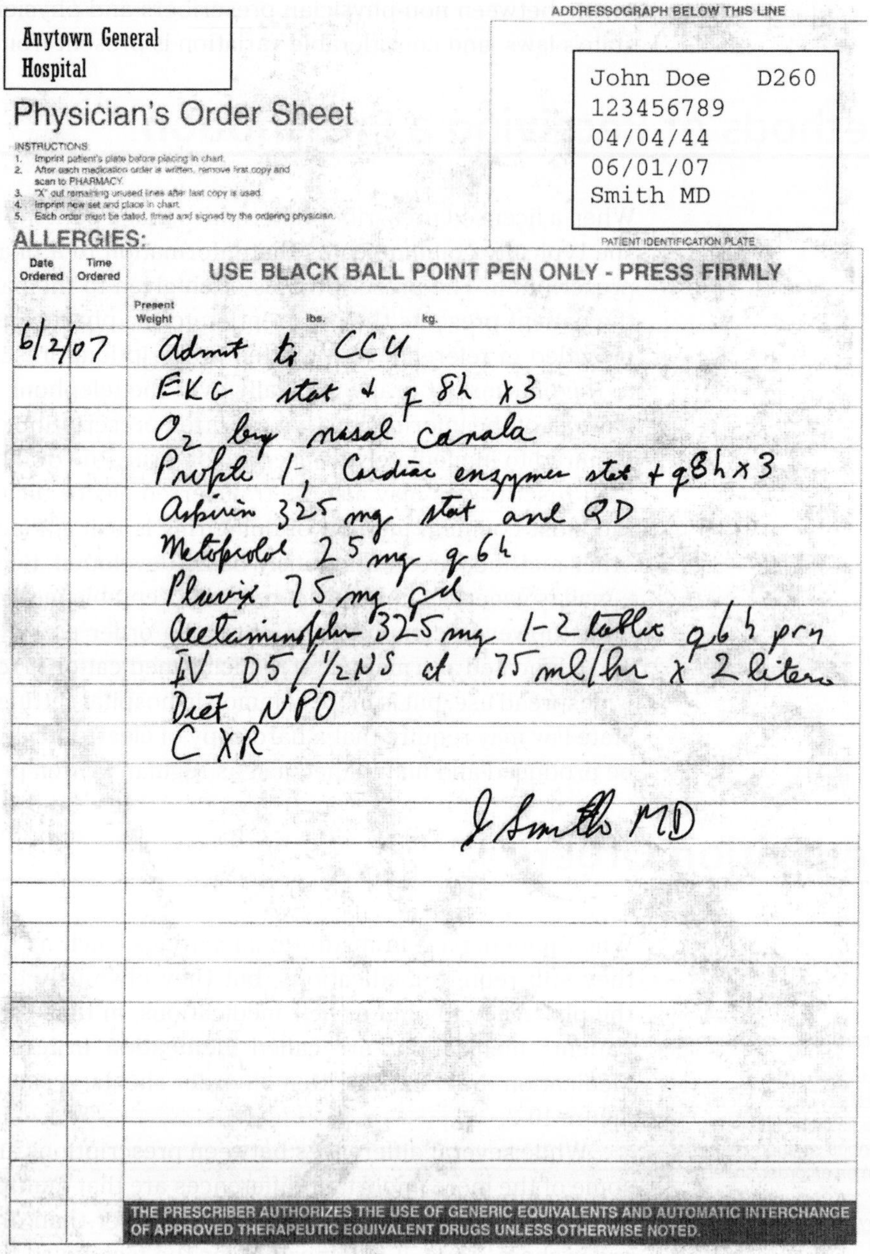

Anytown General Hospital

Physician's Order Sheet

INSTRUCTIONS:
1. Imprint patient's plate before placing in chart.
2. After each medication order is written, remove first copy and scan to PHARMACY.
3. "X" out remaining unused lines after last copy is used.
4. Imprint new set and place in chart.
5. Each order must be dated, timed and signed by the ordering physician.

ADDRESSOGRAPH BELOW THIS LINE

John Doe   D260
123456789
04/04/44
06/01/07
Smith MD

PATIENT IDENTIFICATION PLATE

ALLERGIES:

Date Ordered	Time Ordered	USE BLACK BALL POINT PEN ONLY - PRESS FIRMLY
6/2/07		Present Weight ___ lbs. ___ kg.
		Admit to CCU
		EKG stat & q 8h x3
		O₂ by nasal canula
		Profile 1, Cardiac enzymes stat + q8h x3
		Aspirin 325 mg stat and QD
		Metoprolol 25 mg q 6h
		Plavix 75 mg qd
		Acetaminophen 325 mg 1-2 tablet q6h prn
		IV D5/½NS at 75 ml/hr x 2 liters
		Diet NPO
		CXR
		J Smith MD

THE PRESCRIBER AUTHORIZES THE USE OF GENERIC EQUIVALENTS AND AUTOMATIC INTERCHANGE OF APPROVED THERAPEUTIC EQUIVALENT DRUGS UNLESS OTHERWISE NOTED.

FIGURE 10-2 Medication order.

When a prescriber orders medications in an institutional setting, he or she must often consult a *formulary*, or a list of drugs that the institution has in its inventory. For example, a hospital may decide not to have Lipitor (generic name: atorvastatin), a popular cholesterol-lowering drug, on its formulary and instead have the drug Zocor (generic name: simvastatin), a similar cholesterol-lowering drug. If the prescriber fails to check the formulary, many institutions have a policy of automatic substitution, which allows the pharmacist to automatically substitute the formulary drug for the drug ordered. Committees within the hospital approve

therapeutic substitution the substitution of one drug product with another that differs in composition but is considered to have the same or very similar pharmacologic and therapeutic activity.

dispense as written (DAW) where the medication indicated on the prescription may not be substituted with a generic or other brand drug without the authorization of the prescriber.

such switches, and the change is carried out by the pharmacist. This process is called **therapeutic substitution**. If an institution uses therapeutic substitution, a procedure will exist to indicate that the substitution took place. The technician should be careful to clearly understand this process and realize that the drugs involved in therapeutic substitution may change in different institutions. In the outpatient setting, therapeutic substitution is not routinely used. However, some insurance companies have preferred drugs and will attempt to switch patients to preferred drugs.

This process, therapeutic substitution, should not be confused with generic substitution. *Generic substitution* occurs when a prescription or medication order for one brand name is filled with the same chemical, but one that is sold under either a different brand name or simply by the generic name. In the outpatient or community pharmacy setting, prescriptions may have the notation **DAW (Dispense as Written)** added to prevent generic substitution. In some states, the law may specify that generic drugs must be used unless the letters DAW are added to the prescription.

Medication Errors

Historically, the directions to pharmacists were written in Latin, frequently using abbreviations of Latin instructions and other notations and symbols to indicate quantities. While the use of these Latin abbreviations and notations persists, the use of many such abbreviations is being strongly discouraged due to the tendency toward misinterpreting abbreviations. Misinterpretation occurs because the abbreviations may have two meanings (e.g., MS may mean morphine sulfate or magnesium sulfate) or because the poor handwriting of many prescribers may result in misinterpretation (e.g., when written in script, SC, an abbreviation for subcutaneous (an injection given just under the skin) may appear to be SL, an abbreviation for sublingual (under the tongue)). A list of frequently misinterpreted abbreviations has been prepared by the Institute for Safe Medication Practices. The pharmacy technician should pay particular attention to prescriptions with these abbreviations, as the technician may assist the pharmacist by recalling the potential for misinterpretation.

Summary

The prescription is a legal document that communicates the prescriber's medication treatment to the pharmacist. As a legal document, there are several specific requirements for prescriptions that may vary by state and type of medication. Prescriptions may be written, verbal, or electronic. In the hospital setting, prescriptions are referred to as *medication orders*. *The pharmacy technician should be able to understand the requirements for each type of prescription and recognize whether they are present in a prescription.*

TEST YOUR KNOWLEDGE

Multiple Choice

1. Which of the following elements *cannot* be added to a prescription by the pharmacist?
   a. patient name
   b. patient address
   c. patient date of birth
   d. patient allergies

2. Which of the following is *not* needed to identify the specific patient who will receive a prescription?
   a. patient name
   b. patient address
   c. patient date of birth
   d. indication for drug

3. Which of the following is an acceptable method of delivering a prescription to a pharmacy?
   a. telephone call from the prescriber
   b. fax from the physician's office
   c. written in an e-mail
   d. written prescription delivered by the patient's spouse

4. A difference between a prescription received in a community pharmacy and a drug order received in a hospital pharmacy is that
   a. drug orders do not have patient names.
   b. drug orders do not include directions for administration.
   c. drug orders are not required to have patient addresses.
   d. prescriptions will not have lab tests on them.

5. When a pharmacy technician receives a prescription and notices missing information, which of the following should he or she do?
   a. add the patient's name to the prescription
   b. tell the patient that the prescription cannot be filled
   c. recommend the patient take an over-the-counter medication instead
   d. bring the missing information to the pharmacist's attention

6. The name of the drug, dosage strength, and drug form on the prescription is called the
   a. superscription.
   b. inscription.
   c. subscription.
   d. signatura.

7. Which of the following is a licensed drug prescriber?
   a. pharmacy technician
   b. nurse
   c. physician
   d. nursing assistant

8. What is a list of approved drugs called?
   a. formulary
   b. Kardex
   c. dispensary
   d. index

9. Which of the following is a common reason for medication errors?
   a. following the five rights of medication administration
   b. checking the patient's identification
   c. use of abbreviations
   d. double checking the label against the prescription

Matching

Match the part of the prescription to its description.

1. _____ superscription   a. directions to the pharmacist

2. _____ inscription   b. Rx symbol

3. _____ subscription   c. name, strength, and dose of drug

4. _____ signa   d. directions to the patient

Fill In The Blank

1. When a pharmacist has an arrangement with physicians to prescribe specific drugs under specific conditions, this is called _____.

2. A method being advocated to reduce medication errors is _____.

3. When a pharmacist is allowed to automatically switch a drug to one on a formulary from one ordered by a physician, this is called _____.

4. _____ may appear on a prescription to prevent generic substitution.

5. Misinterpretation of a prescription may occur as a result of the use of _____.

References

Kaushal, R., & Bates, D. W. Chapter 6. Computerized physician order entry (CPOE) with clinical decision support systems (CDSSs). In K. G. Shojania, B. W. Duncan, K. M. McDonald, & R. M. Wachter (Eds.), *Making health care safer: A critical analysis of patient safety practices*. Evidence Report/Technology Assessment: No. 43. AHRQ Publication No. 01-E058, July 2001. Agency for Healthcare Research and Quality: Rockville, MD. www.ahrq.gov/clinic/ptsafety/.

Medical Terminology

Competencies

Upon completion of this chapter, the reader should be able to

1. Recognize word elements and identify word element combinations used in medical terminology.

2. Determine the meaning of common medical terms by evaluating the word elements.

3. Recognize and define several common medical terms related to disease states.

4. Recognize common abbreviations and their meanings.

5. Identify the various components of a prescription.

Key Terms

combining form
prefix
suffix
word elements
word root

Introduction

Understanding the language of medicine or medical terminology is a critical component in the efficient communication with other members of the health care team to facilitate the provision of excellent patient care. The terms used to describe the medical history of a patient provide information about any current transient conditions such as an infection, chronic disease conditions such as hypercholesterolemia, and medical diagnostic or surgical interventions that the patient has undergone, such as angiography and angioplasty.

Medical terminology is a growing body of knowledge that has its roots as early as the first century B.C. and is constantly increasing with the development of new diagnostic methods and the identification of new disease states.

Word Elements

word elements
in medical terminology, made up of word roots, prefixes, and suffixes.

word root a primary building block; the core word used to identify fundamental anatomic and physiologic nomenclature.

combining form a word type that facilitates the attachment of a prefix or suffix; formed when a word root is incorporated into a medical term.

prefix a word element attached to the beginning of a word to modify its meaning.

suffix a word element attached to the end of a word to create a new word with a specific meaning.

Words in the medical vocabulary are constructed with a series of building blocks or **word elements**. The primary building block is the **word root** or core that identifies the fundamental anatomic or physiologic system. The word root is often a Greek or Latin word such as *dermatos* (Greek), meaning skin, or *renes* (Latin), meaning kidney. When the word root is incorporated into the medical term, the word root assumes a **combining form** that facilitates the attachment of a prefix or suffix. For example, *cardi-/o-* (combining form for the Greek word *kardio*) refers to the heart and is found as the word root in disease names and diagnostic procedures associated with the heart. The remaining building blocks, **prefix** (a word element that is not an independent word but is attached to the beginning of a word to modify its meaning) and **suffix** (a word element that is not an independent word but is attached to the end of the word to create a new word or grammatical form) are added to the word root to create a word that carries a very specific meaning.

For example, the term *electrocardiogram* is composed of the prefix *electro-*, relating to electrical activity, the root *cardio-*, which identifies the organ system as the heart, and the suffix *-gram*, which means a graphical representation. Therefore, *electrocardiogram* means "the graphical representation of the electrical activity in the heart." If the root word changes, as in *electroencephalogram*, the prefix *electro-* and the suffix *-gram* indicate that the term still refers to a "graphic representation of the electrical activity," but the organ involved is the brain (*encephal-/o-* = brain). Note that the insertion of a vowel, most commonly *o*, is used to combine the building blocks and make the term easier to pronounce. Root words for some of the major organ structures are presented in Table 11-1.

Prefix

The addition of a prefix will modify the root word by indicating the number of parts, the location or position of an organ or body part, or the time or frequency, or produce a term with the opposite meaning of the root element. For example, the prefix *mono-* means one, while the prefix *bi-* means two. Combination of a prefix with the root element *nuclear* (the nucleus of a cell) produces the words mononuclear (a cell with one nucleus) or binuclear (a cell with two nuclei). Common prefixes that indicate numbers or measurement (such as size) are listed in Tables 11-2 and 11-3.

TABLE 11-1 Root Words for Organ Structures

aden-/o-	glands	my-/o-	muscle
arteri-/o-	arteries	nas-/o-; rhin-/o-	nose
arthr-/o-	joints	nephr-/o-	kidneys
bronch-/o-	bronchial tubes	neur-/o-	nerves
cardi-/o-	heart	ocul-/o-	ear
cephal-/o-	head	oste-/o-	bone
cholecyst-/o-	gallbladder	ot-/o-	ear
col-/o-	colon	pharyng-/o-	pharynx
cyst-/o-	bladder	pneumn-/o-	lungs
cyt-/o-	cell	pulmon-/o-	lungs
dermat-/o-	skin	splen-/o-	spleen
encephal-/o-	brain	thyr-/o-	thyroid
enter-/o-	small intestine	trache-/o-	trachea
esophag-/o-	esophagus	trich-/o-	hair
gastr-/o-	stomach	ur-/o-	urinary
hemat-/o-	blood	uter-/o-	uterus
hepat-/o-	liver	vagin-/o-	vaginal
mamm-/o-	breast	ven-/o-	veins

TABLE 11-2 Common Prefixes for Numbers and Time

mono-	one	re-	again
bi-; di-	two	hemi-	half
tri-	three	multi-; poly-	many
quad-; quadric-	four	ante-	before
nulli-	none	post-	after
pan-	all	neo-	new

TABLE 11-3 Common Prefixes for Measurement

ambi-	both	micro-	small
an-	without	multi-	many
brady-	slow	pan-	all
dipl-/o-	double	poly-	many
hemi-	half	semi-	partial
hyper-	above normal; excessive	super-	above or excess
hypo-	below normal	tachy-	rapid
macro-	large	ultra-	beyond or excess

Prefixes are also used to indicate the position or direction of movement of an organ or body part. The prefix *ab-* means "away from," as in *abduction*, a medical term meaning "away from the midline." The prefix *pre-* indicates "in front of," as in *prefrontal* (in front of the frontal bone), while *epi-* is defined as "upon or over," as

TABLE 11-4 Common Prefixes for Position or Direction

a-; ab-	away from	infra-	under, beneath
ambi-	both sides	inter-	among
ante-; antero-	in front of	intra-	within, inside
circum-; peri-	around	latero-	side
de-	down	medi-; meso-; mid-	middle
dorso-	back	para-	beside
ec-	out, out from	postero-	behind
endo-	within, inner	pre-; pro-	in front of
epi-	upon, over	sinistro-	to the left
ex-	out from	sub-	below
exo-	out	super-; supra-	above
hyper-	over	sym-; syn-	together
hypo-	under, below	trans-	through, across

in *epigastric*, meaning over or above the stomach. Common prefixes that indicate position are listed in Table 11-4.

Some prefixes will reverse, or produce a term with the opposite meaning of the root element. The importance of these terms is to indicate that an ability of the body has been lost or is not functional. For example, the prefix *a-* indicates "without or away from", such that the addition of *a-* to the root element *phagia* (to eat) creates the word *aphagia*. This term indicates that the patient does not have the capability to eat and, specifically, is not able to swallow. The prefix *dys-* means "difficult or painful." The combination of the root element *lexia* (from the Greek for *word*) with the prefix *dys-* creates the term *dyslexia*, which means an impaired ability to understand the written word. Table 11-5 illustrates common prefixes that modify the root element to indicate a lack of ability or poor function, or change the root element to mean the opposite of the original meaning.

Other prefixes impart additional information, such as color. Table 11-6 contains prefixes related to color.

TABLE 11-5 Common Prefixes for Poor Function or Lack of Presence or Function

a-	without; away from
an-	without
anti-	against
contra-	against
dys-	impaired
im-	not
in-	not
mal-	bad; ill
pseudo-	false

TABLE 11-6 Prefixes Related to Color

alb-	white	leuk-/o-	white
chlor-/o-	green	melan-/o-	black
cyan-/o-	blue	purpur-/o-	purple
erythr-/o-	red	rose-/o-	rose; pink
eosin-/o-	rosy	xanth-/o-	yellow

Suffix

In the same manner as a prefix, the addition of a suffix modifies the meaning of the root word to provide a precise medical term. The addition of a suffix such as -ac, -al, -ar, or -ic changes the root word (most commonly a noun) into an adjective meaning "pertaining to" or "resembling." For example, the addition of -ac to the root word *cardio*, meaning "heart," produces the adjective *cardiac*, meaning "pertaining to or resembling the heart." *Cardiac muscle* refers to the muscles of the heart, rather than the muscles of the leg or arm. Other suffixes whose addition forms an adjective are -form, -ic, -ical, -oid, -ory, and -ous. Examples include *multiform, neurologic, anatomical, lymphoid, sensory,* and *venous*.

A suffix may indicate a condition, disease, or procedure. For example, the root word combining form for blood is *hema-*, combined with the suffix meaning "a characteristic of the urine," -uria, produces *hematuria*, which indicates a condition where there is blood in the urine, a symptom which may suggest a bacterial infection of the bladder. If the laboratory results confirm the presence of bacteria in the urine, the resulting term is *bacteruria*. The combination of *myo-* (muscle) and -pathy (disease) results in *myopathy*, or a disease of the muscle usually characterized by muscle weakness, tenderness, and wasting. Table 11-7 indicates common suffixes relating to diseases or conditions.

The names of medical procedures indicate the precise type of procedure that is done at a specific anatomic location or to a certain organ or organs. One of the most common suffixes is -ectomy, indicating the surgical removal of tissue or an organ, such as *gastrectomy* (gastr- = stomach; -ectomy = surgical removal). *Dermatoplasty* and *rhinoplasty* both use the suffix -plasty to indicate a surgical repair, the former being repair of the skin and the latter being repair of the nose. In the same way, diagnostic procedures are constructed using the root word combining form and the appropriate suffix. As discussed earlier, *electrocardiogram* contains the root word combining form *cardio-* and the suffix -gram, meaning a record of the heart; in this case, the electrical activity (prefix: *electro-*). Common surgical and procedural suffixes are found in Table 11-8.

Pharmacy-Specific Medical Terminology

Within each discipline in the medical sciences, there is a specific and precise vocabulary. One of the simplest words with a very complex meaning is the term *drug*. A drug may be defined simply as "an exogenous substance which alters the function of the body, or more specifically in terms of a medical substance, as a material for use in the diagnosis, cure, mitigation, treatment, or prevention of disease in man or other animals as defined in the U.S. Food, Drug, and Cosmetic Act."

TABLE 11-7 Common Suffixes for Conditions or Diseases

-algia; -dynia	pain	-oma	tumor; mass
-blast	immature; embryonic	-osis	unusual or diseased condition
-cele	hernia or protrusion	-paresis	weakness
-ectasis	dilation, expansion	-pathy	disease
-ectopia	displacement	-phobia	abnormal fear
-edema	swelling	-plasm	formation; development
-emesis	vomiting	-plegia	paralysis
-emia	presence in the blood	-ptosis	drooping
-genesis	produces; generates	-rrhage; -rrhagia	excessive; abnormal flow
-genic	producing	-rrhea	flow; discharge
-ia	state; condition	-rrhexis	rupture
-iasis	abnormal condition	-sclerosis	hardening
-ism	state; condition	-sis	condition of
-itis	inflammation	-spasm	involuntary muscle contraction
-lysis	disintegration	-stenosis	narrowing
-malacia	abnormal softening	-uria	a particular substance in urine
-megaly	enlargement	-y	condition of

The U.S. Food and Drug Administration (FDA) is the agency of the government responsible for "protecting the public health by assuring the safety, efficacy, and security of human and veterinary drugs, biological products, medical devices, our nation's food supply, cosmetics, and products that emit radiation. The FDA is also responsible for advancing the public health by helping to speed innovations that

TABLE 11-8 Suffixes of Common Surgical Procedures

-centesis	a perforation or tapping operation	-otomy	cutting into
-clasis	to break; surgical fracture	-pexy	fixation (of an organ)
-desis	binding or fusion (commonly of bone or joint)	-pheresis	removal of blood components
-ectomy	surgical removal	-plasty	surgical repair
-gram	record or picture	-rrhaphy	suture
-graph	instrument for recording	-scope	an instrument for viewing or observing
-graphy	process of recording	-scopy	observation or viewing
-logy	study or science of	-stomy; -ostomy	surgical creation of an artificial opening into a hollow organ or the creation of an opening between two hollow organs
-lysis	destruction; loosening	-tome	an instrument for cutting
-meter	instrument for measuring	-tomy	incision
-metry	process of measuring	-tripsy	crushing

make medicines and foods more effective, safer, and more affordable; and helping the public get the accurate, science-based information they need to use medicines and foods to improve their health." More information on the FDA and the U.S. Food, Drug, and Cosmetic Act can be found on the government Web site at www.fda.gov.

The medications available in the pharmacy are divided into two dispensing categories. Over-the-counter medications (OTC) have been determined to be safe in the hands of the consumer and do not require a prescription to obtain. Prescription medications require a written order signed by an authorized health care provider in order for these drugs to be dispensed to a consumer. A second distinction between drugs is the use of the term *generic name* and *trade name*, *brand name* or *proprietary* drugs. A generic name is usually a version of the official name of the drug and is not capitalized. For example, *acetaminophen* is the generic name for the compound OTC medication to reduce pain and fever, while the same medication is also marketed as an OTC trade name medication under the name of Tylenol®. The symbol ® indicates that the name is a registered trademark. The same generic-name drug may be marketed under different trade or brand names. It is important to note that many drug names, both generic and brand names, have spellings that are very close to being the same and may sound alike. Extreme caution must be used to assure the correct medication is dispensed to the patient.

Most medications fall into one of several categories based on their actions. For example, aspirin is an analgesic, a term that means "to relieve pain," while cortisone is an anti-inflammatory (reduces inflammation). The major categories are listed in Table 11-9.

TABLE 11-9 Categories of Drugs and Their Actions

CATEGORY	ACTION
adrenergics	mimics the action of epinephrine, an agent in the sympathetic nervous system
analgesic	reduces pain
anesthetic	abolishes the sensation of pain
antiarthritic	relieves the symptoms of arthritis
anticoagulant	prevents blood clotting
anticonvulsant	suppresses or reduces number or intensity of seizures
antidiabetic	prevents or alleviates diabetes
antiemetic	prevents or relieves nausea or vomiting
antihistamine	prevents symptoms of allergy, such as runny nose
antihypertensive	lowers blood pressure
anti-inflammatory	reduces inflammation and swelling
antineoplastic	prevents the growth of malignant cells
antipruritic	relieves the symptoms of itching
antipyretic	reduces fever
antitoxin	neutralizes a poison or toxin
antivenin or antivenom	counteracts the action of venom from snakes and other venomous animals
diuretic	increases formation of urine to reduce swelling and blood pressure

(Continued)

TABLE 11-9 (Continued)

CATEGORY	ACTION
hypnotic, sedative, tranquilizer	induces sleep or partial loss of consciousness
proton-pump inhibitor	reduces or blocks secretion of stomach acid
vaccine	produces active immunization in the formation of antibodies

GROUPS OF MEDICATIONS	ACTION
Anti-infective agents	
antiamebic	destroys or suppresses the growth of amoebas
antibacterial	an anti-infective agent directed against bacteria
antibiotic	inhibits the growth and reproduction of bacteria
antifungal	an anti-infective agent directed against fungi
antiparasitic	an anti-infective agent directed against parasites
antiviral	an anti-infective agent directed against viruses
Cardiac drugs	
antiarrhythmic	prevents or corrects irregularities in heart rhythm or force of beat
beta-adrenergic blocker	reduces rate and force of heart contraction
calcium channel blocker	slows heart rate; dilates coronary arteries
hypolipidemic or statin	reduces cholesterol
nitrate/antianginal	dilates coronary arteries; lowers blood pressure
Gastrointestinal drugs	
antidiarrheal	reduces intestinal motility to treat or prevent diarrhea
antiflatulent	reduces intestinal gas
cathartic	produces evacuation of the bowel
emetic	induces vomiting
histamine H_2 antagonist	decreases secretion of stomach acid
laxative	stimulates emptying of large intestine
Psychotropics	
antianxiety agent	alters mental activity; reduces anxiety
antidepressant	raises level of chemicals in the brain to relieve depression
antipsychotic	relieves symptoms of psychoses
Respiratory drugs	
antitussive	suppresses coughing
asthma maintenance	prevents asthma attacks
bronchodilator	relaxes bronchial smooth muscle to prevent spasms
decongestant	opens the air passages of the nose and lungs
expectorant	induces coughing to remove respiratory secretions
mucolytic	loosens mucus to improve elimination

Within the pharmacy, there are many different forms that a drug may take and many different methods for administration of the medication. The most common are the solid forms that include *capsules* (in a gelatin container), *tablets* (solid form), *lozenges* (a medicated tablet or disc), and *suppositories* (a soft substance molded for insertion through a body opening such as the rectum). A semisolid or liquid form of medication that is most often used for *topical* (on the skin) application includes creams, ointments, and lotions. Finally, liquid preparations include *parenteral solutions* (a sterile solution intended for subcutaneous, intramuscular, or intravenous injection or insertion into an IV solution), *aerosols* (medication dispersed in a mist), *elixirs* (sweetened liquid intended for oral use), *tinctures* (medication dissolved in an alcohol solvent), *emulsions* (a mixture of two liquids which do not disperse into each other), and *suspensions* (fine particles of drugs that do not dissolve into the liquid). Due to the lack of mixing, the last two forms must be shaken well immediately before use.

Methods and Delivery Sites

Pharmaceutics is the study of the delivery, absorption (entry into the body through the digestive tract or across another membrane), metabolism, and elimination of drugs by the body. The form and method of delivery is very important for the efficacy of the treatment. The various methods of administration of medications are listed in Table 11-10.

TABLE 11-10   Methods of Drug Delivery

hyperalimentation	administration of a nutritionally adequate solution through a catheter into the vena cava; used in cases of long-term coma, severe burns, or severe gastrointestinal syndromes
infusion	the slow injection of a solution into a vein or subcutaneous tissue
inhalation	administration by breathing in a nebulizer or aerosol
instillation	introduction through a body cavity such as the ear or eye (liquid)
intradermal	into the skin
intramuscular	into the muscle
intraorbital	into the orbit of the eye
intraspinal	into the spine or vertebral column
intrathecal	into the subdural space of the spinal cord
intravenous	into the vein (most often the antecubital area of the arm or the hand)
iontophoresis	process of introducing medication into the tissue using an electric current
subcutaneous	under the skin
sublingual	under the tongue
topical	applied to the skin
transdermal	absorption through the skin; usually in the form of a patch placed on the surface

Pharmacy Personnel and the Science of Pharmacy

The people who work in the pharmacy and as pharmacy representatives throughout the hospital have various backgrounds. The pharmacist is authorized to prepare and dispense the medications ordered for the patient. These individuals have completed a bachelor's degree, master's degree, or PharmD (doctorate in pharmacy) program, passed the national examination, and are licensed by the state in which they practice. The role of the PharmD has expanded through the years, and they are actively involved in the assessment of patients and the development of medication regimens and patient education to achieve the best medical outcome for the patient. The *pharmacy intern* is a student in a pharmacy program who is preparing to complete the requirements. The *pharmacy resident* is a graduate pharmacist who is obtaining additional training and expertise, often in a specialty such as geriatrics (dealing with elderly patients and their medication issues), *nuclear* or *radiopharmacy* (treatment of diseases with radioactive materials), or other disease-specific disciplines such as *nephrology* (diseases of the kidney) or diabetes. The *pharmacy technician* is trained and authorized to prepare and dispense medications under the supervision of a registered pharmacist.

The science of pharmacy involves many individuals who study all facets of drug development, delivery, interactions, and use. *Pharmaceutics* is the study of how to prepare a medication (tablet, liquid, injectable, etc.) for use by the body, while *pharmacokinetics* is the study of the concentration of the drug in a patient's body and how the drug is metabolized and cleared from the body. This is very important to the appropriate treatment of the patient, as the level of medication in the body is critical to achieve the therapeutic outcomes for the patient. *Pharmacotherapeutics* is the study of the use of drugs and the effects on the patient's condition. They also look at patient behavior with respect to medications, such as *compliance* (the act of taking medications according to the instructions). *Pharmacology* is a scientific field that investigates how drugs affect the body systems at the biochemical level. One of the newest areas of interest is *pharmacogenetics*, which is the study of the relationship between the genetic profile of an individual and that individual's response to medication. *Pharmacogenomics* is the biotechnological science that combines the techniques of medicine, pharmacology, and genomics and is concerned with developing drug therapies that are specific to the genetic makeup of an individual patient. The investigation of plants and other natural sources as the origin of new drugs is called *pharmacognosy*.

Medical Vocabulary

Knowledge of the medical vocabulary outside of the discipline of pharmacy is important to achieve effective communication with other health care providers and to begin to understand what medications are appropriate for the condition of the patient. Several common medical terms are presented in Table 11-11 and are grouped into similar concepts.

TABLE 11-11   Medical Terms

Medical assessment	
diagnosis	the identification of a disease from its signs and symptoms
contraindication	any condition that makes a particular medication or form of treatment undesirable or unsafe (such as an allergy to a medication)
etiology	the cause of a disease
prognosis	the expected outcome of the course of the disease
sign	objective evidence of a disease or disorder
symptom	subjective evidence of a disease based on the perception of the patient
syndrome	a group of signs and symptoms that characterize a particular abnormality
Allergies and inflammation	
allergen	an agent that causes the body to respond with the symptoms of an allergy
allergist	a physician with a specialty in the diagnosis and treatment of allergies
allergy	a reaction to a particular antigen (allergen). Allergies can include "hay fever," which results in runny or itchy eyes and nose and sneezing and coughing, contact dermatitis or allergic reactions to substances coming in contact with the skin or mucous membranes, or drug allergies (to ingested agents such as sulfa or penicillin), which can be life threatening
anaphylaxis	a hypersensitive reaction to exposure to an antigen that is immediate, can induce shock-like symptoms, and may be fatal
antibody	a product of the immune system in response to an antigen. Each antibody recognizes a specific antigen. Allergens are a specific type of antigen
antigen	an agent that stimulates the body to produce antibodies
eczema	an inflammatory condition of the skin
hives	an itchy skin eruption characterized by weals (a raised mark on the skin) with pale interiors and well-defined red margins; usually the result of an allergic response to insect bites or food or drugs
pruritic	an intense sensation of itching
psoriasis	a chronic skin disease characterized by dry red patches covered with scales
urticaria	an eruption or rash associated with severe itching
Autoimmune and inflammatory conditions	
arthritis	inflammation of the joints
cystitis	inflammation of the urinary bladder and ureters
gastritis	inflammation of the lining of the stomach; nausea and loss of appetite and discomfort after eating
hepatitis	inflammation of the liver
immunity	resistance to infection
infection	invasion and multiplication of microorganisms in body tissues
inflammation	a localized protective response elicited by injury or destruction of tissues, which serves to destroy, dilute, or wall off (sequester) both the injurious agent and the injured tissue. It is characterized in the acute form by the classical signs of pain (dolor), heat (calor), redness (rubor), swelling (tumor), and loss of function (functio laesa)
meningitis	inflammation of the meninges (the membrane around the brain and spinal cord)
nephritis	inflammation of the nephron (the structure that filters the blood and produces urine) in the kidney
pathogen	any disease-producing microorganism (e.g., bacteria, viruses, etc.)
phlebitis	inflammation of the vein (often seen in the legs)

(Continued)

TABLE 11-11 (Continued)

Autoimmune and inflammatory conditions	
rheumatism	popular name for any of a variety of disorders marked by inflammation, or degeneration, of connective tissue structures of the body, especially the joints and related structures, including muscles, tendons, and fibrous tissue, with pain, stiffness, or limitation of motion
rheumatologist	a physician with specialty training in the diagnosis and treatment of rheumatic disease (those characterized by inflammation such as arthritis)
Cardiovascular system	
aneurysm	a sac formed by the dilatation of the wall of an artery, a vein, or the heart; it is filled with fluid or clotted blood, often forming a pulsating tumor
arteriosclerosis	any of a group of diseases characterized by thickening and loss of elasticity of arterial walls
atherosclerosis	a common form of arteriosclerosis with formation of deposits of yellowish plaques (atheromas), containing cholesterol, in the walls of large and medium-sized arteries
bradycardia	a heart rate that is slower than normal
cardiologist	a physician with specialty training in the diagnosis and treatment of diseases of the heart and vascular system
congestive heart failure	reduced ability or failure of the heart to pump an adequate blood supply to the body
diastolic pressure	the force exerted by the blood on the blood vessels when the heart is at rest (blood is flowing slowly through the vessel)
embolism	the sudden blocking of an artery by a clot or foreign material that has been brought to its site of lodgment by the blood current
fibrillation	rapid, uncoordinated, and ineffectual heartbeat
hemorrhage	severe bleeding
hypertension	high blood pressure
hypotension	low blood pressure
myocardial infarction	injury to the heart muscle (myocardium) due to inadequate oxygen supply caused by the occlusion of a coronary artery
occlusion	blockage of a blood vessel
syncope	fainting; a transient loss of consciousness due to inadequate blood flow to the brain
systolic	the force exerted by the blood when the heart is in a state of contraction (blood is flowing rapidly through the vessel)
tachycardia	rapid heart beat
vasoconstriction	contraction of the smooth muscles surrounding the blood vessels
vasodilation	relaxation of the smooth muscles surrounding the blood vessels
Cancer or oncology	
ascites	fluid that accumulates within the abdominal cavity
basal cell carcinoma	the most common type of skin cancer
benign	the description of tissue that is determined to be normal (not cancerous)
carcinogen	any substance that may cause cancer
carcinoma	a malignant new growth made up of epithelial cells tending to infiltrate the surrounding tissues and give rise to metastases
chemotherapy	the use of chemical agents in the treatment or control of disease; most often associated with the treatment of cancer
leukemia	a malignant disease characterized by an increase in white blood cells
lymphoma	a tumor of the tissue in the lymph glands
malignant	the description of tissue that is cancerous and that will grow out of control

(Continued)

TABLE 11-11 (Continued)

Cancer or oncology	
mastectomy	removal of a breast
melanoma	a cancer of the skin
metastasis	spreading of disease to another part of the body
neoplasm	a new growth of tissue in which the multiplication of cells is uncontrolled and progressive (also called a tumor)
oncologist	a physician with specialty training in the treatment of cancer
tumor	a new growth of tissue in which the multiplication of cells is uncontrolled and progressive (also called a neoplasm)

Clinical and anatomic laboratory testing	
anemia	a reduction in the number or function of the red blood cells. Symptoms include fatigue, weakness, shortness of breath, and pale skin
biopsy	examination of tissues or liquids from the living body to determine the existence or cause of a disease
blood gas	an analysis of the dissolved gases in blood plasma, including oxygen, nitrogen, and carbon dioxide
blood type	the designation of the blood based on normally occurring antigens on the surface of the red blood cell (A, B, O, or AB)
BUN	blood urea nitrogen; nitrogen in the blood that can be measured to determine kidney function
CBC	complete blood count; an analysis of the blood cells to determine number, type, size, shape, and iron content
clinical laboratory technologist	an individual who has obtained the education and training to perform the testing in a clinical diagnostic laboratory
coagulation	the process of blood clotting
creatinine clearance	a test to measure the function of the kidney
cytology	a special area of pathology that studies the structure of cells to determine if they are normal or cancerous
DIC	a condition where the clotting of blood is out of control and results in bleeding (disseminated intravascular coagulation)
erythrocyte	a red blood cell
heparin	a naturally occurring component of the blood that prevents blood clotting; is often given to prevent stroke in patients whose blood clots too fast
liver profile	a group of chemical tests that indicate the function and health of the liver
pathologist	a physician trained in diagnostic laboratory medicine
pathology	the branch of medical science that studies the causes and nature and effects of diseases
plasma	the fluid portion of the blood
PT and PTT	laboratory tests that measure the ability of the blood to clot
serum	the fluid portion of the blood after it has been allowed to clot

Disturbances of metabolism	
acidosis	a condition where the blood pH is too acidic (< 7.4), which impairs body functions such as delivery of oxygen to the tissue
alkalosis	a condition where the blood pH is too alkaline (> 7.4), which impairs body functions such as delivery of oxygen to the tissue
diabetes	a chronic disease where blood glucose does not enter the cells and the blood sugar remains high, causing harm to the tissues
diuresis	increased formation of urine, which is a common symptom of diabetes

(Continued)

TABLE 11-11 (Continued)

Disturbances of metabolism	
glucose tolerance test	a test for diabetes based on the ability of the body to metabolize an induced increase in blood sugar
hypoglycemia	an abnormally low concentration of glucose in the blood
jaundice	yellow appearance of the skin, usually associated with a malfunction or strain on the liver
polydipsia	excessive thirst
polyuria	excessive urine formation
Infection	
amebiasis	an infection caused by an amoeba
antiseptic	an agent that inhibits the growth of a microorganism but does not necessarily kill it
bacteriocide	an agent that will kill bacteria
bacteriostat	an agent that will inhibit the growth of bacteria
decubitus ulcer	a bedsore
febrile	body temperature above normal; fever
impetigo	a very contagious infection of the skin; common in children; localized redness develops into small blisters that gradually crust and erode
incubation	the period between exposure to an infective agent and the appearance of symptoms
pertussis	whooping cough; an acute infectious disease of the respiratory tract
rubella	German measles
sterilization	the process of destroying all microorganisms so that an item is free of contamination
toxin	a noxious or poisonous material
virus	a submicroscopic agent of infectious disease

Common Medical/Pharmacy Abbreviations and Terminology

The medical vocabulary, as in other highly technical fields of science and technology, has many acronyms and abbreviations that are used in everyday conversation. A familiarity with the terms is important to ensure comprehension and smooth communication. Some of these abbreviations are listed in Table 11-12. Asterisked abbreviations should be avoided, as they may be misinterpreted and lead to a medication error. Please refer to Chapter 28, "Preventing and Managing Medication Errors: The Technician's Role."

TABLE 11-12 Common Abbreviations

A–B			
aa	of equal parts	ADH	antidiuretic hormone
AAA	abdominal aortic aneurysm	ADI	American Drug Index
AAD	antibiotic associated diarrhea	ad lib	as much as needed
AAO	awake, alert, and oriented	adm	admission
ABG	arterial blood gas	ADR	adverse drug reaction
ac	before eating	AED	antiepileptic drug

(Continued)

TABLE 11-12 (Continued)

A–B

AFB	acid fast bacillus	ASHD	atherosclerotic heart disease
AHFS	American Hospital Formulary Service	ASHP	American Society of Health-System Pharmacists
AIDS	acquired immunodeficiency syndrome	BBVD	bloodborne viral infection
alb	albumin	BE	barium enema
ALD	alcoholic liver disease	bid	twice a day
ALL	acute lymphocytic leukemia	biw	twice weekly
amb	ambulatory or mobile	BM	bowel movement
AML	acute myelogenous leukemia	BMA	bone marrow aspiration
amt	amount	BMR	basal metabolic rate
ANDA	Abbreviated New Drug Application	BOM	bilateral otitis media (ear infection)
AOB	alcohol on breath	BP	blood pressure
AODM	adult onset diabetes mellitus Type II	BPM	beats per minute
APhA	American Pharmacists Association	BS	breath sounds
APT	Association of Pharmacy Technicians	BUN	blood urea nitrogen
aq	aqueous	BW	body weight
ARDS	acute respiratory distress syndrome	BX	biopsy
ARF	acute renal failure		
ASAP	as soon as possible		

C–E

c	with	C/O	chief complaint
C&S	culture and sensitivity (for identification of bacteria and the appropriate antibiotics)	COPD	chronic obstructive pulmonary disease
		CPR	cardiopulmonary resuscitation
CA	cancer	CSF	cerebrospinal fluid
Ca	calcium	CVA	cerebral vascular accident
CAD	coronary artery disease	CXR	chest x-ray
cath	catheter	DAW	dispense as written
CBC	complete blood count	D&C	dilatation and curettage; a surgical procedure usually performed under local anesthesia in which the cervix is dilated and the endometrial lining of the uterus is scraped away
CC	chief complaint		
ccu	clean catch urine		
CDC	Centers for Disease Control and Prevention		
		D.D.S.	doctor of dental surgery
CF	cystic fibrosis	DDx	differential diagnosis
CHF	congestive heart failure	diag	diagnosis
CI	cardiac index (heart function)	DIC	Drug Information Center
CMV	cytomegalovirus	DICC	disseminated intravascular coagulopathy coagulation
CNS	central nervous system		
CO	cardiac output		

(Continued)

TABLE 11-12 (Continued)

C–E

Disp	dispense	D5W	dextrose 5% in water
DJD	degenerative joint disease	D5/0.33	dextrose 5% in 0.33% sodium chloride
DM	diabetes mellitus	D5/$^1/_2$ Ns	dextrose 5% in 0.45% sodium chloride
DNR	do not resuscitate	D5NS	dextrose 5% in 0.9% sodium chloride
D.O.	doctor of osteopathy	EBL	estimated blood loss
DOE	dyspnea (shortness of breath) on exertion	ECG or EKG	electrocardiogram
		EEG	electroencephalogram
DPT	diphtheria, pertussis, tetanus vaccine	ENT	ears, nose, and throat
DRG	diagnosis related group (billing)	ESR	erythrocyte sedimentation rate
DRL	dextrose 5% in Ringer's lactate	ETOH	ethanol
DTD	let such doses be given	ETT	endotracheal tube
dx	diagnosis		

F–I

FBS	fasting blood sugar	Hgb	hemoglobin
FDA	Food and Drug Administration	HIV	human immunodeficiency virus
FFP	fresh frozen plasma	HLA	histocompatibility antigen
FTT	failure to thrive	HLTV-III	human lymphotropic virus, Type III (AIDS agent, HIV)
FU	follow up		
fuo	fever of unknown origin	HO	history of
Fx	fracture	HR	heart rate
g, gm	gram	HS	at bedtime
g or gtt	drops	HSV	herpes simplex virus
GC	gonorrhea	HTN	hypertension
GFR	glomerular filtration rate	hx	history
GI	gastrointestinal	I&D	incision and drainage
gr	grain	I&O	intake and output
GSW	gunshot wound	ID	infectious disease
GTT	glucose tolerance test	IM	intramuscular
GU	genitourinary	IMV	intermittent mandatory ventilation
GYN	gynecology	IND	investigational new drug
h, hr	hour	INF	intravenous nutritional fluid
HA	headache	IV	intravenous
HBP	high blood pressure	IVPB	intravenous piggyback; small volume parenteral
HCG	human chorionic gonadotropin		
*Hct	hematocrit	IVSS	intravenous soluset; small volume parenteral
HDL	high density lipoprotein		

(Continued)

TABLE 11-12   (Continued)

J–M

JODM	juvenile onset diabetes mellitus Type I	MAO	monoamine oxidase
K	potassium	MAP	mean arterial pressure
KCl	potassium chloride	MAR	medication administration record
kg	kilogram	MBT	maternal blood type
KVO	keep vein open	mcg, ug	microgram
L	left	MCV	mean cell volume
L	liter	MD	medical doctor
lb	pound	mEq	milliequivalent
LDH	lactate dehydrogenase (an indicator of cell death)	Mg	magnesium
LE	lupus erythematosus	MI	myocardial infarction; heart attack
LIH	left inguinal hernia	mL	milliliter
LMP	last menstrual period	mmol	millimole
LOC	loss of consciousness or level of consciousness	MMR	measles, mumps, rubella (vaccine)
		MRI	magnetic resonance imaging
LP	lumbar puncture	MRSA	methicillin resistant staph aureus
LPN	licensed practical nurse	MS	multiple sclerosis
LR	lactated Ringer's solution	MSSA	methicillin-sensitive staph aureus
LVP	left ventricular pressure	mvi	multivitamin injection

N–P

Na	sodium	NSR	normal sinus rhythm
NAD	no active disease	NT	nasotracheal
NCPA	National Community Pharmacists Association	n/v	nausea/vomiting
		O_2	oxygen
NDA	new drug application	OOB	out of bed
NED	no evidence of recurrent disease	*OD	doctor of optometry
NF	National Formulary	OD	overdose/right eye
ng	nanogram	OM	otitis media (ear infection)
ngt	nasogastric tube	OPV	oral polio vaccine
NIDDM	non-insulin dependent diabetes mellitus	p	para or after
NKA	no known allergies	PA	physician assistant
NKDA	no known drug allergies	PAP	pulmonary artery pressure
NMR	nuclear magnetic resonance	pb	piggyback
non rep (nr)	do not repeat	pc	after meals
NPH	neutral protamine Hagedorn insulin	PDR	*Physicians' Desk Reference*
NPO	nothing by mouth	PE	pulmonary embolus/physical examination/pleural effusion
NRM	no regular medications		
NS	normal saline (0.9% sodium chloride)		
NSAID	nonsteroidal anti-inflammatory drug		

(Continued)

TABLE 11-12 (Continued)

N–P

PFT	pulmonary function tests	PR	by rectum
pg	pictogram	PRN	as needed
pH	hydrogen ion concentration (measure of acidity or alkalinity)	Pt	patient
		PT	prothrombin time (measure of clotting system of the blood)
PharmD	Doctor of Pharmacy		
pid	pelvic inflammatory disease	PTH	parathyroid hormone
PMH	previous medical history	PTT	partial thromboplastin time (measure of blood clotting system
PO	by mouth		
POD	postoperative day	PUD	peptic ulcer disease
PP	postprandial (after meals)	PVC	premature ventricular contraction
PPD	purified protein derivative (skin test for tuberculosis exposure)	PVD	peripheral vascular disease
		PZI	protamine zinc insulin

Q–Z

q	every (e.g., q4h = every 4 hours)	SDS	same day surgery
QA	quality assurance	SGA	small for gestational age
qam	every morning	s.i.d.	once a day (semel in dia)
*qd	daily	signa/sig	let it be written or imprinted on the label
qh	every hour	sl	sublingual (under the tongue)
*qhs	every bedtime	SLE	system lupus erythematosus
*qid	four times a day	smo	slips made out
QNS	quantity not sufficient	SOB	shortness of breath
*qod	every other day	sos	if necessary
qs	quantity sufficient	*ss	half/semi
r, rt	right	SSE	soap suds enema
RA	rheumatoid arthritis	SSKI	saturated solution of potassium iodide
rbc	red blood cell	STAT	immediately
RDA	recommended daily allowance	STD	sexually transmitted disease
RIA	radioimmunoassay	Sx	symptoms
RL	Ringer's lactate	tab	tablet
R/O	rule out	T&C	type and cross (blood for transfusion)
ROM	range of motion	TB	tuberculosis
ROS	review of systems	TIBC	total iron binding capacity (blood test for anemia)
RRR	regular rate and rhythm		
RTC	return to clinic	tid	three times daily
Rx	treatment	*tiw	three time weekly
s	without	TLC	total lung capacity
SBE	subacute bacterial	TO	telephone order
*sc, sq, sub Q	subcutaneous (under the skin)	TPN	total parenteral nutrition

(Continued)

TABLE 11-12   (Continued)

Q–Z			
tr	tincture	V fib	ventricular fibrillation
tw	twice a week	VO	verbal order
TWE	tap water enema	VRE	vancomycin-resistent enterococcus
Tx	treatment	VS	vital signs
UA	urinalysis	VSS	vital signs stable
UAO	upper airway obstruction	VT	ventricular tachycardia
UC	ulcerative colitis	WBC	white blood cells
ud	as directed	WDWN	well-developed, well-nourished
*ug	microgram	WNL	within normal limits
ung	ointment	WO	written order
USP	United States Pharmacopoeia	W/U	work up
USPDI	United States Pharmacopoeia Drug Information	XL	extended release
		XS	excessive
ut duct, ud	as directed	YOB	year of birth
UTI	urinary tract infection	Zn	zinc
VA	Veteran's Administration	ZnO	zinc oxide
VC	vital capacity		

Commonly Used Apothecary Symbols

Apothecary symbols are an important part of the history of the practice of pharmacy (Table 11-13). However, many of the symbols have multiple meanings or are easily misinterpreted. Serious medical error can be caused by the misinterpretation of abbreviations, apothecary symbols and dose designations; therefore, caution is

TABLE 11-13   Apothecary Symbols

*ʒ	drachma/dram (1/8 ounce or 60 grains)
ʒ	ounce
ʒss	half ounce, tablespoon
* m	minim (drop)
↑	elevated or increased
↓	depressed or decreased
Δ	change
%	percent
=	equals
°	degree
♀	female
♂	male

advised when confronted with information in this format. See Chapter 28, "Preventing and Managing Medication Errors," for additional information.

The Prescription

To provide patients with medications for home use, a physician or other properly licensed medical practitioner must provide a *prescription* (a written or electronic order for a medication or treatment). An *order* to dispense a medication to an inpatient for immediate use in the hospital is not considered a prescription, but is a written instruction that is documented on the patient's chart. The written or electronic prescription must include the patient's name, name of the medication, the dose and frequency of use, and the number of doses to be dispensed over a period of time. The practitioner's full name, address, and telephone number must be included. Many physicians will use a preprinted or computer-generated form, which contains the standard information and blank spaces for the practitioner to handwrite or electronically complete the information about the patient, the medication desired, and directions for use. Some states have enacted regulations requiring that a generic be dispensed at all times. If a physician wants to ensure his or her patient receives the brand name drug, the prescription should contain the phrase "Brand Name Medically Necessary," "Brand Name Only," "Dispense as Written," or "DAW."

If the prescription is for a controlled substance or narcotic, the practitioner must also provide his or her DEA number. A valid DEA number consists of two letters: the first identifies the type of practitioner, and the second is the first letter of the practitioner's last name. The letters are followed by six numbers and a seventh number (or check digit) determined by a mathematical calculation of the first six numbers. The calculation is to add the first, third, and fifth numbers together. Then add the second, fourth, and sixth numbers together. Double the sum of the second, fourth, and sixth numbers. Add that to the sum of the first, third, and fifth numbers. The last digit of the resulting number is the check digit. For example, the calculation of the check digit for DEA number 123456 would be $1 + 3 + 5 = 9$ and $2 + 4 + 6 = 12$. The sum of the second calculation would be 24. Added together the result is 33, so the check digit is three. The DEA number for Dr. Blake, who is a physician, would appear as CB 1234563.

Summary

Medical terminology is a combination of word elements that describe medical history, medical diagnoses, current medical conditions, surgical interventions, etc., and, as such, the technician's understanding of this language of medicine is essential to effectively communicate with members of the health care team in the provision of patient care.

TEST YOUR KNOWLEDGE

Multiple Choice

1. The term *tracheotomy* indicates
    a. an injectable solution for the throat.
    b. a surgical procedure that involves cutting into the trachea.
    c. a viral infection of the trachea.
    d. a preparation for topical application.

2. The term *mammography* refers to
    a. a surgical procedure on the chest.
    b. a diagnostic term which indicates a malignancy.
    c. a preparation for topical application.
    d. a diagnostic procedure of the breast.

3. The term *cholecystectomy* refers to
    a. a surgical procedure for removal of the gallbladder.
    b. a diagnostic procedure on the gallbladder.
    c. the condition of having two gallbladders.
    d. a solution for irrigation of the gallbladder.

4. The abbreviation *pc*, used in an order or prescription, refers to _____ while *npo* indicates _____.
    a. the patient's compliance; no patient orders
    b. after meals; nothing by mouth
    c. a personal computer; no patient orders
    d. after meals; medication should be taken with meals

5. If a medication is to be given sublingually, it will be
    a. injected under the skin.
    b. instilled into the mouth.
    c. placed under the tongue.
    d. added to an IV preparation.

6. A medication categorized as an *analgesic*
    a. reduces anxiety.
    b. stabilizes a patient's blood sugar.
    c. reduces pain.
    d. increases heart rate.

7. The term *intravenous* refers to
    a. into the spine.
    b. into the vein.
    c. into the skin.
    d. into the mouth.

8. A medication classified as an *antibiotic*
    a. is used to treat a bacterial infection.
    b. is used to treat high blood pressure.
    c. is used to treat diabetes.
    d. is used to treat a heart arrhythmia.

9. If a drug is categorized as *OTC*, it
   a. is used to treat an ear infection.
   b. does not require a prescription for distribution.
   c. requires a prescription for distribution.
   d. must be shaken thoroughly just before use.

10. The term *myopathy* can be broken into the root word *myo-* and the suffix *-pathy*, meaning
    a. a disease of the inner ear.
    b. eye disease.
    c. a disease of the brain.
    d. muscle disease.

Matching

Match the term with its meaning.

1. _____ hepato-	a. false
2. _____ -itis	b. red
3. _____ diuretic	c. liver
4. _____ ad lib	d. tumor or mass
5. _____ signa/sig	e. reduces intestinal motility
6. _____ bronchodilator	f. a sterile solution
7. _____ -algia	g. directions for patient use
8. _____ pneumno-	h. twice a day
9. _____ pan-	i. diagnosis
10. _____ erythro-	j. lungs
11. _____ anesthetic	k. all
12. _____ bid	l. as much as needed
13. _____ intradermal	m. inflammation
14. _____ parenteral	n. state or condition
15. _____ hyper-	o. pain
16. _____ -ectomy	p. increases urine formation
17. _____ melano-	q. reduces symptoms of allergy
18. _____ antihistamine	r. surgical removal
19. _____ dx	s. black
20. _____ intra-	t. relaxes smooth muscle of the lung
21. _____ -ism	u. one
22. _____ pseudo-	v. study of drug delivery
23. _____ topical	w. over
24. _____ -oma	x. within

25. _____ mono-   y.   reduces itching

26. _____ pharmaceutics   z.   abolishes the sensation of pain

27. _____ antipruritic   aa. into the skin

28. _____ -scopy   bb. applied to the skin

29. _____ antidiarrheal   cc. below

30. _____ sub-   dd. diagnosis

Calculation

A prescription for a narcotic pain killer is submitted to the pharmacy. The ordering physician is listed as Dr. Thompson, with a DEA number of CA 4762343. What is wrong with the number? Define the correct number.

References

Dorland. (2007). *Dorland's illustrated medical dictionary*. Philadelphia: W. B. Saunders Co.

Steadman. (2005). *Steadman's medical dictionary*. Philadelphia: Lippincott Williams and Wilkins.

Web Sites

Dorland's Online Dictionary   www.dorlands.com/wsearch.jsp

Merck Source   www.mercksource.com/pp/us/cns/cns_home.jsp

12 Pharmaceutical Dosage Forms

Competencies

Upon completion of this chapter, the reader should be able to

1. Explain the different interpretations of "dosage form" by the patient, by members of the health care team, and by pharmacists.
2. List four physiochemical properties of a drug.
3. Name four formulation aids used in the preparation of a given dosage form.
4. Describe the advantages and disadvantages of the major classes of pharmaceutical dosage forms—namely liquids, solids, semisolids, and aerosols.
5. Differentiate between the characteristics of a solution and a suspension.
6. List five desirable qualities for an external suspension.
7. Name and define four solid dosage forms currently in use.
8. Explain the differences between compressed tablets, sublingual or buccal tablets, and multiple-compressed tablets.
9. Describe an oral osmotic (OROS) drug dosage design and give an example.
10. Outline five advantages of the transdermal patch.

Key Terms

additive	granule	polymorphism
aerosol	heterogeneous	preservatives
anhydrous	homogenous	propellant
anionic	hydroalcoholic	pyrogen
buffer system	hydrophilic	radio-opaque
capsule	hydrous	receptor
cationic	hygroscopic	refractory
delayed-release	intraocular	solution
density	iso-osmotic	suppository
diluent	isotonic	suspension
dosage form	lacrimal fluids	tablet
emulsifying agent	lipophilic	transdermal
emulsion	lotions	volatile
excipient	molecular form	wetting agent
extended-release	percutaneous	

Introduction

A drug or a medicinal agent is seldom administered alone. It is usually administered as a dosage form. A **dosage form** is a system or device for delivering a drug or a medicinal agent to the biological system. Drugs are defined as chemicals of synthetic, semisynthetic, natural, or biological origin. Drugs interact with human or animal biological systems resulting in an action. This action may either be intended to prevent, cure, or reduce ill effects in the human or animal body, or to detect disease-causing manifestations. In actual practice, a pure drug is rarely used. What is generally administered to obtain the desired effect is a drug-delivery system, called the *dosage form*. In a dosage form the active ingredient, referred to as the *drug*, is combined with inert or physiologically inactive materials to enable administration of the drug (e.g., administration of the drug in the form of a tablet, a capsule, or a solution).

The term *dosage form* means different things to different people. To a patient, for instance, the term signifies the gross physical or pharmaceutical form in which the drug is made available for administration or use (e.g., tablet, capsule, solution, injection, ointment). To the members of the health care team, the dosage form of a drug is a drug-delivery system. Any alteration in the system (e.g., a change in the amount or type of inert ingredient) may be expected to alter the delivery rate and the total amount of drug delivered at the site of action. The pharmacist, however, uses the term *dosage form* in a more comprehensive manner to include the physiochemical properties (both the physical properties and the chemical properties) of the drug itself. These properties consist of the particle size of the drug powder, the salt form of the drug substance, the polymorphic state of the drug substance, the dissolution characteristics of the drug, and the nature and quantities of various formulation aids used in the formulation and fabrication of the dosage form.

The *particle size of the drug powder* is important because smaller particles dissolve at a much faster rate than do larger particles. In order for a drug to be absorbed, it has to be in a solution form at the site of absorption. A faster drug dissolution rate assures rapid and complete absorption. Drugs that dissolve slowly tend to exhibit incomplete and/or erratic absorption.

Most drugs are either organic acids (e.g., phenobarbital), or organic bases (e.g., tetracycline, morphine, diphenhydramine). These drugs have poor solubility in the biological fluids. The *salt forms of these drugs* (e.g., phenobarbital sodium, tetracycline hydrochloride, morphine sulfate, diphenhydramine hydrochloride) are generally used because salts dissolve more rapidly in the biological fluids.

Polymorphism means that a compound can exist in more than one crystalline form, called the *polymorphic form of the drug*. The chemical nature (chemical formula and chemical properties) of all crystalline forms of the substance are identical, but the physical properties (crystal shape, melting point or boiling point, solubility, etc.) of the crystalline forms may be different. The manufacturers prefer to use the polymorphic form of the drug that possesses better water solubility and exhibits good stability of the drug.

Dissolution characteristics describe the rate at which the drug dissolves. Drugs that dissolve at a faster rate generally exhibit better reproducible and complete absorption than drugs that dissolve relatively slowly.

The nature and quantities of various formulation aids (inert ingredients used in the preparation of the given dosage form) used in the formulation and fabrication of the dosage form are usually used in the preparation and formulation of a dosage form and include the following:

diluent an agent that dilutes or reconstitutes a solution or mixture.

excipient an inert substance added to a drug to give form or consistency.

- **Diluents**, also called bulking agents, are used to increase the bulk weight of a dosage form so that an acceptable product may be formulated.
- **Excipients** are various formulation aids that must be used to help formulate and prepare the dosage form.
- **Additives** are additional formulation aids, which may be essential to successful formulation and fabrication of the dosage form.
- **Preservatives**, as the name suggests, are substances that retard, minimize, or prevent the growth of microorganisms in the dosage form.

Classification of Dosage Forms

additive an addition of an active ingredient to a solution that is intended for intravenous administration or irrigation.

preservatives substances used to prevent the growth of microorganisms.

While most drugs are synthesized as solid powders or solid crystals, some drugs may exist only in liquid or a gaseous state of matter. A solid drug can be formulated either as a solid dosage form (tablet, powder, or capsule) or as a liquid dosage form (solution or emulsion). A drug existing solely as a liquid can only be formulated as a liquid dosage form (solution or emulsion) because it is difficult if not impossible to prepare a solid dosage form of a liquid substance. However, if the dose of the drug is extremely small (e.g., a few drops), it may be possible to absorb this small amount of the liquid onto a powder and formulate the mixture as a capsule or tablet dosage form. Similarly, a drug that is gaseous in nature can only be formulated as a gaseous dosage form.

Because of the diverse physical nature of drug substances, their mode of action, and the route of administration used for delivery of drugs, dosage forms may be classified in several different ways. However, the major classes of pharmaceutical dosage forms may be broadly categorized into four main classes: (1) liquid dosage forms, (2) solid dosage forms, (3) semisolid dosage forms, and (4) miscellaneous dosage forms.

Liquid Dosage Forms

molecular form the drug form that elicits biological responses regardless of dosage form.

receptor a cell component that combines with a drug or hormone to alter the function of the cell.

Biological responses are elicited by the **molecular form** of the drug (i.e., the drug shows its response when molecules of the drug interact with the **receptors** in the body). The term *receptor* is used to indicate substances in the body that interact with drug molecules and exhibit pharmacologic, therapeutic, or toxic effects. Thus, no matter in what state of matter (solid, liquid, or gas) in which the dosage form a drug is administered, the action at the molecular level will involve interaction of the biological constituents (receptors) with the individual molecules of the drug. Therefore, for a drug to elicit the desired response, it has to be present in the form of a molecular dispersion (solution) at the site of action (Figure 12-1). Thus, liquid dosage forms (solutions, emulsions, or suspensions, etc.) are often the dosage form of choice for the following reasons:

- They are effective more quickly than a solid dosage form (tablets or capsules) because the solid form of the drug will have to dissolve in the gastric fluids after administration of the dose.
- Liquid dosage forms are easier to swallow (especially for pediatric and geriatric patients) than solid dosage forms. Small children and older patients may be afraid that the tablet or capsule may get stuck in their throat.

FIGURE 12-1

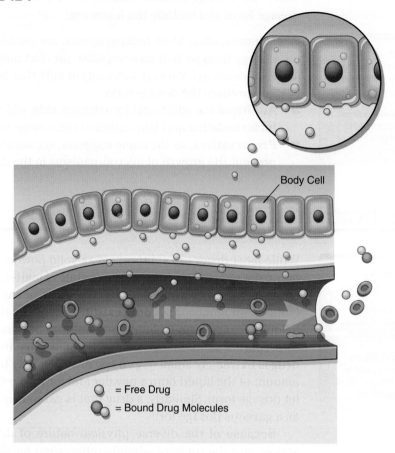

Body Cell

○ = Free Drug
○○ = Bound Drug Molecules

FIGURE 12-1 Drug molecules that attach to plasma proteins in the blood stream render the drug inactive. Unattached drug molecules are free to leave the blood stream and act on cells. The cells contain receptors that attract drug molecules to cross the cell membrane and enter the cell. The drug molecules can then act to stimulate or inhibit cell function.

- Certain substances can be given only in a liquid form because either the character of the remedy or the large dose in any other solid dosage form makes administration of the drug difficult or inconvenient.
- Certain chemical substances may cause pain (e.g., potassium iodide and bromide) or gastric irritation (e.g., aspirin) when administered in a solid state.
- Liquid dosage forms are the dosage forms of choice in certain types of pathological conditions in which absorption of particular ions or molecules is dependent on dissolution of the drug, and the absorption environment is deficient in effecting dissolution. For example, a liquid dosage form provides calcium ions in an absorbable form in patients who lack acidity to dissolve solid calcium compounds (e.g., calcium carbonate powder).

Although liquid dosage forms offer many advantages, they also have some disadvantages. The following disadvantages are most common to almost all liquid dosage forms:

- Liquid dosage forms (especially those that contain water) are liable to undergo deterioration and loss of potency much faster than the corresponding solid dosage forms. For example, when aspirin (acetylsalicylic acid) is dissolved in water, it hydrolyses into salicylic acid and acetic acid (vinegar) in a very short period of time. This is one reason aspirin is not available as a solution dosage form.

■ Liquid dosage forms present many flavoring and sweetening problems. Some drugs are so bitter that it is almost impossible to mask their bitter taste. Similarly, some drugs have an unacceptable odor and present serious problems in masking their odor.

■ Many instances of incompatibility arise because of interaction between dissolved substances in the liquid dosage form.

■ Liquid dosage forms containing water provide an excellent medium for the growth of bacteria and mold. For this reason, substances that prevent or retard the growth of molds and bacteria (called preservatives) are often included in the formulation of such preparations. The most commonly used preservatives in liquid products are methylparaben, propylparaben, benzoic acid, and sodium benzoate. The presence of preservatives in a liquid dosage form may present problems of a diverse nature. The U.S. Pharmacopoeia (USP) discourages the use of antibacterials for products intended for newborns. Liquid preparations for neonates do not necessitate the inclusion of preservatives due to the potential of causing either acute or long-term adverse effects.

■ Inaccuracy in various doses may arise due to the patient measuring the dose with a household measuring device (e.g., a teaspoon). A teaspoonful is supposed to be equivalent to five milliliters, but a "standard" teaspoon is not sold as a "standard" measuring device. Some people think that a teaspoon is the smallest spoon in the kitchen, whereas others may think that a teaspoon is an average-sized spoon. A few years ago, a study was conducted by the outpatient department of a hospital to determine the perception of a teaspoonful dose by an average patient. Patients were given a measured amount of a liquid formulation with instructions to take one teaspoonful twice a day for 10 days and bring the bottle containing unused formulation, as well as the teaspoon used for measuring the dose, back to the hospital. The results demonstrated that the volume of a teaspoonful perceived by the patients ranged between two milliliters and more than seven milliliters.

■ Oral liquid dosage forms are bulkier to carry than oral solid dosage forms and necessitate the use of a measuring device (e.g., a teaspoon). Carrying a bottle containing a liquid medication as well as a teaspoon is considered cumbersome by many people, and this may lead to reduced patient compliance of using the medication.

■ Many interactions arise because of changes in solubility produced by mixing solutions and/or solvent alterations.

Liquid dosage forms are generally classified into two main categories: liquid dosage forms containing soluble matter and liquid dosage forms containing insoluble matter.

Liquid dosage forms containing soluble matter

solution a homogeneous mixture of one or more substances dispersed in a dissolving solvent; clear liquid with all components completely dissolved.

hydrophilic water-loving.

Liquid dosage forms containing soluble matter are called **solutions**. A solution consists of a solute (substance dissolved) in a solvent (liquid in which the solute is dissolved). A liquid dosage form may consist of one or several soluble substances (solutes) dissolved in a suitable solvent (usually water). The solute in a liquid dosage form may be a solid, a liquid, or a gas, and the solvent may be any **hydrophilic** liquid. The term hydrophilic (*hydro-* = water, *-philic* = loving) is used for water-miscible substances. Hydrophilic solvents are preferred because such a solvent system is safe to the human body and is able to mix with body fluids. Examples of hydrophilic solvents include water, glycerin, ethanol, propylene glycol, and polyethylene glycols. Some of the potential problems that one should be aware of in dealing with the solution dosage forms are described next.

Solvent system. Since most drugs are either weak organic acids or weak organic bases, they possess sufficient solubility in organic solvents (e.g., alcohol) but lack adequate solubility in water. Therefore, solutions of such drugs are generally made using a blend (mixture) of solvents. Products intended for oral administration usually utilize a **hydroalcoholic** solvent system. A hydroalcoholic (*hydro-* = *water,* alcoholic = containing alcohol) solvent system is one that contains both water and alcohol. Some hydroalcoholic systems contain more than 20 percent alcohol (e.g., elixirs). Obviously, when a product prepared using a hydroalcoholic solvent is either diluted with water or combined with a product prepared using only water as the solvent, the mixture is likely to cause precipitation of the poorly water-soluble compound or appear milky due to lack of sufficient alcohol in the system.

> **hydroalcoholic**
> a mixture of water and alcohol.

Concern has been expressed over the undesirable pharmacologic and potential toxic effects of alcohol when ingested in pharmaceutical products, particularly by children. The FDA (Food and Drug Administration) has proposed that manufacturers of OTC (over-the-counter) oral products restrict the use of alcohol and include appropriate warnings on the labeling of their products. It should be noted that in the case of neonates, ingestion of alcohol (in a pharmaceutical product) can cause some serious problems. For example, alcohol can alter liver function, cause gastric irritation, and can also affect neurological depression. Neurological depression may cause lethargy and poor feeding (reduced formula intake), resulting in unnecessary workups for suspected sepsis. It is for this reason that the American Academy of Pediatrics Committee on Drugs recommends that, if possible, alcohol should not be included in medicinal products intended for children. The recommended alcohol limit for OTC oral products intended for children is shown in Table 12-1.

pH change. In those instances where alcohol should not be used as a solvent system, the manufacturer uses a salt form of the drug that, unlike the drug itself, possesses good water solubility. For acidic drugs, the salt form is generally the sodium salt or the potassium salt, and for basic drugs, the commonly used salt forms are the hydrochloride or the sulfate salts. Since the combination of a basic drug with a strong acid (e.g., hydrochloric acid or sulfuric acid) or an acidic drug with a strong base (e.g., sodium hydroxide or potassium hydroxide) results in a strongly acidic or a strongly basic solution, the pH of the resulting solution is far removed from neutrality (pH of 7).

Although dilution of these solutions with water does not pose any problems, one must be careful if two such solutions are mixed. For example, a solution con-

TABLE 12-1 Recommended Alcohol Limit for OTC Oral Preparation

CHILD'S AGE	MAXIMUM ALCOHOL CONCENTRATION
Under 6 years of age	0.5%
6 to 12 years of age	5%
12 years of age and adults	10%

taining the hydrochloride of one drug when mixed with a solution containing the sodium salt of another drug is likely to result in the precipitation of both drugs. This is because the hydrochloride and sodium portions mixed together will neutralize each other, resulting in a poorly water-soluble weakly basic drug, and a poorly water-soluble weakly acidic drug.

Buffer system. A number of drug solutions are stable within a given pH range. To ensure maximum stability of the drug and a longer shelf life of such solutions, a **buffer system** is used. A buffer system helps to resist a change in the pH of the solution when a small amount of an acid or a base is added to the solution. Buffer systems used in pharmaceutical dosage forms generally consist of either a mixture of a weak acid and its corresponding salt with a strong base, or a mixture of a weak base and its corresponding salt with a strong acid. The purpose of using a buffer system is to maintain the pH of the solution of the dosage form within the range of its optimal or maximal stability. It should be realized, however, that dilution of a drug product's solution that has been formulated with a buffer system is likely to reduce the capacity (or the strength) of the buffer system, and consequently the ability of the buffer to resist the change in pH.

> **buffer system**
> used to maintain the pH of a drug solution within the range of optimum stability, or when the pH of blood and body fluids are maintained virtually constant although acid metabolites are continually being formed in the tissues or are being lost in the lungs.

Liquid dosage forms containing insoluble matter

Some drugs are insoluble in solvents that are commonly used in the preparation of liquid dosage forms, and therefore these drugs cannot be formulated as solutions. To derive some or all of the advantages of administering a liquid dosage form, insoluble solutes may be suspended in a suitable liquid (vehicle). There are two common dosage forms of the drugs that do not possess adequate solubility to be formulated as solutions: **suspensions** and **emulsions**.

Suspension dosage forms are those dosage forms in which the solid (called the *internal phase* or the *dispersed phase*) is suspended or dispersed in a liquid. The liquid is referred to as the *dispersion phase* or the *external phase*. The dispersed solid is generally in a state of fine subdivision (i.e., the solid particles are very small in size). The liquid phase (external phase) in most pharmaceutical suspensions is water, and the suspension is called an *aqueous suspension*.

A suspension formulation may be preferred over the administration of the solute as a solid dosage form because the solid may have poor solubility. When formulated as a suspension, the solid will generally show a better rate of solubility (dissolution rate) because of two reasons: improved wetting of the drug particles, and increased surface area of the drug particles due to the very small size of the particles.

Pharmaceutical suspensions may be classified into three groups: (1) orally administered mixtures, (2) externally applied lotions, and (3) injectable suspensions.

> **suspension** a liquid containing finely divided drug particles uniformly distributed.
>
> **emulsion** a heterogeneous system of at least one immiscible liquid intimately dispersed in another in the form of droplets, stabilized by the presence of an emulsifying agent.

Orally administered mixtures. Orally administered mixtures may supply insoluble and often distasteful substances in a pleasant-tasting liquid dosage form. Examples of oral suspensions are oral antibiotic syrups, which normally contain 250 to 500 milligrams of the solid material (drug) per 5 milliliters (teaspoonfuls) of suspension. The concentration of the suspended material may be greater in the case of pediatric drops or in antacid preparations and **radio-opaque** suspensions. Radio-opaque suspensions are generally used for diagnostic purposes. For example, barium sulfate suspension is administered before taking an X-ray of the intestinal tract to determine obstructions in the intestines. Barium sulfate is radio-opaque because it does not allow the X-rays to pass through it.

> **radio-opaque**
> having the property of absorbing X-rays.

Externally applied lotions. Lotions are suspension dosage forms intended for external application to the skin or mucus membrane. Externally applied lotions provide dermatological materials in a form that is convenient and suitable for external application to the skin. The concentration of the dispersed phase in such formulations may exceed 20 percent of the total formulation (e.g., calamine lotion).

Injectable suspensions. Injectable suspensions provide an insoluble drug in a form suitable for intramuscular or subcutaneous administration. The concentration of solid particles in these preparations may range from 0.5 percent to 30 percent. These preparations are generally of low viscosity, since viscosity affects the ease of injection. Particle size is another significant factor in these preparations, since particle size of the solids affects the availability of the drug, especially in depot therapy (e.g., Procaine Penicillin G or insulin NPH). The term *depot* signifies that the drug is released over a long period of time. These injectable preparations are formulated to contain the active ingredient in a relatively minute particle size. This enables the suspension to pass easily through the needle of the syringe.

An acceptable suspension should possess the following desirable qualities:

- Since suspensions by definition are unstable disperse systems, the suspended material should not settle rapidly. The particles that do settle down must be readily re-dispersed into a uniform mixture (suspension) when the container is shaken.
- The suspension must not be too viscous, and it should pour freely from the orifice of the bottle or through a syringe needle.
- In the case of suspensions intended for external application (e.g., a lotion), the product must be fluid enough to spread easily over the affected area, yet it must not be so mobile that it runs off the surface of application.
- Suspensions intended for external application should dry quickly after application to the affected area.
- Suspensions intended for external application should provide an elastic protective film that will not rub off easily.
- The suspensions intended for external application should have an acceptable color and odor.

Emulsions consist of a system of at least one immiscible liquid intimately dispersed into another liquid in the form of droplets. Emulsions are not **homogeneous** systems. A homogeneous system is one that contains ingredients that are miscible with each other (e.g., a solution of sodium chloride in water, or a solution of sucrose in water). Emulsions are **heterogeneous** systems (i.e., they contain ingredients that do not mix with each other—for example, a mixture of oil and water). The droplet size of the dispersed phase in most emulsions generally range from about 0.1 to 10 micrometers in diameter (one millimeter = 1,000 micrometers, or one centimeter = 10,000 micrometers).

Emulsions are also by definition unstable dispersions, and the system is stabilized by the presence of one or more **emulsifying agents**. An emulsifying agent is a substance that helps to keep the mixture of immiscible liquids dispersed into each other for a reasonable length of time. Examples of emulsifying agents include gelatin, acacia, and synthetic substances that reduce the tension between the immiscible liquids. The choice of an emulsifying agent(s) is governed by the composition of the emulsion and the intended route of administration of the emulsion. Either the dispersed phase or the continuous phase of an emulsion may range in consistency from that of a free-flowing mobile liquid (e.g., emulsions and lotions of relatively low viscosity) to a semisolid (e.g., an ointment).

Emulsions, in general, are considered dispersions of oil and water. When an oily substance or an oil is the dispersed phase, the emulsion is called an oil-in-water (o/w) emulsion. When water is the dispersed phase, the emulsion is called water-in-oil (w/o) emulsion. More recent in its origin is a third type of emulsion, described as a micro-emulsion or transparent emulsion. Micro-emulsions are also called transparent emulsions because they possess the property of transparency due to the very small size of the dispersed droplets (e.g., Haley's M.O.). The droplet size in micro-emulsions is generally 0.05 micrometers or less.

Medicinal emulsions for oral administration are usually of the oil-in-water type emulsions, requiring the use of o/w emulsifying agents. The common examples of oil-in-water emulsifying agents include synthetic nonionic surface active agents (e.g., Tweens and Spans), acacia (also known as gum arabic), tragacanth, and gelatin. A surface active agent is a substance that has the property of reducing surface tension (tension at the surface of a liquid) and interfacial tension (tension at the interface of immiscible liquids).

An oil-in-water emulsion is a convenient means of orally administering oily liquids, especially those that have an unpleasant taste or odor (e.g., mineral oil and castor oil). Because the oil globules are completely surrounded by an aqueous medium, the taste of the oil droplets is almost completely masked, and the odor is also markedly suppressed. Also, it has been observed that some oil-soluble compounds (e.g., some vitamins) are absorbed more completely when emulsified than when administered orally as an oily liquid or oily solution. This is because, in an emulsion, the very small globule size of the oily substance renders a large surface area of the oily solution (provided by the oil droplets). Therefore, the large surface area of the oily substance is made available for contact at the absorption site, resulting in better and faster absorption of the oily liquid. Similarly, the use of intravenous emulsions has been studied as a means of maintaining debilitated patients who are unable to assimilate materials administered orally. Radio-opaque emulsions have found application as diagnostic agents in X-ray examinations.

Emulsions intended for external application may be either the oil-in-water type or water-in-oil type. An oil-in-water emulsion for external use offers the advantage of being water-washable and non-staining to clothes. In the preparation of such emulsions, the following emulsifying agents (in addition to the ones already mentioned) are used: triethanolamine stearate, sodium lauryl sulfate, and monovalent soaps (e.g., sodium oleate). The water-in-oil emulsions, which are used almost exclusively for external application, contain one or several of the following emulsifying agents: polyvalent soaps (e.g., calcium palmitate), synthetic nonionic sorbitan esters, wool fat, and cholesterol.

In pharmaceutical and cosmetic products for external use, emulsification is widely used to formulate dermatological and cosmetic lotions and creams that have better patient acceptability. For example, in the formulation of foam-producing aerosol products, the liquefied gases that propel the emulsion from within the container (called the **propellant**) form the dispersed liquid phase. When the emulsion is discharged from the container, the liquefied gases vaporize. The vaporization of the gases turns the emulsion into a foam.

Because emulsions are heterogeneous and unstable in nature, they present various stability problems. For example, an improper selection of the emulsifying agent, either in quality or in quantity, may lead to separation of the emulsion during storage. By shaking the container, the emulsion may or may not reform. When the

propellant a substance used to help expel the contents of a pressurized container.

emulsion does not reform on shaking the container, the emulsion is said to have broken. Once the emulsion is broken, it cannot be reformed. Therefore, caution must be exercised when an emulsion is to be diluted or mixed with another liquid. An emulsion may be diluted only with a liquid that is miscible with the external phase. Also, dilution of an emulsion may dilute the concentration of the emulsifying agent, leading to the instability or breaking of the emulsion. If the dilution is done with a liquid possessing characteristics different from those of the external phase of the emulsion, the emulsion can break. The same is true when an emulsion is mixed with another liquid. When two emulsions are mixed, another factor that must be considered is the nature of the emulsifying agent in the two emulsions.

If one emulsion contains an **anionic** (carrying a negative charge) emulsifying agent and the other contains a **cationic** agent (carrying a positive charge), the mixture will tend to produce interaction between the positive charges and the negative charges of the emulsifying agents, and both emulsions may break.

A simple method to determine the type of emulsion (oil-in-water or water-in-oil) is to dilute the emulsion with an equal quantity of water and shake the container. An oil-in-water emulsion will dilute with water and appear homogeneous. A water-in-oil emulsion will not dilute with water and have a non-homogeneous appearance.

anionic carrying a negative charge.

cationic carrying a positive charge.

Gels and jellies

Gels and jellies are also two-phase systems of a solid and a liquid. However, they differ from true suspensions because in these preparations it is difficult to distinguish between the external phase and the internal phase. The particles of the solid phase are interlinked like irregular meshwork; thus, the liquid partly surrounds the interconnected solid particles and is partly occluded by them (e.g., lidocaine gel).

Solid Dosage Forms

Solid dosage forms in current use include powders, granules, capsules, and tablets. Powders and granules constitute a very small portion of the solid dosage forms dispensed today. Capsules and tablets have gained popularity for the following reasons:

- They are easy to package, transport, store, and dispense.
- They offer convenience for self-medication.
- They are largely devoid of taste and odor.
- They are more stable than other solid dosage forms.
- They are pre-divided dosage forms and, therefore, provide an accurate dose.
- They are especially suited for those drugs that are not stable in liquid form and, therefore, provide a longer shelf life for such drugs.
- They are more suited for the formulation of sustained and delayed release of medication because controlled-release techniques are generally more applicable to solid dosage forms than to liquid dosage forms.

Powders

Powders have certain inherent advantages. For example, they give the physician free choice of selecting drugs, the amount of drug in each dose, and the amount of powder to be contained in each dose. They permit the administration of large "bulk" of a medicinal, and they may be administered as a suspension if the patient has difficulty swallowing a tablet or a capsule. However, powders are not the dosage form of choice for drugs that have an unpleasant taste or unacceptable odor, or are not stable when exposed to atmospheric conditions.

Powders are prescribed for both internal use and external application. When intended for internal use, powders may be prescribed as *bulk powders*, as *dispersible powders*, or as *divided powders*. Powders prescribed for external use are generally dispensed as bulk powders (dusting powders).

Bulk powders are supplied as multi-dose preparations. The dose is measured by the patient. This dosage form is used for those drugs administered in a large dose, and the drug possesses very low toxicity. This is because of the variation in dose weight inherent in domestic methods of measurement (e.g., with a household teaspoon). Also, such measurements are volumetric. Therefore, the weight of powder in each dose weight will vary with the bulk **density** of the powder and the degree of fill (depending on whether level or heaped measures are used). Bulk density of a powder is a measure of weight of powder per unit volume. Antacids are frequently prescribed in this manner. Minor differences in the amount of antacid ingested by the patient is of little consequence. Antacids contain substances such as aluminum hydroxide, calcium or magnesium carbonate, magnesium trisilicate, and sodium bicarbonate. Other drugs that may be prescribed as a bulk powder must be those where a small variation in the dose does not have a major influence on the therapeutic effect of the drug. Bulk powders may also be used as antiseptics or cleansing agents for a body cavity. For example, tooth powders generally contain a soft soap or detergent and a mild abrasive. Similarly, douche powders are products that are completely soluble and are most commonly intended for vaginal use, although they may also be formulated for nasal (nose), otic (ear), or ophthalmic (eye) use.

Dispersible powders are readily wetted by water to form an extemporaneous suspension for oral administration. The quantity contained in a dispersible powder may be enough for a single dose, or it may contain a sufficient amount to last two to three days. It is important that the dispersible powder formulation is such that the powder, upon suspending in the liquid vehicle, settles slowly and no foam is produced. For powders not easily wetted by the liquid, a **wetting agent** may be used. A wetting agent is a substance that helps wetting of the particles in a powder. Sodium lauryl sulfate and synthetic surface active agents are generally used as wetting agents. If a wetting agent is used, it must be relatively free from any toxicity. Dispersible powders are used for substances that are unstable in the presence of water, and, therefore, cannot be formulated as liquid dosage forms.

Divided powders are dispensed in individual doses. To achieve accuracy, each dose is individually weighed, transferred to a powder paper, and the powder paper is folded. Divided powders containing **hygroscopic** and **volatile** drugs are packaged in waxed paper, then double-wrapped with a bond paper to improve the appearance of the completed powder. Hygroscopic substances are those substances that absorb moisture when the substance is exposed to humid air. Examples of hygroscopic substances include calcium chloride, ephedrine sulfate, hydrastine, hyoscyamine lithium bromide, pepsin, phenobarbital sodium, physostigmine, pilocarpine, potassium citrate, and sodium iodide. Volatile substances are those substances that evaporate at very low temperatures, such as room temperature. Examples of volatile substances include alcohol, chloral hydrate, and peppermint oil. Hygroscopic and volatile powders may also be dispensed in metal foils, small heat-sealed plastic bags, or other containers that restrict the passage of air through them.

density weight per unit volume.

wetting agent a surface active agent which allows materials to penetrate into a solid surface.

hygroscopic moisture absorbing.

volatile evaporates at low temperature.

Dusting powders are locally applied nontoxic preparations intended to have no systemic action (i.e., they are not absorbed into blood circulation). They are dispensed in a very fine state of subdivision to enhance their effectiveness and minimize irritation. Commercial dusting powders are available in sifter-top cans, in sterile envelopes, or as aerosols in pressurized containers. Foot powders, talcum powders, and antiperspirants available as aerosols are generally more expensive than those marketed in nonaerosol containers, but they offer the advantage of protection of powder from air moisture and contamination, as well as convenience of application.

Absorbent powders are intended to absorb secretions and excretions on the surface of the skin from superficial infections. They usually contain starch, often with zinc oxide, kaolin, or talc.

Antifungal substances, such as salicylic acid and zinc undecylenate, are applied as powders diluted with starch, kaolin, or talc. Insecticides, such as chlorophenothane and benzene hexachloride, are incorporated in dusting powders for the destruction of lice, fleas, ticks, and such.

Granules

granule a very small pill, usually gelatin-coated or sugar-coated, containing a drug to be given in a small dose.

Granules are small, irregular particles. They are used as effervescent granules, or they may be marketed for therapeutic purposes. Effervescent granules derive their name from the fact they produce effervescence when the granules come into contact with water. Effervescent granules are formulated to contain a carbon dioxide-producing combination of a weak acid and a weak base (alkali), in addition to the active therapeutic ingredient(s). On solution in water, carbon dioxide is released as a result of acid-base reactions, causing effervescence, which serves to mask the taste of salty and bitter medications. The base usually employed in effervescent granules is sodium bicarbonate. The weak acid used in these granules may be citric acid, tartaric acid, or sodium biphosphate. In most effervescent granules a combination of citric acid and tartaric acid is used, rather than using either acid alone. When tartaric acid is used alone, the resulting granules readily lose their firmness and crumble. The use of citric acid as the sole acid results in a sticky mixture that is difficult to granulate. The combination of citric acid and tartaric acid results in granules that are neither too sticky nor too soft. Effervescent granules also offer the advantage of quick dissolution of the active ingredient(s) contained in the formulation. Laxative salts, such as magnesium and sodium sulfate, are frequently formulated as effervescent granules.

Capsules

capsule a soluble container enclosing medicine.

Capsules are solid dosage forms in which the drug is enclosed in a "shell" of a suitable form of gelatin. Mothes and Dublanc, two Frenchmen, are generally credited with the invention of gelatin capsules in 1834. The two-piece telescoping capsule was invented by James Murdock of London in 1848 and patented in England in 1865.

Capsule dosage forms offer a wide variety of advantages. Some of these, not necessarily in the order cited, are as follows:

- Easy to carry the day's supply.
- Easy to swallow.
- Easy to identify the product due to availability of capsules in wide range of colors.
- Pharmaceutically elegant.

- Easy to mask undesirable taste and/or odor of the active ingredient(s) because the shell containing the active ingredient is tasteless.
- Flexibility of providing combination drugs.
- Economically produced in large quantities.

Upon administration, the gelatin shell of the capsules softens and begins to partially dissolve within 10 to 20 minutes after the capsule is swallowed, releasing the drug. The capsule shell is eventually digested by proteolytic enzymes and absorbed. Since the capsule shell may not dissolve completely in the gastric fluid, capsules should not be used for substances that may irritate the gastric mucosa, or very soluble compounds. Examples of these compounds include potassium chloride, calcium chloride, potassium bromide, or ammonium chloride. In these cases, when the partially dissolved capsule comes in contact with the stomach wall, the concentrated solution may cause localized irritation and gastric distress.

The capsule dosage form is available as (a) hard gelatin capsules and (b) soft gelatin capsules. Hard gelatin capsules are generally used for dry powders. The contents of these capsules may range from 50 milligrams to 1 gram of powder per capsule. Some manufacturers prefer to seal their capsules to prevent the loss of drug due to accidental opening, or to discourage easy removal of the contents, or as a safeguard against potential tampering. Soft gelatin capsules, also known as *soft shell* or *soluble elastic capsules*, are a one-piece construction with the liquid fill material literally wrapped inside a sealed, gelatin matrix. The contents of the soft gelatin capsule range from one minim (drop) to almost three milliliters. The capsule may be spherical (pearls) or ovoid (globules) in shape. Examples of drugs available as soft gelatin capsules include Digoxin, Ethosuccimide Ranitidine, vitamin E, and Advil Liqui-Gels.

Hard gelatin capsules are two-piece capsules manufactured as empty shells. The contents are filled in the capsule shell either mechanically or manually after the capsule shells are manufactured. Historically, hard gelatin capsules for human use have been available in various lengths, diameters, and capacities. There are eight different sizes. These are numbered as follows: 000, 00, 0, 1, 2, 3, 4, and 5 (Figure 12-2). Capsule Number 000 is the largest size and capsule Number 5 is the smallest size. Capsule size 000 is generally too large to be conveniently swallowed by a patient. However, this capsule size may be used in cases where the contents of the capsule are emptied and mixed with a liquid (e.g., orange juice) or food (e.g., applesauce). Capsule Number 00 is the largest size acceptable to most patients. The most commonly employed capsules for humans range from size 0 to size 5. Size 00 may occasionally be required if the volume of material to be filled into an empty capsule cannot be accommodated into a smaller capsule. Capsule sizes 000 and 00 are generally avoided because they may be too difficult to swallow. However, these sizes are useful when the contents of a capsule are intended

FIGURE 12-2

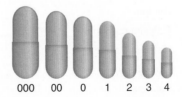

000 00 0 1 2 3 4

FIGURE 12-2 Various capsule sizes.

to be mixed with food for administration of medication to young children. Some patients, especially senior citizens, may find the smaller capsules (Number 5 and Number 4) somewhat difficult to handle.

The numerical designations of the capsule size are not based on any mathematical or scientific basis and do not reflect the capacity of the particular capsule. An arbitrary numerical designation was used when the first manufacturer of the empty gelatin capsules marketed its product, and this designation has been used ever since. Eli Lilly and Parke-Davis were the original pioneers in the manufacture of empty gelatin capsules. Both companies maintained this designation system. In recent years, empty hard gelatin capsules have been marketed by many other manufacturers. While most of the manufacturers have continued to follow the original numerical designation and almost original capsule volume for each capsule size, some manufacturers have not. Since the empty gelatin capsules are produced by various manufacturers, the fill volume of capsules (capacity) of the same designated size is not necessarily identical. Therefore, the volume of powder that can be filled in a given capsule size varies from manufacturer to manufacturer. It should be mentioned, however, that the weight of powder that can be accommodated in a given capsule size depends on two factors: (1) the density of the powder being placed in the empty capsule, and (2) the degree to which the powder can be compacted. A small-sized capsule can accommodate a much larger weight of a dense powder, but it will hold only a smaller weight of a much lighter (less dense) powder.

Empty gelatin capsules for veterinary use are available in three sizes. These are designated as Number 10, Number 11, and Number 12. Veterinarians refer to size 10 as a one-ounce capsule, size 11 as a half-ounce capsule, and size 12 is referred to as a quarter-ounce capsule. In recent years, some manufacturers have developed empty gelatin capsules of varying sizes to meet the needs of researchers using small animals (rabbits, guinea pigs, rats, etc.) or doing clinical research involving therapeutic comparative evaluation of two or more drugs.

Table 12-2 shows the weight of different powders that can be filled in empty gelatin capsules intended for human use.

The moisture content of a hard gelatin capsule ranges between 10 and 15 percent. Therefore, hard gelatin capsules should be stored in tight containers and under controlled conditions of relative humidity. Less than 10 percent moisture in a capsule tends to make the capsules brittle, and moisture content greater than 15 percent makes them stick to each other.

TABLE 12-2 Weight of Powder (mg) for Different Capsule Sizes

POWDER	Capsule Size							
	000	00	0	1	2	3	4	5
Acetaminophen	1100	750	540	420	310	240	180	130
Ascorbic acid	1420	980	700	520	400	310	220	130
Aspirin	975	650	490	325	260	195	130	65
Calcium carbonate	1140	790	600	460	350	280	200	120
Calcium lactate	800	570	460	330	260	210	160	110
Cornstarch	1150	800	580	440	340	270	200	130
Lactose	1250	850	600	460	350	280	210	140
Sodium bicarbonate	1430	975	715	510	390	325	260	130

Empty gelatin capsules are manufactured by dipping thin cylindrical rods in a solution of gelatin in water. The rods are removed quickly, and the gelatin solution adhering to the rods is dried. The capsules thus obtained are transparent. Capsules are usually colored by including a dye in the gelatin solution during manufacture of empty capsules. Colored capsules are used either for aesthetic reasons or to make them distinctive. Incorporation of titanium dioxide in gelatin solution makes the capsules opaque. The addition of sucrose in the gelatin solution increases the hardness of the capsule shell, and incorporation of sulfur dioxide results in transparent capsules.

Soft gelatin capsules are used to fill liquid ingredients in a capsule. The liquid should be nonaqueous, because the presence of water can soften and/or dissolve the gelatin shell. The liquid is filled in the capsules during the manufacture of soft-gelatin capsules (i.e., the capsules are filled with the contents during their manufacture). Soft gelatin capsules cannot be filled after the soft capsules have been manufactured. Soft gelatin capsules do not come in standard sizes. They are more elastic than hard gelatin capsules and contain a relatively larger moisture content. Oil-soluble products, such as vitamin E, or oily solutions of drugs are usually marketed in soft gelatin capsules.

All solid dosage forms, including capsule dosage forms, must meet USP standards for potency (test for content uniformity), the dose contained in each capsule (weight variation test), release of drug from the dosage form (disintegration test), and rate of release of drug from the formulation (dissolution test). If a batch does not meet any one of these tests, the batch cannot be released for sale. In almost all cases, when a batch fails to meet these requirements, the entire batch has to be destroyed.

Tablets

> **tablet** a solid dosage form of varying weight, size, and shape that contains a medicinal substance.

Tablets are solid pharmaceutical dosage forms prepared either by compression or by molding. They are the most popular of all the medicinal preparations intended for oral use. They offer the advantages of accuracy and compactness of dosage, portability of the dosage form, convenience of self-administration, and blandness of taste.

Tablets are available in various shapes and sizes. Although most frequently discoid in form, tablets may be round, oval, oblong, cylindrical, or triangular (Figure 12-3). Manufacturers generally add a colorant to a tablet formulation, either for identification or for aesthetic purposes. Some tablets are scored so that they may be easily broken in halves or in quarters. However, some tablets (e.g., sustained-action, extended release, or controlled-release tablets) should never be broken or crushed unless directed to do so by the manufacturer. This is because the technology used in the manufacture of such tablets may not warrant their breaking or crushing. A majority of tablet dosage forms are embossed with the name of the manufacturer or a tablet code number.

Depending on their method of production, tablets are classified as molded tablets or compressed tablets. Molded tablets were originally made from moist materials on a triturate mold. Later on, molded tablets were made by compression on a tablet machine. Such tablets were intended to be completely and rapidly soluble. Molded tablets are no longer in use.

Compressed tablets are formed by compression in a tablet machine and are made from powdered, crystalline, or granular material, either alone or in combination with excipients necessary to formulate a tablet. Excipients are substances that are "inert materials" and do not possess any therapeutic activity. Most tablet

FIGURE 12-3

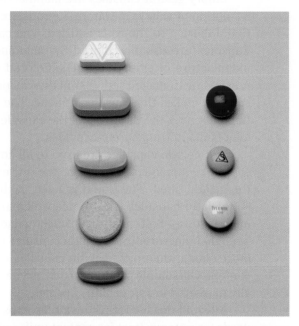

FIGURE 12-3 Various tablet shapes.

formulations contain two types of excipients: (1) those that are necessary to formulate a tablet dosage form, and (2) those that are included in the formulation for aesthetic purposes or to make the product more acceptable to the patient. Examples of some of the "non-essential" ingredients included in the tablet formulation are the following: colorants, flavoring agents, sweetening agents, and tablet coating materials.

- Colorants may be added to a formulation to make the tablet attractive in appearance or to impart identification characteristics to the product. Coloring agents used in pharmaceutical preparations must be those that are approved by the Food and Drug Administration.
- Flavoring agents or sweeteners may be included to make the product more acceptable (e.g., in chewable tablets). Flavoring agents may be natural (e.g., mint, lemon, chocolate, and vanilla), or they may be artificial (e.g., banana or bubblegum).
- A coating of a polymer may be applied to the finished product to make the tablet look glossy and shiny, or to help ease swallowing of the tablet. Some tablets are coated with a polymer to resist or prevent the release of drug in the stomach. Such coatings are called *enteric coatings*. Enteric coating is used for those drugs that are either unstable in the gastric environment or may cause gastric irritation and distress (e.g., aspirin is marketed as an enteric coated tablet [Ecotrin]).

The essential ingredients in a tablet formulation are those necessary for the successful production of the tablet dosage form. These include the following:

- *The drug.* Except for placebo tablets, all tablet formulations must contain the active ingredient.
- *Diluent.* Diluents are inert ingredients that add bulk to the tablet formulation. This ingredient is essential for those tablets that contain a very small amount of the drug. Without the diluent, the tablet will be so small that it could not be

made and could not be handled by the pharmacist or the patient. Examples of drugs that have a very small dose include the following: digoxin, levothyroxine, prednisone, chlorpheniramine, and so forth. Examples of diluents used in tablet formulations include lactose, starch, and cellulose esters.

- ■ *Binder.* A binder is a sticky substance used to hold (bind) the powders together, so that the powders do not segregate (un-mix) during the process of tablet manufacture. Examples of binders used in a tablet formulation include gelatin, starch, and acacia.

- ■ *Disintegrant.* The function of a disintegrant is to help disintegrate (break down) the tablet when it comes into contact with gastric fluids. It will essentially undo what the binder does to the tablet formulation. The most commonly used disintegrant is starch. More recently, some of the manufacturers of tablet dosage forms are using disintegrants that have the ability to disintegrate the tablet in the mouth as soon as it comes into contact with the saliva. These tablets have been variously advertised as rapidly disintegrating, quick dissolving, or rapid release.

- ■ *Lubricant.* A lubricant is included in the tablet formulation to facilitate the flow of tablet formulation through the tablet machine and also to prevent the formulation from sticking to the dies and punches of the machine during tablet compression. Magnesium stearate is the most commonly used lubricant in a tablet formulation. Stearates in general help to grease up the tablet machine to speed up production of the tablets.

Among the various types of compressed tablets available in the market, the following six are most common:

1. *Standard compressed tablets (CT).* These are the conventional tablets we are all familiar with and are compressed on a tablet machine.

2. *Enteric-coated tablets (ECT).* These are compressed tablets coated with a substance (polymer) that resists solution in the gastric fluid but dissolves in the intestinal fluids, thereby allowing the medication to be released in the intestinal tract.

3. *Sugar-coated tablets (SCT).* These are compressed tablets coated with sugar after the tablet has been compressed. Sugar coating is used to cover the objectionable taste and/or odor of the medicinal compound and to protect sensitive materials subject to deterioration due to light, air, oxygen, and so forth. However, sugar is a hygroscopic substance that can absorb moisture, resulting in tablets sticking to each other if they are stored in humid conditions. Also, the coating operation is very time consuming.

4. *Film-coated tablets (FCT).* These are compressed tablets covered with a thin film of a water-soluble polymeric material. Such coverings impart the same general characteristics as a sugar coating, and the coating operation is relatively simple, less time consuming, and much more economical.

5. *Sublingual or buccal tablets (ST).* These are tablets intended to be inserted below the tongue (sublingual tablets) or in the buccal pouch (buccal tablets) where the active ingredient may be directly absorbed through the oral mucosa. This dosage form is primarily used for those drugs that cannot be administered through the gastrointestinal tract due to stability problems. The drug must dissolve in the mouth quickly and should be absorbed very rapidly. Nitroglycerin is an example of such a drug.

6. *Multiple compressed tablets (MCT).* These are tablets made by more than one compression cycle. Multiple compressed tablets may be layered

tablets or press-coated tablets. Layered tablets are prepared by compressing additional tablet granulation on a previously compressed tablet. This tablet is, in fact, a two-layered tablet. The two layers may be of different colors to make the tablet look attractive and to help in its identification. Press-coated tablets are prepared by compressing another layer of tablet around a preformed compressed tablet. Press-coated tablets are often referred to as the "tablet within a tablet."

Miscellaneous tablets. Miscellaneous tablets are those specially formulated or intended for a specific function. There are three common types of miscellaneous tablets: chewable tablets, delayed-release tablets, and sustained-release tablets.

Chewable tablets are compressed and meant to be chewed rather than swallowed. Vitamin C and some antacid tables are marketed as chewable tablets. Chewable tablets are often intended for children. They contain a sweetening agent and a flavoring agent to make the product attractive for chewing. Mannitol is generally used as a sweetener because it has a sweet taste and also produces a cooling effect in the mouth.

Delayed-release tablets are special formulations of tablets in which the active ingredient is released some time after the tablet is ingested. Enteric-coated tablets fall under this category.

Sustained-release tablets are designed to release their active ingredient for a prolonged period of time. They are also variously described as "timed release," "long acting," "prolonged action," "sustained release," or some similar term implying an extended period of action for a given drug.

Table 12-3 lists some of the terms (names) that have been associated in describing commercial sustained release dosage forms. The use of some of these terms is no longer very common because the current USP terminology embodies these terms into one term: "extended release."

TABLE 12-3 A Listing of Some Names Associated with Oral Sustained Release Dosage Forms

constant release	prolonged action
continuous action	prolonged release
continuous release	protracted release
controlled action	repeat action
controlled release	repository
delayed absorption	retard
delayed action	slow acting
delayed release	slow release
depot	slowly acting
extended action	sustained action
extended release	sustained release
gradual release	sustained release depot
long acting	timed coat
long lasting	timed disintegration
long-term release	timed release
programmed release	

The USP definition. It should be mentioned that, based on the release characteristics of a drug from an oral dosage form, the USP (United States Pharmacopoeia) recognizes and defines two terms in solid dosage form technology: (1) immediate release dosage forms, and (2) modified release dosage forms. Rapid release dosage forms are those that release their active ingredient soon after ingestion. Immediate release tablets are designed to disintegrate and release their contents almost immediately after the tablet is ingested. These tablets do not contain any special rate-controlling features (e.g., special coatings or other special techniques that may control the release of an active ingredient(s) from the dosage form).

The USP defines modified-release tablets as dosage forms for which the drug-release characteristics (i.e., the time and location of drug release) are chosen to accomplish convenience or therapeutic objectives not offered by conventional dosage forms such as solutions, ointments, or dissolving dosage forms, such as immediate-release tablets. The USP defines two types of modified-release dosage forms: delayed-release and extended-release.

Delayed-release dosage forms are those dosage forms that release their drug at a time other than promptly after administration. Enteric-coated dosage forms are classified as delayed-release dosage forms.

Extended-release tablets are formulated in such a manner as to make the contained medicament available over an extended period of time following ingestion. Expressions such as "prolonged action," "repeat action," and "sustained-release" have also been used to describe such dosage forms. However, the term *extended-release* is used for pharmacopoeial purposes and designates the pharmacopoeial description of such tablets.

Extended-release dosage forms are dosage forms that allow at least a two-fold reduction in dosing frequency as compared to the conventional-release (immediate-release) dosage forms. For example, if the frequency of administration of the conventional-release (immediate-release) dosage form is every four hours, then the frequency of administration of the extended-release dosage form must be not less than every eight hours. Compared to conventional-release (immediate-release) dosage forms, extended-release dosage forms offer many advantages, including the following:

- Elimination of peak and valley levels of concentration of a drug in the blood during chronic administration.
- Reduction in adverse side effects because of fewer peak concentrations of the drug.
- Reduction in frequency of drug administration.
- Enhanced patient convenience.
- Enhanced patient compliance due to less frequent administration.

To be a successful extended-release dosage form, the drug should possess the following characteristics:

- It should not be absorbed either very rapidly or very slowly.
- It should be administered in relatively small doses and possess a good margin of safety.
- It should be absorbed uniformly from the gastrointestinal tract.
- It should be used in the treatment of chronic rather than acute conditions.

All tablet dosage forms, immediate-release as well as modified-release, must conform to the tests indicated in the USP monograph of the particular tablet dosage

delayed-release specifically formulated pharmaceutical dosage forms in which the active ingredient is released at a constant rate over a specific time period.

extended-release capsules that are formulated in such a way as to gradually release the drug over a predetermined time period.

form. The requirements for each test (content uniformity, weight variation, disintegration, and dissolution) depend on the nature of drug and the type of tablet dosage form.

The final two tablet forms we will discuss are lozenges and pellets. Lozenges, also known as troches or pastilles, are discoid-shaped solids containing the medicinal agent in a suitable flavored base. Lozenges are meant to be placed in the mouth, where they dissolve slowly, liberating the active ingredient. As used now, the term *pellet* signifies small cylinders meant to be implanted under the skin, or in the subcutaneous tissue, for prolonged and continuous absorption of potent hormones, such as testosterone or estradiol.

Semisolid Dosage Forms

Semisolid dosage forms are those dosage forms that are too thick or viscous to be considered a liquid dosage form, yet not solid enough to be considered a solid dosage form. The semisolid dosage forms discussed here are dosage forms intended for topical application. They may be applied to the skin, placed on the mucous membrane of the eye, or used in one of the body cavities (e.g., nasal, rectal, or vaginal). The most commonly used semisolid dosage forms are ointments, creams, pastes, and suppositories.

Ointments, creams, and pastes

Ointments, creams, and pastes are semisolid preparations used mainly for local application to the skin or mucous membrane. Very few ointments are intended to produce systemic effects due to absorption of drug into the bloodstream. Nitroglycerin is the most common example of an ointment that is applied to the skin for absorption into the bloodstream.

Pastes are similar to ointments and creams, except that pastes contain more solids and therefore are firmer (thicker) than ointments and creams. Ointments and creams that contain a medicinal agent (therapeutic ingredient) are called medicated ointments or medicated creams (e.g., nitroglycerin ointment, gentamicin sulfate ointment, nystatin cream, lidocaine ointment, and Tinactin cream). They are intended to deliver the drug or a therapeutic agent to the site of application. Some ointments are used for the physical effects they provide (e.g., emollients, protectants, or lubricants). Most ointment bases are used unmedicated for their physical effects. Ointment bases are classified according to the relationship of water to the composition of the base used to prepare the ointment or paste. The USP classifies ointment bases into four general groups: absorption bases, water-removable bases, oleaginous bases, and water-soluble bases.

The term *absorption* in *absorption bases* does not signify absorption of the drug. Absorption bases have the capability of absorbing water, hence the name "absorption" bases. There are two types of absorption bases: those that are essentially **anhydrous** in nature and those that are **hydrous**. Anhydrous absorption bases are called *anhydrous* because they contain no water. Hydrous absorption bases contain a certain degree of water. Because anhydrous absorption bases do not contain water, they are capable of absorbing more water than do hydrous absorption bases. However, both types of bases are insoluble in water and are not water-washable. These bases are used when either water or an aqueous solution must be incorporated into the ointment. Examples of anhydrous absorption bases include the following: Aquaphor, Aquabase, lanolin (or wool fat), and Polysorb. Included in the examples of hydrous absorption bases are cold cream, Eucerin, Nivea, and hydrous lanolin (or hydrous wool fat).

anhydrous containing no water.

hydrous combined with water, forming a compound with one or more molecules of water.

Water-removable bases are oil-in-water emulsions. Because the external phase of these bases is water, they can be easily washed off from the skin. Hence, they are also referred to as "water-washable" bases. These bases resemble creams in physical appearance. Examples of water-removable bases include hydrophilic ointment, Dermabase, Velvachol, and Vanishing Cream.

Oleaginous bases contain a mixture of high molecular weight and low molecular weight hydrocarbons. Hence, they are also termed *hydrocarbon bases*. High molecular weight hydrocarbons are solids, and low molecular weight hydrocarbons are liquids. A mixture of these two types of hydrocarbons results in a semisolid product that is useful as an ointment base.

Hydrocarbon bases are oily in nature and are insoluble in water. These bases do not contain water, nor do they absorb water. Therefore, these ointment bases are not water-washable. Upon application to the skin, they have an emollient effect and protect the escape of moisture from the skin. Therefore, they are effective as occlusive dressings. Because these bases are hydrocarbons in nature, they do not accept aqueous solutions. As a rule, liquids are generally not added to these bases for fear of making the final product too fluid. Examples of oleaginous bases include Petrolatum USP, Yellow Ointment USP, White Ointment USP, Plastibase, and Vaseline.

Water-soluble bases may be essentially anhydrous or they may contain water. In either case, they absorb water to the point of solubility. Thus, they are water-soluble and completely water-washable. Water-soluble bases are often referred to as *greaseless bases* because they do not contain oily components. Polyethylene Glycol Ointment-NF is an example of a water-soluble base.

Suppositories

suppository solid dosage forms for insertion into body cavities (e.g., rectum, vagina, urethra), where they melt at body temperature.

Suppositories are solid unit dosage forms intended for the application of medication to any of several body orifices, namely the rectum, vagina, or urethra. These dosage forms may exhibit their therapeutic activity locally or systematically, either by melting at body temperature or by dissolving in the aqueous secretions of the mucous membrane of the body cavity. Suppositories intended for administration via the vagina or the urethra are sometimes referred to as "inserts," particularly when the suppository is made by compression as a specially shaped tablet. Melting or dissolution of suppositories in the secretions of the body cavity usually releases the medication over a prolonged period of time. The commonly used suppository bases can be oleaginous (or oily), water-soluble, or hydrophilic (water-loving) solids. Examples of oleaginous bases are cocoa butter (also known as theobroma oil) and mixtures of synthetic triglycerides. Examples of water soluble bases are glycerinated gelatin, polyethylene, and glycol polymers. An example of a hydrophilic solid is polyethylene sorbitan monostearate, Polyoxyl 40 stearate, or a commercial product sold under the trade name Tween 40.

Rectal suppositories for adults are usually between 2.5 and 3.5 centimeters long. They weigh about two grams each and have a tapered shape. The largest diameter of a rectal suppository is about 1.2 to 1.3 centimeters (about 0.5 inch), usually tapered to about six to seven millimeters. For pediatric use, the diameter and the length is less, with reduction of weight to about one gram.

Vaginal suppositories vary in shape from globular or ovoid to modified conical shapes. They weigh between three and five grams and are used primarily for local effects.

Urethral suppositories, like vaginal suppositories, are primarily used for local action. These are slender rods from three to five millimeters in diameter. The female urethral suppositories range in length from 6 to 7.5 centimeters, and the male urethral suppositories range in length between 10 and 15 centimeters (four and six inches). Although somewhat flexible, urethral suppositories are firm enough for insertion.

Miscellaneous Dosage Forms

The dosage forms considered in this section have been classified "miscellaneous" for the sake of convenience. The properties associated with these dosage forms are either unique to them, or represent a combination of the properties of solid and liquid dosage forms.

Aerosols

aerosol finely nebulized medication for inhalation therapy.

Aerosols are systems consisting of a suspension of fine solid particles or liquid droplets in air or in a gas. Aerosols are held in a pressurized container. Pressure is applied to the aerosol system through the use of one or more propellants. A *propellant* is a liquid or gas that pushes the contents of an aerosol from within the container into the atmosphere when actuated by the valve assembly. The pressure exerted by the propellant or the propellants forces out the contents of the package through the opening of the valve. Because an aerosol dosage form is a pressurized package, it should be stored away from heat.

An aerosol dosage form consists of three components: the product concentrate, the container, and the propellant.

Product concentrate. The product concentrate represents the formulation consisting of the active ingredient and other ingredients used in the formulation. These ingredients include buffers, isotonicity-imparting ingredients, antioxidants, preservatives, and so forth that may be necessary to formulate the product.

Container. The container used in an aerosol dosage form may be made of glass, plastic, or metal. Metal containers tend to be relatively more expensive, but they can stand much higher pressures within the container. Plastic containers are relatively cheaper to make, but cannot withstand high pressure and may absorb the active ingredient or other formulation ingredients. Glass containers present fewer compatibility problems than plastic or metal containers, but glass containers are fragile and brittle, and they can break easily. Tin-coated metal containers are the most widely used metal containers for aerosols. Glass and plastic containers can withstand a maximum pressure of about 25 psig (pounds per square inch gauge), but metal containers can hold up to 80 psig.

Propellant. The propellant in an aerosol container is the driving force that propels the formulation from inside the container into the atmosphere. A propellant may be a gas (e.g., carbon dioxide, nitrogen, or nitrous oxide), or it may be a gas that can be liquefied under pressure or by reducing temperature. For many years, propellants widely used in aerosol products were chlorofluorocarbons (CFCs) sold under the trade name of *Freon*. Freons are gases at room temperature, but can be liquefied by cooling below their boiling point or by compression at room temperature. These propellants have been phased out because the chlorine content in their structure was considered to be responsible in reducing the amount of ozone in the stratosphere, resulting in an increased amount of ultraviolet radiation reaching the earth, which has been reported to increase the incidence of skin cancer and other adverse environmental effects.

The currently used propellants in aerosol packages are fluorocarbons that do not contain chlorine in their structures. They are organic compounds that contain carbon, hydrogen, and fluorine, but no chlorine.

Aerosols may be classified as either pharmaceutical aerosols or medicinal aerosols. Pharmaceutical aerosols are intended for topical administration or for administration into one of the body cavities, such as the nose or the mouth. Medicinal aerosols are intended both for local action in the nasal areas, the throat, and the lungs and for prompt systemic effect when absorbed into the bloodstream (e.g., from lungs—inhalation or aerosol therapy).

Aerosols offer convenience and ease of application. If the product is packaged under sterile conditions, sterility can be maintained without danger of contamination. The use of aerosols eliminates the irritation produced by the mechanical application of a medicinal, especially over an abraded area. Medication can also be applied to areas that are difficult to reach otherwise.

Inhalation therapy avoids the trauma of injections and the risk of potential of decomposition of orally administered drugs in the gastrointestinal tract.

The particle size of therapeutic aerosols affects their clinical usefulness. Therefore, it is essential that the aerosol dosage form be formulated with the most effective particle size. The particle size of the drug contained in aerosols is expressed in micrometers (previously referred to as *micron*). One centimeter is equal to 10,000 micrometers. Particles larger than 30 micrometers are most likely to be deposited in the trachea. Particles between the size range of 10 and 30 micrometers may reach the terminal bronchiole, and those between 3 and 10 micrometers may reach the alveolar duct. Smaller particles can penetrate deeper into the pulmonary tract: those between 1 and 3 micrometers may reach the alveolar sac, and particles less than 0.5 micrometers in size may reach the alveolar sac and be exhaled.

Metered dose inhalers. Metered dose inhalers are used in inhalation therapy involving potent medications. In these devices, the amount of drug discharged from the inhaler is controlled by an auxiliary valve chamber. A fixed amount of drug is delivered with a single depression of the actuator. Examples of metered dose inhalers include Advair, Aerobid, and Ventolin.

A unique translingual (*lingual* = pertaining to the tongue) aerosol formulation of nitroglycerin (Nitrolingual Spray) permits a patient to spray droplets of nitroglycerin onto or under the tongue for acute relief of an attack of angina pectoris due to coronary artery disease. Two metered spray emissions deliver 0.4 milligrams of nitroglycerin. Because translingual sprays are intended to deliver the drug on the tongue, Nitrolingual Spray should not be inhaled.

Isotonic solutions

Body fluids, including blood and **lacrimal fluids** (tears), have an osmotic pressure identical to that of a 0.9 percent solution of sodium chloride. Thus, a 0.9 percent solution of sodium chloride is said to be **iso-osmotic** with physiological fluids. *Iso-osmotic* is a physical term that compares the osmotic pressure of two substances. This term is often used interchangeably with the term **isotonic**, which means "having the same tone." A solution is isotonic with a living cell if there is no net gain or loss of water by the cell, or any other change in the cell, when in contact with that

lacrimal fluids tears.

iso-osmotic having the same tone.

isotonic having the osmotic pressure.

solution. Although most iso-osmotic solutions are isotonic, a solution that is iso-osmotic may not necessarily be isotonic. For example, a solution of boric acid is iso-osmotic with blood and lacrimal fluid, but is isotonic only with lacrimal fluids. It causes hemolysis of red blood cells, because the molecules of boric acid pass freely through the erythrocyte membrane regardless of concentration.

When dealing with isotonic solutions, caution must be exercised because any alteration in the composition of the solution (e.g., mixing it with another solution, or dilution with water) may affect the tonicity of the solution.

Parenteral products

Some drugs must be administered parenterally (by injection) because oral administration of these drugs either does not elicit any therapeutic effect, or if a therapeutic effect is elicited, it is less than desirable (i.e., they are not therapeutically effective when administered orally). For these drugs, a parenteral route of administration is one of the few routes that may be available for drug administration.

Parenteral products are dosage forms administered by injection. Hence, they are also referred to as *injectable products*. The most commonly used parenteral products are administered by three routes: (1) intravenously (directly into the bloodstream), either as a rapid bolus (single) dose or as a constant infusion, (2) intramuscularly, and (3) subcutaneously. Examples of parenteral products include the following: lidocaine intravenous injection, warfarin injection, aminophylline infusion, chlorpromazine intramuscular injection, and insulin subcutaneous injection.

Most parenteral products are manufactured on a large scale by the pharmaceutical industry. Many pharmacists, particularly those working in hospitals, home health care practices, or serving long-term care facilities, routinely handle and manipulate intravenous admixtures and injections. A pharmacist practicing in this specialty area has a special responsibility for understanding and implementing the standards of practice for handling sterile drug products.

Sterility is an absolute term. It means the absence of living microorganisms. A sterile product is completely devoid of living microorganisms. Depending upon the nature of the active ingredient(s) and the stage at which the preparation is sterilized, a parenteral product may be sterilized by an established method that assures sterility of the product. The USP recognizes the following five methods for sterilization of compendial articles: (1) steam sterilization, (2) dry-heat sterilization, (3) gas sterilization, (4) sterilization by ionizing radiation, and (5) sterilization by filtration. For home-use sterile products, the USP recognizes *sterilization by filtration* and *terminal sterilization by moist heat*. According to the USP, a home-use sterile product is a drug product requiring sterility that is prepared in and dispensed from a licensed pharmacy for intended administration by the patient or by a family member or other caregiver in a setting other than an organized, professionally staffed health care facility.

In addition to being sterile, injectable products must also be pyrogen-free. **Pyrogens** are products of microbial metabolism. The most potent pyrogenic substances (endotoxins) are constituents of the cell wall of gram-negative bacteria. Endotoxins are high molecular weight (about 20,000 daltons) lipopolysaccharides. The presence of pyrogens in parenteral preparations is considered a contamination because pyrogens should not be present in parenteral drug products. Pyrogens can be destroyed by heating at high temperatures. Glassware and equipment can be de-pyrogenated by maintaining a dry heat temperature of 180°F for 4 hours, 250°F for 45 minutes, or 650°F for 1 minute. The usual autoclaving cycle (moist

pyrogen an agent that causes a rise in temperature. Pyrogens are produced in bacteria, molds, viruses, and yeasts.

heat) does not destroy pyrogens. In general, it is impractical to remove pyrogens from a drug product.

The presence of pyrogens in parenteral drug products and their subsequent injection into the patient can cause fever, chills, pain in the back and legs, and malaise. The intensity of the pyrogenic response and its degree of severity is determined by the following factors:

1. Medical condition of the patient.
2. Potency of the pyrogen injected.
3. Amount of the pyrogen injected.
4. Route of administration of the pyrogen. Intrathecal is the most hazardous route, followed by intravenous, intramuscular, and the subcutaneous route.

Although pyrogenic reactions are rarely fatal, they can cause serious discomfort. In the seriously ill patient, pyrogenic reactions can cause potentially fatal shock-like symptoms.

As with any other route of drug administration, parenteral administration of drugs has some advantages and some disadvantages. In some clinical situations the advantages outweigh the disadvantages, while in other situations neither the advantage nor the disadvantage may outweigh the other.

Among the many advantages of parenteral administration of drugs, the following are noteworthy:

■ Parenteral administration provides a faster physiologic or therapeutic response than can be expected by other routes of administration.

■ Parenteral administration offers an alternative route of drug administration when a patient is unable to take medication by mouth (e.g., when the patient is unconscious, comatose, or cannot retain medication due to vomiting).

■ Parenteral administration offers an alternative route of drug administration to protect the drug from degradation due to liver metabolism and/or due to inactivation of drug in the gastrointestinal tract or first-pass metabolism by the liver.

■ Parenteral administration offers an alternative route of drug administration for those drugs that are destroyed or inactivated by gastric secretions such as hydrochloric acid and/or enzymes.

■ Parenteral administration is used to attain local effects for drugs used in dentistry and anesthesiology.

■ Parenteral administration offers a route to feed patients who cannot be fed by mouth (total nutritional requirements may be provided by parenteral route).

There are some disadvantages associated with parenteral therapy. Some of these disadvantages include the following:

■ Compared to products administered by non-parenteral routes, parenteral products are more difficult to produce.

■ Parenteral products require absolute sterility and must be pyrogen-free.

■ Due to stringent sterility and pyrogen-free requirements, parenteral products are much more costly to produce than nonparenteral products.

■ Parenteral products require special skills, equipment, devices, and techniques for handling and administration of the product.

■ Problems with doses or adverse effects associated with parenteral products may be difficult or impossible to reverse, because, once administered, a parenteral product cannot be removed from systemic circulation.

- Parenteral products may cause discomfort or pain at the site of injection.
- There is always a danger of air embolism by the intravenous route.

Gastrointestinal Therapeutic System

The gastrointestinal therapeutic system (GITS) is based on Alza Corporation's OROS (oral osmotic) design. This dosage form resembles an ordinary tablet, but the characteristics of drug release and drug delivery are very different. The system consists of a drug-containing core surrounded by a semipermeable polymer membrane that is pierced by a small (0.4 mm), laser-drilled delivery orifice. Upon ingestion of the dosage form, water is osmotically drawn through the membrane from the gastrointestinal tract at a constant and controlled rate, thereby creating a drug solution inside the tablet. The influx (intake) of water pushes the drug solution out of the orifice at a constant rate. The system operates on the principle of osmotic pressure.

The first product marketed in this country based on this technology was Ciba-Geigy's Acutrim, an over-the-counter appetite suppressant. Administered once daily, this dosage form delivered 20 milligrams of phenylpropanolamine initially and then 55 milligrams released osmotically for approximately 16 hours. Other examples of products using this technology include Glucotrol XL Extended Release Tablets and Procardia XL Extended Release Tablets.

Fast-Dissolving/Disintegrating Tablets (FDDTs)

Fast-dissolving/disintegrating tablets disintegrate and/or dissolve rapidly in the saliva without the need for water. Some tablets are designed to dissolve in saliva within a few seconds. These are true fast-dissolving tablets. Others contain ingredients that enhance the rate of tablet disintegration in the mouth and are more appropriately termed *fast-disintegrating tablets*. Fast-disintegrating tablets may take up to one minute to completely disintegrate. For a tablet to be considered fast-dissolving or fast-disintegrating, it must disintegrate in the saliva while maintaining a pleasant taste and feel in the mouth to allow maximal patient acceptability.

Examples of products available as FDDTs include the following: Benadryl Allergy & Sinus Fastmelt (OTC), Children's Benadryl Allergy & Cold Fastmelt (OTC), Claritin Reditab, Dimetapp Quick Dissolve Children's Cold and Allergy Tablets (OTC), Feldene Melt, Maxalt-MLT, NuLev, Pepsid RPD, Remeron Soltab, Tempra FirstTabs (currently available in Canada), Triaminic Softchew (OTC), Xyprexa Zydis, Zofran ODT, and Zomig ZMT.

A major claim of the some fast-dissolving/disintegrating tablet manufacturers is that these tablets exhibit increased bioavailability of the drug compared to the traditional compressed tablets. They offer the following reasons: (1) quick dispersion of the drug in saliva while the dosage form is still in the oral cavity can result in pregastric absorption from some formulations. Buccal, pharyngeal, and gastric regions are all areas of absorption of the many formulations. (2) Any pre-gastric absorption avoids first-pass metabolism and can be a great advantage in drugs that undergo a great deal of hepatic metabolism. The major advantage of these formulations is convenience. Pharmacists can expect to see an increase in the number of drug products marketed as FDDT formulations.

Ocular System

Topical application of drugs to the eye is common for eye disorders. The most prescribed ocular dosage form is the traditional eye-drop solution. But the eye-drop solution is not an efficient drug-delivery system because the greater part of the one to two drops (50–100 microliters) of an ophthalmic solution is squeezed out of the eye by the first blink following administration (1,000 microliters = 1 milliliter or 1 cc). The residual volume mixes with the lacrimal fluid (about 7–8 microliters), becomes diluted, and is drained away by the nasolacrimal drainage system until the solution volume returns to the normal tear volume of 7–8 microliters. The initial drainage results in the loss of about 75 to 80 percent of the administered dose within five minutes of instillation. Then drainage stops and the residual dose declines slowly.

The efficiency of an ophthalmic drug-delivery system can be greatly improved by prolonging the contact of drug with the corneal surface. To achieve this purpose, various approaches have been used: (a) preparing a suspension of drug particles in pharmaceutical vehicles, (b) adding viscosity-enhancing agents such as methylcellulose to the eye-drops preparation, or (c) providing the drug as an ointment.

In recent years, it has been shown that drug-presoaked hydrogel-type contact lenses prolong the drug-eye contact time. The Bionite lens, for example, is inserted into the eye after being presoaked in the drug solution. Similarly, Sauflon hydrophilic contact lenses are manufactured from a vinyl pyrrolidone-acrylic copolymer of high water content. These contact lenses have been shown to improve the delivery of fluorescein, phenylephrine, pilocarpine, chloramphenicol, and tetracycline.

More recently, drug-dispersing ocular inserts have been used for the ocular delivery of drugs. The new generation of drug-dispersing ocular inserts consists of a medicated core matrix confined within a pair of flexible, transparent, biocompatible, and tear-insoluble polymer membranes. This polymer membrane provides the required degree of permeability for the drug. When the insert is placed in the conjunctival cul-de-sac between the sclera of the eyeball and the lower lid, the drug is continuously released by diffusion through the membrane as a result of solvation in the lacrimal fluid. Alza Corporation's Ocusert System is a pilocarpine core reservoir sandwiched between two sheets of transparent, **lipophilic**, rate-controlling membranes. The term *lipophilic* means lipid- (or oil-) loving (i.e., the lipophilic rate controlling membranes are not readily soluble in the ocular fluids). When placed in the cul-de-sac, the pilocarpine molecules penetrate through the rate-controlling membranes. This controlled pilocarpine-releasing therapeutic system has several advantages over the conventional eye-drop solution. It provides better patient compliance, less frequent dosing, around-the-clock protection for four to seven days, fewer ocular and systemic side effects, possible delay in the **refractory** state, and a significantly smaller dose of pilocarpine for the effective management of **intraocular** pressure in the treatment of glaucoma. The administration of one Ocusert Pilo-20 insert, for example, delivers a daily dose of only 0.4 to 0.5 milligrams, compared with the four to eight milligrams provided by the instillation of one to two drops of the conventional 2 percent pilocarpine solution administered four times a day.

Transdermal Drug Delivery System

The **transdermal** system is an innovation that employs the skin as a portal of drug entry into the systemic circulation. Using the **percutaneous** route instead of the more conventional oral, parenteral, pulmonary, or rectal routes, this technique is designed to provide systemic therapy for acute or chronic conditions that do not involve the skin.

lipophilic lipid-loving.

refractory resistant to treatment or a stimulus.

intraocular within the eye.

transdermal entering through the dermis or skin, as in administration of a drug applied to the skin in ointment or patch form.

percutaneous through the skin.

Among the most popular and intriguing percutaneously administered drug-delivery systems is the transdermal patch. There are several advantages of transdermal drug-delivery systems. These include convenience, uninterrupted therapy, better patient compliance, accurate drug dosage, and regulation of drug concentration. However, percutaneous delivery is more difficult for those drugs existing as large molecules (i.e., those drugs that have a large molecular weight; for example, insulin) that do not possess adequate lipid and aqueous solubility. Drugs with molecular weights of 100 to 800 and adequate lipid and aqueous solubility can permeate the skin. The ideal molecular weight of a drug for transdermal drug delivery is believed to be less than 400.

The transdermal patch is formulated to deliver a constant and controlled dose of the drug through the intact skin. The drug enters directly into the bloodstream. Although each manufacturer designs its transdermal system based on the technology developed for its individual product, most delivery systems consist of at least three layers: (1) a backing layer, (2) a drug reservoir, and (3) an adhesive layer that incorporates a priming dose of the drug.

Nitroglycerin is available in various forms—sublingual, oral, intravenous injection, topical ointment, and transdermal preparations (Table 12-4). The popular transdermal preparations of nitroglycerin are Ciba-Geigy's Transderm-Nitro, Searle's Nitrodisc, and Key's Nitro-Dur. All nitroglycerin transdermal patches are designed to be applied to the upper arm or chest to provide the drug for 24 hours. Although these patches can be applied anywhere on the body except the distal parts of the extremities, most patients have a tendency to apply these near the thorax, perhaps on the assumption that the medication for the heart should be placed near the heart. Manufacturers do recommend, however, that to avoid irritation each patch should be applied at a site different from that used the previous day.

Transderm-Scop, a scopolamine-containing transdermal delivery system marketed by Ciba-Geigy, is a circular, flat, tan disc, about two millimeters thick and the size of a dime. Each disc contains one to five milligrams of scopolamine and is programmed to deliver 0.5 milligrams of scopolamine over three days. According to Ciba, this delivery system is more effective than the conventional oral dose, which has been reported to cause excessively rapid heartbeat, confusion, and hallucinations. The patch works best when placed behind the ear on a hairless site, delivering scopolamine through intact skin directly into the bloodstream for three days.

Other drugs available as transdermal patches include hormone preparations and nicotine (for smoking cessation). Table 12-5 is a partial listing of some drugs that are available as transdermal delivery systems.

TABLE 12-4 Comparison of Nitroglycerin Dosage Forms

	Antianginal Effect		
DOSAGE FORM	DOSE	ONSET	DURATION
intravenous injection	variable	minutes	minutes
sublingual tablet	0.15 to 0.6 mg every 30 minutes	2 minutes	up to 30 minutes
oral timed-released	2.5 to 9 mg twice a day	0.5 to 1 hour	8 to 9 hours
topical ointment (2%, 15 mg/inch)	1 to 2 inches every 4 hours	30 minutes	3 hours
transdermal	1 patch every 12 to 24 hours	30 minutes	20 to 24 hours

TABLE 12-5 Examples of Transdermal Systems

DRUG	COMMENTS
scopolamine	Used for motion sickness. The patch should be applied to an area where the skin is relatively thin (e.g., behind the ear).
nitroglycerin	Used for angina. Nitroglycerin is deactivated by liver enzymes. The patch should be applied to the chest wall or in the shoulder area. The nitroglycerin patch should be on for 12 hours and off for 12 hours, because the body develops tolerance to nitroglycerin and it does not work well anymore.
clonidine	Used for hypertension. The patch is good for seven days.
nicotine	Used for smoking cessation. The patch can be used for 12 weeks.
fentanyl	Fentanyl is an opioid analgesic for pain (usually used for cancer patients).
lidocaine	Used for relief of pain associated with post-herpetic neuralgia.
estrogen	Estrogen patches are applied to the buttocks or lower abdomen area. They are used for the treatment of (a) moderate to severe vasomotor symptoms associated with menopause, (b) vulval and vaginal atrophy, (c) hypoestrogenism due to hypogonadism, castration, or primary ovarian failure, (d) abnormal uterine bleeding due to hormonal imbalances in the absence of organic pathology associated with hypoplastic and atrophic endometrium, (e) atrophic vaginitis and urethritis, (f) kraurosis vulvae, and (g) prevention of osteoporosis.
testosterone	Used in the treatment of testosterone deficiency.

Intranasal Drug Delivery

The nasal route for drug delivery is becoming popular because of the need to develop a route for newly developed drugs that cannot be administered orally because of lack of their stability in the gastrointestinal tract, and/or due to lack of drug absorption from the gastrointestinal tract due to their molecular weight. Examples of such drugs include newly developed, synthetic, biologically active peptides and polypeptides. Some drugs that are subject to destruction in the gastrointestinal tract (e.g., insulin) are administered by injection. The intranasal route of drug administration is an alternative route for some of these drugs.

The nasal mucosa has been shown to be amenable to the systemic absorption of such drugs as hydralazine, insulin, progesterone, propranolol, and scopolamine. The intranasal bioavailability of those drugs that are relatively small molecular compounds appears to be comparable to the bioavailability of the drugs administered by injection. Some drugs for intranasal delivery are already on the market, while some drugs are under investigation for intranasal delivery. Examples of these drugs are butarphenol, calcitonin, desmopressin, insulin, lypressin, oxytocin, progesterone, and vitamin B_{12}.

Summary

Within the last few years the pharmaceutical industry has made significant progress in the development and manufacture of new dosage forms. The new concepts of bioavailability have made it possible to prepare more efficient delivery systems. The latest developments include such dosage forms as rapid-dissolving tablets, intranasal drug delivery, and metered dose inhalers. More drugs are being made available as transdermal delivery systems (TDS, popularly known as the "patch"), the osmotic pump, the insulin pump, and FDDTs (fast-dissolving/disintegrating tablets. In the future, one can expect dosage forms containing optimal amounts of active ingredients to provide maximal therapeutic benefits, thus markedly reducing or completely eliminating the side effects always associated with therapeutic agents. The current trend appears to be in the direction of development of better drug-delivery systems rather than the development of new compounds as new drugs.

TEST YOUR KNOWLEDGE

Multiple Choice

1. Drugs are defined as chemicals of
   a. natural origin.
   b. synthetic origin.
   c. semisynthetic origin.
   d. all of the above.

2. Which of the following is not a drug dosage form?
   a. brew
   b. tablet
   c. solution
   d. injection

3. Drug formulation aids include
   a. diluents.
   b. excipients.
   c. preservatives.
   d. all of the above.

4. For a drug to elicit the desired response, it is required at the site of action to be in the form of
   a. a soluble gel.
   b. a molecular dispersion.
   c. an isotonic solution.
   d. an acidic vehicle.

5. A soluble substance is called
   a. a solvent.
   b. a solubilizer.
   c. a solute.
   d. none of the above.

6. Medicinal emulsions for oral administration are usually
   a. o/w type.
   b. w/o type.

7. Which of the following is not a solid dosage form?
   a. powder
   b. capsule
   c. suspension
   d. granule

8. The most prescribed ocular dosage form is
   a. eye-drop solution.
   b. drug-presoaked hydrogel-type contact lens.
   c. ocular inserts.
   d. core reservoirs in lipophilic membranes.

9. Advantage(s) of transdermal patches include
   a. convenience.
   b. uninterrupted therapy.
   c. better patient compliance.
   d. all of the above.

Matching

Match the following:

1. _____ medicinal aerosols
2. _____ transdermal patches
3. _____ bionite lens
4. _____ lozenges
5. _____ pellets

a. slowly dissolved in the mouth
b. implanted subcutaneously
c. inhaled through nose or mouth
d. applied to the skin
e. inserted into the eye

Fill In The Blank

1. A _____ is a system or device for delivering a drug or a medicinal agent to the biological system.

2. _____ are various formulation aids that must be used to help formulate and prepare the dosage form.

3. The term _____ is used for substances that are water-miscible.

4. A _____ helps to resist a change in the pH of the solution when a small amount of an acid or a base is added to the solution.

5. An _____ is a substance that helps to keep the mixture of immiscible liquids dispersed into each other for a reasonable length of time.

References

Allen, L. V., Popovich, N. G., & Ansel, H. C. (2005). *Ansel's pharmaceutical dosage forms and drug delivery systems* (8th ed.). Philadelphia: Lippincott Williams and Wilkins.

Gennaro, A. R. (Ed.). (2006). *Remington: The science and practice of pharmacy* (21st ed.). Philadelphia: Lippincott Williams and Wilkins.

Madan, P. L. (1985). Sustained release drug delivery systems: I. An overview. *Pharmaceutical Manufacturing*, 2(2), 22.

Madan, P. L. (1985). Sustained release drug delivery systems: II. Preformulation considerations. *Pharmaceutical Manufacturing*, 2(3), 40.

Madan, P. L. (1985). Sustained release drug delivery systems: III. Technology. *Pharmaceutical Manufacturing*, 2(4), 38.

Madan, P. L. (1985). Sustained release drug delivery systems: IV. Oral products. *Pharmaceutical Manufacturing, 2*(5), 40.

Madan, P. L. (1985). Sustained release drug delivery systems: V. Parenteral products. *Pharmaceutical Manufacturing, 2*(6), 50.

Madan, P. L. (1985). Sustained release drug delivery systems: VI. Special devices. *Pharmaceutical Manufacturing 2*(7), 32.

Madan, P. L. (1990). Sustained release dosage forms. *U.S. Pharmacist,* 15, 39.

Madan, P. L. (2005, Chapter 11). In J. M. Durgin & Z. Hanan (Eds.), *Pharmacy practice for technicians* (3rd ed.). Clifton Park, NY: Thomson Delmar Learning.

Madan, P. L., & Komotar, A. (1979). Quality control in the pharmaceutical industry. *Drug and Cosmetic Industry,* 124, 66.

Parrot, E. L. (1970). *Pharmaceutical technology.* Minneapolis, MN: Burgess Publishing Co.

The United States Pharmacopoeia/National Formulary (2006). The United States Pharmacopeial Convention: Rockville, MD.

Pharmaceutical Calculations

Competencies

Upon completion of this chapter, the reader should be able to

1. Interpret a medication order for calculations and dispensing.
2. Convert quantities stated in apothecary units to their equivalent units in the metric system.
3. Convert quantities within the metric or apothecary systems (e.g., g to mg).
4. Set up proportions to perform calculations required in administering medications.
5. Calculate using alligation to dilute ingredients in formulations.
6. Calculate quantities to be administered when ordered in fractional doses.
7. Calculate dosages for infants and children.
8. Calculate dosages for individual patients given the patient's weight and/or height and the recommended dose.
9. Perform calculations necessary for the preparation and infusion of IV medications.
10. Identify techniques to decrease errors in interpreting the strength of drugs from the written order.

Key Terms

alligation
apothecary system
body surface area (BSA)
grain
gram
International System of Units (SI)
liter
meter
metric system
nomogram
percentage
piggyback
proportion
ratio

Introduction

It is common practice in hospitals for the pharmacist to calculate and prepare or select the drug dosage form administered to the patient. However, this practice does not relieve other health care providers from the legal and professional responsibility of ensuring that the patient receives the correct dose of the correct medication at the correct time in the correct manner. *A pharmacy technician should have every calculation regarding drugs or compounding checked by a pharmacist before preparing or dispensing a medication order.* This chapter will review the necessary calculations involved in the safe administration of drugs to the patient.

Interpreting the Drug Order

The welfare of the patient necessitates proper interpretation of the medication order. While this is the pharmacists' responsibility, it is often the technician who is the first person to screen the order. If any doubt or question exists, or if a particular order appears unusual, it is the pharmacy technician's responsibility to confirm the order with the pharmacist before proceeding (Figure 13-1).

Common Abbreviations

Abbreviations derived from Latin are often used by physicians and pharmacists in writing and interpreting drug orders. Refer to Table 13-1 for common abbreviations regarding quantities and dosages seen in drug orders.

The pharmacy technician must be able to interpret these abbreviations correctly when they are used in a drug order. Some examples of drug orders encountered in practice include the following:

FIGURE 13-1

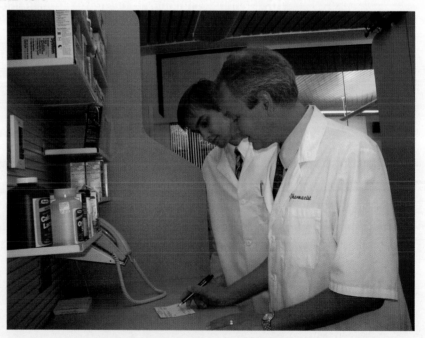

FIGURE 13-1 When in doubt, always verify a prescription with the pharmacist.

EXAMPLE

Benadryl (diphenhydramine) caps 25 mg po q4h

Interpretation

Give the patient one 25 mg capsule by mouth every four hours.

EXAMPLE

Tylenol (acetaminophen) Elixir gtts 20 po tid pc and hs

Interpretation

Give 20 drops of elixir by mouth three times a day after meals and 20 drops at bedtime. (Because of the word *and* in the directions, this does mean a total of four doses per day.)

EXAMPLE

100 mg Demerol (meperidine) IM stat. 50 mg q4h prn pain

Interpretation

Give 100 mg of Demerol intramuscularly immediately, then give 50 mg of Demerol intramuscularly every four hours as needed for pain.

The abbreviation "prn" can often be a source of trouble if not interpreted carefully. In the last example, the medication (Demerol) can be administered if a dosing interval *of at least four hours is maintained*. The nurse assesses the patient's need for the Demerol to control pain, or the patient requests the medication, and

TABLE 13-1 Abbreviations Commonly Seen in Drug Orders

ABBREVIATION	ENGLISH
gal	gallon
qt	quart
pt	pint
oz, ℥	ounce
tbsp, ℥ss	tablespoonful
tsp, ℨ, ℥	teaspoonful
L	liter
mL	milliliter
gtt	drop
lb	pound
gr	grain
kg	kilogram
g	gram
mg	milligram
mcg	microgram
no, #	number
qs	quantity sufficient
s̄s̄ or s̄s̄	one-half

TABLE 13-2 Values of Single Roman Numerals

ROMAN NUMERALS	VALUE
ss or s̄s̄	$\frac{1}{2}$
I or i	1
V or v	5
X or x	10
L or l	50
C or c	100
D or d	500
M or m	1,000

All small Roman numerals may be written with a line above them (see "ss" in table).

it may be administered *only* if it has been *four hours or more* since the previous injection.

Roman Numerals

Most prescriptions today are written using Arabic numerals; however, Roman numerals may still be used by some prescribers. The use of Roman numerals may make it more difficult to alter the quantity of a written prescription. A few of the most common Roman numerals are shown in Table 13-2.

Examples of the use of Roman numerals are as follows:

iv	four
xvi	sixteen
LV	fifty-five
CC	two hundred
CDXV	four hundred fifteen
MMDCXL	two thousand six hundred forty

International System of Units (The Metric System)

International System of Units (SI) commonly known as the Metric System for weights and measures.

metric system a system of weights based on the meter, the gram, and the liter.

gram a base unit of weight in the metric system.

liter a basic unit of measure in the metric system.

The **International System of Units (SI)**, commonly known as the metric system, is the internationally used system of weights and measures. The three basic units of the **metric system** are the gram (weight), the liter (volume), and the meter (length). The technician must be able to convert from one unit to another unit within the metric system.

Gram

The **gram** is the basic unit of weight in the metric system. The gram is defined as the weight of one cubic centimeter of distilled water at 4°C.

Liter

The **liter** is the basic unit of volume used to measure liquids in the metric system. It is equal to 1,000 cubic centimeters of water. One cubic centimeter is considered equivalent to 1 milliliter (mL); thus 1 liter (L) equals 1,000 milliliters (mL).

Meter

meter a basic unit of length in the metric system.

The **meter** is the basic unit of length used to measure distances in the metric system. The meter is 1/10,000,000 distance from the North Pole to the equator (or a little larger than one yard).

Multiples or parts of these basic units are named by adding a prefix. Each prefix has a numerical value, as shown in Table 13-3 and Table 13-4.

TABLE 13-3 Metric Prefixes

PREFIX	NUMERICAL VALUE
mega-	1,000,000
kilo-	1,000
deci-	0.1
centi-	0.01
milli-	0.001
micro-	0.000,001

TABLE 13-4 Common Metric Abbreviations Found in Pharmacy

ABBREVIATION	MEASURE
mcg	microgram
mg	milligram
g	gram
kg	kilogram
mL	milliliter
L	liter
mm	millimeter
cc	centimeter
m	meter

Examples of the use of the metric prefixes are as follows:

- 1 milligram (mg)   1/1,000 gram   0.001 g
- 1 microgram (mcg)   1/1,000,000 gram   0.000001 g
- 1 kilogram (kg)   1,000 grams   1,000 g
- 1 milliliter (mL)   1/1,000 liter   0.001 L
- 1 deciliter (dL)   1/10 liter   0.1 L

Conversions

Conversion of units is a common calculation when working with medications. The metric conversions are depicted in Table 13-5.

TABLE 13-5 Metric Conversions

1,000 g	=	1 kg
1,000 mg	=	1 g
1,000 mcg	=	1 mg
1,000 mL	=	1 L
100 mL	=	1 dL

EXAMPLE

Convert 22 g to milligrams.

Solution by proportion

1 gram is equal to 1,000 mg. It is possible to convert between grams to milligrams using proportions. (Proportions are covered in detail in the next section of this chapter.)

$$\frac{1000 \text{ mg}}{1 \text{ g}} = \frac{X \text{ mg}}{22 \text{ g}}$$

$$X = 22{,}000 \text{ mg}$$

EXAMPLE

Convert 150 mL to liters.

Solution by dimensional analysis

1 liter is equal to 1,000 mL. It is possible to convert from liters to milliliters.

$$150 \text{ mL} \times \frac{1 \text{ L}}{1000 \text{ mL}} = 0.15 \text{ L}$$

Important:

- A 1,000 difference means moving the decimal point three places to the right.
- Approach this logically—milliliters are a smaller unit than liters; therefore, more of them are needed to equal a liter.

Ratio and Proportion

Nearly every calculation involving medications can be broken down to a simple ratio and proportion. Developing skill in setting up ratios and proportions will be a valuable aid to the technician in solving medication problems quickly and accurately.

Ratio

ratio the relationship of two quantities, e.g., 1:10 is read as one part in 10 parts.

A **ratio** is the relationship between two quantities. It may be expressed in the form 1:10 or 1:2,500, or it may be expressed as a fraction—1/10 or 1/2,500. The ratio expression 1:10 or 1/10 can be read as one in ten, one-tenth, or one part in ten parts.

EXAMPLE

A handful of 20 jelly beans contains one red jelly bean.

Interpretation

The ratio of red jelly beans to total jelly beans is 1 in 20 or 1:20 or 1/20.

Proportion

proportion a proportion is formed using two ratios that are equal, e.g., 1/2 = 5/10.

A **proportion** is formed when two ratios are equal (or proportional) to one another. For example, 1:2 = 5:10. When two ratios or fractions are equal, their cross product is also equal. The cross product is obtained by multiplying the denominator of one ratio by the numerator of the other, as follows:

$$\frac{1}{2} = \frac{5}{10} \quad \text{therefore, } 2 \times 5 = 10 \times 1$$

The cross products are equal: 10 = 10. This confirms that the ratio 1:2 is equal (proportional) to the ratio 5:10.

Is 1:3 proportional to 4:12?

$$\frac{1}{3} = \frac{4}{12} \quad \text{yes, } 3 \times 4 = 1 \times 12$$

The cross products are equal: 12 = 12. Therefore, 1:3 is proportional to 4:12.

This characteristic of proportions is very useful in solving problems that arise in drug administration. If any three of the values of a proportion are known, the fourth value can be determined.

EXAMPLE

The prescriber orders 20 mg IM of a drug for a patient. The drug is available in a 10 mL vial which contains 50 mg of drug. How many milliliters will be needed to supply the dose of 20 mg?

Solution

Three things are known from the statement of the problem.

1. The vial contains 10 mL of drug solution.

2. 50 mg of the drug are in the 10 mL vial.

3. 20 mg is the desired dose.

A ratio can be stated for the drug on hand.

$$\frac{50 \text{ mg}}{10 \text{ mL}}$$

A ratio can also be stated for the required dosage.

$$\frac{20 \text{ mg}}{X \text{ mL}}$$

Thus the proportion is

$$\frac{50 \text{ mg}}{10 \text{ mL}} = \frac{20 \text{ mg}}{X \text{ mL}}$$

Note in the proportion that the units are labeled, and like units are located in the same position in each fraction or ratio (mg is in the numerator and mL is in the denominator). It is important to correctly equate the units of the proportion.

Important: Three conditions must be met when using ratio and proportion:

1. The numerators must have the same units.

2. The denominators must have the same units.

3. Three of the four parts must be known.

To solve the last example, equate the cross products and solve for the unknown (X).

$$\frac{50 \text{mg}}{10 \text{mL}} = \frac{20 \text{mg}}{X \text{mL}}$$

$$50 \ (X \text{ mL}) = 10 \times 20$$

$$50 \ (X \text{ mL}) = 200$$

$$X = 4 \text{ mL}$$

Therefore, 4 mL of the solution will supply the 20 mg dose of drug ordered.

It is helpful to note that a proportion is similar to the way we think logically: if this is so, then that will follow. Problems can be analyzed with the "if-then" approach.

In the last example, we could say IF 50 mg of drug are contained in 10 mL of drug solution, THEN 20 mg of drug will be contained in X mL of solution. To use the if-then approach, the first ratio of a proportion is always formed from the quantity and strength (concentration) found on the label of the drug on hand.

EXAMPLE

An ampicillin oral suspension contains 250 mg of the drug in each 5 mL. How many milliliters would be measured into a medication syringe to obtain a dose of 75 mg of ampicillin?

Solution

Step 1. Set up the proportion beginning with the drug on hand.

$$\begin{array}{cc} \text{IF} & \text{THEN} \\ \dfrac{250 \text{ mg}}{5 \text{ mL}} & = \dfrac{75 \text{ mg}}{X \text{ mL}} \end{array}$$

Step 2. Then cross multiply.

$$250 \,(X \text{ mL}) = 5\,(75)$$
$$250 \,(X \text{ mL}) = 375$$
$$X = 1.5 \text{ mL}$$

The Apothecary System

apothecary system an early English system of weights and liquid measure.

The **apothecary system** was the traditional system used in the practice of pharmacy. Today, only components of it may be found on some prescriptions. The fluid dram sign (ʒ or ℨ) is sometimes used by physicians to represent one teaspoonful. The apothecary symbol for one ounce is ℥. Examples of apothecary notations are shown in Table 13-6.

TABLE 13-6 Apothecary Notations

ʒ or ℨ	teaspoonful
ʒ s̄s̄ or ℨ s̄s̄	one-half teaspoonful
ʒ is̄s̄ or ℨ is̄s̄	one and a half teaspoonfuls
ʒ iis̄s̄ or ℨ iis̄s̄	two and a half teaspoonfuls
℥i	one ounce
℥ss	one half-ounce or one tablespoonful
℥iss	one and a half ounces
℥iiss	two and a half ounces

Apothecary System of Volume (Liquid) Measure

The apothecary liquid measures are the same as the avoirdupois measures such as ounces, pints, and quarts. The smallest unit of volume in the apothecary system is the minim (𝕞), which is not in common use today. The minim should *not* be confused with the drop, because they are not equivalent. The size of a drop varies with the properties of the liquid being dispensed or measured. Table 13-7 shows the common units of liquid measure in the apothecary system.

Apothecary System of Weights

grain a base unit of weight in the apothecary system.

The apothecary system of weights is based upon the **grain** (gr), which is the smallest unit in the system. The origin of the grain is uncertain, but it is believed that at one time solids were measured by using grains of wheat as the standard.

TABLE 13-7   Liquid Measures in the Apothecary System

MEASURE	EQUIVALENT
1 tablespoonful (℥ ss)	3 teaspoonfuls (ʒiii or ℥iii)
1 fluid ounce (℥)	2 tablespoonfuls
1 pint	16 fluid ounces
1 quart	2 pints
1 gallon	4 quarts

In practice, the technician will rarely see apothecary units of weight with the exception of the grain, which is still sometimes used in ordering medications such as:

nitroglycerin (1/100 gr, 1/150 gr, 1/200 gr, 1/400 gr)
phenobarbital sodium (1/4 gr, 1/2 gr, 1 gr)
aspirin or acetaminophen (5 gr, 10 gr)

Converting from the Apothecary System to the Metric System

Before reviewing the types of calculations used in determining medication dosages, it is necessary to examine conversions between systems of measurement. It was mentioned previously that nearly all medication orders today are written using the metric system. However, some orders will be written using the apothecary system. The technician must be able to convert from the apothecary system to the metric system and from one unit to another unit within both systems. Table 13-8 provides conversion factors between the apothecary and the metric systems. Many conversions can be readily made by use of the ratio and proportion method.

TABLE 13-8   Conversions Between the Apothecary and Metric Systems

APOTHECARY	METRIC EXACT CONVERSION	METRIC APPROXIMATE CONVERSION
1 teaspoonful, ʒ or ʒ	no longer in use	5 mL
1 tablespoonful (℥ ss)	no longer in use	15 mL
1 fluid ounce (℥)	29.6 mL	30 mL
1 pint	473 mL	480 mL
1 quart	946 mL	960 mL
1 gallon	3,784 mL	3,840 mL
1 grain	64.8 mg	65 mg or 60 mg
1 ounce	28.4 g	30 g
1 pound	454 g compounding 2.2 kg person's weight	no approximate conversion used
1 inch	2.54 cm	no approximate conversion used

EXAMPLE

How many milligrams of nitroglycerin are in one 1/150 gr tablet of the drug?

Solution

This problem requires conversion from the apothecary system to the metric system. Use the equivalent 1 gr = 60 mg. The proportion is:

$$\begin{array}{cc} \text{IF} & \text{THEN} \\ \dfrac{1\ gr}{60\ mg} & = \dfrac{1/150\ gr}{X\ mg} \end{array}$$

Cross multiplying:

$$1\ (X\ mg) = 60\ (1/150)$$
$$X\ mg = 0.4\ mg$$

EXAMPLE

Four fluid ounces are equal to how many mL?

Solution

$$\frac{1\ ounce}{30\ mL} = \frac{4\ ounces}{X\ mL}$$

Cross multiplying:

$$1\ (X\ mL) = 4\ (30)$$
$$X\ mL = 120\ mL$$

Calculations Related to Solutions

Solutions are formed in two ways:

1. By dissolving a solid called the *solute* in a liquid called the *solvent*, or
2. By mixing two liquids together to form a solution.

An example of the first method is adding salt to water to make a normal saline solution. Mixing Zephiran Chloride solution with water to make an antiseptic wash is an example of the second method.

Percentage Solutions

Many solutions are available in or are prepared to a specified percentage strength. To produce a solution of the desired strength, it is necessary to calculate the exact amount of drug to prepare a specified final volume of product. Although most solutions are prepared by the pharmacist if they are not commercially available, the pharmacy technician must understand the concept of percentage to interpret medication labels.

Percentage is defined as the number of parts per hundred and is expressed as follows:

percentage a percent number representing an amount per hundred, e.g., 5 percent represents 5 parts per 100.

$$\text{Percentage (\%)} = \frac{\text{No. of parts}}{100\ \text{parts}} \times 100$$

Parts will refer to grams (in the case of solids) and milliliters (in the case of liquids).

To calculate the percentage of active ingredient in a solution, the amount of active ingredient in grams is divided by the total volume of the solution. To convert the result to a percentage, it is multiplied by 100.

$$\frac{\text{Active ingredient}}{\text{Total quantity of product}} \times 100 = \text{Percentage (\%)}$$

Problems in percentage solutions are generally concerned with three types of percentages:

1. weight to volume (% W/V)
2. weight to weight (% W/W)
3. volume to volume (% V/V)

Weight to volume percentage is defined as the number of grams of solute in 100 mL of solution. Typical % W/V examples include the following:

- 1 L of D5W, which contains 5 g of dextrose in each 100 mL of solution.
- a ¼% solution of pilocarpine HCl, which contains 1/4 g (0.25 g) of pilocarpine HCl in each 100 mL of solution.

EXAMPLE

What is the percentage weight to volume (% W/V) of sodium chloride (solid solute) in normal saline solution, if 9 g of the salt are dissolved in enough water to make 1,000 mL of solution?

Solution

$$\frac{\text{Amount of salt in grams: 9g}}{\text{Total volume of solution: 1000mL}} \times 100 = 0.9\%$$

Percentage weight to weight (% W/W) is defined as the number of grams of solute in 100 g of a solid preparation.

Note: Concentrated hydrochloric and sulfuric acids are two examples of *solutions* given as a weight to weight percentage. Typical % W/W examples include the following:

- a 10% ointment of zinc oxide, which contains 10 g of zinc oxide in each 100 g of ointment.
- hydrocortisone cream ½%, which has 1/2 g (0.5 g) of hydrocortisone in each 100 g of cream.

The third form of percentage is volume to volume (% V/V), which is defined as the number of milliliters of solute in each 100 mL of solution. Examples of this form include the following:

- Rubbing alcohol 70%, which contains 70 mL of absolute alcohol in each 100 mL of the solution.
- A 2% solution of phenol, which contains 2 mL of liquified phenol in each 100 mL of solution.

When the type of percentage is not stated, assume that for solutions of a solid in a liquid the percentage is W/V; for solutions of a liquid in a liquid the percentage is V/V; and for mixtures of two solids the percentage is W/W.

Ratio Strength Solutions

Concentration expressions for weak solutions (or solids) may also be expressed in terms of ratio strength. This is another way of expressing percentage strength. A 0.1 percent solution of drug is interpreted to be 0.1 grams of drug in 100 mL of solution. The ratio strength could be expressed as 0.1:100. However, it is customary to give a ratio strength with the initial part as "1." The correct expression of the 0.1 percent solution as a ratio strength is 1:1,000. This would be interpreted as 1 gram of drug in 1,000 mL of solution. Any concentration can be restated as a ratio strength by using proportions to convert.

> **Important:**
>
> **1.** A ratio strength is written with a colon (1:20) and *not* as a fraction (1/20).
>
> **2.** As with percentages, solids are given in grams and liquids in milliliters.

> **EXAMPLE**
>
> Express the strength of a 2.5 percent solution as a ratio strength.
>
> *Solution*
>
> 2.5 % means 2.5 grams of drug in 100 mL of solution
>
> $$\frac{2.5\ g}{100\ mL} = \frac{1\ g}{X\ mL}$$
>
> $$X = 40$$
>
> The ratio strength is expressed as 1:40 W/V. (This product contains 1 gram in every 40 mL of solution.)

Dilution and Alligation

A physician may order a commercially prepared dosage form to be diluted to a lower strength for a patient. Liquid dosage forms, such as suspensions or solutions, or semisolid dosage forms, such as creams or ointments, may all be diluted with a vehicle (diluent) that is compatible with the original product.

These problems may be solved by:

1. Proportions—as discussed earlier in the chapter.
2. The equation (Q1)(C1) = (Q2)(C2), where Q1 is the original quantity, C1 is the original concentration, Q2 is the final quantity, and C2 is the final concentration.
3. Alligation.

(Q1)(C1) = (Q2)(C2)

> **Important:** Three conditions must be met when using (Q1)(C1) = (Q2)(C2).
>
> **1.** Three of the four parts must be known.
>
> **2.** Each quantity must have the same units.
>
> **3.** Each concentration must be of the same type (i.e., W/W, W/V, V/V).

EXAMPLE

The physician orders 10 percent Coal Tar Ointment be diluted to 2.5 percent Coal Tar Ointment. How many grams of petrolatum (Vaseline) must be added to 30 grams of the 10 percent ointment to correctly dilute this product?

Solution

(Original Quantity) (Original Concentration) = (Final Quantity) (Final Concentration)

(30 g) × (10%) = (X g) × (2.5%)

X = 120 g   Note: 120 g is NOT the correct answer.

Solving for X gives the quantity of 2.5 percent ointment that can be made when 30 grams of 10 percent ointment are diluted with petrolatum. Subtract the weight of the original ointment from the diluted ointment to calculate the amount of petrolatum needed.

120 g − 30 g = 90 g

Therefore, to make this product, 30 grams of 10 percent coal tar ointment is mixed with 90 grams of petrolatum to make 120 grams of 2.5 percent coal tar ointment.

EXAMPLE

How many mL of 5 percent acetic acid solution must be used to make 125 mL of 2 percent acetic acid solution?

Solution

(Original Quantity) (Original Concentration) = (Final Quantity) (Final Concentration)

(X mL) × (5%) = (125 mL) × (2%)

X = 50 mL of 2 percent acetic acid solution.

To make this product, measure 50 mL of 5 percent acetic acid solution and add enough water (75 mL) to make 125 mL of solution, which will have a strength of 2 percent acetic acid.

Alligation

alligation the relative amounts of solutions of different percentages from a mixture of a given strength.

Alligation is a method generally used to solve problems in which two liquids, solids, or semisolids of different strengths are combined to create a final strength. The final strength must be somewhere between the strengths of the two components (weaker than the strongest strength and stronger than the weakest strength). Alligation can also be used in place of the (Q1)(C1) = (Q2)(C2) equation.

EXAMPLE

The physician orders 10 percent Coal Tar Ointment to be diluted to 2.5 percent Coal Tar Ointment. How many grams of petrolatum (Vaseline) must be added to 30 grams of the 10 percent ointment to correctly dilute this product? (This is the same question posed in the first example, but will be solved using the allegation method.)

Note: The final product has a strength of 2.5 percent, which is weaker than 10 percent and stronger than 0 percent (as petrolatum contains no coal tar).

Solution

- Put the percent strengths *available* in the first two columns.
- Put the percent strength *ordered* in the next column.
- Subtract on the diagonal to calculate the *parts* of each component needed in the last column.

10%   2.5 parts (of 10% ointment)

2.5%

0%   7.5 parts (of petrolatum)

(Continued)

Then solve by proportion.

$$\frac{2.5 \text{ parts}}{7.5 \text{ parts}} = \frac{30 \text{ g}}{\text{Xg}}$$

$$X = 90 \text{ g}$$

EXAMPLE

How many mL of 5 percent acetic acid solution must be used to make 125 mL of 2 percent acetic acid solution? (This is the same question posed in the second example, but will be solved using the allegation method.)

Solution

5%   2 parts of 5% solution

   2%

0% $\dfrac{3 \text{ parts of water}}{5 \text{ parts total}}$

The parts must be added because the total amount of the final solution is given.

$$\frac{2 \text{ parts}}{5 \text{ parts}} = \frac{X \text{ mL}}{125 \text{ mL}}$$

$$X = 50 \text{ mL}$$

Calculation of Fractional Doses

Health care professionals encounter fractional or partial medication dosages because physicians often order medication for a patient in a strength that differs from the strength of the commercially prepared product.

The ratio and proportion method can be used to solve all problems of fractional dosages. Since the concentration of the medication on hand is known, it forms the IF ratio of the proportion. The THEN portion allows for calculation of the amount of drug product necessary for the fractional dose.

EXAMPLE

The physician orders 1 million units of penicillin G for a patient. The penicillin G on hand is prepared as a solution containing 250,000 units/mL.

Solution

Find the strength of the product on hand. This expression forms the "if" ratio of the proportion:

Place the number of units wanted in the "then" ratio and solve for the unknown X.

$$\underset{\text{IF}}{\frac{250,000 \text{ units}}{1 \text{ mL}}} = \underset{\text{THEN}}{\frac{1,000,000 \text{ units}}{X \text{ mL}}}$$

$$250,000 \text{ X} = 1,000,000$$

$$X = 4 \text{ mL}$$

Remember to label all parts of the proportion carefully with the appropriate units.

EXAMPLE

The physician orders 250 mcg of cyanocobalamin (vitamin B_{12}) IM daily. The vitamin B_{12} on hand is labeled 1,000 mcg/mL. How many milliliters should be given to the patient?

(Continued)

Solution

The concentration of B_{12} on hand is 1,000 mcg/mL. Placing the number of micrograms needed opposite the micrograms on the "if" side, the "if-then" proportion is:

$$\underset{\text{IF}}{\frac{1000 \text{ mcg}}{1 \text{ mL}}} = \underset{\text{THEN}}{\frac{250 \text{ mcg}}{X \text{ mL}}}$$

Solving for X yields:

$$X = 0.25 \text{ mL}$$

To supply 250 mcg of vitamin B_{12} requires 0.25 mL of the concentrated B_{12} on hand.

EXAMPLE

A patient is to be given 25 mg of diphenhydramine (Benadryl) by mouth. The Benadryl elixir is available in a strength of 12.5 mg/5 mL. How many milliliters should be given to the patient?

Solution

$$\underset{\text{IF}}{\frac{12.5 \text{ mg}}{5 \text{ mL}}} = \underset{\text{THEN}}{\frac{25 \text{ mg}}{X \text{ mL}}}$$

$$X = \frac{125}{12.5}$$

$$X = 10 \text{ mL}$$

EXAMPLE

A medication order calls for 750 mg of calcium lactate to be given tid po. On hand are tablets of calcium lactate 0.5 g. How many tablets should be given for each dose?

Solution

Note: Remember when using ratio and proportion, the units must be alike. Grams cannot be used in a proportion opposite milligrams. Therefore, in this example, the grams must be converted to milligrams or the 750 mg converted to grams. Changing the grams to milligrams yields:

$$0.5 \text{ g} = 500 \text{ mg}$$

The "if-then" proportion would read:

$$\frac{500 \text{ mg}}{1 \text{ tab}} = \frac{750 \text{ mg}}{X \text{ tab}}$$

$$X = 1.5 \text{ or } 1\tfrac{1}{2} \text{ tablets}$$

Calculation of Dosages Based on Weight

The recommended dosages of drugs are often expressed in literature as a number of milligrams per unit of body weight per unit of time (refer to package inserts, *Physicians' Desk Reference*, or other standard drug references). Such dosage expressions are commonly used for pediatric doses. For example, the recommended dose for a drug might be 5 mg/kg/24 hours (either given all at once or in divided doses each day). This information can be utilized by the pharmacist to:

- Calculate the dose for a given patient.
- Evaluate doses ordered that are suspected to be significant over- or underdosages.

EXAMPLE

The physician orders Mintezol tablets for a 110-pound child. The recommended dosage for Mintezol is 20 mg/kg per dose. How many 500 mg tablets of Mintezol should be given to this patient for each dose?

Solution

Step 1. Since the dose provided is based on a kilogram weight, convert the patient's weight to kilograms by proportion. Since 1 kg = 2.2 lb, then:

$$\frac{1\ kg}{2.2\ lb} = \frac{X\ kg}{110\ lb}$$

$$X = 50\ kg$$

Step 2. Calculate the total daily dose using the recommended dosage information: 20 mg/kg. This is interpreted as, "For each one kilogram of body weight, give 20 mg of the drug."

$$\frac{20\ mg}{1\ kg} = \frac{X\ mg}{50\ kg}$$

$$X = 1,000\ mg$$

Step 3. Calculate the number of tablets needed to supply 1,000 mg per dose. The concentration of tablets on hand is 500 mg/tablet.

$$\frac{500\ mg}{1\ tab} = \frac{1000\ mg}{X\ tab}$$

$$X = 2\ tablets\ per\ dose$$

EXAMPLE

The recommended dose of meperidine (Demerol) is 5 mg/kg/24 h for pain. It is given in divided doses every four to six hours. How many milliliters of Demerol injection (50 mg/mL) should be administered to a 35-pound child as a single dose every six hours?

Solution

Step 1. Calculate the daily dose for a 35-pound child.

$$\frac{5\ mg}{1\ kg\ (2.2\ lb)} = \frac{X\ mg}{35\ lb}$$

The calculation can be done in one step by inserting the conversion unit 2.2 lb for 1 kg in the ratio.

$$X = 79.5\ mg\ (or\ 80\ mg)\ of\ Demerol\ per\ day\ (24\ hours)$$

Step 2. Calculate the number of mg of Demerol needed for one dose.

$$\frac{80\ mg}{24\ h} = \frac{X\ mg}{6\ h}$$

$$X = 20\ mg\ per\ dose$$

Step 3. Calculate the number of milliliters to be given per dose.

$$\frac{50\ mg}{1\ mL} = \frac{20\ mg}{X\ mL}$$

$$20 = 50\ (X\ mL)$$

$$X = 0.4\ mL$$

Pediatric Dosage Calculations

nomogram a chart that determines body surface area from height and weight.

The **nomogram** is a chart that uses the weight and height (size) of the patient to calculate his or her **body surface area (BSA)** in square meters (m^2). The body surface area (BSA) is then placed in a proportion with the dose when it is ordered per meter squared (m^2).

body surface area (BSA) the measurement of the height and weight of the patient to establish an estimate of his or her body surface.

To determine BSA, the weight and height of the patient must be known. The nomogram scales contain both metric (cm, kg) and avoirdupois (inches, pounds) values for height and weight. Thus, the BSA can be determined for pounds and inches or kilograms and centimeters without making conversions. Figure 13-2 contains the nomogram "Body Surface Area of Children." (A different nomogram is available for adults.) Note the three columns labeled height, body surface area, and weight. Also note that the height and weight scales show both metric and avoirdupois values.

FIGURE 13-2

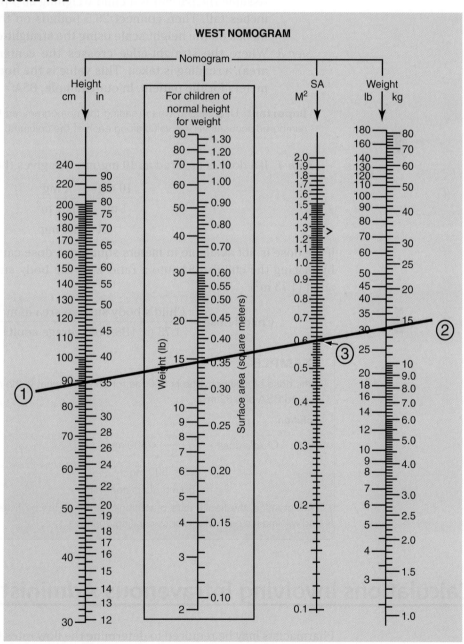

FIGURE 13-2 The West Nomogram (from Behrman, R. E., Kliegman, R. M., & Jenson, H. B. (Eds.). *Nelson textbook of pediatrics* (16th ed.). Philadelphia: W.B. Saunders, 2000. Reprinted with permission).

To determine the body surface area, a ruler or straight-edge is needed. (A piece of paper can be used if there is at least one even, straight edge.) The following steps demonstrate the use of the nomogram.

Step 1. Determine the height and weight of the patient. This information may be given in metric values (e.g., height 84 cm, weight 12 kg) or in avoirdupois values (height 33.5 inches, weight 26.5 pounds). Mixed values can also be used (height 85 cm, weight 26.5 pounds). Be very careful to use the intended scale for each.

Step 2. Place the straight-edge on the nomogram connecting the two points on the height and weight scales that represent the patient's values. Assume the patient is a child weighing 26.5 pounds and standing 33.5 inches tall. Then connect 26.5 pounds on the weight scale and 33.5 inches on the height scale using the straight-edge.

Step 3. Where the straight-edge crosses the center column (body surface area), a reading is taken. This value is the body surface area in square meters for the patient. In our example, BSA = 0.52 m^2.

> **Important:** Use caution when reading the nomogram, as the divisions between the numbered sections vary in value along each of the columns.

Step 4. If a dose is ordered as 10 mg/m^2, this gives the proportion:

$$\frac{10 \text{ mg}}{1 \text{ m}^2} = \frac{X \text{ mg}}{0.52 \text{ m}^2}$$

$$X = 5.2 \text{ mg}$$

If the dose is not available in meters squared, a dose can be estimated for a child by placing the child's BSA into a ratio with the body surface area of an average adult (1.73 m^2).

$$\text{Child's dose} = \frac{\text{Child's body surface area in m}^2}{1.73 \text{ m}^2 \text{ (BSA of average adult)}} \times \text{Adult dose}$$

> **EXAMPLE**
>
> If the dose of aminophylline is 500 mg for an adult, what is the dose for a child with a calculated BSA of 0.52 m^2?
>
> **Solution**
>
> $$\text{Child's dose} = \frac{0.52 \text{m}^2}{1.73} \times 500 \text{ mg}$$
>
> $$= 0.3 \times 500 \text{ mg}$$
>
> $$= 150 \text{ mg of aminophylline}$$
>
> With practice, the health care practitioner can become proficient in using the nomogram and will find it a useful tool for calculating dosages.

Calculations Involving Intravenous Administration

Pharmacists may be required to determine the flow rates for intravenous infusions and to calculate the volume of fluids administered over a period of time. Infusion solutions may be large volume and run continuously at a specified rate, or smaller volume and run intermittently (for a certain period of time and repeated at intervals throughout the day). Sometimes a second IV solution is run through the line of a primary solution. These are known as **piggyback** or secondary solutions. The calculations necessary to perform these tasks can all be accomplished by the use of ratio and proportion.

Chapter 15 provides information on the techniques involved in IV administration, the equipment used, and the documentation to be prepared by the nurse administering IV solutions. The calculations required for IV administration are detailed in the following sections.

> **piggyback** refers to a small-volume IV solution (25–250 mL) that is run into an existing IV line over a brief period of time (e.g., 50 mL over 15 minutes).

Calculating the Rate of IV Administration

When the physician orders intravenous solutions to run for a stated number of hours, the pharmacist may have to compute the number of drops per minute to comply with the order.

To calculate the flow rate using the ratio and proportion method, one must determine the following three steps:

Step 1. The number of milliliters the patient will receive per hour.

Step 2. The number of milliliters the patient will receive per minute.

Step 3. The number of drops per minute that will equal the number of milliliters computed in Step 2. The drop rate specified for the IV set being used must be considered in this step. The drop rate is expressed as a ratio of drops per mL (gtt/mL).

Since it is not possible to obtain a fraction of a drop, always round off the number of *drops per minute* to the nearest whole drop.

EXAMPLE

The physician orders 3,000 mL of dextrose 5 percent in water (D5W) IV over a 24-hour period. If the IV set is calibrated to deliver 15 drops per milliliter, how many drops must be administered per minute?

Solution

Step 1. Calculate mL/hr.

$$\frac{3,000 \text{ mL}}{24 \text{ hr}} = \frac{X \text{ mL}}{1 \text{ hr}}$$

$$X = 125 \text{ mL/hr or}$$
$$= 125 \text{ mL/60 min}$$

Step 2. Calculate mL/min.

$$\frac{125 \text{ mL}}{60 \text{ min}} = \frac{X \text{ mL}}{1 \text{ min}}$$

$$X = 2.1 \text{ mL/min}$$

Step 3. Calculate gtt/min using the drop rate per minute of the IV set.

$$\frac{15 \text{ gtt}}{1 \text{ mL}} = \frac{X \text{ gtt}}{2.1 \text{ mL (amt needed/min)}}$$

$$X = 32 \text{ gtt/min}$$

EXAMPLE

The physician orders 2 L of Lactated Ringer's solution (LR) to be administered over a 12-hour period. The IV set is calibrated to deliver 10 gtt/mL. How many drops per minute should the patient receive?

(Continued)

Solution

Step 1. Determine the number of milliliters to be administered in one hour. Since the answer requested is in milliliter units, first convert liter quantity to milliliters.

$$2 L = 2,000 mL$$

$$\frac{2000 \ mL}{12 \ hr} = \frac{X \ mL}{1 \ hr}$$

$$X = 167 \ mL/hr \ or$$

$$167 \ mL/60 \ min$$

Step 2. Calculate the number of milliliters per minute.

$$\frac{167 \ mL}{60 \ min} = \frac{X \ mL}{1 \ min}$$

$$X = 2.8 \ mL/min$$

Step 3. Calculate the number of drops per minute.

IV set drop rate = 10 gtt/mL

$$\frac{10 \ gtt}{1 \ mL} = \frac{X \ gtt}{2.8 \ mL}$$

$$X = 28 \ gtt/min$$

The following example shows how to calculate the time required to administer an IV solution when the volume and flow rate are known.

EXAMPLE

How many minutes will it take to complete an IV infusion of 1.5 L of D5W being administered at the rate of 45 drops/minute? The IV set is calibrated to deliver 15 drops/mL. This problem is a variation of the flow rate problem considered earlier.

Solution

Step 1. Determine the number of milliliters/minute being infused.

$$\text{Drop rate of IV set} = \frac{15 \ gtt}{1 \ mL} = \frac{45 \ gtt}{X \ mL}$$

$$15X = 45 \ gtt$$

$$X = 3 \ mL/min$$

Step 2. Calculate the number of minutes required to administer the total volume of the solution.

$$\frac{3 \ mL}{1 \ min} = \frac{1,500 \ mL}{X \ min}$$

$$X = 500 \ min$$

EXAMPLE

A patient is ordered to receive 0.9 percent sodium chloride solution with 10 mEq potassium chloride per liter at a rate of 125 mL per hour. How many liters of solution must be provided to cover a 24-hour period?

Solution

$$\frac{125 \ mL}{1 \ hr} = \frac{X \ mL}{24 \ hr}$$

$$X = 3,000 \ mL \ or \ 3 \ liters \ of \ solution \ per \ 24\text{-hour period}$$

Calculations Involving Piggyback IV Infusion

The physician may order medications to be run piggyback with the IV electrolyte fluids. The medications are usually dissolved in 50 or 100 mL of an IV solution and run for short periods of time through the open IV line. The flow rate for these piggy-back infusions is calculated the same way as the rate for the regular IV solutions.

EXAMPLE

An IV piggyback of cefazolin sodium (Ancef, Kefzol) 500 mg in 100 mL/hour is ordered. The piggyback IV set is calibrated to deliver 10 gtt/mL. How many drops/minute should be administered?

Solution

Step 1. The entire 100 mL is to be infused in 1 hour. Calculate the number of milliliters/minute.

$$\frac{100 \text{ mL}}{60 \text{ min}} = \frac{X \text{ mL}}{1 \text{ min}}$$

$$60X = 100$$

$$X = 1.7 \text{ mL/min}$$

Step 2. Calculate the flow rate.

$$\text{Drop rate} = \frac{10 \text{ gtt}}{1 \text{ min}} = \frac{X \text{ gtt}}{1.7 \text{ mL/min.}}$$

$$X = 17 \text{ gtt/min}$$

It may be necessary for the volume of the piggyback and the time of its administration to be accounted for in calculating the daily fluid requirements, or fluid intake, of the patient.

When fluids are not restricted, calculating daily fluid intake simply involves adding all of the volumes administered to a patient in a 24-hour period. Flow rates are determined by each fluid/drug and an ordered infusion rate.

- cefazolin 100 mL q.i.d. 100 mL × 4 = 400 mL.
- Standard hydration fluid D5W at 75 mL/hr = 1,800 mL in 24 hours.
- Add to determine total intake = 1,800 mL + 400 mL = 2,200 mL in 24 hours if the piggyback is run in concurrently.

OR

- 75 mL/hr × 20 hours (if the standard fluid is stopped when giving the piggyback) = 1,500 mL,
- Plus 400 mL from piggyback cefazolin,
- Total = 1,900 mL in 24 hours.

Prevention of Medication Errors

Medication errors fall into several categories, such as omitting the dose, administering the wrong dose, administering an extra dose, administering an unordered drug, administering by the wrong route, and administering at the wrong time. The focus here will be to consider the errors that occur when the drug order is misinterpreted. The pharmacist and all personnel assisting them (technicians) are vital in catching, preventing, and correcting medication errors.

Very often, the way the amounts are expressed in the original order for weights, volumes, and units can cause interpretational errors. For instance, writing .5 instead of 0.5 can result in a tenfold error if the decimal point is missed. To reduce the possibility of errors, the following rules should be adhered to in transcribing orders. These are important for all health care professionals to follow (physicians, nurses, pharmacists, technicians, etc.):

- Never leave a decimal point "naked." Always place a zero *before* a decimal expression less than one. Example: 0.5 is correct; writing .5 is incorrect.

- A whole number should be shown with no decimal point or "trailing" 0. The decimal may not be seen and result in a tenfold overdose. Example: 2.0 mg is incorrect, as it may be read as 20 mg. The correct way is to write this is simply 2 mg.
- Avoid using decimals when a whole number can be used as an alternative. Example: 0.5 g should be expressed as 500 mg, and 0.4 mg should be expressed as 400 mcg.
- A space should be left between a number and the units for clarity in reading the number.
- Use the metric system; convert when necessary.
- Always spell out the word *units*. The abbreviation "U" for unit can be mistaken for a zero. Example: 10 U interpreted as 100 if the U is unclear. The better way is to write 10 *units*.

Summary

Accuracy in pharmaceutical calculations is one of the most critical and important functions in the profession of pharmacy. *A pharmacy technician should have every calculation regarding drugs or compounding checked by a pharmacist before preparing or dispensing any medication order.* Pharmacists frequently double-check each other in this important matter, because life and death can hinge on a proper or improper dose being administered. Emergency situations or other life-threatening situations are never an excuse for undue haste and lack of sufficient double-checks. Care and vigilance are required whenever drug doses or formulations are calculated.

TEST YOUR KNOWLEDGE

Convert the following to Arabic numbers.

1. viii

2. xxiv

3. XLV

4. CXXV

5. DCCL

Convert the following:

6. 2,500 mg = _____ g

7. 7.5 g = _____ mg

8. 0.3 L = _____ mL

9. 250 mcg = _____ mg

10. 1.5 kg = _____ g

11. 0.05 g = _____ mcg

12. 1.5 L = _____ mL

Solve the following problems by setting up the proportion and finding the unknown quantity.

13. Digoxin Elixir contains 50 mcg of digoxin in each milliliter. How many micrograms of the drug are in 0.3 mL of the elixir?

14. A solution of gentamycin contains 3 mg of gentamycin per milliliter. How many micrograms of gentamycin are in 0.2 mL of the solution?

15. Benadryl Elixir contains 12.5 mg per 5 mL (teaspoonful). How many milliliters are needed to provide 30 mg of the drug?

16. The physician orders 24 mg of theophylline to be administered orally to a pediatric patient. If theophylline solution contains 80 mg of theophylline per 15 mL (tablespoonful), how many milliliters of the solution should be administered?

17. A bottle of erythromycin suspension contains 250 mg of erythromycin in every 5 mL of suspension. How many grams of erythromycin are in a 200 mL bottle?

Convert the following:

18. 2 fluid ounces (℥ii) contain how many teaspoonfuls?

19. 24 pints equal how many gallons?

20. 1.5 quarts contain how many fluid ounces?

Convert the following:

21. Convert a patient's weight of 138 pounds to kg.

22. Convert 2.5 pounds of ointment to grams.

23. Convert ℥ iiss to mL.

24. Convert 2 quarts to liters.

25. Convert 5 g to mg.

26. If a doctor orders ℨ ii three times a day for 10 days, how many mL of solution must be dispensed to fill the prescription?

27. Calculate the percent strength of a solution made from 102 g of sucrose and enough water to make 120 mL of solution.

28. How many grams of hydrocortisone are present in 40 g of a 2.5 percent hydrocortisone ointment?

29. How many mL of alcohol are in 30 mL of a mouthwash made with 18 percent V/V alcohol?

30. How many grams of dextrose does a patient receive from 3 liters of 5 percent dextrose in water?

Calculate the following using the equation $(Q1)(C1) = (Q2)(C2)$.

31. How many grams of petrolatum must be added to 15 grams of 20 percent ichthammol ointment to dilute it to a 12 percent ichthammol ointment?

32. To make 240 mL of a solution that contains 20 percent alcohol, how many mL of 70 percent alcohol must be used?

33. How many grams of 1.5 percent Bactroban ointment can be made from 30 grams of 2 percent Bactroban ointment?

34. How many mL of 17 percent benzalkonium chloride solution must be diluted to make 480 mL of 2 percent benzalkonium chloride solution?

Using alligations, recalculate questions 31–34 and calculate the following:

35. How many mL of 70 percent dextrose solution must be diluted to make 2 liters of 20 percent dextrose solution?

36. To make 120 g of 1.5 percent hydrocortisone ointment, how many grams of the following must be weighed?
    a. 5 percent hydrocortisone ointment
    b. petrolatum

37. How many grams of 3 percent Coal Tar Ointment can be compounded by adding petrolatum to one pound of 5 percent Coal Tar Ointment?

38. How many mL of water must be added to 120 mL of 95 percent alcohol to dilute it to 75 percent alcohol?

39. A patient is to receive a 120 mg dose of gentamicin. The drug is available in a vial containing 80 mg/2mL of the drug. How many mL should be given to the patient to obtain the correct dose?

40. After reconstitution, a multiple-dose vial of a penicillin G potassium solution contains 100,000 units per mL. How many mL of this solution must be administered to a patient who requires a 450,000 unit dose?

41. A physician orders 40 mg of Demerol IM for a patient. How many mL of a Demerol solution with a strength of 100 mg/mL should the patient receive?

42. The nurse is asked to administer an intramuscular dose of 0.45 mg of an investigational drug. How many mL must be withdrawn from a vial containing 200 mcg/mL of the drug?

43. An elderly patient is to be given a 120 mg dose of phenytoin by administering an oral suspension containing 50 mg/5 mL of phenytoin. How many mL of the suspension should be administered for each dose?

44. The recommended dose of cefuroxime (Ceftin) for a pediatric patient is 20 mg/kg/day. How many milligrams must be given daily to an 80-pound child?

45. Acyclovir (Zovirax) is administered in a dose of 15 mg/kg/day. How many mg of the drug must be administered for each dose to a 175-pound adult if the drug is to be given three times a day?

46. The recommended dose for methotrexate is 2.5 mg/kg once every 14 days. How many milligrams of this drug must be administered to a 125-pound adult for each dose?

47. Chlorpromazine HCl is to be administered in a dose of 0.25 mg/lb. How many 25 mg tablets of chlorpromazine HCl should be administered for each dose to a 91-kg patient?

48. A new drug is to be dosed at 40 mg/kg/dose. Calculate the number of mg a 48-kg adult should receive for each dose.

Solve the following problems using the nomogram.

49. Find the BSA for the following children:
a. 9 pounds, 23 inches
b. 3.2 kg, 50 cm BSA
c. 15 kg, 40 inches BSA

50. If the adult dose of amoxicillin is 500 mg, what should the dose be for the child in problem 49c?

51. If the adult dose of furosemide (Lasix) is 40 mg, what is the dose for a child whose BSA is 0.62 m²?

52. If a dose of drug is ordered at 5 mg/m², what is the dose for a child who weighs 55 pounds and who has a height of 41 inches?

53. If a dose of drug is ordered at 25 mg/m², what is the dose for a child who weighs 8 kg with a height of 68 cm?

54. The physician orders 1,500 mL of D5W solution to be administered over a 12-hour period. The IV set is calibrated to deliver 20 gtt/mL. Calculate the number of drops per minute the patient must receive.

55. An IV infusion containing 500 mL is to be administered at a drop rate of 40 gtt/min. The IV set is calibrated to deliver 20 gtt/mL. Calculate the number of minutes it will take to administer the entire infusion solution.

56. A physician orders a solution to be run continuously at 75 mL/hr.
a. How many 500 mL bags must be prepared for the patient to cover a 24-hour period?
b. An IV set is being used, calibrated to deliver 15 gtt/mL. At how many drops per minute must it be set to infuse the solutions?

57. An IV piggyback of cefazolin containing 1 g of drug in 100 mL is to be infused over one hour. The IV set being used is calibrated to deliver 15 gtt/mL. How many drops/minute should be administered?

58. A piggyback infusion solution of heparin sodium containing 25,000 in 500 mL is to be infused at a rate of 1,000 units per hour. The IV set is calibrated to deliver 30 gtt/mL. How many drops/minute should be administered?

59. What should the rate be (in drops per minute) to infuse a piggyback solution of 300 mg of cimetidine in 50 mL of normal saline (0.9 % sodium chloride solution) over 45 minutes? The set being used delivers 25 drops/mL.

References

Ansel, H. C., & Stoklosa, M. J. (2006). *Pharmaceutical calculations* (12th ed.). Philadelphia: Lippincott Williams & Wilkins.

Capriotti, T. (2004). Basic concepts to prevent medication calculation errors. *MEDSURG Nursing 04*, 13(1), 62–65.

Cohen, M. R. (2007). *Medication errors* (2nd ed.). Washington: American Pharmacists Association.

Kelly, L. E., & Colby, N. (2003). Teaching medication calculation for conceptual understanding. *Journal of Nursing Education* 03, 42(10), 468–471.

Preston, R. M. (2004). Drug errors and patient safety: The need for a change in practice. *British Journal of Nursing* 04, 13(2), 72–78.

Richardson, L. I., & Richardson, J. (2004). *The mathematics of drugs and solutions with clinical applications* (6th ed.). New York: Pearson Publishing Co.

Trim, J. (2004). Clinical skills: A practical guide to working out drug calculations. *British Journal of Nursing 04*, 13(10), 602–606.

Web Sites

Institute for Safe Medication Practices (ISMP)   www.ismp.org

Extemporaneous Compounding

Competencies

Upon completion of this chapter, the reader should be able to

1. Define a Class A prescription balance, a counter balance, and a solution balance.

2. Describe what is meant by extemporaneous compounding.

3. Explain the circumstances that may require the extemporaneous compounding of a drug dosage form.

4. Outline the steps required to accurately weigh a pharmaceutical ingredient.

5. Describe the meaning of the term *geometric dilution.*

6. Explain the difference between a solution and a suspension; an ointment and a cream.

7. Describe the process of levigation.

8. List some of the steps involved in the process of compounding suppositories.

9. Give an example of the ingredients found in an enteral solution.

10. List the essential equipment used in the compounding process.

Key Terms

chemical sterilization
Class A prescription balance
counter balance
electronic balance
extemporaneous compounding
filtration
geometric dilution
graduate
levigation
meniscus
radiation
solution balance
suspending agent
tare
taring
thermal sterilization
triturate

Introduction

This chapter will familiarize students with terminology, equipment, and principles of extemporaneous compounding and their role in providing this service. The student should understand this to be an introduction to compounding; experience is needed to develop this valuable skill. While it is beyond the scope of this chapter to review all types of compounding, the most common and relevant practices are reviewed. The student is referred to compounding textbooks for more detailed knowledge.

Extemporaneous compounding is a true pharmaceutical service, not simply the redistribution of a commercially available commodity. This service requires a specialized knowledge of physical and chemical properties of drugs and their vehicles. This knowledge is based on sound scientific principles; however, the practice is closer to an art.

Extemporaneous Compounding

extemporaneous compounding prepared at the time it is required, with materials on hand.

Extemporaneous compounding may be defined as the timely preparation of a drug product according to a physician's prescription, a drug formula, or a recipe in which the amounts of the ingredients are calculated to meet the needs of a particular patient or group of patients.

Although demand is less, the need for extemporaneous preparations continues. Extemporaneous pharmaceutical compounding is among the most exciting, challenging, and rapidly expanding areas in pharmacy today. Practically every medical discipline incorporates these dosage forms in their everyday practice. Many pharmaceutical products are either no longer produced, or for some reason become temporarily unavailable. Many commercially available products are in dosage forms that may not be convenient for dosing a specific patient. These are some of the challenges that are overcome by modern compounding techniques. Veterinary medicine, sports medicine, ophthalmology, and pain management have opened up vast new areas for the compounder. The compounding of sterile products such as ophthalmics, injectables, and intravenous prescriptions, when done following proper procedure, is both very challenging and professionally rewarding. With the development of modern equipment and devices, the properly equipped compounding pharmacy is capable of delivering the highest quality specialty dosage forms.

Traditional Equipment

Class A prescription balance has a sensitive balance of 6 mg.

solution balance a single unequal arm balance used for weighing large amounts.

The tools of pharmaceutical practice are those used to measure, transfer, transform, and handle medications in any way desired. Those involved in non-sterile compounding are classic, and every pharmacy technician should be familiar with their proper handling.

Every pharmacy is required to have a **Class A prescription balance** (Figure 14-1a). Class A balances have a sensitivity requirement of 6 mg. A scale's sensitivity is the smallest weight required to move the indicator at least one degree.

A **solution balance** is a single-pan instrument with an unequal arm that acts as a compound lever (Figure 14-1b). These balances are less accurate than Class

FIGURE 14-1

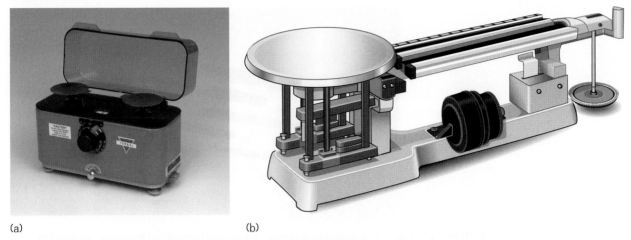

(a)   (b)

FIGURE 14-1 a. The Class A prescription balance. b. Solution balance.

counter balance
a double-pan balance
capable of weigh-
ing relatively large
quantities.

A balances, but are useful for measuring large masses with a weighing capacity of
about 20 kg.

   Counter balances are double-pan balances also capable of weighing large
quantities, but again are not intended for small weights, having a sensitivity of 100
mg and a limit of about 5 kg.

   Weights used with the balances should be of good quality and stored well.
Weights made of corrosion-resistant metals such as brass are preferred (Figure
14-2). Metric weight sets are commonly available in a range from less than 1 g to
50 g. Always use forceps to transfer the weights, and take care not to drop them.
Keep the weights covered in their original case when not in use.

   Spatulas (Figure 14-3) are used to transfer solid ingredients to weighing pans.
They are the preferred mixing instruments with semisolid dosage forms such as
ointments and creams. These are available in stainless steel and hard rubber or
plastic. Care must be used with materials that corrode metals, such as iodine, salts
of mercury, or tannins. Use rubber spatulas for these agents. Check that spatulas
are clean.

   Weighing papers, preferably nonabsorbable paraffinic glassine paper, should
always be used to weigh powders and other solid and semisolid pharmaceuticals

FIGURE 14-2

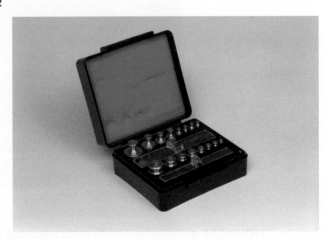

FIGURE 14-2 Pharmaceutical weights should be corrosion-resistant and handled with forceps.

FIGURE 14-3

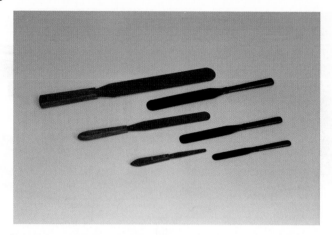

FIGURE 14-3 Spatulas, available in stainless steel and hard rubber or plastic, are used to transfer solid ingredients to weighing pans.

to prevent contamination or damage to the weighing pans. For small amounts of powders, the paper should be creased diagonally from each corner and then flattened and placed on the pans. This ensures a collection trough in the paper. Discard the paper after each product to prevent contamination.

Essential equipment that technicians must be familiar with include the mortar and pestle, commonly available in three types: glass (Figure 14-4), Wedgwood, and porcelain (Figure 14-5), which is quite similar to Wedgwood in use and appearance. Wedgwood and porcelain mortars are relatively coarse and are used to grind **triturate** crystals and large particles into fine powders. Both are earthenware and are somewhat porous, and will easily stain. Glass mortars are preferable for mixing liquids and semisoft dosage forms.

When mixing ingredients, always place the most potent drug, which is usually the smallest amount, into the mortar first. Then add an equal amount of the next most potent ingredient and mix thoroughly. This process is repeated until

triturate to reduce particle size and mix one powder with another.

FIGURE 14-4

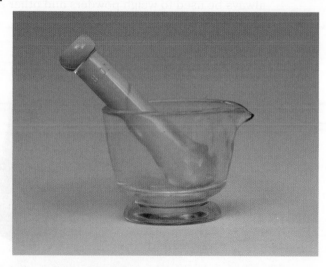

FIGURE 14-4 A glass mortar and pestle is preferable for mixing liquids and semisoft dosage forms.

FIGURE 14-5

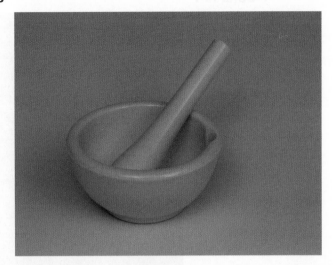

FIGURE 14-5 A porcelain mortar and pestle is used for trituration of crystals and large particles.

geometric dilution the addition of approximately equal amounts of the prescribed drugs when mixing in a mortar.

graduate a marked (or graduated) conical or cylindrical vessel used for measuring liquids.

all ingredients are added. Because each addition is approximately equal to the amount in the mortar, the process is called **geometric dilution**.

Ointment slabs are ground glass plates, often square or rectangular, that provide a hard, nonabsorbable surface for mixing compounds. When combining creams and ointments, spatulas are used to spread the material, using a shearing force to mix ingredients. Some pharmacists use disposable, nonabsorbent parchment paper to cover the work area, which is not as durable as the ointment slabs, but saves time in cleaning.

Accurately measuring liquids is an essential skill technicians must master. Equipment consists of conical **graduates** (containers marked with degrees of measurements) (Figure 14-6), cylindrical graduates (Figure 14-7), and syringes. Beakers are generally not accurate enough for prescription work.

Conical graduates are the easiest to use, with wide mouths and narrow bases, and are the easiest to clean. Liquids may be stirred in them with the aid of a stirring rod. As the diameter of the graduate increases, the accuracy of the measurement

FIGURE 14-6

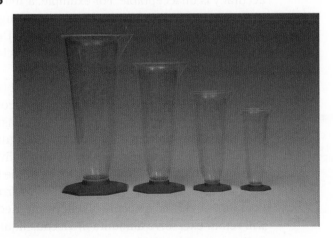

FIGURE 14-6 Conical graduates have a wide mouth and a narrow base.

FIGURE 14-7

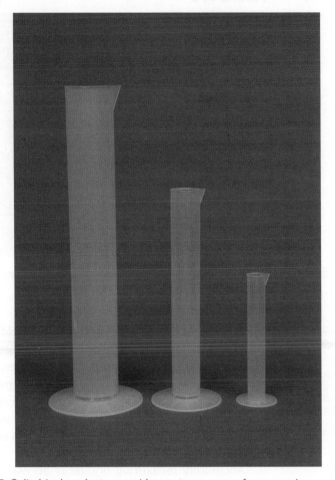

FIGURE 14-7 Cylindrical graduates provide greater accuracy for measuring.

decreases. This design makes the narrow-diameter cylindrical graduates preferable when greater accuracy is desired. Graduates are available in sizes ranging from 10 mL to 4,000 mL. When selecting a graduate, always choose the smallest graduate capable of containing the volume to be measured. Avoid measurements of volumes that are below 20 percent of the capacity of the graduate, because the accuracy is unacceptable. For example, a 100 mL graduate cannot accurately measure volumes below 20 mL. When measuring small volumes, such as 30 mL and less, it is often preferable to use a syringe. Disposable plastic injectable and oral syringes are readily available in all pharmacies and have essentially replaced the use of smaller-sized graduates.

When measuring liquids in a graduate, it is important that the reading be done at eye level. The surface of the liquid has a concave or crescent shape that bulges downward, called the **meniscus**. When measuring liquids, the correct reading is the mark at the bottom of the meniscus (Figure 14-8).

Most graduates are marked "TD" (to deliver). They are calibrated to compensate for the excess of fluid that adheres to the surface after emptying the graduate. Caution must be used to differentiate this from older glassware marked "TC" (to contain), or errors in accuracy will result. Keep in mind that even "TD" glassware will retain excessive amounts of viscous liquids if not drained completely. Essentially, no liquid should remain in the graduate after emptying.

meniscus the outer surface of a liquid having a concave or crescent shape, caused by surface tension.

FIGURE 14-8

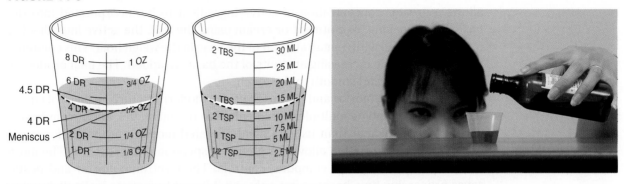

FIGURE 14-8 When measuring liquids, the correct reading is the mark at the bottom of the meniscus.

Modern Equipment

Modern pharmacy compounding labs are equipped with digital electronic balances. These balances greatly increase the ease and accuracy of the weighing process. These balances do away entirely with the need for the counterweights that were used with the earlier torsion balances. Because they are self-leveling and self-calibrating, they remove a great deal of potential error and stress from the weighing process. They allow for greater accuracy and improved recordkeeping, due to their ability to be interfaced with printers and computer software programs that enable the retention of a record of weights and calibrations. The more sophisticated software programs will actually enable the weights to be applied directly to log the formula being prepared.

Electronic balances will vary based upon their purpose. Bulk balances are used to weigh quantities greater than 1 g. Standard prescription balances are accurate to 1 mg, while analytical balances are accurate to 0.001 mg.

Since chemicals are never weighed directly onto the table of the balance, different receptacles are used to contain the chemicals being weighed. The most common receptacles have been glassine weigh papers; however, most compounders now use different types of weigh boats. Weigh boats come in several shapes, sizes, and materials, depending on their use. Some have an octagonal shape, allowing several chemicals to be weighed into the same weigh boat into separate corners, making the process more efficient. Electronic balances allow this process because they can be reset to a zero reading, which is known as **taring**, with each chemical added.

A formula with six chemicals can be weighed into one weigh boat by taring the balance after each chemical has been weighed. Weigh boats also allow more efficient transportation of chemicals from the balance to the processing area.

The recent development of the *mini-ointment mill* has added a whole new dimension to semisolid compounding. The ointment mill allows the incorporation of solid ingredients into cream, gel, and ointment bases by milling the active ingredients to minute particle size and efficiently incorporating and dispersing the active ingredient throughout the base. This process is similar to methods used in the commercial manufacture of creams, gels, and ointments, and enhances the effect of the active ingredients in the base. The old method of using the ointment tile or pad along with geometric dilution, although effective, could not result in

electronic balance a balance scale that varies based on its purpose; can be used to weigh bulk quantities greater than 1 g. Standard prescription balances are accurate up to 1 mg or smaller quantities down to 0.001 mg.

taring resetting an electronic balance to a zero reading.

the same particle size and distribution of active ingredient. The ointment mill also allows a greater concentration of active ingredient to be incorporated into the base. When making an ointment or cream using the mill, the active ingredient is usually combined with a small amount of the base in the weigh boat. This combination is milled while increasing amounts of the base are added. The final product is evenly dispersed and smooth to the touch.

The electronic mortar and pestle (EMP) is a modern, motorized piece of equipment used to combine multiple ingredients into ointment, gel, and cream bases. It is far more efficient than using a hand-operated mortar and pestle for many reasons. Its rapid rotation allows for greater dispersion of ingredients. The more elaborate EMPs can have computer controls. The electronic mortar and pestle saves processing time because not only can it be set to operate by itself, but it is able to produce a large quantity of product in one single operation. Many finished products are both mixed and blended in their final dispensing container, thus reducing handling and preserving the purity of the final product. The newest of the EMPs allows the mixing of up to 500 g of finished product.

Today, basic compounding equipment will always include a combination thermostatically controlled hot plate and magnetic spinner. This combination allows semisolids and liquids to be heated and stirred at the same time. It also allows the heating of viscous liquids without burning. A magnetic stirring rod is placed in the bottom of the holding vessel, and it is spun by a magnet within the hot plate. The speed of the stirring rod is controlled by a rheostat.

New pressure-driven tube heat sealers and tube-filling devices allow the compounder to package creams, gels, and ointments in collapsible plastic tubes and seal them in much the way a manufacturer would. The final product is elegantly presented. In instances where products must be packaged in metal tubes, modern crimping devices allow the application of a professional-looking seal. The most popular tube sizes range from 3 g to 120 g. Tubes can also be filled from the large-size electronic mortar and pestle jar or by using special tube-filling devices.

Homogenizers are used to both reduce particle size of active ingredients and to disperse and emulsify them into suspensions, emulsions, and low viscosity lotions. Homogenizers are necessary in the compounding of sterile suspensions in ophthalmics and sterile injectables where particle size and dispersion are critical to the efficacy of the dosage at the site of use.

Traditional Weighing Techniques

The critical first step in any pharmaceutical dispensing is the selection of the proper drug and dose. Qualitative and quantitative accuracy is the hallmark of our profession. Technicians given the responsibilities of compounding must learn the skills and work carefully under the supervision of a pharmacist.

Prior to weighing with a Class A balance, the technician should gather and organize all materials in a level, well-lighted, draft-free area. The balance should be leveled by adjusting the thumbscrew at the base of the legs until the pointer rests at zero. Place weighing papers on each pan and adjust the balance again if necessary. The beam weight should be all the way to the left and set at zero. When equilibrium is reached, the balance is arrested in place by a lock screw. The desired weights are placed in the right pan using forceps. The desired material is placed on the left pan using a spatula. When weighing less than a gram, one may wish to shift the weight beam to the appropriate weight. The balance is carefully unlocked to observe the movement of the pointer, which will shift to the side with the greater weight. Relock the balance and use a spatula to subtract or add material being weighed. This process is repeated until equilibrium is reached and the indicator is at the zero point. The balance is then locked, the lid closed, and the lock released one final time to verify the equilibrium. The weight should be checked by a pharmacist. If it is correct, the material can be removed from the balance in the cradle of the folded weighing paper. Weights should be checked three times: when selected, when resting on the pan, and when returned to the kit.

When weighing, the sensitivities and limitations of the balance used must be kept in mind.

Compounding Liquids

Liquids are probably the most common form of compounded medications. Extemporaneous, non-sterile compounds most often involve solutions and suspensions, whereas emulsions and lotions are less popular. Solutions are clear liquids in which the drug is completely dissolved. The simplest compound solution involves the addition of a drug in liquid form to a vehicle such as water or syrup. This involves careful liquid measurement of the drug, using graduates or syringes, and then dilution to the final volume desired. Gentle shaking effects thorough dispersion of additives.

Compounding Solids

When solids are required in solution, they must be carefully weighed, using a prescription balance. Most solids dissolve readily in a solvent, but others require intervention. Some solids may be reduced in size by grinding in a mortar to increase dissolution rates. Other times, the vehicle is heated to enhance dissolution, but care must be used since some drugs decompose at higher temperatures. Dissolution of a solute may require vigorous shaking or stirring.

Compounding Suspensions

Suspensions are liquid preparations of drugs containing finely-divided drug particles distributed uniformly throughout the vehicle. Suspensions appear cloudy in nature, and shaking is often required to resuspend drug particles that have settled. Depending on particle size, some suspensions settle so rapidly that a uniform dispersion cannot be maintained long enough for an accurate dose to be withdrawn. Such preparations require a **suspending agent**, a thickening agent that gives some structure to a suspension. Typical agents are carboxymethylcellulose, methylcellulose, bentonite, tragacanth, and others. Some suspending agents may bind the drug, limiting availability, so these agents should be carefully selected.

suspending agent a chemical additive used in suspensions to "thicken" the liquid and retard settling of particles.

While some solid drugs may be added directly to a suspending vehicle, some agents need to be "wetted" first. That is, the powder to be added is first mixed with a wetting agent, such as alcohol or glycerin, in a mortar with a pestle. This displaces the air from the particles of the solid and allows them to mix more readily with a suspending vehicle. Next, the vehicle is added in portions and mixed with mortar and pestle until a uniform mixture results. This mixture is then blended into the remaining vehicle. The mortar and pestle can be rinsed with small portions of the vehicle and added until the final volume is reached. Suspensions should be dispensed in tight, light-resistant containers that contain enough air space for adequate shaking. The bottle should contain the auxiliary label "Shake well." Refrigeration may be used to slow separation.

Compounding Ointments and Creams

These two semisolid external dosage forms are still popular choices for extemporaneous compounds and share common preparation techniques. Ointments are oil-based in nature, whereas creams are water-based. Given the commercial availability of unmedicated cream and ointment bases, their preparation is more of historic interest, but we will focus on the addition of drugs to these bases. In the simplest cases, physicians often desire the combined effects of two or more ointments or creams in a specified proportion. This usually involves the thorough mechanical mixing of the weighed bases on an ointment slab using a spatula until a uniform preparation has been obtained. Using the spatula, transfer the material into an ointment jar just big enough for the final volume. When filling the ointment jar, use the spatula to bleed out air pockets. Tapping the jar on the countertop will settle the contents. Wipe any excess material from the outside of the jar, including the cap screw threads. Cover the jar and label it appropriately.

Drugs in powder or crystal form, such as salicylic acid, precipitated sulfur, or hydrocortisone, are often prescribed to be mixed into cream or ointment bases. Large particles should be reduced to fine powder with a mortar and pestle. The ointment base may be placed on one side of the working area, with the powders to be incorporated on the other. Using a spatula, mix a small portion of powder with a portion of the base on an ointment slab (Figure 14-9). Repeat this until all powder is incorporated into the base and a uniform product is produced.

Occasionally, the direct mixture method results in a gritty product with poorly dispensed clumps of powder that fail to blend in despite vigorous mixing. Here, it is desirable first to reduce the particle size of the powder by levigating it. **Levigation** is the mixing of powder with a vehicle in which it is insoluble to produce a smooth dispersion of the drug. The dispersion is then mixed with the base. When

levigation the mixing of particles with a base vehicle, in which they are insoluble, to produce a smooth dispersion of the drug by rubbing with a spatula on a tile.

FIGURE 14-9

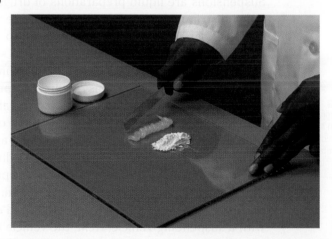

FIGURE 14-9 Gradually mix the medication and base until the substance is uniform.

using ointments, mineral oil is a good levigating agent. When working with creams, glycerin or water can often be used.

Compounding Transdermal Gels

Ointments and creams are used to introduce and maintain the presence of drugs to the body topically. Their effectiveness is usually limited to the drug's ability to pass through the skin barriers. Transdermal gels are able to disrupt the lipid layers of the stratum corneum of the skin without damaging it the way harsher agents can. The most popular form of transdermal gel is the pleuronic lecithin organogel, or PLO gel.

PLO allows the medication to slip through the stratum corneum into systemic circulation via dermal-epidermal blood flow. PLO gels are used in all disciplines of compounding. These gels are extremely effective for the delivery of pain management drugs to local sites with excellent results and decreased liver absorption. Combinations of localized pain trigger receptor agonists (i.e., drugs that block pain) can be incorporated into a single gel and applied with excellent results. These gels have many positive uses. They are used in veterinary medicine to allow ease in dosing. Cats, which can be difficult to medicate, will respond extremely well to PLO gels administered to the pinna or inner flap of the ear. They can also be used to deliver drugs to pediatric patients who might otherwise be difficult to dose. A good example of this is the dosing of the drug Secretin to treat autism. It replaces the need for daily injections and the absorption is equivalent.

These gels are easily compounded using the ointment mill or the EMP. The active ingredient is dissolved in a solvent and combined with isopropyl palmitate and Pluronic-127. They are then blended and mixed to allow the formation of small emulsion units called *micelles*, which transport the drug across the skin barrier.

There are many other new forms of gels, such as aqueous gels, which are water miscible and easily washable and act as effective carriers for drugs across the skin barrier. Though not every drug can be introduced in gel form and the expiration dating of gels is usually less than six months, they have proven to be a valuable tool for compounding.

Compounding Troches, Lollipops, and Gummy Bears

Pharmacists had always compounded pastilles and troches by using a hand-rolling technique. They incorporated certain types of drugs into a candy base and were able to produce a hard disc or barrel-shaped troche or pastille that would be placed in the cheek and allowed to dissolve. Modern compounders are able to produce troches that can contain a much wider array of active ingredients and can be sugar-free and elegantly colored and flavored. The advent of the troche mold allows the active ingredient to be calculated and combined into a pre-measured amount of base to make a much more uniform product. There are many troche bases, such as soft, chewy, and hard, which allow for greater flexibility in dosing. The different bases are used to adjust the time that the drug takes to be absorbed, along with adapting to the personal preference of the patient. The recent development of lollipop molds now allows medication to be incorporated in this very attractive and fun dosage form. Actiq, which is a commercial pain medication with the active ingredient fentanyl, started out as a custom-compounded product. It was designed to allow the pleasant dosing of a narcotic analgesic to both children and hospice patients. Lollipops are a good dosage form for ease of compliance. As with troches, they can be made sugar-free and in literally 101 flavor combinations.

Gummy Bears are another dosage form used to deliver medication to children. The same base is used in their formulation as is used for soft troches. The base is melted and the active ingredient, suspending agents, sweetener, and choice of flavors are combined and introduced into a pre-calibrated mold. Children particularly like this dosage form.

Flavoring

The development of modern flavoring techniques, along with a multitude of different flavors, sweeteners, and flavoring vehicles, has added a great deal of flexibility to modern compounding. There are flavors that are either oil-soluble or water-soluble. There are powdered flavorings that can be added to dry bulk powders for veterinary use, such as apple flavor for horses. There are specific flavors for either level of pH balance. There are flavors to enhance most dosage forms. The development of more sweetening products now allows the compounder to make a greater assortment of sugar-free products. Flavoring is very important in medication dosing compliance. Very bitter drugs can be made more palatable. Dosage forms can be changed; for example, tablets can be pulverized, suspended, and flavored, creating a different dosage form of the same drug. This is especially useful in dosing children and also those patients who have difficulty swallowing. Commercially-available liquid products can be flavor-enhanced to make them taste better. Prescriptions can be flavored for animals based on preference. Cats like tuna fish, while dogs like liver flavors. Small birds like tutti-frutti flavors. Hundreds of bases, flavors, and flavor combinations are now available.

Compounding Suppositories

Suppositories are solid dosage forms intended for insertion into body orifices, predominantly rectal or vaginal, where they melt or dissolve to release their active ingredients. Extemporaneous manufacture of suppositories remains a vital art today for several reasons. Industrial manufacturers market relatively few products in suppository form in this country, in part because rectal administration is not socially popular. So, although the products are limited, there is a subgroup of patients who cannot tolerate oral medications, but who also are not candidates for parenteral drug therapy.

Suppositories must be manufactured so that they remain solid at room or refrigerated temperatures, yet melt readily at body temperature—a fine line indeed. This process is accomplished by using special bases, such as cocoa butter or polyethylene glycol. Polyethylene glycols are available in various molecular weight ranges. Those of 200, 400, or 600 are liquids; those over 1,000 are solid and wax-like. Often, combinations of liquid (low molecular weight) and solid polyethylene glycol are used to achieve a suppository that melts as desired. By increasing the waxy portion of the blend, we gain a suppository that melts more slowly and provides more sustained action.

To prepare suppositories, the base material is melted and the active ingredients are added. The material is poured into molds and chilled until congealed. Then they are removed from the mold.

FIGURE 14-10

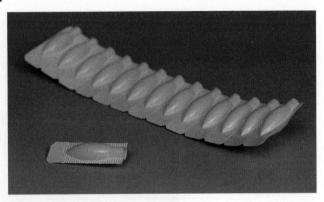

FIGURE 14-10 Suppository molds.

Most modern compounding labs will tend to use disposable suppository strip molds (Figure 14-10). These are pre-calibrated to the specific bases, are easier to fill and dispense, and can be heat-sealed to present a far more elegant and professional-looking product. Modern compounders melt the base by placing it in a beaker with a magnetic stirrer at the bottom, then heating it on an electric hot plate with a stirrer. The mixture must be allowed to cool almost to the point of congealing, so as not to melt the plastic molds and also to properly fill the mold cavity.

Suppositories (both commercial and extemporaneous sources) are still commonly used to deliver analgesics, hormones, antiemetics, laxatives, and vaginal anti-infectives.

Compounding Capsules

Extemporaneous capsule manufacturing remains a popular means of providing unusual (and often low) doses of oral medication. You may recall that commercially available capsules cannot be divided. Tablets can only be reliably broken in quarters at best and usually only halves. A typical situation for capsule compounding may be when a drug is only available in 50 mg tablets or capsules, but the prescribing physician desires 12.5 mg doses, or what would amount to a one-quarter dose. If crushed, the resulting powder would be too small to handle accurately.

To facilitate measuring, first dilute the crushed tablet (or emptied capsule) with inactive filler and measure a portion containing the desired amount. Select empty, hard gelatin capsules (available in eight sizes, with 000 being the largest and 5 the smallest). In general, the smallest capsule capable of containing the final volume is used because patients often have difficulty swallowing large capsules. To fill each capsule, place the powder on a tile or paper and press the body of the capsule repeatedly into the powder until it is filled (Figure 14-11).

Be careful not to touch the powder with your fingers. This is called the *punch method* of capsule filling. Place the cap onto the body and weigh the result, using an empty capsule the same size as the **tare**. Adjust the weight, if needed, by adding or removing powder. To keep the capsule clean during the process, the compounder may wear rubber gloves or finger cots. Since some material is lost in the process, always calculate a little extra material to compensate for this loss.

tare a weight used to counterbalance the container holding the substance being weighed.

FIGURE 14-11

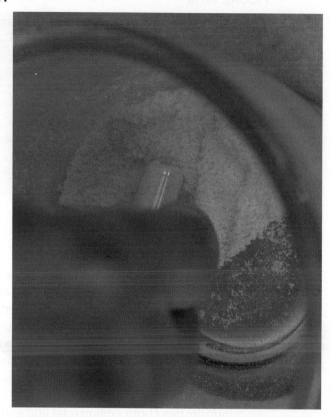

FIGURE 14-11 The punch method is used to fill the capsule with the prepared medication.

In this example, select a #3 capsule and set the final weight at 200 mg. To make 10 capsules, three 50 mg tablets are needed, which would produce 12 doses, in theory. Twelve doses of 200 mg require 2,400 mg of final powder. Three tablets might weigh 700 mg, to which we would add 1,700 mg of diluent, such as lactose powder, by trituration. We would pack 200 mg of this powder into each capsule to yield the 12.5 mg dose.

The use of capsule-filling machines can greatly facilitate the capsule-filling process. These machines vary from a strictly manual to a highly-automated process. The use of a machine requires the prior development of a formulation that will deliver a given dose of a drug in a pre-calculated volume of powder. As such, they are useful for manufacturing batches of a standard formula.

The machines require the loading of capsules into a molded plate. The capsule bodies may be separated by hand or by an automated process, leaving the capsule openings aligned with the surface of the plate. The formulated powder is poured over the plate, and spreaders are used to fill the capsules. The capsules are then closed by hand or by an automated process. The machine is inverted to release the filled capsules. The machines are useful for filling many capsules in a timely manner, because they are designed to fill from 50 to 300 capsules with each operation.

Compounding Lotions

Lotions are liquid preparations intended for external application. The most common lotions are "shake" lotions, in which insoluble substances are dispersed by agitation. Often, gums or other agents are used as suspending agents to prevent rapid settling of suspended particles. To prepare shake lotions, place the measured powders of the formula into a mortar and triturate until well blended. Slowly add a liquid levigating agent and triturate to form a smooth paste, free of gritty particles. Add the vehicle in small portions with continued trituration. After roughly two-thirds of the vehicle has been added, transfer the solution to a graduated vessel and rinse the mortar with remaining vehicle to bring the lotion to its final volume. Transfer this to a well-sealed bottle and label "Shake well."

Compounding Enteral Preparations

Pharmacy departments may also prepare enteral nutrition products. Although enteral literally means "in the intestine," the term is commonly used to mean a refined liquid diet, often administered by nasogastric tube to patients unable to eat solid foods.

Preparation of enteral products usually involves simple dissolution of pow-dered material in a blender, following package directions. But there are times when there is a need for varied dilutions of feedings to match a patient's clinical state. We use pharmaceutical calculations to prepare a two-thirds- or three-fourths-strength formula. For example, suppose a package of powdered dietary supple-ment is normally diluted to 500 mL. To prepare a two-thirds-strength enteral formula, we divide 500 mL by two-thirds to yield 750 mL. Each packet should be dissolved to 750 mL to yield the more diluted two-thirds mixture required.

At times, these oral feedings are supplemented with additional electrolytes, such as sodium chloride or potassium chloride. The pharmacy technician may be required to convert weight in milligrams to milliequivalents (mEq).

The use of clean equipment, precise measurement, and proper packaging, labeling, and storage of enteral nutrition products is important. They often require refrigeration after preparation, and each product has a recommended expiration period.

Sterile Compounding, On-Site Sterility, and Pyrogen Testing

Many compounding labs are equipped to prepare sterile compounds, including ophthalmic drops and ointments, injectable solutions and suspensions, and intra-venous drugs. This is an area of practice where many drugs must be prepared near to the time of actual use due to the instability of the final products. Great care must be taken to ensure the integrity of these compounds. The products must be prepared in a sterile environment. Special equipment is required to prepare these compounds. The creation of new on-site testing for selective impurities and steril-ity allows for the proper compounding of the products.

Pyrogens, dead cell particles that can cause fevers if allowed to exist in the sterile product, are easily prevented by proper techniques and can now be tested on-site prior to the release of the drug to the patient. One such test is *Pyro Test*, which can give a final result within one hour of preparation. Sterility can also be verified by the use of similar on-site tests, such as *Q-Test*. These tests are designed to use only minute volumes of the finished product. There are also products that test the accuracy of the person performing these procedures. Periodic testing of personnel is necessary to maintain the standard of the compounding facility. Most responsible compounders will send a specified percentage of their products for outside testing to ensure the integrity of their procedures.

Sterilization

When talking about sterilization, understanding the concept of maintaining the integrity of the pharmaceutical product to be dispensed is vital. Proper sterilization techniques start with using betadine scrub to wash hands and nails thoroughly under the sink for several minutes before applying gloves, arm sleeves, hairnets, and lab coats to ensure aseptic procedure is intact. Technicians can spread microorganisms into the laminar hood by wearing jewelry, coughing, sneezing (and not wearing a mask), or having loose facial hair. No food, beverages, or gum should be allowed in the sterile area. The hood should always be cleaned properly with alcohol after each compounded prescription is completed. There are four methods of sterilization we will discuss in this chapter: thermal, chemical, filtration, and radiation.

> **thermal sterilization** heat; moist heat and dry heat are methods of heat or thermal sterilization.

There are two types of **thermal sterilization**: moist heat and dry heat. Moist heat is used to coagulate the protein contained in microorganisms. Dry heat causes death by oxidation. Microorganisms need protein to survive, and thermal sterilization prevents this organism from surviving. Moist heat sterilization is performed in an autoclave, which uses steam under pressure for a specified period of time. Dry sterilization is performed in an oven between 140°C to 260°C to kill spores and other microorganisms. This method of sterilization is preferred for products such as mineral oil, paraffin, and zinc oxide.

> **chemical sterilization** process of completely removing or destroying all microorganisms by exposure to a chemical.

Chemical sterilization uses chemical agents to prevent microorganism proliferation. The most common chemical agent used in this process is ethylene oxide. This chemical only requires a temperature of 54°C for approximately 4 to 16 hours, and can be used for rubber and plastic items. This type of sterilization can never be used in IV solutions due to possible chemical reactions.

> **filtration** the process of passing a liquid through a porous substance that arrests suspended solid particles.

Filtration, aside from being the easiest, is the most often-used form of sterilization in most pharmacies. In order for a filter to prevent passage of all bacteria, it must be no more than 0.22 microns in size. Filters are used for IV, IM, and ophthalmic preparations, since heat and chemicals often damage these solutions. Filter sizes range from 0.025 to 14 microns. The smallest bacteria can be eliminated using a 0.22-micron filter. This filter is widely used as a standard in a majority of compounding procedures.

> **radiation** use of X-rays, ultraviolet or short radio waves for treatment or diagnosis.

Radiation is a form of sterilization normally used in hospitals, laboratories, and large institutions. This method is largely used to sterilize hospital supplies, vitamins, antibiotics, steroids, plastic syringes, and needles.

Most pharmacies will prepare sterile products in either a horizontal or vertical air flow hood; each provides a Class 100 clean environment. The horizontal laminar flow hood consists of three major components: a pre-filter, a HEPA filter, and the work surface. The horizontal hood blows clean air from the back of the hood to the front, maintaining a clean area within three inches of its outside boundaries. The constant air flow through the HEPA filter prevents all particles greater than 0.3 microns in size from entering the sterile area. The vertical air flow hood sends the sterile filtered air from the top of the cabinet to the base and recirculates it within the cabinet. It is a closed system that better protects the person performing operations within the clean barrier. Vertical flow hoods can be used for those products toxic to humans and the environment, such as chemotherapeutic drugs. Both types of hoods must be cleaned with the proper chemical compounds before each operation. A more detailed and thorough discussion of laminar air flow hoods is presented in Chapter 15.

Labeling of Finished Products and Recordkeeping

Extemporaneous products should be labeled with neat, well-designed labels, in accordance with hospital policy. Outpatient prescription labels must contain all information required by state and local laws. Auxiliary labels should be affixed if applicable. The label should contain the ingredients and proportions of the compounded prescription. If a master compounding form was used, the internally assigned lot number should appear on the label.

In general, no specific expiration date can be assigned to an extemporaneous compound unless the institution has a policy for assigning reasonable expiration dates. Even with such a policy, some judgment is needed on the part of the supervising pharmacist. It may suffice to list the date of preparation on the label.

Accurate recordkeeping is essential in extemporaneous compounding. Master formula records (Figure 14-12) are excellent sources for both directions for compounding and uniform recordkeeping. When using a master form, record all lot number information on the form, and use the internal lot number on the prescription label. These master records also contain the amount of ingredients used, initials of the pharmacy technician or preparer and the pharmacist who checked the finished product, and all measurements. All work sheets should be filed as permanent records.

For single extemporaneous compounds without master records, such as those involving outpatient prescriptions, the lot numbers and manufacturers of the ingredients can be recorded on the prescription.

Cleaning Equipment

Cleaning the equipment is as important as the preparation and labeling of the product. It should not be overlooked. Improperly cleaned equipment can contaminate the next preparation and be dangerous to the patient. Cleaning is sometimes not as simple as washing dishes because oily residues, such as ointments, often must be dissolved. Proper cleaning may require a rinse with organic solvents, such as alcohols or acetate, to facilitate removal. When working with these volatile solvents, the student must be aware of their flammable nature as well as the risk of inhaling fumes. Although these fumes are generally safe for limited exposure, care must be taken to wash solvents down the drain with cold water to limit exposure. Occupational safety data sheets should be available in every pharmacy, outlining the hazards of each substance.

FIGURE 14-12

EXTEMPORANEOUS PREPARATION
GENTIAN VIOLET 10%

MATERIALS
- 1 glass flask 600ml
- Absolute alcohol 300ml
- Gentian Violet 30gm
- Stirring rod
- 1 oz. amber dropper bottle

LABEL
- Gentian violet solution
- 10% W/V
- In 95% absolute alcohol
- Volume: 300 ml
- Control # _____
- Tech/R.Ph. _____ Exp. date _____

Procedure
1. Clean all materials to be used and rinse with absolute alcohol.
2. Weigh out 30 gram gentian violet and have pharmacist check it.
3. Measure out 300ml absolute alcohol and have pharmacist check it.
4. In glass flask, dissolve the gentian violet in the absolute alcohol. Stir well until in solution.
5. Measure out 30ml and put in 1 oz. glass amber dropper bottle.
6. Have pharmacist check label.
7. Put label on product.
8. Have pharmacist check final product.

Date Prepared	Control #	Ingredients	Mft. & Lot #	Amt. Used	Check by R.Ph	Expiration Date of Prod. Made	Quant. Prep.	Sample Label	Tech.

FIGURE 14-12 Master formula record.

Summary

Bulk compounding by pharmacy technicians should be viewed as a challenge and a rewarding skill. The student can readily appreciate the necessity of competence in other aspects of pharmacy, such as calculation, dose forms, and pharmaceutical terminology. The responsibility of bulk compounding should not and will not be required of technicians who are not trained or not competent with these skills. Any bulk compounding must be done only under close supervision of a licensed pharmacist, and in some states, must be done only via master manufacturing records.

Bulk compounding is a difficult art to master, but it is one of the most rewarding. It remains one service no other health care profession can provide.

TEST YOUR KNOWLEDGE

Multiple Choice

1. The concave surface of a liquid in a graduate is called the
   a. sight line.
   b. metric point.
   c. meniscus.
   d. tare.

2. Clear liquids in which drugs are completely dissolved are called
   a. suspensions.
   b. emulsions.
   c. lotions.
   d. solutions.

3. The hazards of using organic solvents are
   a. their flammability.
   b. their lack of odor.
   c. their explosive nature.
   d. their acidity.

4. A packet of external nutrition supplement diluted to what strength would yield the greatest volume?
   a. full strength
   b. three-fourths strength
   c. two-thirds strength
   d. none of the above

5. A master formula record should contain
   a. directions for compounding.
   b. a record of lot numbers.
   c. the initials of preparer and checking pharmacist.
   d. all of the above.

6. What type of balance can weigh large quantities?
   a. Class A prescription balance
   b. solution balance
   c. counter balance
   d. electronic balance

7. A thickening agent that gives some structure to a suspension is called
   a. gel agent.
   b. cream agent.
   c. suspending agent.
   d. soluting agent.

8. The punch method is used to compound
   a. capsules.
   b. suppositories.
   c. solids.
   d. ointments.

9. What piece of equipment is used to transfer solid ingredients to weighing pans?
   a. graduate
   b. syringe
   c. spatula
   d. beaker

10. The device used to reduce the particle size of active ingredients is the
    a. homogenizer.
    b. electronic mortar and pestle.
    c. hot plate.
    d. ointment mill.

Matching

Match the piece of equipment to its use.

1. _____ Class A prescription balance
2. _____ mortar and pestle
3. _____ spatula
4. _____ graduate
5. _____ ointment slab

a. used to measure liquids
b. used to grind large particles
c. used to mix and transfer ingredients
d. used to weigh small quantities
e. used to mix ointments

Fill In The Blank

1. The timely preparation of a drug product according to a prescribed recipe is called _____.

2. The correct reading of a liquid is at the bottom of the _____.

3. The mixing of a powder into a vehicle in which it is insoluble to produce a smooth dispersion is called _____.

4. The resetting of a balance to a zero reading is known as _____.

5. _____ are dead cell particles that can cause a fever.

References

Ansel, H. H. (1986). *Introduction to pharmaceutical dosage forms* (4th ed.). Philadelphia: Lea & Febiger.

Gennaro, A. R. (Ed.). (1990). *Remington's pharmaceutical sciences* (18th ed.). Easton, PA: Mack Publishing Co.

Parrot, E. L. (1970). *Pharmaceutical technology*. Minneapolis, MN: Burgess Publishing Co.

Shrewsburg, R. (2001). *Applied pharmaceutics in contemporary compounding*. Englewood, CO: Morton Publishing Co.

Sterile Preparation Compounding

Competencies

Upon completion of this chapter, the reader should be able to

1. List three routes of administration and give an example.
2. List several advantages of administering a drug by the parenteral route.
3. Define an ISO Class 5 area.
4. Define a buffer area.
5. Define an antearea.
6. Understand and explain the difference between a vertical flow hood and a horizontal flow hood.
7. Describe the proper order for garbing and entering the clean room.
8. Understand and describe the concept of unidirectional air flow and "first air."
9. Understand and explain the difference between compounding a Low-Risk versus a Medium-Risk, or a High-Risk Level preparation.
10. Understand and describe the appropriate steps in compounding sterile preparations.

Key Terms

admixture
antearea
aseptic processing
aseptic technique
buffer area
compounded sterile preparation (CSP)
critical area
critical site
direct compounding area (DCA)
hypertonic
hypotonic

intermittent infusion
intra-arterial
intra-articular
intracardia
intradermal (ID)
intramuscular (IM)
intraperitoneal
intrapleural
intrathecal
intravenous (IV)
intraventricular
intravesicular

intravitrial
ISO Class 5 area
ISO Class 7 area
ISO Class 8 area
parenteral
primary engineering control (PEC)
sterile
sterilizing filter
subcutaneous (SC)
unidirectional flow
validation
verification

Introduction

A **parenteral** (*para* + *enteron*) product is an example of a sterile preparation. Parenteral products are products that bypass the gastrointestinal (GI) tract. They are administered by injection through some other route, thereby bypassing the gastric mucosa, the skin, and other membranes. Hence, parenteral products must be **sterile** (free from living microorganisms), free from particulate matter, and free from bacterial endotoxins. *Bacterial endotoxins* are a type of pyrogen. A *pyrogen* is any fever-causing substance.

Administration of a sterile preparation by injection might be necessary because the drug is destroyed when taken orally, inactivated in the gastrointestinal (GI) tract, or poorly absorbed. An injection may also be used when the patient is unable to swallow or take anything by mouth, is unconscious, or is uncooperative. Administering a drug by the parenteral route is also used when rapid drug absorption is essential, such as in emergency situations.

According to the U.S. Pharmacopoeia (USP), **compounded sterile preparations (CSPs)** are parenteral products and include diagnostic agents, radiopharmaceuticals, inhalation solutions, baths and soaks for live organs, irrigations for wounds and body cavities, ophthalmic drops and ointments, and tissue implants.

Parenteral Routes of Administration

The route of administration chosen depends on the drug characteristic, the effect desired, and the required site of action.

Intravenous Route

An **intravenous (IV)** injection is administered directly into the vein. Because the medication is rapidly diluted with blood, a rapid effect of the drug, along with a predictable response, is seen. Drugs may be given by IV bolus, a continuous infusion, or an intermittent infusion. A *bolus* is used to deliver a relatively small volume of drug over a short time and is often written as "IV push." This is useful in emergency situations where a rapid therapeutic effect is desired. For some drugs that cannot be given quickly without causing adverse effects to the patient, **intermittent infusions** are sometimes used. Intermittent infusion is also used for drugs that require being given at defined intervals over a specific amount of time in order to be most effective. They are used to deliver a relatively small volume of solution. When the patient has an established IV administration set, the intermittent infusion is piggybacked through the established primary IV administration set. A *piggyback* is a second medication that is infused through the primary IV administration set and is usually 250 mL or less. This eliminates the need for another needle stick and also dilutes the medication to reduce irritation of the vein (see Figure 15-1).

Intramuscular Route

An **intramuscular (IM)** medication is injected deep into a large muscle mass, such as the upper arm, thigh, or buttocks. Typically, no more than 2.5 mL (but up to 5 mL depending on muscle mass) of medication may be administered IM as a solution or suspension. Sterile preparations given by the IM route act more quickly than when given by the oral route, but not as quickly as if the drug was given by the IV route.

FIGURE 15-1

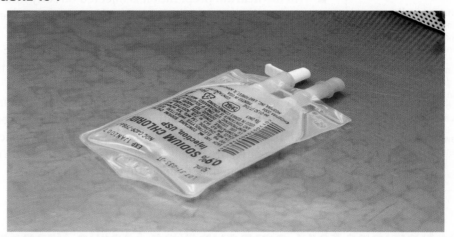

FIGURE 15-1 A continuous infusion allows for the introduction of larger volumes of solution, usually run at a constant rate and given over an extended period of time (Courtesy of the University of Tennessee Parenteral Medications Lab).

Depending on the solubility of the drug and the vehicle it is in, a sustained-release action can be achieved as the drug is released from muscle tissue at a prolonged rate. IM injections are often painful, and if an adverse effect occurs from the sterile preparation, reversing the effect can be difficult.

Subcutaneous Route

subcutaneous (SC) under the skin.

Sterile preparations given by the **subcutaneous (SC)** route can be solutions or suspensions. They are given beneath the surface of the skin. The volume of medications administered by this route must be not more than 2 mLs. SC injections are not absorbed as well and have a slower onset of action than injections given by the IV or IM route.

Intradermal Route

intradermal (ID) situated or applied within the skin.

Sterile preparations given by the **intradermal (ID)** route are injected into the top layer of the skin. The injection is not as deep as a SC injection. Preparations used for diagnostic purposes, such as an allergy test or a tuberculin test, are often given by the ID route. The volume of solution is limited to 0.1 mL, and the onset of action and rate of absorption from this route are slow.

Intra-arterial Route

intra-arterial the injection of a sterile preparation into an artery.

The **intra-arterial** route of administration occurs when the sterile preparation is injected into the artery and thus delivers the medication directly to the desired location. A preparation used for diagnostic purposes, such as radio-opaque materials for an arteriogram, is one example. Another example of this route of administration is for the delivery of cancer chemotherapy directly to the desired site of action.

Other Parenteral Routes of Administration

intra-articular the injection of a sterile preparation in a joint such as the elbow or knee.

Other parenteral routes of administration are as follows:

- An **intra-articular** preparation is injected into a joint such as the elbow or knee.

intracardia the injection of a sterile preparation directly into the heart.

intraperitoneal a sterile preparation is injected into the peritoneal or abdominal cavity.

intrapleural a sterile preparation is injected into the sac surrounding the lungs.

- An **intracardia** preparation is injected directly into the heart muscle.
- An **intraperitoneal** preparation is injected into the peritoneal or abdominal cavity.
- An **intrapleural** preparation is injected into the sac surrounding the lungs.
- An **intraventricular** preparation is injected directly into a ventricle of the brain.
- An **intravesicular** preparation is instilled into the urinary bladder.
- An **intravitrial** preparation is injected into the vitreous humor of the eye.
- An **intrathecal** preparation is injected into the space around the spinal cord. Preservative-free drugs must be used for this route of injection, as the preservative system may damage the nervous system.

Definitions for Compounding Sterile Preparations

intraventricular the injection into a ventricle of the brain or heart.

intravesicular a preparation instilled into the urinary bladder.

intravitrial a sterile preparation is injected into the vitreous chamber of the eyeball behind the lens.

intrathecal within the subdural space of the spinal cord.

admixture the term used to denote one or more active ingredients in a large-volume parenteral solution.

antearea an ISO Class 8 or better area where personnel perform hand hygiene and garbing procedures, staging of components, order entry, CSP labeling, and other high-particulate generating activities.

aseptic processing a method to assure that no contamination of compounded sterile products will occur during their compounding.

aseptic technique a method of preparation that will prevent contamination of a site (e.g., wound) or product (e.g., IV admixture).

The following are definitions you will need to know for compounding sterile preparations:

- **Admixture**—parenteral dosage forms are combined for administration as a single entity.
- **Antearea**—an ISO Class 8 or better area where personnel perform hand hygiene and garbing procedures, staging of components, order entry, CSP labeling, and other high-particulate generating activities. Such an area is maintained under positive pressure in comparison to the rest of the pharmacy, but negative to the buffer area. The antearea is supplied with HEPA-filtered air.
- **Aseptic processing**—product components, containers, and closures, and the product itself, are sterilized separately and then brought together and assembled in an aseptic environment; the primary objective of aseptic processing is to create a sterile product.
- **Aseptic technique**—a means of manipulating sterile products without contaminating them.
- **Buffer area**—usually an ISO Class 7 area where the laminar flow hood is located. It has positive pressure to the rest of the pharmacy and is supplied with HEPA-filtered air.
- **Critical area**—an ISO Class 5 area.
- **Critical site**—any opening or surface that can provide a pathway between the sterile product and the environment (e.g., the hub of the needle, the tip of the syringe, the open neck of the ampoule, the top of the vial closure, the ribs of the plunger on a syringe).
- **Direct compounding area (DCA)**—a critical area within the ISO Class 5 primary engineering control (PEC) where critical sites are exposed to unidirectional HEPA-filtered air, also known as "first air."
- **Hypertonic**—a solution containing a higher concentration of dissolved substances (hyperosmotic) than the red blood cell, which causes the red blood cell to shrink.
- **Hypotonic**—a solution containing a lower concentration of dissolved substances (hypoosmotic) than the red blood cell, causing the red blood cell to swell and possibly burst.
- Isotonic—a solution with an osmotic pressure close to that of body fluids. This minimizes patient discomfort and damage to red blood cells. Dextrose 5

buffer area usually an ISO Class 7 area where the laminar flow hood is located.

critical area an ISO Class 5 area.

critical site any opening or surface that can provide a pathway between the sterile product and the environment.

direct compounding area (DCA) a critical compounding area meeting ISO 5 specifications.

hypertonic having a higher osmotic pressure than a reference solution, usually referring to blood plasma or lacrimal fluid.

hypotonic having a lesser osmotic pressure than a reference standard, usually referring to blood plasma or lacrimal fluid.

percent in water and sodium chloride 0.9 percent solutions are approximately isotonic.

- **ISO Class 5 area**—the air in the area has no more than 3,520 particles per cubic meter of air 0.5 microns and larger. This is equivalent to the air in a Class 100 area, which is the number of particles per cubic foot of air 0.5 microns and larger.

- **ISO Class 7 area**—the air in the area has no more than 352,000 particles per cubic meter of air 0.5 microns and larger. This is equivalent to a Class 10,000 area.

- **ISO Class 8 area**—the air in the area has no more than 3,520,000 particles per cubic meter of air 0.5 microns and larger. This is equivalent to a Class 100,000 area.

- **Primary engineering control (PEC)**—a device such as a laminar air flow workbench (LAFW), biological safety cabinet (BSC), or compounding aseptic isolator (CAI) that provides an ISO Class 5 environment for the exposure of critical sites when compounding sterile preparations.

- **Sterilizing filter**—a filter that, when challenged with the microorganisms *Brevundimonas diminuta*, at a minimum concentration of 10^7 organisms per cm^2 of filter surface, will produce a sterile effluent; a sterilizing filter has a pore size rating of 0.2 or 0.22 microns.

- **Unidirectional flow**—air flow moving in a single direction, in a robust and uniform manner, and at sufficient speed to reproducibly sweep particles away from the critical processing area.

- **Validation/verification**—establishing documented evidence that provides a high degree of assurance that a specific process will consistently produce a product meeting predetermined specifications and quality attributes.

United States Pharmacopoeia 31/National Formulary 26

ISO Class 5 area International Organization of Standardization (ISO) Classification of Particulate Matter in room air, with no more than 3,520 particles per cubic meter of air 0.5 microns and larger.

ISO Class 7 area International Organization of Standardization (ISO) Classification of Particulate Matter in room air, with no more than 352,000 particles per cubic meter of air 0.5 microns or larger.

The new Chapter <797> Pharmaceutical Compounding—Sterile Preparations, became official on June 1, 2008. The chapter has four specific risk levels of CSPs: Low-Risk Level, Medium-Risk Level, High-Risk Level, and Immediate-Use.

Low-Risk Level CSPs

Compounding is classified as *low-risk* under these prevailing conditions:

1. CSPs are compounded using only sterile ingredients, product, components, and devices entirely within an ISO Class 5 environment or better.
2. Compounding involves simple aseptic manipulations with not more than three manufactured products, including an infusion or diluent solution.
3. Manipulations are limited to penetrating stoppers on vials with sterile needles and syringes, opening ampoules, and transferring sterile liquids in sterile syringes.
4. In the absence of passing a sterility test, the storage periods cannot exceed the following time periods before administration:
   a. stored for not more than 48 hours at controlled room temperature.
   b. stored for not more than 14 days at a cold temperature of 2 to 8 degrees C.

c. stored for not more than 45 days in a solid frozen state between −25 and −10 degrees C.

Medium-Risk Level CSPs

Medium-risk level CSPs are compounded under low-risk conditions, and one or more of the following exists:

1. Compounding requires pooling of sterile products that will be administered to either multiple patients or to one patient on multiple occasions.
2. Compounding involves complex manipulations.
3. In the absence of passing a sterility test, the storage periods cannot exceed the following time periods before administration:
   a. stored for not more than 30 hours at controlled room temperature.
   b. stored for not more than nine days at 2 to 8 degrees C.
   c. stored for not more than 45 days in a solid frozen state between −25 and −10 degrees C.

Compounding a total parenteral nutrition solution or filling reservoirs of injection and infusion devices with more than three sterile drug productions are examples of medium-risk level compounding.

High-Risk Level CSPs

The following compounding conditions may result in contamination or leaves the products at high risk to become contaminated:

1. Compounding with non-sterile ingredients or a non-sterile device before sterilization.
2. Sterile ingredients or components are exposed to air quality inferior to ISO Class 5; this includes storage in environments inferior to ISO Class 5 of opened or partially-used packages of manufactured sterile products with no antimicrobial preservative system.
3. Non-sterile preparations containing water that are stored for more than six hours before being sterilized.
4. Compounding personnel are observed to be improperly garbed and gloved.
5. No examination of labeling and documentation from suppliers or direct determination that the chemical purity and content strength of ingredient meet their original or compendia specification.
6. In the absence of passing a sterility test, the storage periods cannot exceed the following time periods before administration:
   a. stored for not more than 24 hours at controlled room temperature.
   b. stored for not more than three days at 2 to 8 degrees C.
   c. stored for not more than 45 days in a solid frozen state between −25 and −10 degrees C.

An example of high-risk level compounding is preparing a CSP from non-sterile ingredients.

Immediate-Use CSPs

The immediate-use CSPs category is intended only for a situation where there is an emergency, or immediate patient administration of a CSP is needed. It may be used for only low-risk level CSPs and may not be used for any hazardous drugs. Immediate-use CSPs are exempt from the requirements of low-risk level CSPs only if:

1. The compounding process is continuous and does not exceed one hour.
2. The finished product is compounded with good aseptic technique and is under continuous supervision until administered.
3. Administration begins not later than one hour after the start of preparation.
4. Unless administered immediately by the person who prepared it, the CSP bears a label listing patient identification information, ingredients and amounts, the name or initial of the person who prepared it, and the exact one hour beyond-use time and date.

Sterile Product Preparation Area

The horizontal LAFW draws air in through a pre-filter (Figure 15-2). The pre-filtered air is pressurized in the plenum for even distribution of air to the high efficiency particulate air (HEPA) filter. Pre-filters should be checked regularly and changed as needed. A record of these checks and changes of the pre-filter should be kept. The *plenum* of the hood is the space between the pre-filter and the HEPA filter. The air is blown across the work surface toward the operator. The air from the HEPA filter is unidirectional (laminar-flow) and should have uniform velocity. Federal Standard 209E recommends airflow from the filter of a velocity of 90 feet per minute, plus or minus 20 percent. USP 31/NF26 Chapter <797> states that the air flow must be sufficient to sweep particles away and provide an ISO Class 5 environment. The pre-filter in the laminar flow workbench protects the HEPA filter

FIGURE 15-2

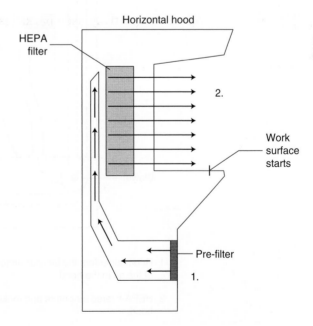

1. Room air enters, is filtered and drawn up to the top of the hood, where it is filtered through a HEPA filter.

2. Filtered air is directed out over the work surface.

FIGURE 15-2 Horizontal laminar flow workbench (HLFW).

from premature clogging. The HEPA filter consists of banks of filters, separated by corrugated aluminum pleats. The HEPA filter is 99.97 percent efficient at removing particles 0.3 microns and larger. To put this in perspective, the smallest particles visible to the human eye are about 40 to 50 microns in size. When working in horizontal flow, the compounding personnel must be careful to never put their hand behind an object. In other words, nothing must come between the critical site and the HEPA filter.

A vertical laminar flow workbench (VLFW) works similarly to the horizontal flow hood in that air is drawn in through the pre-filter and pressurized in the plenum (Figure 15-3). The main difference is the air is blown down onto the work surface instead of at the operator. This means the operator, when working in a vertical flow hood, will modify his or her aseptic technique so that his or her hands and any objects are never above an object in the hood. Nothing should come between the HEPA filter and the critical site.

The biological safety cabinet (BSC) is a type of vertical laminar flow workbench that provides protection to the product by having vertical HEPA-filtered air, protection to the operator by having the air intake at the open front of the hood, and protection to the environment by having the exhausted air pass through a HEPA filter (Figure 15-4). Ideally all of the exhaust should be directed outside to the roof.

FIGURE 15-3

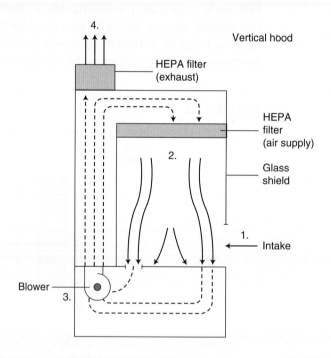

1. Room air enters the laminar airflow. This makes up about 30% of the air in the hood.

2. HEPA-filtered air enters and makes up 70% of the air in the hood.

3. Air from the work area is drawn down into the base and pulled back through the unit.

4. Air is exhausted after being filtered through carbon or HEPA filters.

FIGURE 15-3 Vertical laminar flow workbench (VLFW).

FIGURE 15-4

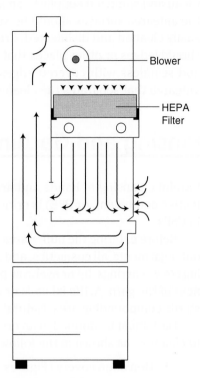

Blower

HEPA
Filter

FIGURE 15-4 Biological safety cabinet (BSC).

Buffer Area

Primary engineering controls (PECs) must maintain an ISO Class 5 environment while compounding of the sterile preparation occurs (e.g., under dynamic conditions). It usually must be kept in the buffer area, located away from excess traffic, doors, air vents, or anything that could produce air currents greater than the velocity of the air flow from the HEPA filter. The buffer area should be an ISO Class 7 area with positive pressure of 0.02 to 0.05 inches of water between this area and the antearea. ISO Class 7 areas must be supplied with HEPA-filtered air and achieve 30 air changes per hour. A recirculating PEC may supply 15 of those 30 air changes per hour.

Certification of all ISO-classified areas needs to be done no less than every six months. This includes testing the integrity of the HEPA filter, determination of air changes per hour in the classified rooms, and the total particle counts of the ISO 5, 7, and 8 areas.

The buffer area should be enclosed from other pharmacy operations. Surfaces should be smooth, nonporous, nonshedding, and able to be easily cleaned and disinfected. Cracks, crevices, and seams should be avoided, as should ledges or other places that could collect dust. The floor of the buffer area should be smooth and seamless with covered edges. There should be no sink or floor drains in the buffer area. Access to the buffer area should be restricted to only qualified personnel.

Antearea

The antearea should be enclosed from other pharmacy operations, supplied with HEPA-filtered air, and able to attain an ISO Class 8 environment under dynamic conditions. A barrier separates it from the buffer area. The antearea is used to decontaminate supplies, equipment, and personnel. The antearea is the support area for performing hand hygiene, gowning, and unpacking supplies from cardboard boxes.

Clean and sanitized supplies can also be stored in this area. As in the buffer area, the antearea surfaces should be smooth, nonporous, nonshedding, and able to be easily cleaned and disinfected. Cracks, crevices, and seams should be avoided, as should ledges or other places that could collect dust. The floors should be smooth and seamless with covered edges. There should be a line of demarcation in the antearea that separates the clean side from the dirty side.

Personnel Cleansing and Garbing

Careful cleansing of hands and arms and correct donning of garb (personal protective equipment, or PPE) is critical in the prevention of microbial contamination in CSPs.

Before entering the buffer area, compounding personnel must remove personal outer garments, all cosmetics, and all hand, wrist, and other visible jewelry or piercings (e.g., earrings, lip or eyebrow piercings), as they can interfere with the effectiveness of the garb. Artificial nails or extenders may not be worn while working in the sterile compounding area. Natural nails must also be kept neat and trimmed.

Garb must be donned in an order that proceeds from those considered dirtiest to cleanest, as shown in the following figures:

1. Don shoe covers (Figures 15-5a and b).
2. Don hair covers and beard covers (if necessary) (Figures 15-5c and d).
3. Don face mask (Figure 15-5e).
4. Perform a hand-cleansing procedure by removing debris from underneath fingernails using a nail cleaner under running water (Figure 15-5f).
5. Wash hands and forearms to the elbows with soap and water for at least 30 seconds while in the antearea (Figure 15-5g).
6. Completely dry hands and forearms, using either lint-free disposable towels or an electronic hand dryer (Figure 15-5h).
7. Don a nonshedding gown with sleeves that fit snugly around the wrists and closes at the neck (Figure 15-5i).
8. Once inside the buffer area, prior to donning sterile, powder-free gloves, use a waterless, alcohol-based surgical hand scrub with persistent activity to cleanse hands again. Allow hands to dry before donning sterile gloves.
9. Sterile gloves should be the last item donned before compounding begins. The appropriate size gloves should be opened, removed from the package, and the inner package unfolded (Figures 15-5j and k).
10. The first glove should be picked up by the folded-down cuff of the gloves. The hand should now touching the inside of the glove (Figure 15-5l).
11. The ungloved hand should never touch the outside of the glove. The cuff of the glove should not be fully pulled up at this time (Figure 15-5m).
12. Next, two fingers of the gloved hand should be inserted into the cuff of the other glove such that the gloved hand is now touching the outside of the glove (Figure 15-5n).
13. The glove should be pulled on and the cuff pulled up over the sleeve of the gown. The cuff of the second glove should be pulled over the coat (Figures 15-5o, p, and q).
14. Routine application of sterile 70 percent IPA throughout the compounding process and whenever non-sterile surfaces are touched is essential (Figure 15-5r).

FIGURE 15-5

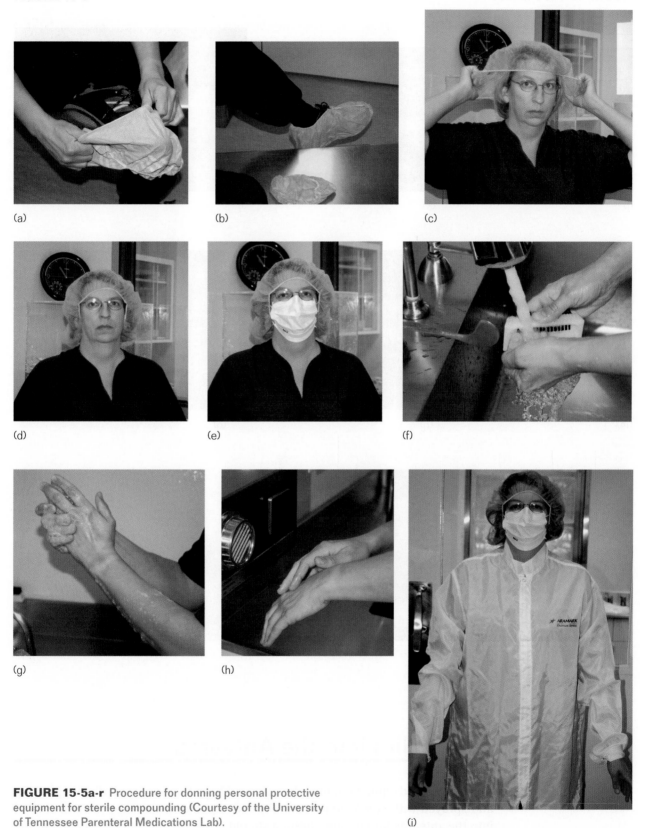

(a)   (b)   (c)

(d)   (e)   (f)

(g)   (h)

(i)

FIGURE 15-5a-r Procedure for donning personal protective equipment for sterile compounding (Courtesy of the University of Tennessee Parenteral Medications Lab).

(Continued)

FIGURE 15-5 (Continued)

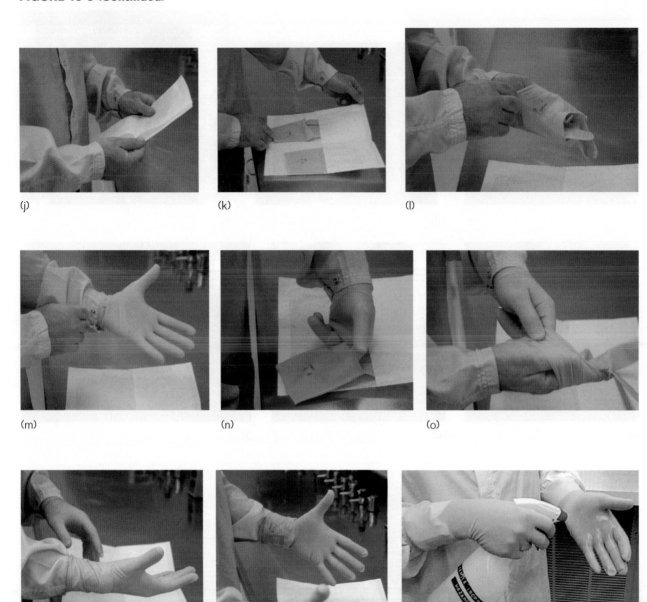

(j)

(k)

(l)

(m)

(n)

(o)

(p)

(q)

(r)

Introduction of Supplies into the Antearea

All supplies and equipment must be removed from their outer cardboard packing and sprayed with sterile 70 percent IPA and wiped down as they are transferred into the antearea for storage. Nothing should cross the line of demarcation in the anteroom without being sanitized.

Training of Compounding Personnel

All personnel who prepare CSPs must be thoroughly trained by expert personnel in the principles and practical skill of garbing procedures, aseptic work practices, achieving and maintaining ISO Class 5 environmental conditions, and cleaning and disinfecting procedures. This training should be completed and documented before any compounding personnel begin to prepare CSPs. Compounding personnel must complete didactic training, pass written competence assessments, and undergo skill assessment using observational audit tools, such as a checklist and media fill testing.

Compounding personnel must also demonstrate proficiency of proper hand hygiene, garbing, and cleaning procedures. The personnel should be observed during the process of performing hand hygiene and garbing procures. This should be documented using a checklist format, allowing for the maintenance of a permanent record of training. After completion of garbing, a gloved fingertip sample should be taken, using sterile contact agar plates. The evaluator will collect a gloved fingertip and thumb sample from both hands of the compounding personnel onto Trypticase Soy Agar (TSA) with lecithin and polysorbate 80, which will be incubated at 30 to 35 degrees C for 48 to 72 hours. This evaluation process must be successfully completed three times before the compounding personnel are allowed to perform the initial media fill. Reevaluation of all compounding personnel for this competency must occur at least annually for low- and medium-risk levels and semiannually for high-risk levels, using one or more sample collections during the media-fill test procedure, before being allowed to continue compounding CSPs for human use.

The risk of contamination of a CSP is highly dependent on proper hand hygiene and garbing practices, compounding personnel's aseptic technique, and the presence of surface contamination, assuming that all work is performed in a certified and properly functioning ISO Class 5 PEC with secondary engineering controls, an ISO Class 7 buffer area, and an ISO Class 8 antearea. Sampling of compounding personnel glove fingertips is performed for all CSP Risk Level compounding, because direct touch contamination is the most likely source of introduction of microorganisms into CSPs prepared by humans. This sampling is used to evaluate the competency of personnel in performing hand hygiene and garbing procedures, in addition to educating compounding personnel on proper work practices, which includes frequent and repeated glove disinfection using sterile 70 percent IPA during actual compounding of CSPs. However, disinfecting gloves immediately before sampling will provide false negative results and is not allowed.

Media fill testing to evaluate aseptic work skills should be performed initially before beginning to prepare CSPs and at least annually thereafter for low- and medium-risk level compounding, and semiannually for high-risk level compounding. The media test is done by using a growth-promoting media, such as Soybean Casein Digest, in place of the drug product. The test should mimic as closely as possible the most complicated procedure the compounding personnel perform, and should be done under worst-case conditions. Sterile media may be purchased for use in low- and medium-risk level media fills. For high-risk level compounding, the media used is commercially available, non-sterile Soybean Casein Digest Medium, made up to a 3 percent solution. Normal processing steps should then be mimicked. The purpose of any media fill is to evaluate the compounding personnel's aseptic technique, the compounding process used, and the environment of the facility.

Surface Cleaning and Disinfection

A major source of contamination can be the clean-room environment. Therefore, careful attention to cleaning and disinfecting is required. Compounding personnel are responsible for assuring that the frequency of cleaning is in accordance with what is stated in USP <797>. All cleaning and disinfection procedures must be written as standard operating procedures and followed by all compounding personnel. The ISO Class 5 environment must be cleaned and disinfected frequently, at a minimum at the beginning of each shift, before each batch is prepared, every 30 minutes during continuous compounding of CSPs, when there are spills, or when surface contamination is known or suspected. Work surfaces in the ISO Class 7 buffer area and in the ISO Class 8 antearea should be cleaned and disinfected at least daily, and dust and debris must be removed when necessary from storage sites for compounding supplies. Floors in the buffer area and antearea must be cleaned and disinfected daily when no compounding activities are occurring. The walls, ceiling, and shelving of the buffer area and antearea must be cleaned and disinfected on at least a monthly basis. All cleaning materials, such as mops, sponges, and wipes must be nonshedding and used in the clean room only.

Visual observations of cleaning and disinfection competency should occur during initial training and at the end of any media fill test. This should be documented by using a checklist format and the documentation maintained in the personnel's training file.

Surface sampling using contact plates is useful for evaluating the cleaning and disinfection procedures, personnel work practices as far as component/vial disinfection, and the overall state of the facility. Surface sampling using a contact plate filled with Trypticase Soy Agar, which has polysorbate 80 and lethicin added as neutralizing agents, should be done periodically in all ISO classified areas. Sampling should only be done at the conclusion of compounding.

Working in the Primary Engineering Control (PEC)

One must always use good aseptic technique when compounding sterile preparations. Compounding personnel must be careful not to get a false sense of security concerning the sterility of the products just because they were prepared in the primary engineering control (PEC). The ISO Class 5 environment does not remove particulates or microbial contamination from the surfaces of the containers or other items being placed in the PEC. The laminar flow workbench is not a sterilization device; it must be properly used and maintained to provide the ISO Class 5 environment.

Products and supplies not in an overwrap are first wiped with a nonshedding wipe soaked with sterile 70 percent IPA before being placed in the PEC. Items should be checked for cracks, tares, and particles before use in compounding sterile preparations. If items are in a protective overwrap, the overwrap may be removed at the edge of the hood and the item placed in the hood in uninterrupted unidirectional air flow. One exception to this practice is the needle. It should not be opened until immediately before use. Needles in the wraps are placed within the first six inches of the hood.

Compounding materials in a horizontal flow workbench are placed to the right or left of the direct contiguous work area (DCA). Critical sites must be in uninterrupted air flow at all times. The operator must work without placing a hand or object behind a critical site. The operator must work at least six inches inside the horizontal flow workbench. As the unidirectional air flow hits the operator, it must split and go around him or her. This can create turbulence, allowing an ingress of air from the buffer area into the PEC. Remember, the PEC is not a means of sterilization. It can only provide an ISO Class 5 environment when properly maintained, cleaned and disinfected, and used by the operator with good aseptic technique. A PEC will not compensate for bad technique. The most common method of contamination of a compounding sterile preparation is touch by the operator.

When an item is in a horizontal laminar flow workbench, it disturbs the unidirectional flow of the air behind the object, approximately three times the diameter of the object. If the vial or bottle is placed next to the side wall of the hood, it disturbs the air flow behind it, approximately six times the diameter of the object. Therefore, any non-sterile item has the potential to contaminate articles downstream with particles or microorganisms. Once again, it is very important that first air is maintained.

When working in a vertical laminar flow workbench, supplies must be placed so the compounding personnel may work without putting their hands or an item over the top of a critical site. Movements in and out of the VLFW should be minimized. Articles to be thrown away can be dropped over the edge into the trash or left in the first six inches of the hood until the manipulations are completed.

Needles

Sterile and pyrogen-free needles are wrapped in plastic with a twist-off top or wrapped in paper. Whatever the type of wrap, it should be inspected before using, as tares or pinholes in the wrapping materials will compromise the sterility of the needle. Needles come in various sizes—the larger the gauge of the needle, the smaller the bore of the needle. Many facilities use an 18-gauge to 21-gauge needle. The needle length is measured in inches, with the most common lengths for pharmacy being 1-inch to 1.5-inch lengths.

The basic parts of the needle are the bevel tip, the bevel, bevel heel, shaft, and hub. The needle shaft is encased in a rigid plastic sheath to cover the needle and allow for ease in handling. This sheath is left on until the needle is ready to be used. The entire needle is considered a critical site (Figure 15-6).

Syringes

Sterile and pyrogen-free disposable plastic syringes are packed in either paper or rigid plastic. Before using, the wrap should be inspected carefully for holes or tears to assure the syringe is intact and sterile. The basic parts of the syringe are the barrel, piston, top collar, plunger, flange, and tip—either a slip tip where the needle is held on the friction, or a Leur Lok Tip, where the needle is screwed into place (Figure 15-7). The critical sites on the syringe include the tip of the syringe and the ribs of the plunger. There are calibration marks on the syringe that allow the technician to estimate accurately to one-half of the interval marked. The larger the syringe, the larger the intervals marked on the syringe area. The final edge of the rubber tip

FIGURE 15-6

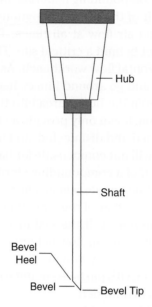

FIGURE 15-6 Parts of a needle.

FIGURE 15-7

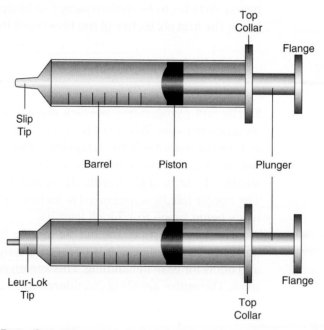

FIGURE 15-7 Parts of a syringe.

of the plunger that comes in contact with the syringe side wall is lined up with the calibration mark corresponding with the volume of solution desired.

Preparing the Horizontal Laminar Flow Workbench (HLFW)

The hood is disinfected with sterile 70 percent isopropyl alcohol (IPA). The sterile IPA is poured onto the surface of the workbench. This allows for better wetting of the

FIGURE 15-8

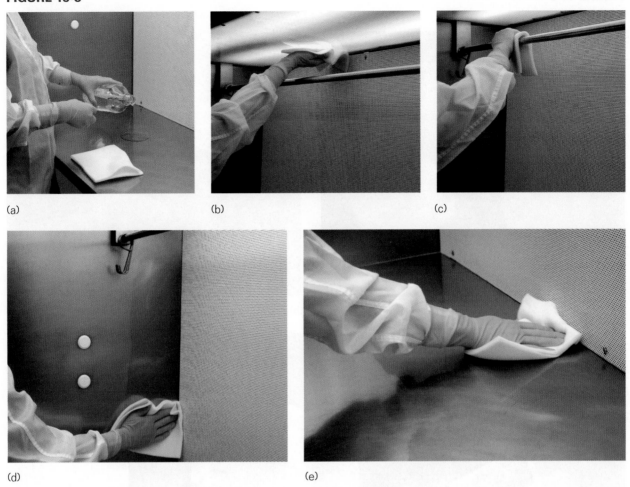

(a)　　　　　　　　　(b)　　　　　　　　　(c)

(d)　　　　　　　　　(e)

FIGURE 15-8a-e Preparation of a horizontal laminar flow workbench (HLFW) (Courtesy of the University of Tennessee Parenteral Medications Lab).

surfaces than using a spray bottle (Figure 15-8a). Wet nonshedding wipes with 70 percent sterile IPA. Wipe the light cover, then the IV bar (Figures 15-8b and c). Next, wipe the side walls. The technique is to wipe up and down, working out from the HEPA filter. Do not go from the edge of the hood back in over wiped surfaces (Figure 15-8d). Wipe the workbench in the same manner. Start at the back on one side by the HEPA filter, and wipe from side to side, moving the wipe forward the width of your hand each time. The last place to be wiped is the front edge (Figure 15-8e). Discard the wipes into the trash, being careful not to touch the trash container.

Aseptic Technique: Using a Needle and Syringe

(The following instructions are given for a right-handed person. If the operator is left-handed, the directions should be reversed.)

1. Select an appropriately-sized syringe, one large enough to contain the volume of solution desired.
2. Inspect the integrity of the outer wrap for defects such as pinholes, tears, or breaks in the wrap.

FIGURE 15-9

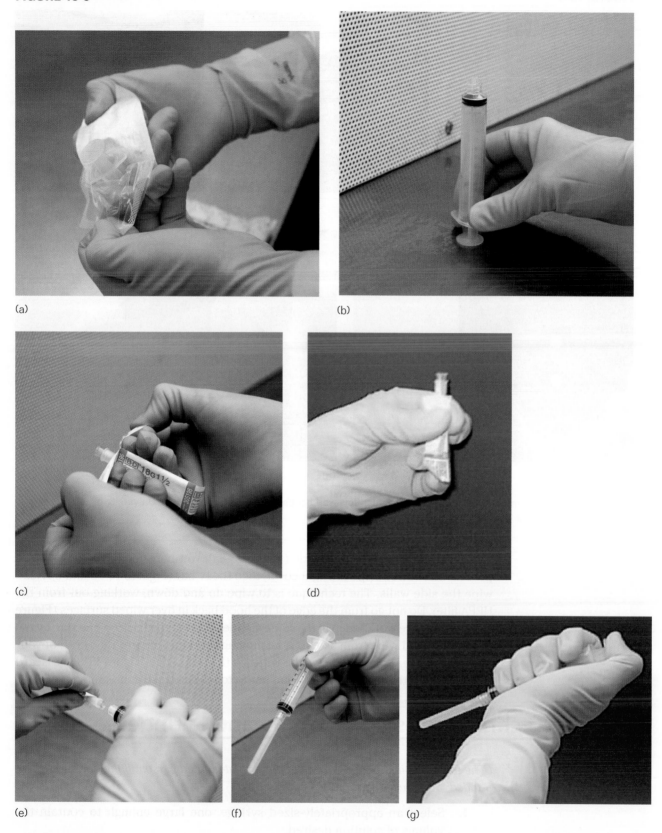

(a)

(b)

(c)

(d)

(e)

(f)

(g)

FIGURE 15-9a-g Aseptic technique—using a needle and syringe (Courtesy of the University of Tennessee Parenteral Medications Lab).

3. At the edge of the hood (in the six-inch supply staging area) peel back the paper on the syringe or remove the syringe from a plastic container (Figure 15-9a).

4. Place the syringe in the hood. Do not push the syringe through the paper wrap (Figure 15-9b).

5. Select a wrapped needle and peel back the paper tabs while not touching the needle hub. Keep the hub in uninterrupted HEPA-filtered air (Figure 15-9c).

6. Holding back the paper, hold the needle in a vertical position in the unidirectional air flow (Figure 15-9d).

7. Hold the syringe in a horizontal position, roll the left hand containing the needle to the right, and connect the needle hub to the syringe (Figure 15-9e).

8. Turn the syringe counterclockwise to lock the needle on the syringe (Figure 15-9f).

9. Hold the syringe by the barrel (a noncritical site) firmly with four fingers. Push the plunger in to seat and loosen the plunger (Figure 15-9g).

Using Ampoules, Filter Needles, and an Intravenous Solution

Ampoules are single-dose containers. Once the tip is broken, you have an open system with a large critical site. The contents of the ampoule should be used immediately and may not be stored for any length of time.

The ampoule should be wiped with a nonshedding wipe soaked in 70 percent IPA before being placed in the PEC (Figure 15-10a).

The neck of the ampoule should be wiped with a sterile alcohol wipe, as glass particles will fall into the solution when the ampoule is broken. The ampoule must be dry so the hands do not slip while attempting to break it open (Figure 15-10b).

Open the ampoule toward the side wall of the laminar flow hood, because glass particles and small amounts of fluid are dispersed when the ampoule is broken. Do not wrap the ampoule in gauze to open it, as this could allow particles to fall into the ampoule. Position the thumbs about a half inch apart on either side of the constricted neck of the ampoule to apply pressure with the fingers, as if breaking a pencil in half. You may use an ampoule breaker if you prefer. If the ampoule does not break easily, rotate it a quarter of a turn before trying again (Figures 15-10c and d).

Once the ampoule is broken, place the top to the side, and place the ampoule in uninterrupted unidirectional air flow (Figure 15-10e).

The needle cover (a noncritical site) is removed by grasping the needle cover between two fingers of the left hand and pulling the needle cover off. Do not twist the needle cover, as this will unscrew the needle from the syringe. The needle cover may also be placed on a sterile alcohol prep pad pointing toward the HEPA filter (Figures 15-10f and g).

The bevel of the needle is inserted into the shoulder of the ampoule, with the bevel down. The ampoule is tilted to pool the drug solution into the shoulder of the ampoule. When inserting the needle into the ampoule, the needle should not touch the outside edge of the ampoule. If this does happen, the contaminated needle should be replaced with a new needle on the syringe. The opening of the

FIGURE 15-10

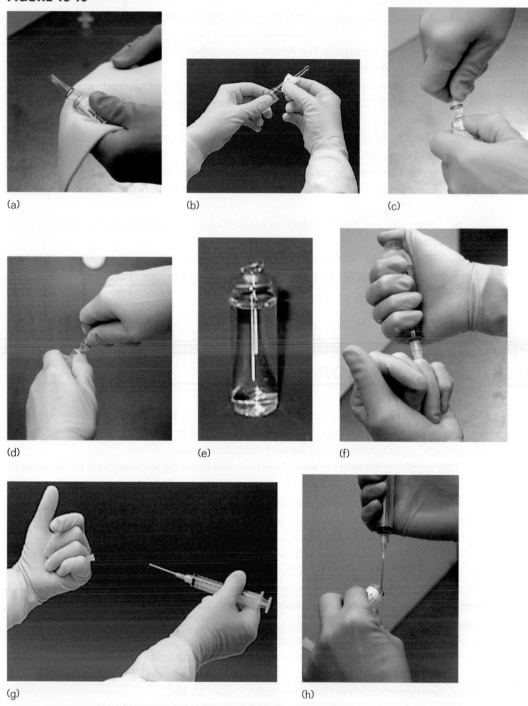

(a)

(b)

(c)

(d)

(e)

(f)

(g)

(h)

FIGURE 15-10a-aa Using ampoules, filter needles, and an intravenous solution (Courtesy of the University of Tennessee Parenteral Medications Lab).

ampoule and the needle are critical sites, so care must be taken to keep them in uninterrupted unidirectional air flow (Figure 15-10h).

The solution is withdrawn, using the thumb on the plunger end plate and withdrawing the plunger. If the thumb is not long enough to withdraw the solution into the syringe, the first finger can be used to extend the length of the plunger withdrawal (Figures 15-10i and j).

FIGURE 15-10 (Continued)

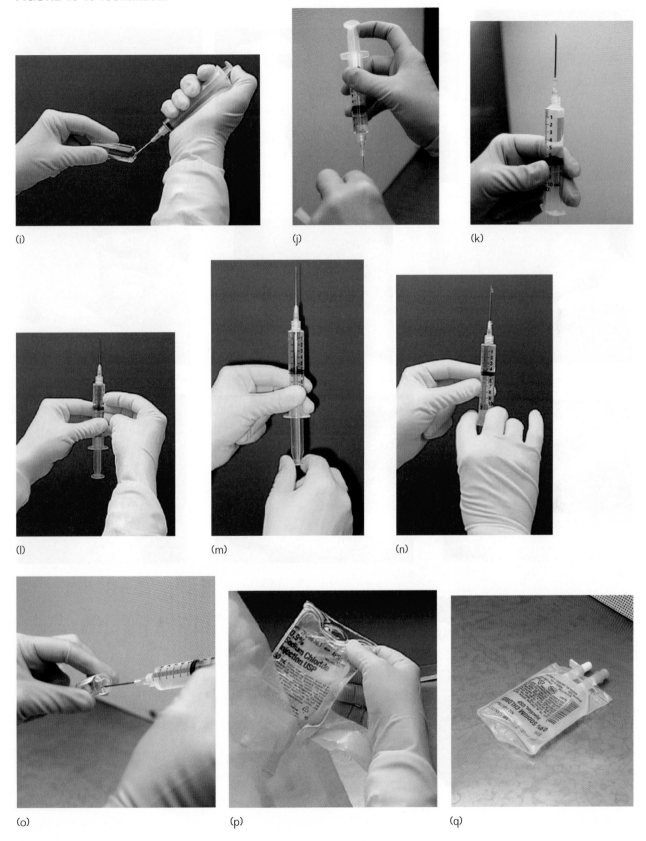

(i)

(j)

(k)

(l)

(m)

(n)

(o)

(p)

(q)

(Continued)

FIGURE 15-10 (Continued)

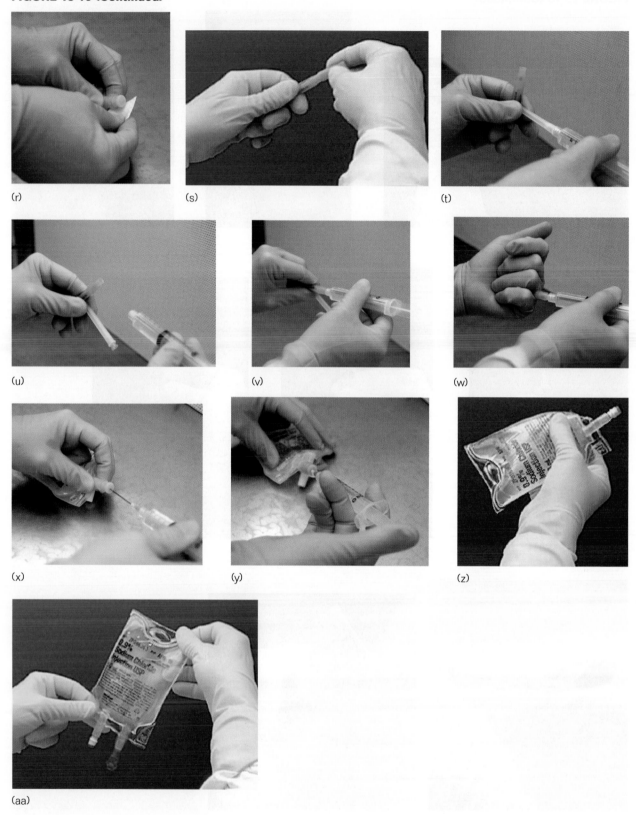

(r)   (s)   (t)

(u)   (v)   (w)

(x)   (y)   (z)

(aa)

Any unused solution in the ampoule should be discarded.

If air is in the syringe, it must be removed to have an accurate measure of the volume of solution. Turn the syringe to a vertical position with the needle pointing up, and tap the syringe firmly with the fingertips to loosen air bubbles from the plunger and side walls (Figures 15-10k and l).

The plunger is drawn back to pull any solution in the needle shaft back into the barrel of the syringe. The plunger is then pushed in slowly to expel the air until the first drop of solution appears on the bevel of the needle. Do not spray drug solution into the hood. Any excess solution is put back into the ampoule (Figures 15-10 m, n, and o).

Open the outer wrap for the intravenous solution bag and place it in the PEC. Position the bag so the injection port is facing the unidirectional air from the HEPA filter (Figures 15-10p and q).

Wipe the injection port with a sterile alcohol prep pad in one direction to remove particles and disinfect the injection port (Figure 15-10r).

Any solution taken from an ampoule must be filtered with a 5-micron filter, because glass particles can fall into the ampoule when it breaks open. Most often, a filter needle is used. The filter needle may be used for withdrawing the solution from the ampoule. This filters the solution as it enters the syringe. A regular needle must then be put on the syringe before the solution can be injected into the IV bag. Another method used is withdrawing the solution with a regular needle and then putting on a filter needle before injecting the solution into the IV bag. This method is described next.

A filter needle is a sterile needle that contains a 5-micron filter to remove glass particles (Figure 15-10s).

To filter the solution in the syringe as it is injected into the IV bag, the filter needle is attached to the syringe after the regular needle is removed. Holding the filter needle, the regular needle is removed by unscrewing the syringe from the needle (Figure 15-10t).

The left hand is rolled 90 degrees to the right, the filter needle is aligned with the syringe tip, and the syringe is screwed onto the filter needle (Figures 15-10u and v).

The cover of the filter needle is removed. The filter needle is inserted into the center of the injection port of the IV bag. Care must be taken so the needle does not penetrate the side of the injection port of the IV bag itself (Figures 15-10 w, x, and y).

The IV solution is mixed by kneading the bag. The compounded IV solution must be checked for precipitates, particulates, undesirable color changes, and gas evolution before release to the nurse or patient (Figures 15-10z and aa).

Vials

Vials can be glass or plastic containers with rubber closures and aluminum or flip top seals crimped in place to secure the closure. They can be filled with sterile solution, lyophilized powder (freeze-dried), dry powders, or be empty, evacuated containers. Vials may be single-dose or multiple-dose. Multiple-dose containers can have product removed from them on multiple occasions. They contain a pre-servative system and may be used for up to 28 days after the initial entry or opening, unless otherwise specified by the manufacturer. Single-dose containers may

FIGURE 15-11

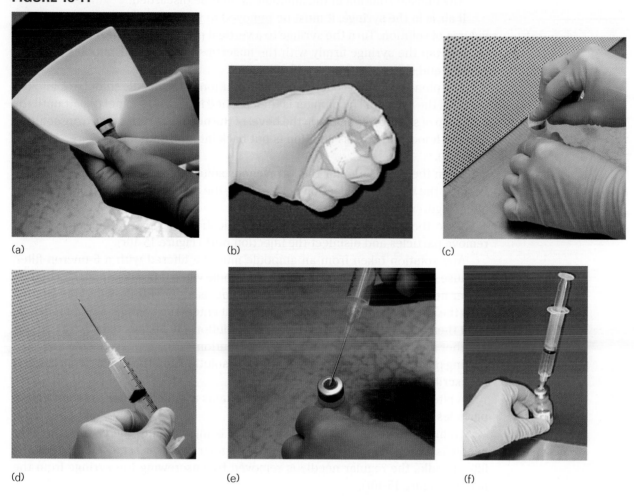

(a)

(b)

(c)

(d)

(e)

(f)

FIGURE 15-11a-l Withdrawing solution from a vial (Courtesy of the University of Tennessee Parenteral Medications Lab).

be used for up to one hour if opened or entered in worse than an ISO Class 5 environment. If entered or opened in an ISO Class 5 environment, the contents of the single-dose container may be used for six hours. However, opened ampoules may not be stored for any length of time. The first person using a vial or other container must label the container with the date, time of the initial entry, and their initials.

Withdrawing Solution from a Vial

The vial must be wiped with a non-shedding wipe wet with sterile 70 percent IPA before being placed in the hood (Figure 15-11a).

Once placed in the hood, the flip top of plastic cap is removed to reveal the rubber closure (stopper) (Figure 15-11b).

The top of the closure is wiped in one direction with a sterile alcohol wipe. Wiping in one directions helps to remove particles, and the alcohol disinfects the closure. This minimizes the chance of contaminating the drug when the needle is pushed through the rubber closure. While the alcohol is drying, the needle and syringe should be put together as described in the ampoule section above (Figure 15-11c).

Remove the needle cover placed between the ring finger and the little finger, or on a sterile alcohol pad with the opening pointing toward the HEPA filter. Draw

FIGURE 15-11 (Continued)

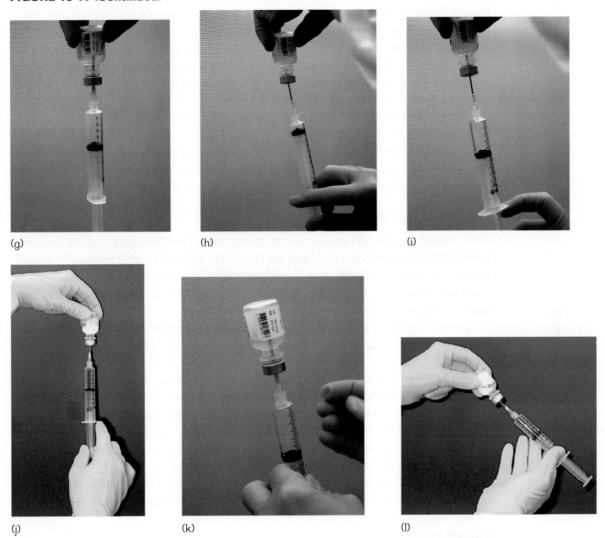

(g)   (h)   (i)

(j)   (k)   (l)

in a volume of air equivalent to the amount of drug solution that will be withdrawn from the vial. Since the vial is a closed system, to get solution out you must put air in (Figure 15-11d).

While holding the base of the vial with one hand, the needle is placed in the center of the rubber closure, bevel up, at approximately 45 degrees. This is to help prevent coring of the stopper when the needle is inserted through the closure. Do not touch the aluminum seal with the needle. As the closure is penetrated, the needle is elevated to a vertical position while exerting pressure laterally on the needle. Make sure the critical sites stay in uninterrupted unidirectional air flow (Figures 15-11e and f).

Invert the syringe and needle. Do not place a gloved hand between first air and the critical sites (Figure 15-11g).

Inject the air into the syringe, creating positive pressure in the vial. This will help push the drug solution back into the syringe when the pressure on the plunger is released (Figure 15-11h).

Withdraw the needle tip to just above the inside of the rubber closure to keep the tip of the needle in solution. Allow the positive pressure inside the vial to push the liquid back into the syringe. If more solution is needed, pull back on the plunger slowly. Place the middle finger and thumb on the flat top of the plunger and push against the collar of the syringe with the index finger to pull back on the plunger. The plunger should be pulled back to an amount slightly larger than desired. Take care not to touch the ribs of the plunger, as this is a critical site (Figures 15-11i and j).

Invert the vial and syringe. Tap on the syringe with the fingertips to dislodge any air bubbles from the plunger and side walls. Push up the plunger to inject the air back into the vial, and adjust the plunger until the appropriate amount of solution is in the syringe (Figure 15-11k).

While holding the inverted vials with one hand, hold the syringe barrel with the other and turn vial and syringe over, taking care to protect the critical sites. The needles and syringe are then withdrawn from the vial (Figure 15-11l).

Reconstitution

Vials containing lyophilized drugs or sterile drug powder must first be reconstituted with a diluent to put the drug into solution. When the drug product is lyophilized or in a powder form, it is usually because the drug has limited stability in solution. Sometimes the drug will come with a special diluent for reconstitution, and the diluent is specified on the label or in the product information. The label of the vial should be read to determine the proper diluent and the volume needed before reconstituting. In this example, sterile water for injection is used as the diluent.

Air is injected into the sterile water for injection vial, and the correct volume needed for reconstitution is withdrawn (Figure 15-12a).

The water is then injected into the vial, reconstituting the lyophilized drug. The excess air should be allowed to go back into the syringe so the vial will not contain positive pressure. If this is not done, some of the drug may be forced out of the vial when the needle is removed (Figure 15-12b).

The vial should be shaken and checked for clarity, particulates, unexpected color changes, extra long dissolution time, and gas evolution before withdrawing

FIGURE 15-12

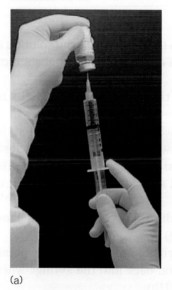
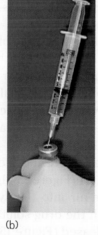
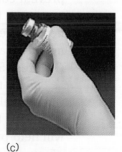

(a) (b) (c)

FIGURE 15-12a-c Reconstitution (Courtesy of the University of Tennessee Parenteral Medications Lab).

the necessary amount of drug solution. The reconstituted solution does not need filtering unless a particle or a rubber core is found floating in solution upon inspection of the vial (Figure 15-12c).

Visual Inspection of Parenteral Solutions

Each completed sterile preparation must be inspected and verified by the pharmacist. The operator also must check the completed sterile preparation immediately after compounding it. It must be checked for:

■ Correct labeling.
■ Correct intravenous solutions, including strength and quantity.
■ Correct drug additives, including strength and quantity.
■ Particulate matter, crystals, and precipitates.

Sterilization Methods

The pharmacist is responsible for choosing the appropriate sterilization method for high-risk level CSPs and the necessary equipment. There are three commonly used methods: filtration, steam sterilization, and dry heat sterilization.

Filtration

Filtration is the most common method of sterilization of CSPs in the pharmacy. Care must be taken to choose the correct filter. One must take into consideration the volume that is to be filtered and the temperature and pressure at which filtration will occur. Filters used to sterilize CSPs must be sterile, pyrogen-free, and have a nominal porosity of 0.2 or 0.22 microns. Filtration occurs by a combination of mechanisms: sieving, adsorption, and entrapment. Filter manufactures have compatibility data on their membrane and housing types with various solvent systems. They are a great source of information when selecting a filter.

Hydrophilic filter membranes wet spontaneously with water and are used to filter aqueous solutions, and aqueous solutions contain water-miscible solvents.

Hydrophobic filter membranes do not wet spontaneously with water and are used to filter gases and solvents.

Filter integrity test

All sterilizing membranes must undergo a filter integrity test after filtration has occurred (bubble point test). This test is a simple, nondestructive test that checks the integrity of the filter membrane and of the housing. It is based on the fact that liquid is held in the capillary structure of the membrane by surface tension. The minimum pressure required to push the liquid from the largest pores in the membrane is the *bubble point*.

The test is performed by wetting the filter with water and applying pressure on the upstream side. The pressure is increased until bubbles are seen coming out the downstream side of the filter. The typical water bubble point for a pore size rating of 0.2 microns is > to 50 psig (pounds per square inch gauge). If the bubble point of the filter is 50 psig as stated on the certificate of quality, to pass the integrity test you cannot exceed the bubble point at a pressure less than 50 psig.

Heat Sterilization

Moist-heat sterilization is a common method of terminally sterilizing the product in its final container. However, it can only be used to sterilize products that are aqueous. Steam (at 121 degrees C and 15 psig), when it comes in contact with a cooler object, condenses and loses heat to the object, which releases about 524 kcal/g. This kills the microorganisms. In order for steam sterilization to work, the steam must contact the object or be made inside the closed vial or ampoule from the water that is in the CSP. This is why items like oils or powders that don't wet cannot be sterilized by steam. Steam sterilization also does not destroy bacterial endotoxins.

Dry-heat sterilization requires higher temperatures and longer exposure times than moist-heat sterilization. Dry-heat sterilization can be used to sterilize oils and powders. It should be used only on products that cannot be sterilized by steam. The commonly used temperature for dry heat is 170 degrees C.

Dry-heat depyrogenation is used to sterilize and destroy bacterial endotoxins on equipment. A cycle of 30 minutes at 250 degrees C is usually adequate.

Summary

The pharmacy technicians who prepare CSPs must be highly motivated and very conscientious. They must be thoroughly trained and follow the written procedures at all times. Due to the possibility of microbial contamination or errors in compounding, all personnel must pay attention to every detail and thoroughly document the compounding process they followed. The pharmacist is responsible for double-checking and supervising all compounding activities. Quality must never be compromised. The pharmacy technician fulfills an important roll in compounding sterile preparations.

TEST YOUR KNOWLEDGE

Multiple Choice

1. When working in a horizontal laminar air flow hood, you must work at least _____ in from the outside edge of the work surface.
   a. 2 inches
   b. 4 inches
   c. 6 inches
   d. 8 inches

2. Which of the ISO classifications listed below is equivalent to a Class 100 area?
   a. ISO Class 3
   b. ISO Class 5
   c. ISO Class 6
   d. ISO Class 7

3. Please choose the correct answer. When working in a laminar flow hood:
   a. You must protect all critical sites by never putting your hand or an object between the critical site and the HEPA-filtered air.
   b. You must never put your hand behind an object in a vertical flow hood.
   c. You must always spray your vials thoroughly with 70 percent IPA before placing them in the hood.
   d. You should always unwrap your needles and lay them down in the hood before attaching them to the syringe.

4. In the definition of Class 100, Class 10,000, and Class 100,000 rooms, we are always talking about total particles _____ microns in size and larger.
   a. 0.3
   b. 0.5
   c. 1.2
   d. 5

5. A tuberculin skin test is given by which route of administration?
   a. intravenous
   b. intrapleural
   c. intradermal
   d. intramuscular

6. The compounding of a total parenteral nutrition solution would be an example of
   a. low-risk level compounding.
   b. medium-risk level compounding.
   c. high-risk level compounding.
   d. immediate-use CSPs.

7. When choosing a sterilizing filter, which of the following items must be considered?
   a. the volume of product to be filtered
   b. the compatibility of the membrane with the product to be filtered
   c. whether the solution to be filtered is hydrophobic or hydrophilic
   d. all of the above

8. Concerning the placement of items in the laminar flow workbench and working in the laminar flow workbench, choose the correct answer.
   a. Items should be placed in a horizontal flow hood to the right or left of the work area.
   b. Items in a vertical laminar flow hood should be placed so that when working in the hood, your hand never goes over the top of a critical site.
   c. An object placed in a horizontal flow hood disturbs the air flow three times the diameter of the object downstream of the object.
   d. All of the above.

9. The pore size of a sterilizing filter is
   a. 0.2 microns.
   b. 0.45 microns.
   c. 0.12 microns.
   d. 5.0 microns.

10. A sterile product is one that is
    a. free from all pyrogens.
    b. free from all viruses.
    c. free from all living microorganisms.
    d. free from all endotoxins.

11. Please choose the correct statement concerning USP media transfers.
    a. An operator must successfully complete one media fill before compounding any sterile products.
    b. An operator who passes a written exam may compound sterile products until the chief pharmacist gets time to watch his or her aseptic technique.
    c. An operator who has successfully completed a media fill must re-qualify semi-annually if the operator is preparing low-risk level products.
    d. Once an operator successfully completes one media fill for high-risk compounding, the operator needs to revalidate quarterly by completing one media fill.

12. Choose the *most correct* answer about transferring products into the antearea.
    a. Bottles, bags, and syringes must be removed from brown cardboard boxes before being brought into the antearea.
    b. Vials stored in laminated cardboard may not be brought into the antearea.
    c. Stainless steel carts may be used to transfer items into the antearea directly from the storage area.
    d. Large volume parenteral bags of IV solution must be removed from their protective overwrap before being brought into the antearea.

13. Please choose the *most correct* conclusion to this statement. The plenum in a laminar flow workbench is
    a. where the air is pre-filtered.
    b. the area where air is pressurized for distribution over the HEPA filter.
    c. the area where compounding takes place.
    d. an area that serves no purpose.

References

Buchanan, E. C., & Schneider, P. J. (2005). *Compounding sterile preparations.* Bethesda, MD: American Society of Health-System Pharmacists, Inc.

CETA applications guide for the use of compounding isolators in compounding sterile preparations in healthcare facilities, CAG-001-2005. Controlled Environment Testing Association (CETA), November 8, 2005.

International Organization for Standardization. (May 1, 1999). ISO 14644-1:1999. *Cleanrooms and associated controlled environments—Part 1: Classification of air cleanliness.*

U.S. Food and Drug Administration, Guidance for Industry. *Sterile drug products produced by aseptic processing: Current good manufacturing practice.* September 2004.

U.S. Pharmacopoeia USP 31/NF 26 Chapter <797>. *Pharmaceutical compounding—Sterile preparations*, available on the Web at www.usp.org/USPNF/pf/generalChapter797.html.

Other Recommended Readings

Agalloco, J., & Akers, J. E. (2005). Aseptic processing: A vision of the future. *Pharmaceutical Technology.* Aseptic Processing supplement, s16.

Eaton, T. (2005, Sep/Oct). Microbial risk assessment for aseptically prepared products. *American Pharmaceutical Review.* 8(5): 46-51.

Guideline for hand hygiene in health care settings. MMWR, October 25, 2002, vol. 51, No. RR-16. Available on the Internet at www.c.c.gov/handhygiene/.

NIOSH alert: Preventing occupational exposures to antineoplastic and other hazardous drugs in health care settings. Atlanta, GA: Centers for Disease Control and Prevention, National Institute for Occupational Safety and Health. 2004 DHHS (NIOSH) publication 2004–2165.

Power, L., & Jorgenson, J. (2006). *Safe handling of hazardous drugs.* Bethesda, MD: American Society of Health-System Pharmacists, Inc.

Trissel, L. A. (2005). *Handbook on injectable drugs* (13th ed.). Bethesda, MD: American Society of Health-System Pharmacists, Inc.

Administration of Medications

Competencies

Upon completion of this chapter, the reader should be able to

1. Specify the drug information that should be reviewed by the health care practitioner prior to administering a drug to a patient.

2. Describe the clinical and technical concerns required for administering medications by the following routes: oral, topical, rectal, vaginal, intraocular, intranasal, and into the ear.

3. Identify five methods in which the person administering medications can reduce medication errors.

4. Discuss the characteristics and professional concerns of a drug administrator or drug technician.

5. Differentiate the directions that should be given to a patient receiving a buccal tablet and a gelatin capsule.

6. Differentiate between labeling requirements for internal and external drug preparations.

7. List five situations in which a drug is discontinued or drug administration is interrupted.

8. Describe the procedure to be followed if a patient states, "I cannot swallow that large tablet."

9. Discuss some causes of medication errors. Explain the universal policy to be observed if a medication error is detected.

10. List the requirements for each health care practitioner who accepts the responsibility for the administration of medications.

Key Terms

dosage schedule
hypoglycemic
medication administrator
nosocomial infection
prn (pro re nata) order
STAT order
systemic action
verbal order

Introduction

This chapter focuses on the clinical, professional, and technical aspects of medication administration. While policies and procedures vary from institution to institution (and the institution's policy takes precedence over what is written here), the person who administers medications must always respect the dignity, privacy, safety, and autonomy of the patient. Patient cooperation is essential to the administration of most forms of medications. Even those patients who appear comatose, confused, or otherwise compromised should have the proposed procedure explained to them. Each health care practitioner who accepts the responsibility for the administration of medications must become familiar with the patient population, the institution's policies concerning medications, the approved methods of medication administration, the formulary and other resources that are available for reference and information, and the institution's expectations of the person who administers medications. All are very serious responsibilities.

Medication Orders

verbal order an order for a drug or other treatment that is given verbally to an authorized receiver by an authorized prescriber.

Drug administration is initiated with the physician's (prescriber's) *medication order*. No drug is given to a patient without physician authorization. Numerous kinds of medication orders exist. Orders written in the chart at the time of admission, which may be subsequently increased, decreased, or deleted, are the most common type of medication orders. Another type of drug order is a **verbal order** that may be given by the physician to a nurse or pharmacist, usually via the phone, when an emergency or unusual circumstance arises. Prior to initiation, verbal orders should be repeated to the prescriber. Verbal orders are always transcribed in the patient's chart, signed by the order taker, and cosigned by the physician on the next visit to the hospital. Verbal orders should be cosigned by the physician within 24 hours or as specified by hospital policy. Medication orders are also written upon transfer and discharge of patients and upon changes in the patient's condition or required medical therapy.

STAT order to be given immediately.

Orders for drugs that should be immediately administered are called **STAT orders**. The immediacy relates to the patient's condition, such as the need for pain relief, when the patient is experiencing clinical distress, or when the patient has a drug or allergic reaction. The person administering drugs always gives top priority to making sure the patient receives a STAT drug in timely fashion. Orders written by the physician (to be given to the patient only if required by the patient's condition) are **prn (pro re nata) orders**. One-time orders are written for specific circumstances, such as patient sedation for a test or procedure. Standing orders sometimes accompany a patient on admission to the hospital, or may be the printed drug regimens prescribed by the physician or a physician group to treat particular conditions (e.g., women who are admitted to the obstetrical unit preceding childbirth). These orders may be prewritten and signed by the physician or stamped on the chart with the physician's signature. Medication orders may also be included in physician, unit, or patient-specific protocols, pathways, and standards of care.

prn (pro re nata) orders drugs to be given as needed when a clinical situation arises.

Institutional policy may permit drug orders to be written by persons other than physicians, including doctors of osteopathic medicine, physician assistants, clinical nurse practitioners, dentists, podiatrists, and in some states, pharmacists. These policies must be known and observed.

Information Needed on Drug Orders

To properly administer a drug, the following information is needed for each drug order:

- Patient's full name.
- Room number, bed number, and other identifiers required by hospital policy (e.g., medical record numbers, ID bar codes).
- Name of drug (clearly written).
- Dosage strength (e.g., 10 mg).
- Dosage schedule (e.g., STAT, t.i.d.).
- Route of administration (e.g., sublingual, subcutaneous, instill in left eye).
- Length of time drug is to be given (e.g., for 24 hours, one week, length of hospital stay, as needed).
- Prescriber's signature.

The drug order is entered into the patient's medication order forms (this can be done by hand or as part of a computerized physician order entry [CPOE] system) and transmitted to the pharmacy to be filled. Illegibility of handwritten physician orders has been identified as a key contributor to medication errors, which is leading to the development and implementation of CPOE systems. The person who administers the drug verifies the label on the drug by comparing it with the order on the patient's medication record. Computerized medication systems are being used more and provide additional levels of automated checking—from the time of drug order, to delivery to the patient, to the drug being administered. A rule of thumb—never administer a medication without checking it three times against the order or medication administration record (MAR). Leave all medications fully labeled in their unit-dose packages until they are at the bedside. The last check just prior to administration is the most important, because it is the last chance to pick up an error.

The Medication Administrator

medication administrator the person who administers or gives medication to patients.

The **medication administrator** (nurse or other authorized health care practitioner) should appreciate the responsibility inherent in their role. This person should be knowledgeable about the responsibilities of the other members of the health team regarding drug administration and communicate effectively with them. The medication administrator should always give priority to patient care, treating each patient with dignity and professional concern regardless of physical or mental impairment, lifestyle orientation, religious beliefs, or cultural background. The medication administrator must be totally familiar with the policies and procedures that prevail in a particular hospital and always know the physician, nurse, or pharmacist to whom he or she directly reports. Any unusual physical or emotional change noted by the medication administrator during medication rounds should be immediately reported to the charge nurse. Professional confidentiality regarding any patient is of prime importance. Patients have, at all times, a right to have personal matters respected and held in confidence. Technicians should report to work dressed in appropriate hospital attire, with a name identification badge, in keeping with the dignity of the position and the respect they should expect from others.

The individual administering medications should be in good health, free of communicable infections (e.g., a head cold, a sore throat, an open lesion). This is of importance for both the patient and the drug administrator. Patients are susceptible to **nosocomial infections** (infections incurred in the hospital). Often the patient is weak, has had surgery or radiation therapy, and the immune system may be compromised for these or other reasons (e.g., aging process, malnutrition). The drug administrator who is at a low physical ebb due to exhaustion or poor health is more likely to make a drug administration error than a person who is well, alert, and fully attentive. In addition, a drug administrator (e.g., nurse) who is in poor health is more apt to pick up an infection from a patient. Any person who gives direct patient care must ensure and maintain good health through proper nutrition, exercise, and healthy living habits. In case of an upper respiratory infection or other indisposition, the drug administrator should inform the supervisor for a change of assignment away from direct patient care for the duration of the illness. Personal protective devices to ensure standard precautions for bloodborne disease transmission must be used during medication delivery as required. If the patient is in isolation due to an infectious, transmittable disease, the drug administrator should follow hospital policy regarding protection.

In all events, persons who are about to administer drugs should thoroughly wash their hands before handling any drugs and rewash their hands between patients when hospital policy or aseptic technique requires it. Hand hygiene is the single most effective infection control measure.

> **nosocomial infections** an infection or illness that occurs as a result of the patient's stay in the hospital or health facility.

Administration of the Drug

Prior to drug administration, the medication administrator should become familiar with the following information regarding the drug:

- General and special uses or indications.
- Usual dose or dosage range.
- Special precautions (e.g., do not give with food, observe patient for rash).
- Side effects that may occur.
- Foods or other drugs that should not be given with the drug.
- Time when onset of action is expected.

By reviewing this information before administering the drug, mistakes and errors can be avoided and the patient's well being better ensured. Hospital policy will indicate how involved the medication administrator becomes in providing this information to the patient. Generally, the registered nurse or the pharmacist has the responsibility to answer drug information questions and to counsel the patient on proper drug use.

Patient Rights

Nearly every patient in the hospital will receive drugs during their stay. Each patient is entitled to the "five rights" for safe, appropriate drug administration. Drug rights of the patient include the right drug, right dose, right route (or right dosage form), right time, and right patient. These rights should be memorized and checked prior to each drug administration.

The Right Drug

The right drug is verified by checking the physician's (prescriber's) order sheet and the nurse's (or pharmacist's) drug administration form, drug Kardex, or drug summary on the patient's computer profile. Thousands of drugs are available and many sound alike, are spelled alike, and look alike. Abbreviation of drug names has become a risky practice, and many hospitals are limiting or eliminating the use of medication abbreviations entirely as a risk reduction strategy. One or two letters in a name can mean an entirely different drug (e.g., Zantac or Zyrtec, Lasix or Luvox). Capital letters are now used to differentiate between like-sounding drugs (e.g., vinCRISTINE, vinBLASTINE). The prescriber must be contacted if there are any questions or doubts concerning the order. Most drugs used in hospitals today are in unit-dose packages. The name is clearly visible on each drug dosage form.

Labels should be checked *three times* before the drug is administered. The expiration date should also be checked. The Institute for Safe Medication Practices (ISMP) has identified top high-risk drugs. These are medications that have been involved frequently in serious errors. Examples include insulin and chemotherapy drugs. It is important to follow the hospital's special safety precautions when administering these high-alert drugs.

The Right Dose

Accurate dosage strength is critical to beneficial drug administration. Giving the wrong strength, particularly to children or infants, can be and has been fatal. The right dose is further checked with special care given to decimal points. A zero before the decimal, called a *leading decimal* (e.g., 0.1 mg), should be noted. Care should be taken if there is a zero after the decimal, called a *trailing zero*, which can be misleading and can be misread, leading to a 10 times greater dosage error (e.g., 1.0 is one, not ten). Orders for units must always be written out. The abbreviation *u* for units can be misread as a *0*, or *10, 4*, and lead to a 10 times greater dosage error.

Proper dosage strength should never be presumed by anyone in the prescribing, dispensing, or administering process. Physicians must clearly indicate the desired strength on the medication order, pharmacists are expected to further verify dosage to be sure it is within appropriate therapeutic limits, and nurses are expected to further check that the dosage strength ordered by the physician was accurately dispensed by the pharmacist. After the drug and dosage strength has gone through these three checkpoints, the last checkpoint resides with the person who administers the drug to the patient. If any dosage changes have been made along the way, the change should be clearly indicated on the patient's chart and other medication records. Children, the elderly, and patients with impaired liver and kidney function are at the greatest risk of adverse drug events related to medication dosage.

The Right Route/Dosage Form

In addition to ensuring that the right drug in the right strength has been selected, it is important to check and be sure that the drug is given by the right route in the right dosage form. Drugs come in many different dosage forms. Liquids come as solutions, tinctures, suspensions, syrups, and elixirs. Oral solid dosage forms come as tablets, gelatin capsules, caplets, enteric-coated tablets, extended-release capsules, sublingual tablets, and buccal tablets. External preparations include creams, ointments, and lotions. Some medications in ointment form contain potent active ingredients. The length of the ointment strip must be carefully measured by the drug administrator. Injectable medications must be carefully checked to be sure whether the injection should be administered by an intramuscular route, intravenous route, subcutaneous route, or other route of administration. Drop-type drugs must be checked and used only as indicated for the eye, ear, or nose. There are many suppository dosage forms, such as rectal, vaginal, and urethral. Dosage forms are *not* interchangeable, so it is important that it is the right drug, administered in the right dosage form. It is also important to note when a drug dosage form has been changed by the prescriber (e.g., an injectable drug [IM] is changed to an oral dosage [po]). Every drug order should include the route of administration. If a question arises, the proper dosage form should be confirmed before the drug is administered.

The Right Time

dosage schedule
the determination and regulation of the size, frequency, and number of doses.

hypoglycemic a drug that lowers the level of glucose in the blood; used primarily by diabetics.

Time of drug administration (i.e., **dosage schedule** or frequency) is an important factor in pharmacotherapy. Drugs should be given at the time ordered, allowing for an ordinary deviation of a half hour, unless timing is critical. Diabetic patients may receive their **hypoglycemic** drugs a half hour before meals, unless otherwise specified. Patients on therapeutic drug monitoring are involved in pharmacokinetic laboratory studies. Dosage time is related to drug half-life and the time the phlebotomist will draw blood for the serum analysis. Time of drug administration can be a critical factor in pharmacokinetic laboratory results. Time of drug administration can be of great concern to the patient who is waiting. A patient who has been ordered an analgesic for pain relief to be given every four hours for the first 24 hours after an operation should receive this drug on time. Delays for this patient increase the pain and anxiety and slow the recovery process. Many drugs are now administered per parameters. An example is a cardiac medication that is administered if the heart rate and blood pressure are within a certain range and held if outside the range. Knowledge of when the physician wants the medication administered, any hospital-, unit-, or physician-specific per parameters policy applicable, and the actual monitoring required prior to administration are required. It is less confusing for the patient if, when possible, drug administration times in the hospital are kept close to when the patient would normally take them at home, being considerate of the patient's individual waking and sleeping times. This also facilitates an accurate assessment of therapeutic effects.

The Right Patient

The last requirement is to verify that the right patient is the one to receive the drug. The patient should be asked, "Please tell me your name and date of birth"; this is checked against the patient's armband (Figure 16-1). Just addressing the person by name is not sufficient. People may respond positively even if they have not clearly heard their name, due to distractions, deafness, or language barriers. Beds are often shifted to different positions in the room, so identifying a person as the patient in Room 120, Bed 3 is insufficient information and may be misleading. Hospitals are implementing computerized medication systems that utilize bar coding or other methods of patient verification, and compare this information to the actual medication order or medication profile.

FIGURE 16-1

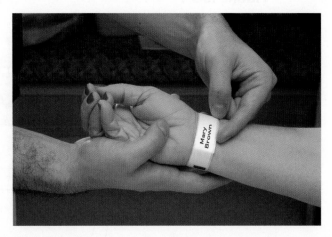

FIGURE 16-1 It is critical to be certain that medications are being delivered to the correct patient. The medication administrator must always verify the patient's identity.

Oral Drug Administration

After the patient has been properly identified, the patient is either given the medication to swallow, to place under the tongue (sublingual tablets), or to place between the cheek and the gum (buccal tablets). If the patient is to self-administer an oral tablet, the nurse or medication administrator should remain with the patient until the drug has been swallowed. Drugs are never left at the patient's bedside without a doctor's order. Drugs left at the bedside may be forgotten, discarded, or hoarded for future use. The patient should be instructed to place a sublingual tablet under the tongue and leave it there until it dissolves (Figure 16-2). A patient ordered a buccal tablet should be told to place the tablet between the gum and the cheek and allow it to dissolve (Figure 16-3). Throat and mouth troches or lozenges should not be swallowed or chewed but allowed to remain in the oral cavity until dissolved. In the case of a medicated mouthwash used for oral and throat infections, the patient should be told to swish the liquid around in the

FIGURE 16-2

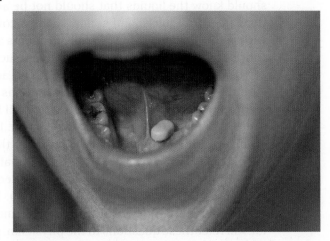

FIGURE 16-2 A sublingual tablet is placed under the patient's tongue to dissolve.

FIGURE 16-3

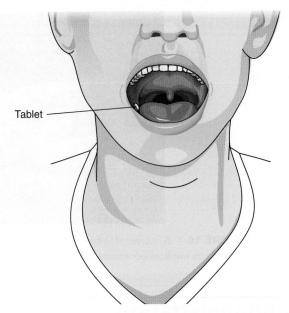

Tablet

FIGURE 16-3 A buccal tablet is placed between the patient's cheek and gums to dissolve.

mouth and then either swallow or expectorate (spit out) according to the nature of the substance and the dosage directions.

Usually, the patient should be given an adequate amount of water (at least four ounces or a full 8-ounce glass of water if possible) to allow for easy swallowing, dissolution of the tablet or capsule, and prevention of esophageal erosion. Esophageal erosion can occur when an oral medication lodges and remains in the esophagus and does not move into the stomach. Particular care must be given to tablets with a corrosive potential, such as a compressed potassium chloride tablet.

The exceptions to the rule for administering sufficient water with an oral dosage form are in the cases of cough syrups intended to soothe and work in the throat area, medicated mouthwashes intended to be swallowed or expectorated, and after administering either a buccal or sublingual tablet. There are times when a liquid other than water may be indicated. If there is no contraindication, the patient may prefer to follow the drug with a drink of milk or fruit juice. However, there are some definite contraindications. The person administering the drug should know the liquids that should not be administered with particular medications (e.g., fruit juices and sodas, such as cola beverages, should never be given with penicillin tablets; milk or milk products should not be given with certain categories of antibiotics or certain laxatives, such as Dulcolax™).

Before leaving the patient, the person administering the drug should make sure the patient has taken the drug and has had no difficulty in swallowing the medication or following other instructions. If the patient asks questions about the drugs, an adequate answer should be given. If the person administering the drug is limited either on time or knowledge when the question is asked, a follow-up visit should be made. Such answers as "that is what the doctor ordered" or "this is given to you to make you feel better" are not adequate. This is in fact dismissing the patient's questions and need for information. The patient is entitled to information regarding the drugs he or she is ordered. In most cases the medication administrator will refer these questions to the physician, nurse, or pharmacist responsible for the care of the patient, who will further discuss the question. Medication administration must be documented immediately *after* the drug is taken. Documentation should never be done prior to administration, because the person administering the drug could be called away from the bedside unexpectedly.

Topical Drug Administration

A topical drug is one applied to the skin or mucous membranes. Topical medications are intended to either produce local effects or provide a sustained release (e.g., transdermal patches). The person applying an ointment should wear disposable gloves and explain the procedure to the patient. The area should be cleaned and any remaining ointment removed. Ointments should be applied in thin layers using cotton swabs or a tongue depressor. Liquid medications, such as lotions and suspensions, should first be shaken well and then applied as directed with quick sprays. Both the patient and the drug administrator should be careful not to inhale the aerosol spray. In some cases, directions may require that the area be covered with sterile gauze after application. Special care should be given to burn-injured patients because they are most susceptible to infections. Generally, absorption of topically applied medications is less predictable than other routes.

Eye Drop and Eye Ointment Application

Always aseptically clean hands by scrubbing well or wearing disposable gloves before instilling eye drops. To preserve the cleanliness of the delivery orifice, do not touch the tip of the dropper or container to the patient's eye or an external surface. Position the patient with his or her head tilted back. The lower eyelid can be gently pulled forward to create a well into which the drop or drops can be inserted (Figure 16-4). Be careful not to touch the eye or conjunctival sac with the medication dispenser.

FIGURE 16-4

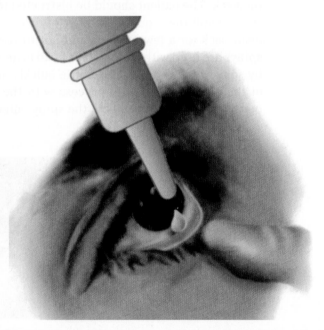

FIGURE 16-4 It is important to make sure you are using proper techniques for instilling eye drops to avoid causing infection or damage to the eye.

Accurately apply the drop or number of drops as directed. Many eye drops have systemic effects; therefore, additional drops should not be given. Before the drops are administered, check the label for the drug name, strength, and directions for use, including which eye (or, if directed, both eyes) should be treated. Check labels for an expiration date. Never use any expired drug. If an ointment is used, discard the first bead (as it is considered contaminated), instruct the patient to look up, and then apply a thin line of ointment to the slightly retracted lower eyelid without allowing the tip of the tube to touch the eye. After instillation of either eye drops or ointment, instruct the patient to close the eye for a few minutes to permit the dispersion of the drug through the eye. If a tear appears, wipe it away with sterile gauze. If there is any noticeable change in the eye (e.g., increased redness, discharge, signs of irritation), report it right away to the supervising nurse or pharmacist.

Administration of Ear and Nose Preparation

To instill ear drops, the patient should be sitting with the unaffected ear resting on the shoulder or lying down with the affected ear facing up (Figure 16-5). It will be more comfortable for the patient if the solution to be instilled is warmed slightly with your hand or by placing the solution under warm water for a few minutes prior to instillation. For an adult or a child older than three, the ear should be gently pulled up and back, and for a child younger than three, the ear should be gently pulled down and back to make the ear canal more accessible. Drops are inserted directly into the canal without touching the tip of the dropper or nozzle to the ear. The patient should remain positioned for a few minutes to keep the drops from running out of the ear. If a cotton plug is ordered, it should be sterile and gently placed just at the opening of the canal. Administer only the prescribed number of drops after carefully reading the label.

Nose drops should be applied with the patient's head resting on the back of the neck. The patient should be instructed to breathe through the mouth (Figure 16-6). Instill the required number of drops, and instruct the patient to keep the head back for a few minutes and not to blow the nose for a few minutes. Nose sprays are used with the patient's head in an upright position. The spray is applied by squeezing the applicator bottle quickly and firmly while it is placed in the tip of the nostril. Repeat the process with the other nostril. Use only as directed, because active ingredients in the spray enter directly into the circulatory system

FIGURE 16-5

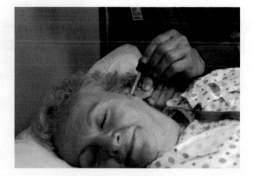

FIGURE 16-5 Instillation of ear drops requires proper positioning of the patient for the medication to work effectively.

FIGURE 16-6

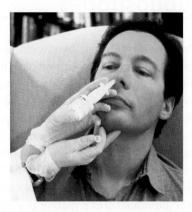

FIGURE 16-6 Instillation of nose drops is accomplished with the patient sitting upright with the head resting on the back of the neck.

and may have untoward systemic effects. Other drugs in nebulizer form come with specific instructions in the package insert. These should be carefully followed to properly administer the drugs.

Application of Transdermal Drugs

systemic action
affects the body as a whole.

Transdermal drugs, often called drug patches, consist of an active drug ingredient inside a patch held in place by adhesive (Figure 16-7). The drug is applied externally for internal or **systemic action**. A drug such as nitroglycerin (for chest pain) is placed in a transdermal patch on the skin where it is picked up by the bloodstream for action over a sustained period of time. The area where the patch is applied should be clearly dry and free of hair (e.g., upper arm). The patch should not be applied to any irritated, callused, or scarred area. The location of the patch should be rotated when a new patch is applied. Do not place the patch below the knee or elbow. Care should be taken that the patch does not come off at night or during bathing. If the patch does fall off, check with the supervisor. The location of the patch needs to be documented.

FIGURE 16-7

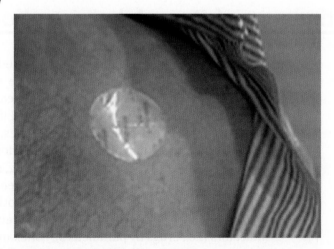

FIGURE 16-7 Transdermal patch (Courtesy of 3M Pharmaceuticals).

Insertion of Suppositories

Prepare a treatment by checking the label on the box. Make sure the suppository feels firm. The cocoa-butter base may begin to soften or melt at warm temperatures. If this occurs, briefly place the suppository, with foil wrapper intact, in cold water to increase firmness. Have a tube of lubricating ointment available, and use a pair of disposable gloves. Inform the patient concerning the drug administration procedure, and position the patient as instructed. Drape the patient and provide for privacy. For rectal insertion, the patient should be on one side (generally the left side unless contraindicated) with one leg extended and other leg flexed at the knee. Don gloves, unwrap the suppository and lubricate the rounded end (or follow more specific manufacturer's instructions), and lubricate your gloved index finger. Instruct the patient to take slow, deep breaths to aid relaxation. Insert the suppository into the rectum beyond the anal sphincter (approximately the length of your index finger for an adult, less for a child), and encourage the patient to retain it for at least 30 to 40 minutes. For vaginal insertion, encourage the patient to void, then position her on her back with knees flexed and legs spread apart. The drug administrator should put on gloves and remove the suppository foil wrapper. Rectal ointment and vaginal suppositories and ointments are inserted using an applicator that accompanies the suppository or cream. Further directions for use are found in the package insert.

Injectable Drug Administration

Many techniques and various routes exist for the use of injectable medications. Injectable drugs can be given directly into a blood vessel (intravascular), into a vein (intravenous), into an artery (intra-arterial), into select muscles (intramuscular), under the skin (hypodermic or subcutaneous), or into the skin (intradermal) by medication administrators, and into the spinal cord (intrathecal) or the heart (intrapericardiac) by practitioners specially trained in these techniques.

Many of these injection techniques require special manipulative skill. They are considered invasive procedures, frequently using very potent drugs. Information and competency development is beyond the scope of this manual.

Discontinuance of Drug Administration

Persons involved in drug administration need to be very alert to the times when drug discontinuance, interruption of dosage schedules, or modification of scheduled dosage patterns are prescribed or indicated.

Drug administration should be withheld if the patient gives evidence of experiencing an adverse drug reaction (e.g., hives; a rash occurring on the body, face, neck, arms, or legs; difficulty in breathing; double vision or seeing various colors that are not objectively present). If the drug administrator observes any of these conditions or the patient speaks about them, the supervising nurse should be contacted before the next dose is given. In other clinical situations, there may be hospital policy or physician orders that direct stoppage of a drug due to certain indicators (i.e., drugs by parameters). For example, do not give digoxin if the apical pulse rate falls below 60 beats per minute.

Surgeons and anesthesiologists usually give specific orders for medication immediately before and after surgery. Many times, physicians or hospital policy will instruct that all or certain drugs be given with a sip of water prior to surgery even if the patient is NPO ("nothing by mouth"). An example would be to continue blood pressure medication even though the patient is NPO for surgery, to ensure the blood pressure remains within normal limits pre- and intraoperatively. Some physicians or hospital policies may discontinue all standing medication orders prior to the patient going to surgery. At that time, drugs needed prior to, during, and immediately after surgery are reordered. All health professionals involved in medication dispensing and/or administration must carefully scrutinize the pre-operative and postoperative drug orders for the surgical patient. Mistakes in this area could jeopardize the surgical outcome.

The patient may be scheduled for physical therapy, X-rays, or other activities that take the patient off the floor during the scheduled times of medication admin-istrations. If this occurs, the supervising nurse should be contacted as to the appro-priate action to take regarding giving the medication when the patient returns.

Other interruptions of drug administration can occur when the patient's orders read "nothing by mouth," and the patient is on oral drug therapy. And in some situa-tions, for various reasons, the patient may refuse to take the drug. In each case, the supervising nurse, the pharmacist, or the prescribing physician must be contacted to clarify the appropriate action to be taken regarding drug administration.

If a patient is in a program for therapeutic drug monitoring (TDM), the drug dosage schedule or laboratory phlebotomy schedule may have to be modified according to the half-life of the drug to obtain the accurate drug blood serum levels that are required for optimum drug therapy dosing. These patients may require an individualized drug dosage administration schedule to be planned by the phy-sician, pharmacist, and medical technologist. Information regarding interrupted drug administration, refusal of the patient to take one drug, and modified drug schedules should always be charted in the medication records and reported to the supervising nurse.

Unit-Dose Drug Administration

A unit-dose drug comes individually packaged and labeled and requires no further packaging or labeling. This system cuts down on the problem of medication errors and preserves the integrity and safety of the product. In a unit-dose drug delivery system, a pharmacist checks every drug order prior to the administration of the drug. The unit-dose system provides each patient with a storage bin, usually in a medication cart, in which no more than a 24-hour supply of drugs is available for the individual patient. The package is opened at the patient's bedside, and the name, label, strength, and patient are checked against the medication administra-tion record. Now, unit doses frequently include drug-specific bar codes to facilitate automation of the medication system (see Chapter 18).

Crushing Medications

Crushing medications to assist patients who have difficulty swallowing pills or cap-sules is recommended only after serious consideration and consultation between the physician and the pharmacist. Medications are designed in tablet or capsule form to ensure their absorption in the correct area of the gastrointestinal tract and to eliminate or minimize digestive problems. Crushing may seriously interfere with these safety measures. Crushing cannot be used for enteric-coated or sustained action medications (e.g., Pronestyl-SR). Notify the pharmacy about the need to crush specific medications, and follow the pharmacist's advice regarding the safety of this action.

If crushing is necessary and approved by institutional policy, each medication must be crushed individually, mixed with a palatable food (e.g., applesauce, Jell-O), and given to the patient separately. Attempt to give the patient as much of the drug in the first spoonful so that very little is wasted if the patient refuses the remainder. Never mix all of the patient's medications in one cup.

Internal and External Medications

Any caregiver who has been in practice for an extended period of time can cite examples of inaccuracies that they read about, heard about, or were involved in. One that comes to mind is that of an elderly monk admitted to the hospital for a severe scalp burn. Someone attempting to dry a wet lesion dropped a sunlamp on his head. The burn became infected, and he was admitted to the hospital. His first morning in the hospital, his caregiver poured out and left at the bedside two ounces of mouthwash in a small waxed paper cup, the same cup as the one the patient had received a liquid medication in the previous evening. When the caregiver returned to assist him with oral hygiene, she asked what happened to the mouthwash. She got the simple answer, "I swallowed it." The aide reported the incident; the patient was carefully monitored, and outside of excessive urination, was fortunately discharged with no other apparent side effects. This story illustrates the fact that one cannot be too careful in providing medications for hospitalized persons.

Internal medications (to be swallowed, ingested, or injected) and external medications (to be applied to the outside of the body or an adjoining orifice) should always be stored separately. These drugs are labeled differently. External preparations require a red external use label. Black or another color is used for internal medications. Drugs labeled for topical use are also external preparations and usually carry a red-lettered label.

Ancillary labels should be carefully read and followed (e.g., "Shake well before using," "Refrigerate," "Do not refrigerate," "For external use only").

Medication Teaching

Patients and families knowledgeable about their drug regimes can be important links in ensuring safe medication administration, understanding the individual therapeutic medication effect, attaining the intended medication effect, and limiting untoward effects. It is key that as part of the medication team, the pharmacist or medication administrator consistently involve the patient and family in the medication process and provide them as much information as appropriate. Active participation and an individualized approach based on patient needs are the standard. Remember that patients will be administering their own medications upon discharge. Listen carefully to patients and families during medication administration. If they question a medication or a dose, double-check it with a supervisor. Many errors have been prevented by an astute patient or family member, and there is the potential for anyone to make a mistake.

The provision of medication information to patients and their families takes some preparation and planning. The patient's physician, pharmacist, and nurse are responsible for establishing the teaching need and priorities, developing the teaching plan, and evaluating learning outcomes. The medication administrator's role is to participate in this process as requested and as appropriate. As the medication administrator administers medications, he or she will learn helpful information that will be important to communicate to the patient care team. This individual will also have a unique opportunity to participate in the teaching process. Information on the patient's readiness to learn, education level, best learning method (e.g., verbal, written, demonstration), and time available for teaching (i.e., expected discharge date) is needed to prepare to teach. It is always best to start with finding out what the patient knows and what the patient would like to know about the medications. There are many excellent sources of medication teaching materials, and every hospital will have many resources available.

Readiness to Learn

With today's shorter lengths of stay, the best time for patient teaching may be a narrow window. Signs of readiness to learn include stable physical condition, pain control, patient alertness and the ability to concentrate for at least short periods of time, and patient interest in learning about medication. When the time frame available for teaching is particularly short, the teaching plan may include instruction done by others along the patient's "continuum of care," including long-term care facility staff, a home care or visiting nurse, the outpatient pharmacy, and family.

Age and Education Level

Age, developmental level, and educational level will all be considered as a teaching plan is formulated by the nurse or pharmacist. Age and years of schooling alone may not be the only guides to how to deliver information, but they do provide a starting point. When the patient's education has been of a basic level, it is best to address the teaching at an eighth-grade level. In many parts of the country, significant numbers of patients cannot read at all or have a very limited reading ability. Generally, patients will not share this type of information and do well covering up their limitations. It is a good rule of thumb to avoid the use of scientific or medical terminology, and give examples to support and reinforce learning. Take clues from the patient; this is ultimately the best guide on patient understanding, application, and retention. Examples of different teaching approaches based on developmental stages are asking adolescents if they want their parents present during the teaching session and providing elderly patients with memory aids such as medication calendars or pill boxes.

Learning Method

How a person learns is a complex and individual process, but learning is facilitated when a number of methods and senses are involved. A good plan includes the methods of instruction. These may include a combination of the following: written materials, verbal instruction, demonstration, providing examples, video or audio tapes, and a question-and-answer session. Information is best absorbed when given over a period of time (e.g., give written material to the patient to read in the morning, and return later in the day to discuss the information and answer questions). Many patients now have access to the Internet at home, and they can be given hospital or general Web sites that include patient educational materials on medication. Clear discharge instructions, medication information leaflets, and providing a number for the patient to call with questions after discharge are all standard ways to reinforce valuable information given to the patient under the stressful circumstances of illness, hospital discharge, or transfer to another facility.

Teaching Plan

The patient's nurse and/or pharmacist in collaboration with the physician will develop the teaching plan. Formation of a teaching plan focuses on the needs of the patient and the information to be taught. The plan will include learning objectives stated as outcome objectives (i.e., what the patient will learn by the completion of instruction). Objectives should be practical, achievable, and measurable. Include the patient's objectives in the plan when possible. Examples of teaching and learning objectives are as follows:

- The patient will be able to list three signs of digitalis toxicity that require physician notification.
- The patient will describe rotation of sites for insulin injection.
- The patient's son will demonstrate correct insulin injection technique.

Objectives provide a basis for evaluating the effectiveness for teaching. The ultimate objective is that the patient has the information and skills necessary for safe medication administration.

Teaching Process

Try to select the most suitable and comfortable location to provide instruction. A comfortable location with limited distractions will allow the patient to concentrate on the information and ask questions. Prior to initiating teaching, the teaching plan and the objectives should be reviewed. It is then important to communicate what will be covered with the patient to the other team members and ensure it is documented. At least two methods of instruction are recommended to improve understanding and retention.

When possible, provide the patient with written material from a patient teaching text, from a computerized program, or from the instructor. When a preprinted text is used, it needs to be reviewed for content, education level, size of type, and so forth, prior to giving it to the patient. Teaching of complex information is generally done by the physician, nurse, or pharmacist, and should be given in more than one session. The definition of "complex" information will vary according to the patient, but any learning that requires cognitive and psychomotor capabilities is considered "complex." Examples of complex learning include self-injection, taking radial pulse prior to cardiac medication, and taking a child's temperature. In each of these situations, the patient or family members need to have information on the reason for the procedure, how to perform the skill or procedure, and what action they are to take based on the results. When participating in teaching complex information, a second or third teaching session should be scheduled to provide the patient with an opportunity to absorb the information, formulate questions, and give a return demonstration as indicated.

Reinforcement

Provide patients with praise and encouragement during their learning process. Describe their progress in terms of readiness for discharge, self-independence, accomplishment of a skill, or being knowledgeable about their medication.

Evaluation of Learning

Since the ultimate goal of the teaching process is to effect learning and change behavior, the evaluation of learning is the final stage of the teaching/learning process. According to the nature of the information, the evaluation method may include a short written test, requesting the patient to verbally state the information, or giving a return demonstration (e.g., taking a pulse).

Professional Responsibility for Drug Administration

Drug administration is the shared privilege and responsibility of different health disciplines, each one with carefully delineated functional activities. Medication administration is just one part of the medication process, which includes prescribing, dispensing, administering, monitoring, and systems and management control. Physician's delegates, such as physician assistants and nurse practitioners, have the responsibility to prescribe rational and selective drug therapy that is dependent upon the patient's medical profile and the drug's therapeutic characteristics.

The pharmacists are responsible to screen these orders for rational drug therapy and appropriateness in particular, individualized cases. In some instances, the pharmacist is invited to participate in the multidisciplinary planning of a particular patient's drug regimen. The pharmacist evaluates the choice of a drug for a particular pathology, and if doubt arises, the physician is contacted. Further consideration is given to the drug dose, the time intervals between doses, and the patient's past drug history regarding allergies, drug sensitivities, and past untoward drug reactions. The pharmacist further considers the drug benefit/risk ratio regarding the possibility of a drug-drug interaction, a drug-food interaction, or a drug-laboratory test interaction. If there is apparent serious drug risk involvement, the pharmacist further consults with the physician regarding appropriate drug administration. If the pharmacist evaluates the regimen to be within the bounds of sound therapy, the drug is dispensed, for an inpatient, through the nursing service in most situations. If the pharmacy completely controls the drug-use process, a medication administrator (technician) may then assume the final responsibility for proper drug administration. However, in most institutions, the nursing department in collaboration with the pharmacy department is responsible for the final step in the drug-use process (i.e., administration of the drug and observation of the patient regarding the therapeutic outcome of the drug action).

According to hospital policy, the task of actually giving the medication to a patient may be delegated to a trained medication technician. Yet the responsibility of the drug's outcome remains with the licensed health professionals involved. Basically, the right drug, for the right reason, must be given to the right patient at the right time in the right dosage strength and in the right drug dosage form. This is the core responsibility of the drug administration process. Responsibility for the outcome is shared by the professionals of medicine, nursing, and pharmacy.

Legal Responsibilities in Drug Administration

Many states and many health care institutions have very specific policies and procedures that must be carried out exactly as written. Presently, many states require a registered nurse to administer all medications. At the same time, other states and health institutions, due to fiscal, technical, personnel, and patient loads, are changing or modifying existing regulations. Basic requirements do not change, even if the assigned or designated personnel change.

Every hospital is required to have a policy and procedural manual to ensure patient safety and patient care. The persons involved in drug administration activities must know and observe these policies and procedures. When medication errors are made, they are usually related to the patient's five rights. To prove negligence, it must be established that drug administration policy was not followed, careless shortcuts were taken, or the medication order and administration procedure were not adequately checked by the responsible licensed professional.

For many years, health care has assumed a myth of infallibility. Errors have been underreported and covered up. Given the dramatic increase in prescription drugs, the toxicity of many medications, and the fact that health care professionals are human and do make mistakes, errors are a reality. The current thinking is that much will be gained in error reduction by refocusing from a culture of blame to one of systems improvement. The systems improvement approach recognizes that there are conditions and environments in which humans are more likely to err and that those conditions can be modified to reduce error. By having more errors and near-misses reported, and by conducting studies to improve those environments, medication systems can be rewired for error prevention. Where do you fit in medication error prevention?

- Be aware of the risk and reality of medication errors. It is unrealistic to believe you will never be involved in an error.
- Report all errors and near-misses consistently based on your hospital's policies and procedures.
- Utilize medication resources, and attend in-service education programs. Recognize it is no longer possible to be knowledgeable on every medication—there are just too many new drugs and too much new information constantly available.
- Know your patient's allergies.
- Be alert to high-risk medications, safe medication practices, and specific safety protocols.
- Recognize the role certain practices have in errors: illegible handwriting, trailing zeros, leading decimal points, abbreviations, use of the abbreviation *u* for units, and so forth.
- Practice meticulous medication administration practices, such as identification of every patient every time, stating the drug-dose-reason for every drug every time, and always listening to patients and families.
- Provide information to patients and families, and facilitate their active involvement in care.
- Participate in performance improvement activities, the implementation of computerized medication systems, and other medication safety improvements.

Please refer to Chapter 28, "Preventing and Managing Medication Errors," for a thorough discussion of this topic.

Adequate patient drug use control, drug use evaluation, and drug use surveillance must be top priorities to ensure patient safety. Detected errors must be reported immediately to the licensed supervisor. The goal of the performance improvement process is to identify individual and system problems that, if corrected, will help to avoid future errors.

Trends in Drug Administration

Drug administration methods are frequently called *drug-delivery systems*. Drug firms have made large investments in researching and developing new methods to target drug administration dosage forms to maximize effectiveness and to limit unwanted systemic effects. The future may see pharmacy technicians specializing in the maintenance, utilization, and monitoring of these new and often unique devices and drug administration delivery systems.

If contemporary trends, particularly the working definition for pharmaceutical care, continue to prevail, pharmacy technicians of the future may require specific knowledge, judgment, techniques, and skills to participate in the health care team as competent pharmacy medication technicians.

Summary

The administration of medication is a serious responsibility, requiring the possession of clinical information and skills. It includes not only information about the drugs being given, but also the proper procedures for safe administration, communication with team members, and documentation. Skills in administration ensure that the patient receives medication in the safest and most therapeutic manner with the least chance of mistakes, untoward reactions, or spread of infection.

TEST YOUR KNOWLEDGE

Multiple Choice

1. The drug administration process begins with
   a. the physician's prescription.
   b. the pharmacist dispensing the drug.
   c. the nurse evaluating the patient.
   d. the request for a drug.

2. Medication orders include
   a. drugs ordered by the physician after medical rounds.
   b. telephone drug orders in emergencies.
   c. standing drug orders for particular patient categories.
   d. all of the above.

3. A prn drug is administered
   a. routinely.
   b. at night before sleep.
   c. before meals.
   d. when the patient asks for the medication, or the patient's condition requires it.

4. Patient rights include the
   a. right drug.
   b. right time.
   c. right route.
   d. all of the above.

5. Prior to administering a drug, the medication administrator should
   a. check the patient's correct identification using two identifiers.
   b. check the drug against the order three times.
   c. leave the medication in the unit-dose package and check the expiration date.
   d. all of the above.

6. A drug may be left at the patient's bedside if
   a. the patient requests that the drug be left.
   b. the patient is asleep.
   c. the patient wants to discuss the drug with the pharmacist.
   d. none of the above.

7. At least four ounces of water should be given following the drug administration of
   a. a buccal tablet.
   b. a medicated mouthwash.
   c. an aspirin tablet.
   d. a sublingual tablet.

8. Sufficient water given after administration of a solid oral dosage form
   a. assists the patient in swallowing.
   b. prevents esophageal irritation.
   c. aids drug solubility.
   d. all of the above.

9. After administration of eye drops, the patient should be advised to
   a. not move the head.
   b. not sneeze.
   c. close the eye(s) for a few minutes.
   d. immediately wipe away any tears.

10. Transdermal drug patches are placed
    a. on the upper arm or inside the forearm.
    b. below the knee.
    c. directly above the wrists.
    d. on the most accessible spot.

11. Outcomes of the performance improvement process for medication errors include
    a. identifying problems in the medication administration process.
    b. determining the need for staff education.
    c. reducing the possibility of future errors.
    d. all of the above.

12. When administering an enteric-coated medication to a child or geriatric patient, the administrator may take the following action(s):
    a. give the medication crushed in applesauce.
    b. dissolve the medication in water.
    c. give the medication with sufficient juice.
    d. none of the above.

Matching

Determine if the following dosage forms are internal or external:

1. _____ ointment
2. _____ topical preparation
3. _____ tablet
4. _____ elixir
5. _____ intramuscular injection

a. internal drug
b. external drug

Fill In The Blank

1. An order for a drug that must be administered immediately is called a _____ order.

2. Never administer a medication without checking it _____ times against the MAR.

3. An infection incurred in the hospital is called a _____ infection.

4. A _____ medication is one that is given under the tongue.

5. A _____ focuses on the needs of the patient and the information to be presented to the patient.

References

Gourley, D. R., Wedemweyer, H. F., & Norvell, M. (2006). Administration of medications. In T. R. Brown & M. C. Smith (Eds.), *Handbook of institutional pharmacy practice* (4th ed.). Baltimore: Lippincott Williams & Wilkins.

Drug Information Centers

Competencies

Upon completion of this chapter, the reader should be able to

1. Describe and perform the steps of the systematic approach to answering a drug information question.
2. Describe the characteristics of tertiary, secondary, and primary resources.
3. Differentiate between reputable and questionable Web sites.
4. Identify useful tertiary resources and Web sites.
5. Devise a system to keep yourself current in pharmacy practice.
6. List and describe the responsibilities of the pharmacy technician working in a drug information center.
7. Explain the qualities and skills that a pharmacy technician must have in order to contribute significantly to the functions of a drug information center.

Key Terms

drug information
drug information centers (DIC)
primary resources
secondary resources
tertiary resources

Introduction

Over the centuries, pharmacy practice has evolved from a more product-oriented profession to a more patient-oriented profession. Traditionally, pharmacists focused primarily on compounding and dispensing medications. This changed as mass-manufacturers of drug products reduced the need for pharmacists to compound drugs. More recently, technological advancements and the addition of pharmacy technicians allowed pharmacists to focus more time on improving patient outcomes through the provision of pharmaceutical care. To meet the demands of their profession, pharmacists had to develop and maintain effective drug information skills. The public and health care professionals turn to pharmacists for accurate and unbiased drug information. Today, the management of vast amounts of information and the provision of evidence-based drug information continues to be the most essential responsibility of all pharmacists.

Pharmacy technicians who have effective drug information skills can assist the pharmacist in improving patient outcomes in a variety of practice settings. In a community pharmacy, technicians can assist in researching questions asked by the customers who walk into the pharmacy or by the physicians who call into the pharmacy. In a hospital setting, a technician can assist in researching acute care questions that originate from the many health care professionals working within the hospital. A technician may also choose to work in a drug information center, which will be discussed in greater detail in this chapter. Regardless of the practice setting in which a pharmacy technician works, the efficient and correct use of drug information is crucial in the prevention of medication errors and will help the technician remain current with the profession.

This chapter will introduce the pharmacy technician to evidence-based drug information practice and will outline the pharmacy technician's role. The content of this chapter may or may not be in compliance with all states' laws and regulations. The pharmacy technician is strongly encouraged to review the laws that govern the state in which he or she practices to determine what activities can be delegated by the pharmacist to the pharmacy technician.

Definition of Drug Information

drug information
information about drugs and the effects of drugs on people, the provision of which is a part of each pharmacist's practice.

The term **drug information** simply means information pertaining to drugs. The more contemporary term *medical information* is often used alternatively to also encompass information pertaining to health, but not directly related to medications. For the purposes of this chapter, the more traditional term *drug information* will be used, although one should realize that the knowledge and expertise of pharmacists extends beyond medications. For example, pharmacists are often consulted on dietary supplements, nonpharmacological methods of managing illness, dietary modifications, and disease prevention.

The provision of drug information can be grouped into two categories: patient-specific or population-based. Pharmacists and pharmacy technicians most often receive patient-specific drug information requests. For example, a woman suffering from postpartum depression needs an antidepressant medication that would allow her to continue to safely breastfeed her infant. In this specific situation, patient-specific information is needed, such as the woman's past medical history including information on her recent pregnancy, her medication history, and any allergies she may have. The patient's values and beliefs regarding the importance of breastfeeding her infant should also be taken into consideration. Information about the infant will also be necessary. Once all of this information has been collected, the pharmacist will perform an extensive search for drug information and subsequently provide an individualized, evidence-based recommendation.

On the other hand, population-based drug information involves researching and evaluating drug information as it relates to a group of patients in general. When providing population-based information, the pharmacist focuses on the general use of a drug in a group of patients and not in an individual patient. For example, a physician requests that the pharmacy department consider adding a particular drug to the hospital formulary. A pharmacist in turn would retrieve and evaluate all of the research that has been performed on the drug and subsequently compare this drug to other similar drugs that are already on the formulary. The pharmacist would then develop an evidence-based decision on whether the drug would potentially benefit future patients admitted to the hospital.

The drug information activities and responsibilities of a pharmacist are outlined in the American Society of Health-System Pharmacists (ASHP) Guidelines in the "Provision of Medication Information by Pharmacists" section. The pharmacy technician should become familiar with this document before aiding pharmacists in answering drug information requests. One can find these guidelines (as well as many other important ASHP policy positions, statements, and guidelines) for free on the ASHP's Web site (www.ashp.org).

Drug Information Specialists

Although all pharmacists are responsible for providing drug information, some pharmacists have chosen to undergo extensive training and specialization in the field of drug information practice. These pharmacists are referred to as *drug information specialists*. Drug information specialists have extensive knowledge of drug information resources, strong literature evaluation skills, problem-solving skills, expertise in information technology, and are effective communicators of verbal and written drug information.

Drug Information Centers

drug information center (DIC) a center directed by a drug information specialist, most commonly funded by or located in a hospital, academic institution, or pharmaceutical company, that provides information and education on drugs, develops policies or guidelines for appropriate use of medications, and coordinates medication error programs.

Drug information centers (DIC) are usually directed by drug information specialists. The first DIC was established in 1962 at the University of Kentucky Medical Center. Ever since then, the number of drug information centers has increased across the United States. The purposes of a DIC vary and depend on the practice setting in which the drug information center is located. A DIC is most commonly funded by or located in a hospital, academic institution, or pharmaceutical company. Some drug information centers provide free drug information services, while others provide drug information for a fee (fee for service). A client could pay an annual fee to contract with a particular drug information center regardless of the number of times the client uses the DIC. Alternatively, the client may pay for each individual question answered or every project (i.e., formulary monograph) completed by DIC personnel.

A function common to all drug information centers is the handling of drug information requests. Requests can be received via the telephone, e-mail, regular mail, or in person. Requestors of information can be physicians, nurses, pharmacists, and patients. Other functions of a drug information center include, but are not limited to, the provision of education through lectures and newsletters, development of policies or guidelines for appropriate use of medications, management of formularies and quality assurance activities, and coordination of adverse drug reaction and medication error programs. Pharmacy technicians can support the drug information specialist in performing all of these activities. Specifically, the pharmacy technician may be expected to collect statistics on the number of drug information requests received, the profession of the requestor using the drug information center, the type of questions asked, and the time spent answering questions on a monthly basis. The technician may assist in maintaining a filing system of old requests and a filing system of important information collected on medications or medical topics of interest to allow for rapid and easy access. In certain drug information centers where computerized databases are used to document and store drug information questions for subsequent easy retrieval, the technician can assist in maintaining and updating the database. The pharmacy technician can help compile information to be published in a newsletter. A pharmacy technician with effective technological skills can help edit the newsletter to allow it to have a consistent appearance. The technician can also assist in the collection of data for research projects, adverse drug reactions, medication errors, quality assurance projects, and formulary management activities.

A directory of drug information centers in the United States can be located in Thompson's *Red Book* and the *Physician's Desk Reference* (PDR). These references can be ordered by visiting www.pdrbookstore.com. A directory of drug information centers has also been published by Koumis, et al., in the *American Journal of Health-System Pharmacy* (see references in the back of this chapter).

The Systematic Approach to Answering a Drug Information Question

The pharmacy technician working in a drug information center, community pharmacy, or hospital pharmacy should have an understanding of the systematic approach to answering a drug information question, originated by Watanabe and colleagues in 1975. The systematic approach was later modified to involve a total of seven steps:

1. Determine the demographics of the requestor.
2. Obtain background information.
3. Determine and categorize the ultimate question.
4. Develop a search strategy and conduct search.
5. Evaluate, analyze, and summarize the information obtained.
6. Formulate and provide a response.
7. Conduct a follow-up, and document the question from beginning to end.

Requestor Demographics

Usually, requestors of information approach or call the pharmacist or drug information center and immediately provide an initial question. One should proceed by quickly writing down the initial question and then asking for the requestor's full name (first names alone are not sufficient), profession, specialty, address, phone numbers, fax numbers, e-mail, and any other contact information thought necessary.

Understanding the requestor's profession or specialty is important in determining the depth and complexity of information needed. For example, a physician's question would most often require extensive research and a detailed scientific response, while a patient's inquiry could usually be answered rapidly without as much extensive research. In addition, when communicating with a patient, it is necessary to use lay terms to ensure that the patient understands the information provided. A pharmacy technician may perform the first step of documenting the information obtained on a drug information request documentation form (Figure 17-1) and should then arrange for the pharmacist or drug information specialist to perform the next step of obtaining background information, especially if the question appears to be of an urgent nature or of high complexity.

Background Information

Obtaining background information is the most important step in the systematic approach and requires effective communication and listening skills. To perform this step well, an extensive knowledge base is needed of different medical conditions and medications. This step generally should be performed by the pharmacist or drug information specialist. If this step is not performed appropriately, serious consequences may occur in that inaccurate or irrelevant information may be provided and valuable time may be wasted. During this step, the pharmacist or drug information specialist will determine if the request is patient-specific or population-based and will proceed to ask important relevant questions to determine the true drug information need. Pharmacy technicians with extensive experience working in a pharmacy or drug information center may also perform this step if the question is deemed not urgent or is easily understood by the technician. An experienced technician will be able to use judgment to determine whether the question needs the attention of the pharmacist or drug information specialist. The experienced technician must demonstrate effective listening, communication, and interviewing skills to perform this step. The technician must also have an extensive knowledge base of drugs and diseases.

Determination and Categorization of the Ultimate Question

Determining the ultimate question (true drug information need) is accomplished easily once sufficient background information is obtained. Often, the initial question differs significantly from the ultimate or final question. Once the ultimate question is identified and clear, the pharmacy technician or the drug information specialist can then quickly categorize the request and the next step can begin. The question should be categorized by type. For example, the question can be categorized as a drug interaction question or a drug identification question. For a list of possible categories of drug information questions, see the drug information request documentation form in Figure 17-1. Categorization of the request is important in that it helps direct one to the resources that would best answer the question (e.g., a drug interaction textbook).

FIGURE 17-1

Date: _____ Time: _____ Received by: _____

Requestor's Demographics

Name: _____ Hospital Location: _____

Affiliation: _____

Address: _____
        Street address

_____
City   State   Zip

Phone Number: ( )   -   Fax Number: ( )   -

Pager Number: ( )   -   E-mail Address:

Profession:
MD   RPh   PharmD   RN   PhD
Consumer/Patient

Specialty _____
Other _____

Background Information:

Patient Specific?   Yes   No   If Yes, fill out below:
MR#_____ **Location:** _____ **Gender:** Female   Male **Age:**_____
Height: _____ **Weight:** _____ **Allergies:** _____
Relevant PMH / HPI / Diagnosis (including organ fxn):

Medications:

Initial Question:

Ultimate Question:

Classification of Request:

Product Availability	Compatibility/Stability	Reference Material
Pharmacokinetics	Dosage/Administration	Drug Interactions
Adverse Reactions/Toxicity	CAM/Dietary Supplements	Product Identification
Pregnancy/Lactation/Repro	Therapeutic Use	Compounding
Other _____		

Urgency of Response: STAT   Other _____
Method of Request: Phone   In Person   E-mail   3rd Person   Other

---

FIGURE 17-1 Drug information request form.

FIGURE 17-1 (Continued)

Actual Response Provided (attach continuation of response and support materials if necessary):

All References Used (indicate whether information found or not):

Response Information

Date: _____ Time: _____ ☐ Verbal   ☐ Written

Answered by: _____ Approved by: _____

Response given via: ☐ Phone   ☐ Letter   ☐ In Person   ☐ Fax   ☐ E-mail   ☐ Other

Total time needed to complete request: _____

Search Strategy and Information Collection

The pharmacy technician can contribute significantly to the development of a search strategy and collection of pertinent information. The technician must first develop a search strategy starting with general resources (**tertiary resources**) and work toward more specific resources (**primary resources**) through use of indexing and abstracting services (**secondary resources**). These three different types of resources will be described later in this chapter. The experienced technician should be able to identify when a search through secondary and primary resources is needed for a given question (e.g., physician inquiry, detailed or complex question) and when tertiary resources would be sufficient to answer the question (e.g., patient or nurse inquiry, general question). The pharmacy technician must have good knowledge of all the resources available to answer drug information questions in the drug information center, pharmacy, affiliated medical library (if applicable), and on the Internet.

The technician must also be proficient in conducting literature searches, using computerized databases, and in the proper use of print resources. Once the necessary resources have been consulted and the information collected, the technician should then promptly provide this information to the pharmacist or drug information specialist for evaluation. The pharmacy technician must also remember to anticipate other questions that must be answered to provide a complete response. For example, if a requestor of information needs the drug of choice to treat a patient's community-acquired pneumonia, the drug name will most likely not be sufficient to completely answer the request. The drug dosing regimen, route of administration, duration of therapy, monitoring parameters, common side effects, and potential drug interactions would be additional information needed by the requestor, although the requestor did not specifically ask for it.

Evaluation, Analysis, and Synthesis of Information

This step requires strong literature evaluation skills and, therefore, should be left to the pharmacist or drug information specialist. Knowledge of study design, research, and statistical concepts is essential to be able to evaluate the medical literature and apply the information to clinical practice and patient-specific situations. The pharmacy technician's involvement in this step would depend upon the training and experience of the technician.

Formulate and Provide Response

After careful analysis and synthesis of information, the pharmacist or drug information specialist will formulate a response and then accurately convey the response back to the requestor of information. This requires strong verbal and written communication skills. If a written response is required, the pharmacy technician may assist in drafting and referencing the response. However, ultimately the pharmacist or drug information specialist must review the written response for accuracy and completeness.

Follow-Up and Documentation

The pharmacy technician can assist in following up on all completed requests to determine whether the information provided was appropriate, recommendations provided were actually followed, and if the response was adequate to meet the requestor's needs. This process ensures and documents the quality of services provided by the drug information center. The pharmacy technician is also responsible for assisting in the appropriate documentation of all requests from beginning to end, and should make sure all references used were properly documented on the drug information request documentation form and/or computerized database.

Drug Information Resources

One of the technician's primary responsibilities in a pharmacy or drug information center is managing the inventory of all resources. Resources should be stored in an organized fashion and kept up-to-date. The technician is responsible for ordering references, keeping track of subscription expiration dates, and ensuring that ordered resources are actually received by the pharmacy or drug information center. The technician is also responsible for maintaining a filing system of important information for easy and rapid access by all pharmacy or drug information center personnel.

The pharmacy technician should also have knowledge of all of the available resources in the pharmacy, drug information center, nearby medical libraries (if applicable), and on the Internet. The technician must be proficient in the retrieval of drug information, whether it comes from the shelves of a library or a computerized database. The technician may also assist in the printing and photocopying of necessary information.

The experienced technician should also be able to differentiate between reputable resources and those of questionable quality. There are three different types of drug information resources: tertiary, secondary, and primary resources. Each type has advantages and disadvantages that the pharmacy technician should be able to describe and keep in mind when researching drug information requests.

Tertiary Resources

A list of tertiary resources (i.e., general resources) is provided in Table 17-1. Tertiary resources are package inserts, textbooks, compendia, computer databases, and review articles. These resources are best if peer-reviewed, authored by an expert in the field to which the resource pertains, and easy to navigate. Tertiary resources can allow for rapid comprehensive access to information, are commonly consulted when initiating a search strategy, and are usually used to educate oneself on a medical condition or medication.

One of the significant disadvantages of tertiary resources is that they are usually somewhat out-of-date by the time they are published. This is due to the significant amount of time that elapses between when the resource is written and when it is actually published (i.e., long lag time). Therefore, one must always take into account the resource's date of publication when using it for drug information. Review articles published in journals and certain references published in update-able binder format (e.g., *Drug Facts and Comparisons*) do not have as significant a lag time. Also, one must keep in mind that the information provided in a tertiary resource is subject to the author's interpretation of the primary literature (i.e., original research) on the topic. Sometimes the author's opinion may not necessarily be accurate or complete. Since tertiary resources are general resources, they usually lack specific details, forcing the reader to conduct further research of the primary literature for more information.

A discussion on tertiary resources would not be complete without discussing package inserts. Before a medication can be made available to the public for use,

TABLE 17-1   Tertiary Resources Listed by Information Provided

ADVERSE DRUG REACTIONS

Anne Lee's *Adverse Drug Reactions*
Aronson's *Side Effects of Drugs*
Davies's *Textbook of Adverse Drug Reactions*
Meyler's *Side Effects of Drugs*

COMPATIBILITY AND STABILITY

Bing's *Extended Stability for Parenteral Drugs*
Gahart's *Intravenous Medications*
King's *Guide to Parenteral Admixtures*
Trissel's *Handbook of Injectable Drugs*
Trissel's *Stability of Compounded Formulations*

COMPLEMENTARY AND ALTERNATIVE MEDICINE

AltMedDEX System, published by Micromedex (www.thomsonhc.com – subscription required)
The Complete German Commission E Monographs
PDR for Herbal Medicines
Rakel's *Integrative Medicine*
The Review of Natural Products
Tyler's *Herbs of Choice*
Tyler's *Honest Herbal*

COMPOUNDING

Allen's *The Art, Science, and Technology of Pharmaceutical Compounding*
Allen's *Compounded Formulations: The Complete U.S. Pharmacist Collection*
Trissen's *Stability of Compounded Formulations*

DRUG AVAILABILITY

American Drug Index
Drug Facts and Comparisons
Drug Topics Red Book
Thomson's *Red Book*

DRUG IDENTIFICATION

Ident-A-Drug Reference
IDENTIDEX System, published by Micromedex (www.thomsonhc.com – subscription required)

DRUG INFORMATION AND LITERATURE EVALUATION

Ascione's *Principles of Scientific Literature Evaluation: Critiquing Clinical Drug Trials*
Dawson's *Basic and Clinical Biostatistics*
De Muth's *Basic Statistics and Pharmaceutical Statistical Applications*
Malone's *Drug Information: A Guide for Pharmacists*
Riegelman's *Studying a Study and Testing a Test: How to Read the Medical Evidence*
Snow's *Drug Information: A Guide to Current Resources*

DRUG INTERACTION RESOURCES

Drug Interaction Facts
DRUG-REAX System, published by Micromedex (www.thomsonhc.com – subscription required)
Hansten and Horn's *Drug Interaction Analysis and Management*

(Continued)

TABLE 17-1 (Continued)

FOREIGN DRUGS

European Drug Index

Index Nominum: International Drug Directory

Martindale's *The Complete Drug Reference*

USP Dictionary of United States Adopted Names (USAN) and International Drug Names

GENERAL DRUG INFORMATION REFERENCES

American Hospital Formulary Service (AHFS) Drug Information

Drug Facts and Comparisons

Drug Information Handbook, by Lexi-Comp Inc. (also available online at www.online.lexi.com – subscription required)

DRUGDEX System, published by Micromedex (www.thomsonhc.com – subscription required)

Mosby's GenRx

Physician's Desk Reference (PDR)

Remington's *The Science and Practice of Pharmacy*

Thomson's *Red Book*

USP DI Volumes I (health care professional), *II* (patient), and *III* (legal requirements)

GERIATRIC RESOURCES

Brocklehurst's *Textbook of Geriatric Medicine and Gerontology*

Cassel's *Geriatric Medicine: An Evidence-Based Approach*

Geriatric Dosage Handbook, by Lexi-Comp Inc. (also available online at www.online.lexi.com – subscription required)

The Merck Manual of Geriatrics

IMMUNOLOGY

Concepts in Immunology and Immunotherapeutics

ImmunoFacts

INFECTIOUS DISEASE

Mandell, Douglas, and Bennett's *Principles and Practice of Infectious Diseases*

INTERNAL MEDICINE

Cecil's *Textbook of Medicine*

Conn's *Current Therapy*

Harrison's *Principles of Internal Medicine*

The Merck Manual of Diagnosis and Therapeutics

LABORATORY DATA INTERPRETATION

Laboratory Test Handbook

Traub's *Basic Skills in Interpreting Laboratory Data*

MEDICAL DICTIONARIES

Davies's *Medical Abbreviations*

Dorland's *Illustrated Medical Dictionary*

Stedman's *Medical Dictionary*

NEPHROLOGY

Drug Prescribing in Renal Failure: Dosing Guidelines for Adults

NONPRESCRIPTION PRODUCTS

Facts and Comparisons' *Nonprescription Drug Therapy Guiding Patient Self-Care*

Handbook of Nonprescription Drugs

(Continued)

TABLE 17-1 (Continued)

NONPRESCRIPTION PRODUCTS
Facts and Comparisons' *Nonprescription Drug Therapy Guiding Patient Self-Care*
PDR for Nonprescription Drugs and Dietary Supplements
Pray's *Nonprescription Product Therapeutics*

ONCOLOGY/HEMATOLOGY
DeVita's *Cancer: Principles and Practice of Oncology*
Dorr's *Cancer Chemotherapy Handbook*
Hoffman's *Hematology: Basic Principles and Practices*

PEDIATRIC RESOURCES
Nelson's *Textbook of Pediatrics*
Neofax
Pediatric Dosage Handbook, by Lexi-Comp Inc.
Teddy Bear Book: Pediatric Injectable Drugs

PHARMACEUTICAL CALCULATIONS
Stoklosa and Ansel's *Pharmaceutical Calculations*
Zatz's *Pharmaceutical Calculations*

PHARMACOKINETICS
Applied Pharmacokinetics: Principles of Therapeutic Drug Monitoring
Winter's *Basic Clinical Pharmacokinetics*

PHARMACOLOGY AND THERAPEUTICS
DePiro's *Pharmacotherapy: A Pathophysiologic Approach*
Goodman and Gilman's *The Pharmacological Basis of Therapeutics*
Katzung's *Basic and Clinical Pharmacology*
Koda Kimble's *Applied Therapeutics: The Clinical Use of Drugs*
Melmon and Morrelli's *Clinical Pharmacology*

PHARMACY LAW
Abood's *Pharmacy Practice and the Law*
Pharmacy Law Digest
Reiss and Hall's *Guide to Federal Pharmacy Law*

REPRODUCTION, PREGNANCY, AND LACTATION
Briggs's *Drugs in Pregnancy and Lactation*
Chemically Induced Birth Defects
REPRORISK System, published by Micromedex (www.thomsonhc.com – subscription required)
Shepard's *Catalog of Teratogenic Agents*

TOXICOLOGY
Casarett and Doull's *Toxicology: The Basic Science of Poisons*
Clinical Toxicology of Commercial Products
Ellenhorn's *Medical Toxicology: Diagnosis and Treatment of Human Poisoning*
Goldfrank's *Toxicologic Emergencies*
Material Safety Data Sheets (MSDS) from the USP
POISONDEX System, published by Micromedex (www.thomsonhc.com – subscription required)
TOMES System, published by Micromedex (www.thomsonhc.com – subscription required)

VETERINARY MEDICINE
Merck Veterinary Manual

the medication must be evaluated for efficacy and safety in animal and human studies. If the medication is reasonably effective and safe, the Food and Drug Administration will grant approval for the manufacturer to market the drug. In this process, the manufacturer compiles a package insert, which is a document that provides prescribing information and other data derived from premarketing studies. The package insert (i.e., product information, prescribing information, etc.) is usually the first comprehensive source of information one can obtain on a drug as it is first marketed. The package inserts provide the following information on the drug: pharmacology, pharmacokinetics, summary clinical studies, indications for use, contraindications, warnings, precautions, adverse effects, dosage and administration, overdosage, how supplied, preparation instructions, patient information, and so forth.

The pharmacy technician should know how to access the most up-to-date package insert of all drugs. The best method is to obtain a package insert from the manufacturer's Web site (e.g., www.pfizer.com). The prescribing information available from the manufacturer's Web site will be the most recently revised. Usually, one may obtain the prescribing information by simply typing "www.brandname .com" (e.g., www.zyvox.com). A package insert can also be found attached to the drug product itself at the point of dispensing. The *Physician's Desk Reference* may also be used to obtain a package insert; however, the information may not be as current as that obtained from the manufacturer's Web site or on the product package itself. Package inserts for older or generic drugs can be obtained by calling the manufacturer.

Secondary Resources

Secondary resources are indexing and abstracting services such as MEDLINE (www.pubmed.gov), International Pharmaceutical Abstracts (IPA), Iowa Drug Information Service (IDIS), EMBASE (European Medline), and Journal Watch. Secondary resources are usually available electronically and quickly link the reader to the primary literature. The pharmacy technician must undergo training in properly searching secondary resources such as MEDLINE and IPA. This training will allow the technician to perform appropriate literature searches and identify useful information. The pharmacist or drug information specialist may either train the pharmacy technician on the proper use of secondary resources or inform the pharmacy technician of available educational programs. It is important to understand that each secondary resource indexes different journals and meeting abstracts; therefore, it is often necessary to search more than one secondary resource to perform a thorough literature search. Some secondary resources can be expensive to subscribe to (e.g., IPA, IDIS) while others are free (e.g., MEDLINE).

Primary Resources

Primary resources are the original research articles, published in journals such as the *Annals of Pharmacotherapy*, *American Journal of Hospital Pharmacy*, and the *Journal of the American Medical Association*. The primary literature also includes descriptive patient case reports, observational studies (i.e., cohort, case-control, cross-sectional studies), and experimental studies (i.e., clinical trials, crossover trials).

The primary literature is the most current source of information and provides a very detailed description of a study (i.e., objective, methods, statistics, results, and conclusion). This allows the reader to make his or her own evaluation and interpretation of the study, compare it to the results of other studies, and apply the study results to patients encountered in practice. Excellent literature evaluation skills are necessary to critically evaluate each study and to be able to apply it to clinical practice. The pharmacy technician should be familiar with all components of an original research article to facilitate communication between the technician and other health care professionals. When answering a drug information request, it often requires a significant amount of time to collect pertinent primary literature and evaluate all of the primary literature on a particular topic.

The Internet

A discussion on drug information practice would not be complete without a discussion of the Internet and how it has changed the provision of drug information. Tertiary (e.g., most Web sites), secondary (e.g., MEDLINE, Internet subscriptions to computerized databases), and primary literature (i.e., electronic full-text articles) may be found on the Internet. Medication package inserts can be downloaded easily off the Internet (e.g., a package insert for metformin may be easily found at www.glucophage.com). The Internet allows for rapid and easy access to a wealth of information. It may help save space in the drug information center by allowing for electronic subscriptions. It also allows for rapid dissemination of important information to others through e-mail.

One must, however, be cautious when using the Internet for drug information. Anyone can create a Web site, and many Web sites may provide false or misleading information. Each site providing drug or medical information must be carefully evaluated for reliability and accuracy. More reliable Web sites should provide balanced information (benefits and risks of medications), author's qualifications and expertise, protection of patient confidentiality, references, the date information provided was last revised, and contact information for the site's creator. The funding sources of the Web site should be clearly stated so one can identify any possible conflicts of interest. In general, Web sites that sell products or advertise products are more likely to provide biased information. Even if a site provides all the above stated information, professional judgment and knowledge must always be used to determine whether information provided on the site is accurate and reliable. A list of reputable Web sites including governmental sites is provided in Table 17-2. Pharmacy technicians should always encourage patients to consult a pharmacist and/or a health care professional prior to following any medical advice obtained from a Web site.

Necessary Skills for the Pharmacy Technician

In order to work in a drug information practice setting, the pharmacy technician must have effective communication and listening skills, should be able to properly pronounce medical and technical terms, and should be able to communicate on a level that is appropriate to the drug information requestor. The technician must have a strong knowledge base of medical conditions, medications, resources, and strong research and technical capabilities. The technician must follow all ethical principles and always behave in a courteous, professional, and caring manner.

The pharmacy technician is also expected to stay current with advances in pharmacy practice. The technician should participate in the pharmacy or drug information center's methods for staying current (e.g., journal clubs, educational conferences, continuing education, journal circulation).

TABLE 17-2 Useful Web Sites

ADVERSE REACTION REPORTING
Food and Drug Administration MedWatch Program *(www.fda.gov/medwatch)*

DIETARY SUPPLEMENTS
Center for Food Safety and Applied Nutrition *(www.cfsan.fda.gov)*
ConsumerLab.com—subscription required for full information *(www.consumerlab.com)*
International Bibliographic Information on Dietary Supplements (IBIDS)—secondary resource *(ods.od.nih.gov/ health_information/ibids.aspx)*
National Center for Complementary and Alternative Medicine *(nccam.nih.gov)*
Natural Medicines Comprehensive Database—subscription required *(www.naturaldatabase.com)*
Office of Dietary Supplements *(ods.od.nih.gov)*
USP-verified dietary supplements *(www.usp.org/uspverified)*

HEALTH-RELATED NEWS AND UPDATES
CNN Health *(www.cnn.com/health)*
Medscape—free registration *(www.medscape.com)*
New York Times—Health *(www.nytimes.com/pages/health/index.html)*
The Pharmacist's Letter—subscription required *(www.pharmacistsletter.com)*
Reuters Health—subscription required *(www.reutershealth.com)*
Yahoo! Health News *(health.yahoo.com/news)*

INTERPRETING MEDICAL ABBREVIATIONS/ACRONYMS
Medi-Lexicon *(www.pharma-lexicon.com)*

MEDICAL DICTIONARIES
Medi-Lexicon *(www.pharma-lexicon.com)*
PubMed MeSH Database *(www.ncbi.nlm.nih.gov/sites/entrez?db=mesh)*

SELECT MEDICAL WEB SITES
American Academy of Geriatric Psychiatry *(www.aagpgpa.org)*
American Academy of Ophthalmology *(www.aao.org)*
American Academy of Pediatrics *(www.aap.org)*
American Cancer Society *(www.cancer.org)*
American College of Allergy, Asthma, Immunology (ACAAI) *(www.acaai.org)*
American College of Emergency Physicians *(www.acep.org)*
American College of Obstetricians and Gynecology *(www.acog.org)*
American College of Physicians *(www.acponline.org)*
American College of Surgeons *(www.facs.org)*
American Dental Association *(www.ada.org)*
American Diabetes Association *(www.diabetes.org)*
American Gastroenterological Association *(www.gastro.org)*
American Geriatrics Society *(www.americangeriatrics.org)*
American Heart Association *(www.americanheart.org)*
American Hospital Association *(www.aha.org)*
American Lung Association *(www.lungusa.org)*
American Medical Association *(www.ama-assn.org)*
American Medical Informatics Association *(www.amia.org)*
American Neurological Association *(www.aneuroa.org)*
American Psychiatric Association *(www.psych.org)*

(Continued)

TABLE 17-2 (Continued)

SELECT MEDICAL WEB SITES (Continued)

American Psychological Association (www.apa.org)

American Urological Association (www.auanet.org)

Association of American Medical Colleges (www.aamc.org)

Institute for Healthcare Improvement (www.ihi.org)

Joint Commission (www.jointcommission.org)

World Health Organization (WHO) (www.who.int)

MEDICATION ERROR REPORTING

Institutes for Safe Medication Practices (ISMP) (www.ismp.org)

National Coordinating Counsel for Medication Error Reporting and Prevention (NCCMERP) (www.nccmerp.org)

USP Medication Error Reporting Program (www.usp.org/hqi/patientsafety/mer/?howdoi)

PATIENT HEALTH INFORMATION WEB SITES

ASHP's Safe Medication (www.safemedication.com)

MedlinePlus (www.medlineplus.gov)

PHARMACY TECHNICIAN WEB SITES

American Association of Pharmacy Technicians (www.pharmacytechnician.com)

National Pharmacy Technician Association (NPTA) (www.pharmacytechnician.org)

Pharmacy Technician Certification Board (www.ptcb.org)

PHARMACY WEB SITES

American Association of Colleges of Pharmacy (www.aacp.org)

American College of Clinical Pharmacy (www.accp.com)

American Council on Pharmaceutical Education (www.acpe-accredit.org)

American Pharmacists Association (www.aphanet.org)

American Society of Consultant Pharmacists (www.ascp.com)

American Society of Health-System Pharmacists (www.ashp.org)

American Society for Pharmacy Law (www.aspl.org)

National Association of Boards of Pharmacy (www.napb.net)

National Association of Chain Drug Stores (www.nacds.org)

REPRODUCTION, PREGNANCY, AND LACTATION

Agency for Toxic Substances and Disease Registry (www.atsdr.cdc.gov)

Center for Evaluation of Risks to Human Reproduction (CERHR) (cerhr.niehs.nih.gov)

Center for Food Safety and Applied Nutrition (www.cfsan.fda.gov/~pregnant/pregnant.html)

Clinical Teratology Web Site (depts.washington.edu/terisweb/)

FDA Pregnancy Exposure Registries (www.fda.gov/womens/registries/)

Drugs and Lactation Database (LactMed) (toxnet.nlm.nih.gov/cgi-bin/sis/htmlgen?lact)

March of Dimes (www.marchofdimes.com)

MOTHERISK (www.motherisk.org)

National Center on Birth Defects and Developmental Disabilities (NCBDDD) (www.cdc.gov/ncbddd/)

Organization of Teratology Information Specialists (OTIS) (www.otispregnancy.org)

REPROTOX—subscription required (www.reprotox.org)

The Teratology Society (www.teratology.org)

(Continued)

TABLE 17-2   (Continued)

SECONDARY RESOURCES (INDEXING AND ABSTRACTING SERVICES)
EMBASE—subscription required *(www.embase.com)*
Google Scholar *(www.scholar.google.com)*
International Bibliographic Information on Dietary Supplements (IBIDS) *(ods.od.nih.gov/health_information/ibids.aspx)*
International Pharmaceutical Abstracts (IPA)—subscription required *(scientific.thomson.com/products/ipa/)*
Iowa Drug Information Service—subscription required *(www.uiowa.edu/~idis/)*
National Library of Medicine Gateway *(gateway.nlm.nih.gov)*
PubMed *(www.pubmed.gov)*
ToxSeek *(toxseek.nlm.nih.gov/toxseek/)*

ADDITIONAL GOVERNMENTAL WEB SITES
Agency for Healthcare Research and Quality (AHRQ) *(www.ahrq.gov)*
Center for Food Safety and Applied Nutrition (CFSCAN) *(www.cfsan.fda.gov)*
Centers for Disease Control and Prevention (CDC) *(www.cdc.gov)*
Centers for Medicare and Medicaid Services *(www.cms.hhs.gov)*
ClinicalTrials.gov *(www.clinicaltrials.gov)*
Department of Health and Human Services (DHHS) *(www.dhhs.gov)*
Directory of Health Organizations Online (DIRLINE) *(dirline.nlm.nih.gov)*
Food and Drug Administration (FDA) *(www.fda.gov)*
Household Products Database *(householdproducts.nlm.nih.gov)*
National Cancer Institute (NCI) *(www.nci.nih.gov)*
National Center for Complementary and Alternative Medicine *(nccam.nih.gov)*
National Guidelines Clearinghouse *(www.guidelines.gov)*
The National Institute for Occupational Safety and Health (NIOSH) *(www.cdc.gov/niosh/)*
National Institutes of Health (NIH) *(www.nih.gov)*
National Library of Medicine (NLM) *(www.nlm.nih.gov)*
Occupational Safety and Health Administration (OSHA)> *(www.osha.gov)*
Surgeon General Reports *(www.surgeongeneral.gov/library/reports.htm)*
United States Pharmacopoeia (USP) *(www.usp.org)*

WEB SITE EVALUATION TOOL
Health on the Net Foundation (HON) *(www.hon.ch)*

Summary

With the increasing complexity of information management and expanding responsibilities of the pharmacist or drug information specialist, pharmacy technicians are essential in assisting with the daily functions of a community pharmacy, hospital pharmacy, or drug information center. Regardless of the practice setting in which a pharmacy technician works, the efficient and correct use of drug information is crucial in the prevention of medication errors and will help the technician remain current with the profession.

TEST YOUR KNOWLEDGE

Multiple Choice

1. Place the following steps of the systematic approach to answering a drug information question in the order in which they should be performed.
   i. Develop a search strategy and conduct search.
   ii. Secure the demographics of the requestor.
   iii. Document and conduct follow-up.
   iv. Obtain background information.
   v. Formulate and provide a response.
   vi. Perform evaluation, analysis, and synthesis of information.
   vii. Determine and categorize the ultimate question.
      a. ii, iv, vii, i, vi, v, iii
      b. ii, iv, vii, vi, i, v, iii
      c. ii, iv, vi, vii, v, i, iii
      d. ii, vii, iv, i, vi, v, iii

2. Although all the steps of the systematic approach are important, which of the following steps is the most important?
   a. Secure the demographics of the requestor.
   b. Obtain background information.
   c. Formulate and provide a response.
   d. Perform evaluation, analysis, and synthesis of information.

3. Which of the following resources provides you with a general overview of a topic?
   a. tertiary resources
   b. secondary resources
   c. primary resources
   d. none of the above

4. Which of the following resources suffers the most from a long lag time (i.e., is somewhat outdated by the time it is published)?
   a. tertiary resources
   b. secondary resources
   c. primary resources
   d. none of the above

5. Which of the following statements regarding the use of the Internet for drug information are true?
   i. Web sites that sell or advertise products are more likely to provide biased or misleading information.
   ii. Governmental Web sites are reputable and can be used for drug information with confidence.
   iii. Patients should be encouraged to follow any medical advice obtained from a Web site without the need to consult with a health care professional.
   iv. The Internet allows for rapid and easy access to a wealth of information and allows for rapid dissemination of information through e-mail.
   v. You may find tertiary, secondary, and primary resources on the Internet.

a. i, ii, iii, iv, v
b. ii, iii
c. i, ii, iv, v
d. iii, v

6. More reputable Web sites should
    a. provide balanced information.
    b. provide references.
    c. provide the author's qualifications and expertise.
    d. all of the above.

7. A useful tertiary resource to answer a drug information question on the safety of a certain medication during pregnancy is
    a. *American Drug Index.*
    b. *Index Nominum.*
    c. *Ident-A-Drug.*
    d. Brigg's *Drugs in Pregnancy and Lactation.*

8. A useful tertiary resource to identify a medication is
    a. *Index Nominum.*
    b. *Ident-A-Drug.*
    c. Brigg's *Drugs in Pregnancy and Lactation.*
    d. *Geriatric Dosage Handbook.*

9. Which of the following is/are responsibilities of the pharmacy technician working at a drug information center?
    a. maintain a filing system
    b. maintain inventory of all informational resources held by the center
    c. perform literature searches
    d. all of the above

10. Which of the following is/are necessary skills a pharmacy technician must possess to work effectively in a drug information center?
    a. effective verbal and written communication skills
    b. correct pronunciation of medical terms
    c. ethical and professional behavior
    d. all of the above

Fill In The Blank

1. Package inserts, textbooks, and computer databases are examples of _____ resources.

2. Indexing and abstracting services provide _____ resources.

3. Original research articles published in journals are examples of _____ .

4. Drug information can be grouped into two categories: _____ information and _____ information.

References

American Society of Health-System Pharmacists. (1996). ASHP guidelines on the provision of medication information by pharmacists. *American Journal of Hospital Pharmacy*, 53, 1843–1845.

Koumis, T., Cicero, L. A., Nathan, J. P., & Rosenberg, J. M. (2004). Directory of pharmacist-operated drug information centers in the United States—2003. *American Journal of Health-System Pharmacy*, 61, 2033–2042.

Malone, P. M., Wilkinson Mosdell, K., Kier, K. L., & Stanovich, J. E. (2001). *Drug information: A guide for pharmacists* (2nd ed.). New York: McGraw-Hill.

Rosenberg, J. M., Koumis, T., Nathan, J. P., Cicero, L. A., & McGuire, H. (2004). Current status of pharmacist-operated drug information centers in the United States. *American Journal of Health-System Pharmacy*, 61, 2023–2032.

Watanabe, A. S., & Conner, C. S. (1978). *Principles of drug information services: A syllabus of systematic concepts*. Hamilton, IL: Drug Intelligence Publications, Inc.

Watanabe, A. S., McGart, G., Shimomura, S., & Kayser, S. (1975). Systematic approach to drug information requests. *American Journal of Hospital Pharmacy*, 32(12), 1282–1285.

18

Drug Distribution Systems

Competencies

Upon completion of this chapter, the reader should be able to

1. Outline the responsibility of the pharmacist and the current and possible future role of the pharmacy technician in the various medication distribution functions.

2. Differentiate among the four major distribution systems.

3. Describe the purpose, functions, and advantages of the unit-dose drug distribution system.

4. Distinguish the main difference between a decentralized and a centralized drug distribution system.

5. Explain why the pharmacist must review a direct physician's order entry for a medication.

6. Briefly explain the methods by which a physician's original orders are transmitted to the pharmacy.

7. List the drug distribution activities that can be generated through computer technology.

8. Describe various ways in which the pharmacy technician is directly involved in the computerization process.

9. List the checkpoints required by the pharmacist and by the pharmacy technician when a physician's order is received in the pharmacy.

Key Terms

centralized dispensing system
decentralized dispensing system
dumbwaiters
floor stock system
individual prescription system
medical information system (MIS)
pneumatic tube system
robotics
unit-dose distribution system

Introduction

Drug control, monitoring utilization, and assisting in the distribution of medications to patients are among the pharmacist's most important contributions to health care. With the advent of new regulations and the constantly changing health care environment, methods of distributing and controlling drugs must undergo continuous reevaluation and review. Only then can effective and efficient systems that meet the changing requirements be ensured. Advancing technology permits the pharmacist to move from the traditional product-focused dispensing to that of a patient advocate and provider of clinical services. As the pharmacist assumes a larger role in improved therapeutic outcomes in disease management, greater efficiency and economy in disease therapy will be realized.

The technician's role in the area of dispensing and drug distribution is to assist the pharmacist. Technicians are an integral and important component of the health care team. However, the legal responsibility for dispensing still remains with the pharmacist. In order to free up time for pharmacists to be more actively involved in clinical functions, some states are looking at the "tech-check-tech" proposals for the more routine distribution functions that consume pharmacist's time. Preliminary studies have shown that technicians checking other technicians in the area of cart fill, for example, scored better than the traditional pharmacist check. This can be rationalized that a technician is interrupted less and thereby focuses totally on the job at hand. More studies are being conducted, with the results being evaluated by the individual state boards of pharmacy, for possible implementation.

After reviewing this chapter, the student should have a good understanding of various drug distribution systems. The technician should be able to distinguish between the different types of distribution systems and clearly define the technician's role in drug distribution. This will allow the technician to actively participate in system planning and development.

Drug Distribution Systems

In most hospital settings, the Pharmacy and Therapeutic Committee is responsible for the development of broad policies and procedures that provide for the proper distribution of medications and pharmaceutical aids to the nursing staff for administration to patients. The currently employed drug distributions are variations of four concepts: floor stock, patient prescriptions, combined floor stock and patient prescription, and unit-dose. Additional components of the drug distribution system are covered in other chapters of this manual and include but are not limited to intravenous admixtures, controlled drug distribution, and interdepartmental requisitions.

floor stock system medications are provided to the nursing unit for administration to the patient by the nurse, who is responsible for preparation and administration.

Floor Stock System

In the **floor stock system** of distribution, all medications are stocked on the nursing unit, with the possible exception of some rarely used or very expensive medications. Medications that require an expanded level of professional supervision and control, such as antineoplastic agents and antibiotics, may also be excluded from floor stock supplies. The nurse is totally responsible for all aspects of preparation and administration of medications. This is *not* the preferred drug distribution method for hospitals and long-term care facilities and should be strongly discouraged because of several inherent disadvantages:

- An increased potential for medication errors exists because a pharmacist does not review medication orders. Thus a nurse may select the wrong medication to administer from a vast array of drugs and dosage forms.
- Economic loss may occur because of misappropriation or diversion by hospital personnel or lost medication charges. Expired, contaminated, and deteriorated drugs remaining on the unit may also mean loss and possible patient harm if administered from the floor stock supply.
- Increased drug inventory is necessary because of multiple inventories on each nursing unit. Thus, drug inventory control is poor.
- Storage and control problems occur because of limited storage facilities on nursing units.

Individual Prescription System

individual prescription system a multiple-day supply of each medication is dispensed for the patient upon receipt of prescriptions or medication orders.

In the **individual prescription system**, a multiple-day supply of each medication is dispensed for the patient upon receipt of prescriptions or medication orders. The nurse transcribes and prepares individual prescriptions or an order from the physician's original written order and forwards the request to the pharmacy for filling. Commonly, a three- to five-day supply is provided by the pharmacy. When the original supply is exhausted, the nurse prepares another request, and the whole process is repeated. An enormous amount of time and manpower is required. Maintenance of drug containers by the nursing staff in an organized, easily-accessible method is wasteful of nursing time. The pharmacy is usually responsible for charges and credits, which are individually entered into the patient's account or forwarded to the business office for processing. Altogether, much time is required of all participants. Although this system is an improvement over the floor stock system, it is not an efficient or practical method of drug distribution. It is also not a preferred drug distribution method for hospitals or long-term care facilities.

Combined Floor Stock and Patient Prescription System

When the previous two systems are combined, the primary method of dispensing medications is the individual prescription order, supplemented with a limited number of floor stock items. The use of the combined systems hopefully increases the benefits of both systems. The floor stock items are generally over-the-counter medications (e.g., aspirin, acetaminophen, laxatives, and vitamins) and selected controlled drug medications. Although this combined system is far superior to the previous individual systems discussed, it also exhibits the disadvantages of both methods.

Unit-Dose Drug Distribution System

unit-dose distribution system the medication is distributed in single dose or unit-dose form from the pharmacy for use by the individual administering the drug.

The **unit-dose distribution system** represents a significant refinement of the individual prescription order system and is considered the safest, most economical method of distributing drugs in health care institutions. It is considered to be a hospital system, not simply a pharmacy system, because it involves many departments and disciplines in its planning, development, and operation.

The unit-dose system has been preferred to the floor stock or individual prescription systems of drug distribution by the federal government and nonfederal

FIGURE 18-1

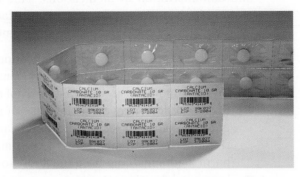

FIGURE 18-1 Examples of unit-dose packaging (Courtesy of AutoMed Technologies, Inc.).

regulatory agencies, including the Joint Commission, the Institute for Safe Medication Practices (ISMP), the Centers for Medicare and Medicaid Services (CMS), and state and local regulatory agencies. It has been proven to be the most effective drug distribution system available today. Following are the advantages of this type of system over antiquated approaches:

- Reduction in medication errors.
- Improved drug control.
- Decrease in the overall cost of medication distribution.
- More precise medication billing.
- Reduction of medication credits.
- Reduced drug inventories throughout the institution.

Numerous variations of the unit-dose system have been implemented throughout the world but all share several common, basic features. In all of the systems, the nurse who administers the medications receives unit-dose packages from the pharmacy in a ready-to-use form that requires no additional manipulation, measurement, or preparation.

A large- or small-volume injection may be considered a unit dose, but it is not normally distributed in the same manner. Virtually all other medications can be dispensed as a unit dose, which is defined as containing the particular dose of the drug ordered for the patient. For example, a unit-dose liquid may contain from a fraction of a milliliter to 60 or more milliliters, but it is the exact amount ordered by the physician. A unit dose of a solid oral medication (tablets, capsules) may contain a fraction of one or more of the particular drugs, but it is the amount to be administered. The term *single-dose package* contains one discrete form, such as one tablet, five milliliters of a liquid, or a prefilled syringe containing a standard strength per milliliter (Figure 18-1). A single-unit package may be a unit-dose package if it contains the prescribed dose. In the event that the dose prescribed and the dose sent vary, an auxiliary label "Note Dosage Strength" should be applied to the package to alert the nursing staff of the difference.

> **centralized dispensing system** a system of distribution in which all functions, processing, preparation, and distribution occur in a main area (e.g., the main pharmacy).

Centralized Dispensing

In **centralized dispensing systems**, all activities in the preparation and distribution of medications take place within the main pharmacy area. Unit-dose medications are made available on the nursing floor one or more times daily, depending on the staff available and the logistics of moving supplies to and from the pharmacy and nursing locations. Patients' drugs are generally dispensed in amounts needed for the next 24 hours. In some long-term care institutions, a 48-hour cart fill is deemed appropriate. Acute care facilities often have multiple pharmacy deliveries throughout the day to insure the patients' needs are being met. Some drugs that require special handling (e.g., antineoplastics, very expensive medications, medications with a very short stability, or items that are too large or unsafe to ship via pneumatic tube) must be carried by hand to the specific nursing unit at the time of administration.

The greatest number of technicians is usually involved in the unit-dose distribution. The technician assists in preparing all medication doses and fills the acabinets, carts, or cassettes. The technician utilizes the patient medication profile, which has been generated by either a manual or computerized system, to prepare and deliver the medications to the patient care areas.

A pharmacist must check all medications before they are distributed to the patient care area. During this process, the pharmacist ensures that the correct drug and the correct number of doses have been prepared. By visually inspecting the total drug supply for each patient, the pharmacist has another opportunity to confirm the absence of drug-drug interactions. The pharmacist is also able to assess the completeness of labeling, look for outdated supplies, and lastly, take full responsibility for the accuracy of the filling and distributing process.

This operation has come under scrutiny in recent years as a possible area where highly-trained technicians would be allowed to check other technician's work. This "Tech-Check-Tech" or "T-C-T" is a two-pronged study that has looked at the quality of one technician checking another technician's cart fill, in conjunction with the drug interventions that are initiated during the time the pharmacist would normally be checking the technician. The data was so overwhelming that California became the first state to pass legislation allowing T-C-T. As the results of this major change in pharmacy unfold, many more states will likely pass similar legislation.

Decentralized Dispensing

decentralized dispensing system a system of distribution in which all functions (processing, preparation, and distribution) occur on or near the nursing unit (e.g., satellite pharmacy).

In a **decentralized dispensing system**, unlike a centralized system with a main pharmacy, the doses are prepared in a satellite pharmacy located in or near the nursing unit. The satellite may serve several nursing units or even one or more floors. Generally, the centralized pharmacy allows for somewhat greater management efficiency and control; the decentralized pharmacy allows closer pharmacist-physician-nurse-patient relationships. In addition, decentralization provides pharmacy services to the nursing unit quicker.

Physician's Order Entry Process

Medications are dispensed only on the written order of a licensed physician or other licensed prescriber such as a physician's assistant, nurse practitioner, or dentist. The prescriber must also be certified by the institution as qualified and having privileges in the institution. Studies have shown the value of a physician order entry system and enhancements are being made to existing hospital information systems so that this may be accomplished. Some of the beneficial effects of a computerized physician order entry (CPOE) in the reduction of medical errors are as follows:

- Elimination of illegible errors.
- Complete and accurate information.
- Automatic dose calculation.
- Clinical decision support at the point of care.

Applications may include the following:

- Formulary status of drug.
- Cost considerations.
- Drug-drug interactions.
- Allergy checking.
- Standardizing ordering, supported by evidence-based medicine.

These processes and systems help ensure the equitable delivery of quality care, minimize human error, improve medication management, facilitate reporting and decision-making, and improve resource utilization. All of these, while offering timely access to information and supporting compliance management and quality assurance initiatives, have the final goal of enhanced positive patient care and associated positive outcomes of therapy.

Transmittal of Orders to Pharmacy

Multiple methods are presently in use for obtaining the physician's order. The Joint Commission and most state boards of pharmacy require that the pharmacy receive the physician's original prescription—or a copy of the original prescription—when filling medication orders. A direct copy of the order is most frequently utilized. This procedure eliminates transcription errors, which are a frequent source of medication errors. It is the pharmacist's responsibility to review, interpret, and evaluate the medication order.

Traditionally, the nurse was given the responsibility of transcribing the doctor's orders as written in the patient's chart onto a pharmacy order form. However, the more people involved in reviewing, evaluating, and transcribing an order, the greater potential for error. By receiving a direct copy of the physician's original order, the pharmacist can review, clarify, and interpret the order, which is the pharmacist's legal and ethical responsibility. This process is now almost universally accomplished by the use of no carbon required (NCR) physician order forms. A direct copy of the original order is available and can easily be transmitted to the pharmacy for immediate processing. The orders may be hand carried to the pharmacy, sent via a pneumatic tube system, or by electronic facsimile (fax).

Electromechanical Systems

Several electronic methods are utilized to transmit orders from the nursing unit to the pharmacy. Electrostatic copying machines (photocopiers) and facsimile transmitting equipment (fax machines) can be used to copy or transmit orders. Evolution in computer/digital technology has reduced paperwork by being able to transmit orders electronically from one computer directly to another via scanners. Scanner technology has made the pharmacist's job easier, since an order may be easily enlarged for clarity, or easily stored for retrieval in the future for reference. A physician is able to chart the patient's progress and order new medications and then have them transmitted instantly to the pharmacy for review and input. The pharmacist utilizes the patient's profile to evaluate any potential problems before a new order is filled. Like any mechanical equipment, provisions must be made for backup systems in the event of mechanical failure.

Computerization

medical information system (MIS) state-of-the-art clinical information that may include anything from drug information applications to video conferencing between other hospitals.

Arguably, the most significant development that has changed drug distribution systems is the utilization of computer technology. A **medical information system (MIS)** has been developed to varying degrees based on the diverse needs of the pharmacy and other departments. There are therefore multitudes of pharmacy-specific computer systems available today. Different hardware items, software programs, and the need to interface with other hospital departments must be considered in the selection of any pharmacy support system.

Computerization offers the pharmacist a systematized method of order entry, patient profile development, label production, fill lists, and reports. It also provides clinical cross-checking mechanisms for allergy and sensitivity detection, dosage verification, drug interaction, and food-drug interactions.

Currently, numerous programs providing comprehensive drug information can be easily accessed during order entry. These allow the pharmacist to confirm the accuracy of drug use and dosage while checking for side effects, contraindications, laboratory test interferences, and so forth. This information may be printed immediately to assist in the education of the pharmacy staff, physicians, or other professionals within the institution.

An efficient computerized order entry system can generate patient profiles for a pharmacist, nurse, or physician to utilize. The profile includes all information necessary for adequately supervising appropriate drug usage within the institution. This information includes *complete* patient demographics, all scheduled and unscheduled (e.g., prn [as needed]) drugs, frequency, and appropriate cautionary statements. The profile is used to generate the medication administration record (MAR) for the nurse. This tool allows the nurse to administer the drug at exactly the prescribed time for which it was intended. The MAR is essential for the accurate administration of medication to patients. A daily check of the MAR by nursing or pharmacy staff is essential and will help validate all changes on the patient's profile within the past 24 hours. Therefore, it is essential to ensure that the MAR is up-to-date. The goal of a paperless online MAR (e-MAR), along with an automated patient profile, is to have ready access for the review of a pharmacist, nurse, or physician.

Other applications that can be derived from the computerized profile include dispensing orders or fill lists, from which the technician fills patients' cassettes or drug drawers for the next 24 hours. If the facility has invested in automated dispensing cabinets (ADCs), lists of drugs needing to be replaced can be generated. This list allows the technician to fill the cabinet, so the appropriate drug and strength are available for the nurse to procure as needed.

The computerized profile should also be capable of transferring charges to the patient's account by a direct interface with the institution's financial system. Credits for drugs not used are also applied in the same manner.

Inventory control is managed by the computerized system by deleting items dispensed and their cost. Unused drugs returned to the pharmacy are credited to the inventory and to the patient simultaneously. Financial status is enhanced, and the pharmacy administration is provided with valuable reports, which may be of importance to upper-level management.

The technician becomes directly involved in all aspects of computerization in most institutions. Order entry may be performed conditionally by the technician. The pharmacist validates the technician's entry before the order is activated. Other areas in which the technician's computer prowess is utilized include floor stock entry, special patient charges and credits, labeling, report generation, and end-of-day functions. In other words, the areas of computerization and the technician's involvement are limitless.

Receiving the Medication Order

The pharmacist and the technician have differing roles when it comes to receiving the medication order. The responsibilities, while clearly defined presently, are being evaluated to determine if some of the routine functions that pharmacists have performed in the past can be shifted to specially trained technicians.

The Pharmacist's Role

It is the legal and ethical responsibility of the pharmacist to review and interpret every medication order prior to dispensing the medication. With the use of computerized patient profile, the pharmacist is able to review the patient's complete medication regimen.

The patient profile

A patient profile is a complete listing of the patient's medications. For those institutions that do not utilize computers, the profile is designed to list all medications, strengths, directions, and patient data, in addition to quantities and the date dispensed. Depending on the institution, some profiles contain clinical data such as laboratory results, antimicrobial culture results, and sensitivity reports. Previously used but discontinued drugs may also be visible.

When the unit-dose distribution system is employed, a profile must be maintained so that the pharmacist may schedule—and the technician may prepare and distribute—individual medication doses according to the appropriate dosing schedule. The drug profile system enables the pharmacist to identify potential drug interactions, dosage changes, drug duplications, overlapping therapy, and any drug that is contraindicated because of allergy or sensitivity. A complete patient profile should include but not be limited to the following information:

- Patient's full name, age, weight, sex, hospital identification number, bed location, and admitting physician's name.
- Provisional diagnosis, secondary diagnosis, and confirmed diagnosis, if available.
- Allergies (e.g., food, drug, latex), sensitivities, and idiosyncrasies.
- Drug history from patient interview.
- Names of medications dispensed, dosage, directions for use, quantity dispensed, date, and initials of pharmacist.
- IV therapy (e.g., large- and small-volume intravenous solutions) with or without additives, hyperalimentation fluids, chemotherapy, and so forth.

- Laboratory data, if known (e.g., electrolytes, creatinine, cultures, sensitivities).
- Diet (e.g., low-sodium diet).
- Selected diagnostic data related to coronary disease, diabetes, hypertension, and the like.

By receiving a copy of the complete physician's order, the pharmacist is able to seek information concerning laboratory test results, nursing procedures, and dietary intake that might have been ordered. The pharmacist can then monitor possible drug-laboratory interactions, food-drug interactions, and other aspects of the patient's therapeutic program.

The pharmacist is also responsible for checking the technician's work in all aspects of the dispensing procedure, including but not limited to the following:

- Verify the order entry on the patient's profile to ensure that transcription or entry of the physician's order is correct.
- Verify drug selection to be certain that the proper medication was set up for dispensing.
- Check the drug label and contents to make sure that the finished product is complete, accurate, and ready for use.
- Check unit-dose cassettes against the profile-generated fill list to verify that the drugs dispensed are correct and properly labeled. This process allows the pharmacist to conduct a final check of all unit-dose drugs that the patient will be administered. This process is currently being studied as a possible area that highly trained technicians can oversee other technicians, thereby freeing up additional time for the pharmacist to engage in more clinical activities.
- The pharmacist will also take into consideration the patient's medical history, if available. (The policy in some hospitals is to have a pharmacist interview patients upon admission to obtain a drug history to assist in evaluating the patient's drug therapy.)

The Technician's Role

The technician who receives a written prescription order is responsible to prepare the medication for dispensing. When the physician's order copy is received in the pharmacy, the technician must confirm that all necessary information pertaining to the patient's identification is available in the computer or on the patient profile (e.g., patient name, age, room number or location, hospital identification number, patient weight, allergies and sensitivities, the name of the physician). If a nurse has received a verbal or telephone order, the nurse's name should follow the name of the prescribing physician.

If all necessary information is present, the technician will enter the order into the computerized profile or transcribe it to a hand-generated profile if that system is in use (Figure 18-2). The pharmacist is responsible to review the order and the technician's order entry to validate its completeness and accuracy. The responsibility of allowing a technician to perform order entry functions rests with the particular facility to have policies and procedures written that set the criteria for technicians to serve in this capacity. The pharmacist must have the validation and final check of the entry.

Following order entry and validation, the technician prepares the drug for dispensing. The proper medication is selected from the appropriate storage site in either unit-dose or bulk form. The technician prepares the label and counts or pours the designated quantity of the drug. Once the pharmacist has checked the

FIGURE 18-2

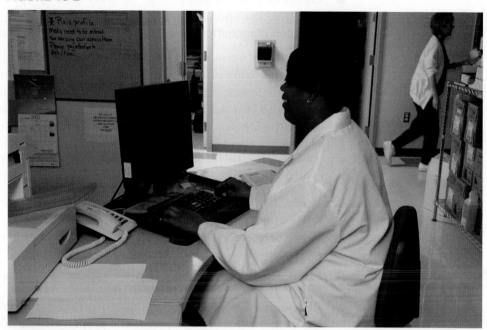

FIGURE 18-2 The pharmacy technician may be responsible for creating and maintaining the patient profile.

medication, a positive, proactive practice would be to deliver the checked medications to the nurse taking care of that patient.

Answering the telephone is another important function of the technician. The technician screens the phone calls and refers callers to the appropriate individuals. All questions of a clinical or drug-action nature should be directed to the supervising pharmacist for his or her professional judgment.

Compounding procedures

Qualified technicians may be allowed to conduct less critical compounding and manufacturing procedures under the pharmacist's direction and supervision. If two or more drugs are mixed together or prepackaged, it may be considered "compounding." If more than a single dose of a compounded product is prepared for future dispensing, it is known as "manufacturing" and requires the use of a manufacturing worksheet on which all components are identified by name, manufacturer, lot number, and quantitative amounts.

Compounding directions are written or printed. A new lot number is assigned from a master control record. An expiration date is applied and should, where possible, be based on published stability information. Packaging information is also documented. The pharmacist must check all weights, measures, processes, and the completed product for uniformity and accuracy. The names of the technician and supervising pharmacist are recorded on the worksheet. After the procedure is completed and checked, the technician performs all necessary maintenance, housekeeping, and recordkeeping duties.

Labeling and dispensing medications

The technician, in most cases, will be responsible for labeling medications. Labels may be computer-generated, typed, or machine-printed. Handwritten labels with pen, pencil, or marker are absolutely prohibited. One label should never be superimposed over a previous label. The label should be clear, legible, and free from erasures and strikeovers. It should be firmly affixed to the container. The pharmacist confirms the original physician's order with the drug and label prior to dispensing.

Patients frequently judge the efficacy of a drug by the appearance of the label attached to the container. A neat label may signify to the patient that the drug is effective and will be beneficial. A sloppily printed label would indicate lack of concern by the pharmacy and its staff. The patient (as well as nursing and medical staffs) may interpret this indifference as a lack of effectiveness of the drug or lack of concern for the patient's well being. Careful attention to the label indicates that careful attention has been given to preparing the medication as well.

With the exception of unit-dose or single-use products, the label should bear the name, address, and the telephone number of the institution or pharmacy. Medications should never be relabeled by nursing personnel or anyone other than personnel supervised by a pharmacist.

Here are other points to consider in labeling:

- The metric system, rather than the apothecary system, should be utilized (e.g., 65 milligrams rather than 1 grain).
- When dispensing medications, the technician should be aware of any needed auxiliary labels, which should be attached to the container (Figure 18-3). These may include, but are not limited to the following:
  - "For the Eye"
  - "Keep in the Refrigerator"
  - "Shake Well Before Use"
  - "Swallow Whole: Do Not Crush, Break, or Chew"
  - "For the Ear"
  - "Poison: Not for Internal Use"
  - "Take with a Full Glass of Water"
- A multitude of auxiliary labels are available, and every pharmacy should have a representative supply on hand to assist patients in understanding the appropriate use of the medication.

FIGURE 18-3

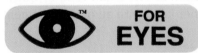 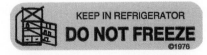 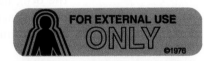

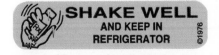 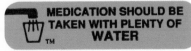 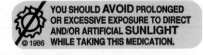

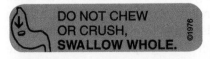 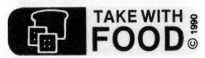 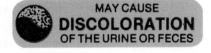

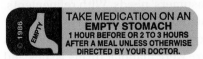 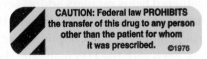

FIGURE 18-3 Examples of auxiliary labels.

- When labeling a compounded prescription for inpatient use, the name and amount or percentage of each active ingredient should be indicated on the label. Prescriptions for outpatients should indicate the name of each therapeutically active ingredient.

- In the event the medication being labeled requires further dilution or reconstitution, the label should provide the appropriate directions. (*Note:* Effective unit-dose distribution systems should not require the nurse to conduct these operations; only in cases of extremely limited stability should this be allowed.)

- Expiration dates should always appear on both unit-dose and prescription labels. Little scientific information is available to assist the pharmacy in determining how long the effectiveness of a medication can be ensured once it is removed from the manufacturer's original container. Many institutions will apply a 12-month expiration date, unless the manufacturer's date precedes the usual one-year date. In *no* case should the expiration date exceed that of the original container. Special circumstances will require that a specific expiration date be assigned. For example, many antibiotics for oral suspension when reconstituted are stable for no longer than 7 to 14 days. Packaging materials, storage conditions, light conditions, and other factors must be considered in assigning an appropriate expiration date. The primary or a secondary label should indicate the following: "Expiration Date: _____" or "Use Before _____."

- Parenteral medications may require special labeling in that the route of administration should be indicated (e.g., "For IM Use Only" or "Not for IV Use").

- Labels for large- and small-volume intravenous solutions should be placed on the container to allow visual inspection of the solution, and they should not cover the original solution (carrier) labeling. Remember to place the label so that it is readable in the hanging position of the container.

- If the medication is an oncology or chemotherapeutic medication, an auxiliary label must be attached indicating "Special Handling—Chemo Hazard—Dispose of Properly." This label should be applied to all forms of chemotherapeutic drugs, whether they are oral, topical, or injectable.

Those containers that present difficulty in labeling, such as small tubes or bottles, must be labeled with a minimum of the patient's name and location. If possible, the drug name and strength should also be included. The small tube or bottle can be placed in a larger container bearing another label with all of the pertinent information.

Bar Code Applications

The use of bar code technology began with the general retail industry. The retail applications, which have been widespread for many years, are mainly for pricing and inventory control. Preferred customer cards issued by some retailers are also used for customer identification and to collect demographic information. The information gathered helps retailers address consumers' needs. With refinements, these applications are being used to enhance the health care industry.

An FDA rule change in 2003 required bar coded labels on all human drugs and biologicals. Even with the FDA mandate, there were manufacturing issues and delays, along with shifts in product availability that slowed down the process.

Such delays should not preclude health systems from adopting bar code-enabled point-of-care systems to achieve gains in patient safety. Bar code technology is an enhancement from the traditional keyboard data entry by a technician. The information embedded in the bar code will help promote an increased level of patient and medication safety. Verification of the right patient, right drug, right dose, right route, and right time will diminish mistakes. The health system must first establish a reliable process and procedure for identifying the correct patient and the identification of the caregiver. Then every medication *must* have a unique bar code identifier to ensure the remaining Five Rights of Medication Administration are met.

When medications are not available from a manufacturer in an appropriate unit dose, other means of applying a suitable bar code must be applied. This is most often accomplished by the use of unit-dosing packaging equipment (either manual or automated) that produces a readable bar code. It is imperative that pharmacies evaluating unit-dose packaging systems ensure that the bar codes produced will, in fact, be compatible with existing systems already in use throughout the health care system. Overwrapping with a manual bar code and even outsourcing some medications to be bar coded in order to have every drug packaged with a readable and suitable bar code is an option for every facility that desires this technology. This must be addressed prior to the implementation of an electronic point-of-care system. The use of these point-of-care systems with their reliable patient and caregiver identification and medication descriptions within a health care system can substantially increase the safe use of medications. This is the ultimate goal for all health care professionals.

Medication Delivery Systems

There are a variety of medication delivery systems as well as equipment used in the medication delivery process. A brief overview of these systems and equipment follows.

Transportation Courier

Some institutions have a centralized transportation courier system that delivers and transports medications, laboratory specimens, and supplies. In other hospitals and institutions, pharmacy technicians transport medications by providing order pickup and delivery. In a unit-dose exchange system, a technician uses a mobile cart to deliver medications in cassettes to the patient care area. Technicians will exchange full cassettes for those used during the previous 24-hour period and return the used cassettes to the pharmacy for crediting unused medications and refilling.

Equipment

pneumatic tube system a method of sending medication orders through the hospital by placing it in a "tube" and sending it to a dispatcher, who then forwards it to the specific location.

Various types of delivery equipment have been utilized to transport medications. The **pneumatic tube system** utilizes carrier cartridges that are sent from the pharmacy department to the terminal at the designated patient care area (Figure 18-4). This system is similar to what banks use to handle drive-through transactions, by creating a vacuum to pull the carrier to its destination. All departments may be served, depending on the location and number of terminals. In the event of mechanical problems, a backup system must be available to ensure rapid transfer of needed medications to the area or patient. Delays in drug delivery have been a major source of irritation for nurses and may result in medication errors when the delivery time is excessive. A *significant drawback* to this system is the limitation of sending fluids because of weight and/or breakage.

Dumbwaiters or elevators can also be used to transport medications. Unfortunately, these move in only a vertical direction. Personnel must then move the materials from the elevator's destination to the patient care area. Fortunately, more efficient methods are replacing these antiquated means of drug transportation. Elevators and dumbwaiters are also subject to mechanical failures and may impose the need for technicians to use stairways to deliver medications to the nursing staff.

Robotics are utilized in some institutions. These mobile, computerized mechanical devices are programmed to move throughout the facility and deliver medications. They are able to detect and move around obstacles. The robot can call elevators in order to deliver medications to all floors of the hospital. Other hospitals have found small, track-mounted carts that move to and from patient care areas to be useful. The big advantage to this type of transport is that it can handle bigger and heavier loads than virtually any other system.

It must be remembered that all mechanical systems are subject to failures, and provisions must be made for alternate delivery methods when breakdowns occur. Drug security and control during transfer is a major concern that must always be considered in the selection and use of any transportation method. Pilferage, loss, and waste may create significant legal and financial problems.

dumbwaiter an in-house elevator used to transport medications and supplies.

robotics technology based on a mechanical device, programmed by remote control, to accomplish manual activities, such as picking medications according to a patient's computerized profile.

FIGURE 18-4

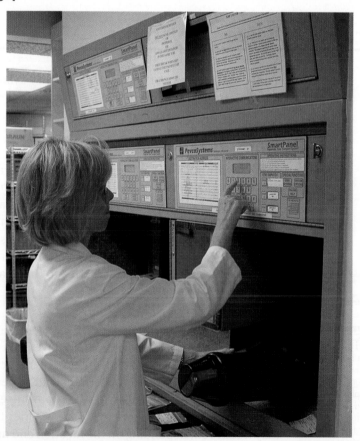

FIGURE 18-4 Pneumatic tube system.

Unit-Dose Picking Area

The area in the pharmacy where unit-dose carts are filled usually consists of slanted shelves on which plastic or cardboard bins are arranged to permit easy access by the technician's hands to select the doses needed (Figure 18-5). Bins are labeled in large letters showing the drug name; if possible, both the generic and brand name are posted, as well as strength. Circular shelves permitting multiple technicians to work with minimum movement are most efficient. Shelves should be within easy reach and should require minimal stooping or stretching. Adequate lighting is essential, along with rubber mats on the floor to reduce the strain and fatigue of standing too long in one place.

One or more computer terminals and printers need to be located in the picking area to permit technicians to generate fill lists, post charges and issue credits, and review patient profiles. Sufficient space should be available outside the immediate picking area for storage of the transfer carts. This will allow the pharmacist to conduct the checking process with little distraction. A telephone is essential, and a small compounding area and packaging area with a sink and running water should be immediately adjacent to the picking area.

The number and variety of drug bins in the picking area are never stagnant. Change is constant, and it is incumbent upon the technicians to ensure that the most frequently needed drugs are the most readily retrievable. Infrequently used items should be relegated to the general stock area. Return of stock to drug bins when patients are discharged or the drug is discontinued is a major source of

FIGURE 18-5

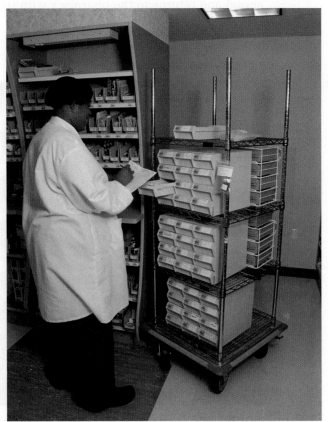

FIGURE 18-5 Unit-dose picking area.

error. Drugs in opened containers are never reissued. Unopened, expired drugs are segregated for return to the manufacturer. Unit-dose packages may be dropped in the wrong bin and, if the technician becomes complacent and does not read the label carefully, the wrong drug or dose may be used in another cart fill operation. The area should be kept free of clutter and trash. Maintaining a clean and orderly picking area is absolutely necessary for optimum efficiency. Food or beverages should never be consumed in the picking area.

Medication Dispensing Units

Medication dispensing units or carts are available in many different configurations. They are designed to be wheeled from the nursing station to the patient's bedside, where the medication is administered directly to the patient.

Single-sided or double-sided carts may contain as many as 60 patient-identified drawers that contain those medications needed for each patient. The drawers may vary in length, width, and depth to accommodate the different needs of specific patient care areas.

Newer carts may also have a computer terminal attached, which enables the nurse to document the administration of each drug removed from the patient's drawer. This information may then be transmitted to the institution's mainframe for charging purposes, inventory control, and to update the patient's profile.

Individual patient bins or drawers are stored in portable cassettes. Each cassette may hold up to 30 drawers. The pharmacy technician uses a mobile cart to transport filled cassettes to the nursing station, unlocks the medication cart, and removes the cassette holding the empty drawers from the previous day's delivery (Figure 18-6). The technician then inserts a filled cassette for the next 24-hour period and returns to the pharmacy with the empty drawers to repeat the filling process.

FIGURE 18-6

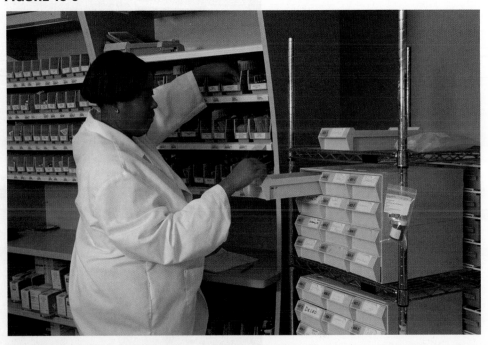

FIGURE 18-6 Delivering medications to fill the medication cart may be performed by the pharmacy technician.

Proper maintenance of patient bins is an important responsibility of the technician. Each drawer or bin must be properly labeled with a computer-generated, typed, or machine-printed label showing the patient's name, room number, and physician's name. Due to patient confidentiality, care must be taken to prevent a patient's identity from being observed during the transport through facility corridors. Sufficient dividers should be available to separate unit-dose packages and provide for efficient organization. In some institutions, drawer dividers serve to identify those drugs to be given at different dosing periods. For example, drugs prescribed to be given early in the morning are located in the front of the drawer; those in the middle are given during the day, while those in the rear are scheduled for late evening or at bedtime. A final section might contain prn (as needed) drugs. Dividers of different colors may also be used to further distinguish administration periods.

Carts and bins should be cleaned frequently. When possible, bins should be taken at regular intervals, or when conditions indicate, to a location where they can be thoroughly washed and sanitized.

Current Automation Systems

The National Association of Boards of Pharmacy (NABP) has adopted a definition of automated pharmacy systems. The policy states, ". . . include, but are not limited to mechanical systems that perform operations or activities, other than compounding or administration, relative to the storage, packaging, dispensing, or distribution of medication, and which collect, control and maintain all transaction information."

With the advancements in technology and the increases in computerization, there have been monumental changes to the pharmacy profession. A pharmacist's clinical knowledge will be drawn upon to provide information to ensure the best clinical outcome for the patient. Technology allows the pharmacist to move from labor intensive medication distribution into a clinical resource position for optimal patient care. Highly-trained and motivated pharmacy technicians are needed to handle the complex distribution of medications.

Also, with the advent of diagnosis-related groups (DRGs), patients will be receiving very intensive short-term care, with the pharmacist's role more firmly involved in therapeutic decision-making to ensure a rapid recovery with minimal adverse effects.

Automation had promised to decrease the number of pharmacists and technicians involved in the drug distribution process. In reality, those claims have not been realized. Automated systems require monitoring, preventative maintenance, upgrades, and database refinements, besides the normal operation of restocking.

Robotics

Many forms of robotic devices are currently available, with others being rapidly developed or improved, to mechanize the medication distribution process. Of primary concern with all products is medication safety and security. Mundane, repetitive tasks can be significantly reduced by the technology of these machines. The major advantage to automation is the increase in the output with a notable decrease in medication errors. However, it must be remembered that restocking one of these machines with a wrong medication will cause multiple errors before it is detected and corrected. Undivided attention must be maintained when restocking. Checking and double-checking is a must to ensure that this type of error is not committed.

In facilities that continue to have a cart exchange, the FastPak™ 330/520 by AutoMed Technologies can be a substantial time-saver. Up to 520 of the most common oral drugs that are used in the facility are stored in individual canisters. The machine is interfaced with the main pharmacy computer system. This allows the bulk drugs to be unit-dosed on the patient's profile in the order in which the drugs will be administered. For example, drug A is to be given at 0800, 1400, and 2000; drug B is to be given at 1200; and drug C is to be given at 0700 and 1900. The drugs are packaged in a strip with all of the patient's information. Drug C would be the first drug packaged, followed by drug A, drug B, another drug A, then drug C, and finally the last dose of drug A. The use of this type of machine assists the health care provider with the proper sequence for drug administration and virtually eliminates cart fill errors, and unit doses lower cost bulk medications so that unopened doses maybe reissued. However, if charges are generated at the time of filling, crediting for unused medications must be done manually.

McKesson is one of the innovators in the automated filling of carts. McKesson's solution to cart fill is the Robot-Rx® (Figure 18-7). This product differs from the FastPak™ 330/520 in that it can select items other than oral medications for filling. A three-axis robot moves horizontally and vertically along rows of bar coded prepackaged solid oral medications or small-volume vials or ampoules. These are selected based on the patient's profile that is interfaced from the main pharmacy computer system to the robot's computer. Another advantage of the Robot-Rx is the ability to issue credits on unused doses and return them to stock for reissue.

As many facilities move to e-MAR and bedside verification routines for medication administration, charges are often generated at administration. This eliminates the need for crediting unused medication, since a charge was not produced.

FIGURE 18-7

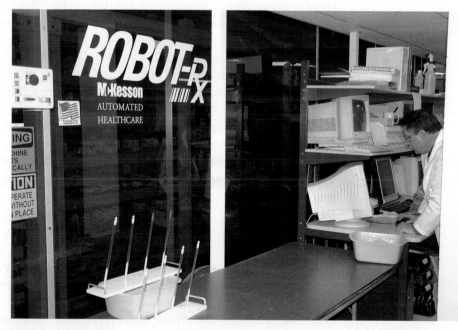

FIGURE 18-7 Robot-Rx.

FIGURE 18-8

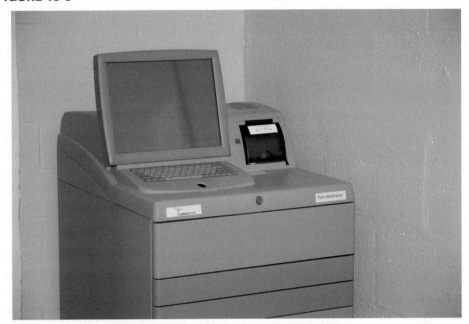

FIGURE 18-8 Pyxis MedStation™.

Automated Dispensing Cabinets

Pyxis, Omnicell, and McKesson are three of the leading companies that supply decentralized medication technology to hospitals and other facilities. Medstation® 3500 by Pyxis (Figure 18-8), OmniRx® by Omnicell, and AcuDose-Rx® by McKesson are similar in that medications are securely stored at remote sites throughout an institution. After pharmacy has reviewed and entered a physician's order on the patient's profile, the drug is available at the patient care unit for administration.

Authorized users, using a login and password, have access via a color touch screen computer terminal. Once a patient has been identified, his or her profile is displayed, and the health care professional can choose the needed medication. A drawer opens, and the drug is easily removed. Updates to the patient's profile are done instantaneously via an interface with the main hospital computer software. Charges and credits are also issued via another interface to the financial department. Documentation of every aspect of the process is maintained, and a variety of reports can be generated. The advantages of these systems are the elimination of end-of-shift counts for controlled substances; no need to have keys for medications locked in cabinets; and missing doses are becoming a thing of the past.

The Future

In order to reduce medication errors, the demand for technology has been under enormous strain to develop better, faster, and quicker ways to ensure patient safety. Direct physician order entry, verification at the patient's bedside, bar coding of medications, faster computers, and more efficient machinery are the current and future requirements. The goal is to provide a safe environment for a speedier recovery for the patient.

The pharmacy profession must look to technicians to assume more of the distribution workload and responsibilities in order to allow pharmacists to participate in clinical evaluations. This ultimate shift in roles will ultimately decrease medication errors, increase interventions, and thereby improve patient outcomes.

The time is coming for technicians to become involved in clinical roles. Experienced technicians could be trained to follow the pain management therapy of patients. This will assist the pharmacist in evaluating drug therapy, while also spotting potential diversion of controlled substances. Identifying patients on IV therapy and being able to switch them to a more economical oral medication would be a major cost-containment process. Another function of the technician could be interviewing patients at the time of admission to document medical history. This would allow the pharmacist to analyze what therapy might be appropriate during the hospital stay. As the procurement of medications becomes more challenging, analyzing drug use and alternative therapies would assist the department's buyer and could reap monumental cost savings.

The underlying factor that will impede the growth of the pharmacy technician is the current lack of standards for technician education and training. Empowering a single nationwide body, such as the Accreditation Council for Pharmacy Education (which performs similar functions for pharmacist education), will benefit the technician, rather than relying on the thousands of employers setting the standards. Once there is standardization in education and a meaningful testing of these competencies, then and only then will the role of pharmacy technician be allowed to move forward. This will also increase the confidence and respect by pharmacists toward technicians and their profession.

A Caveat

None of the current high-tech equipment briefly highlighted here, nor any future product, is immune to hardware failure, power failure, and software glitches. Humans still make mistakes when operating these sophisticated systems, maintenance is sometimes overlooked, or the equipment may be misused. All of this can lead to medication mistakes. Backup systems must be provided for when and if these systems fail to function properly. The pharmacist, along with the help of technicians, will have to return to manual processes to ensure that patients receive the right drug at the right time, in the right dose, and by the right route. A machine will *never* replace humans.

Summary

In this chapter, the technician's role in drug distribution has been generally described. The functions depicted are broad in nature and not all-inclusive. Only a small segment of duties has been outlined. Because each pharmacy is an entity of its own, it would be unrealistic or even undesirable to delineate a structured description of a technician's role in this very important process. After thorough orientation and training, the department's policy and procedure manual should be frequently consulted and followed throughout the technician's employment.

Because pharmacy is a dynamic and not a static profession, the roles of pharmacists and technicians are evolving from a product-oriented profession to a patient-oriented focus. The technician must be willing to continue the learning process, be open to innovative ideas, and be willing to assume newer responsibilities, which may be required as the profession of pharmacy advances.

TEST YOUR KNOWLEDGE

Multiple Choice

1. All of the following are acceptable methods to distribute medications to nursing stations *except*
    a. pharmacy courier.
    b. dumbwaiter.
    c. patients picking up their own medications.
    d. pneumatic tube system.

2. When using a pneumatic tube system, what precautions should first be considered?
    a. weight of item being sent
    b. possibility of breakage
    c. both a and b
    d. none of the above

3. Telephone orders should be handled by
    a. the senior technician.
    b. a pharmacist.
    c. both a and b.
    d. none of the above.

4. Identify the tool that allows the data from one computer system to be processed by a different computer system.
    a. modem
    b. mouse
    c. Internet connection
    d. interface

5. Which of the following is *not* a major vendor in pharmacy automation?
    a. Omnicell
    b. Pyxis
    c. Novation
    d. McKesson

6. The organization that sets practice standards and evaluates accreditation of health care facilities is the
    a. FDA.
    b. Joint Commission.
    c. DEA.
    d. EPA.

7. Dumbwaiters are limited in their usefulness because of their
    a. horizontal movement only.
    b. vertical movement only.
    c. weight restrictions.
    d. noisiness during operation.

8. When two or more compounds are mixed together to make a multiple-dosing unit, the procedure is called
   a. manufacturing.
   b. compounding.
   c. mixing.
   d. titration.

9. Compounding may only be performed by a
   a. registered pharmacist.
   b. a pharmacy technician under the supervision of a pharmacist.
   c. both a and b.
   d. none of the above.

Matching

Match the following:

1. _____ ASHP
2. _____ robotics
3. _____ MAR
4. _____ technician order entry
5. _____ pneumatic tube
6. _____ dumbwaiter
7. _____ NCR
8. _____ facsimile equipment

a. no carbon required
b. used by banks and hospitals for transportation
c. national organization of pharmacists and technicians
d. computerized robot for cassette filling
e. medication administration record
f. must be validated by a pharmacist
g. elevator for transporting medications or orders
h. fax

Fill In The Blank

1. The type of distribution system in which all medications are stocked on each nursing unit is called the _____ system.

2. When all activities that take place in the preparation and distribution of medications are in one main pharmacy area, this is an example of a/an _____ dispensing system.

3. The elimination of errors resulting from illegible information, automatic dose calculation, and clinical decision-making support at the point-of-care are all benefits of _____.

4. All information about a patient is maintained in the _____.

5. "Shake Well Before Use," "For the Eye," and "Keep Refrigerated" are all examples of _____.

References

Desselle, S. (2005). Certified pharmacy technician's views on their medication preparation errors and educational needs. *American Journal of Health-System Pharmacy*, 62, 1992–1997.

Keresztes, J. (2006). Role of pharmacy technicians in the development of clinical pharmacy. *The Annals of Pharmacotherapy*, 40, 2015–2019.

Lefkowitz, S., Cheiken, H., & Barnhart, M. R. (1991). A trial of the use of bar code technology to restructure a drug distribution and administration system. *Hospital Pharmacist*, 26, 239–242.

Mansfield, B. The role of pharmacy technicians with reducing medication errors. *RXinnovate Healthcare Consulting*. Available at: www.continuingeducation.com. Accessed May 2007.

Paoletti, R., Suess, T., et al. (2007). Using bar-code technology and medication observation methodology for safer medication administration. *American Journal of Health-System Pharmacy*, 64, 536–543.

Poon, E., Cina, J., et al. (2006). Medication dispensing errors and potential adverse drug events before and after implementing bar code technology in the pharmacy. *American College of Physicians*, 145, 426–434.

Skibinski, K., White, B., et al. (2007). Effects of technological interventions on the safety of a medication-use system. *American Journal of Health-System Pharmacy*, 64, 90–96.

Weber, E., Hepfinger, C., & Koontz, R. (2005). Pharmacy technicians supporting clinical functions. *American Journal of Health-System Pharmacy*, 62, 2466–2472.

Manufacturers

Automed, 875 Woodlands Parkway, Vernon Hills, IL 60061. Phone: (888) 537-3102   www.automedrx.com. Accessed May 2007.

McKesson Automation, 700 Waterfront Drive, Pittsburgh, PA 15222. Phone: (412) 209-1400   www.mckesson.com. Accessed May 2007.

Omnicell, 1101 East Meadow Dr., Palo Alto, CA 94303. Phone: (800) 850-6664 www.omnicell.com. Accessed May 2007.

Pyxis Corporation, 3750 Torrey View Ct., San Diego, CA 92130. Phone: (800) 367-9947   www.pyxis.com. Accessed May 2007.

Infection Control and Prevention in the Pharmacy

Competencies

Upon completion of this chapter, the reader should be able to

1. List four general causes of contamination of pharmaceuticals and sterile pharmacy products.

2. List three principal goals for infection control and prevention programs.

3. List three basic principles of asepsis.

4. Name the precautions used by health care workers to protect themselves and others from exposure to bloodborne and other pathogens.

5. Name three bloodborne pathogens of most concern to health care workers and for which OSHA exposure control plans are designed.

6. Recognize the routes of transmission of microorganisms.

7. List several components of the routine precautions used by health care workers to protect themselves and others from infections.

8. Describe what health care workers do when there is a possible occupational exposure to bloodborne pathogens.

Key Terms

agent
airborne droplet nuclei
airborne transmission
asepsis
bacteria
bloodborne pathogens
chain of infection
cohorting
colonize
contact transmission
direct-contact transmission

droplet transmission
exposure control plan
fungi
indirect-contact transmission
infection
mode of transmission
multidrug-resistant organism (MDRO)
pathogen
personal protective equipment (PPE)

portal of entry
portal of exit
protozoa
reservoir
rickettsia
standard precautions
susceptible host
tuberculin skin test (TST)
vector-borne transmission
vehicle transmission
virus

Introduction

infection the state or condition in which the body (or part of it) is invaded by an agent (microorganism or virus) that multiplies and produces an injurious effect (active infection).

pathogen any virus, microorganism, or other substance causing disease.

bacteria small, one-celled microorganisms that need a nourishing environment to survive.

viruses a submicroscopic agent of infectious disease that is capable of reproduction.

The infection control and prevention practices essential to ensure safe pharmaceuticals for patients are fundamentally rooted in good hygiene and sanitary practices. For example, hand hygiene is considered the single most important infection control measure practiced by health care workers. To prevent the spread of infection to themselves and to others, however, pharmacy workers need additional infection control education. Fortunately, the principles of infection control and prevention, once learned, are relevant to any health care setting. The information presented here is applicable to a freestanding pharmacy, acute-care hospital, skilled nursing facility, home-care program, or any other setting where pharmacy personnel work. Pharmacy personnel are responsible for ensuring that drugs and solutions are handled in a manner that prevents contamination and protects sterility when indicated. The pharmacy is responsible for the preparation and storage of most sterile medications and, in more and more instances, for managing intravenous therapy admixtures and enteral nutritional products. The pharmacist and pharmacy staff need knowledge of infection control and prevention first and foremost, because patient morbidity (sickness) and mortality (death) can result from contaminated pharmaceuticals. Meticulous attention is needed to prevent the introduction and transmission of germs.

Infections

fungi yeasts or molds that obtain food from living organisms.

protozoa single-celled parasitic organisms with the ability to move.

rickettsia intercellular parasites that need to be in living cells to reproduce.

chain of infection the elements needed to take place in order for an infection to occur.

agent disease-causing; may be biological, such as a bacteria or virus, chemical, such as medications or pesticides, or physical, such as radiation or heat.

reservoir a place where an agent can survive.

An **infection** is the damaging of bodily tissues or organs by the introduction of a **pathogen** (disease-causing organism). There are five types of pathogenic organisms responsible for causing disease:

- **Bacteria**: small, one-celled microorganisms that need a nourishing environment to survive. Examples of diseases caused by bacteria are pneumonia and urinary tract infections.
- **Viruses**: organisms that can only live within another cell. Examples of viruses are the common cold, hepatitis, and genital herpes.
- **Fungi**: yeasts or molds that obtain food from living organisms. An example of a fungus is athlete's foot.
- **Protozoa**: single-celled parasitic organisms with the ability to move. An example of a protozoal infection is malaria.
- **Rickettsia**: intercellular parasites that need to be in living cells to reproduce. Lyme disease and Rocky Mountain spotted fever are caused by rickettsia.

Infection is an interactive process involving the agent, host, and environment. For an infection to occur, several essential elements need to take place; this process is often referred to as the **chain of infection** (Figure 19-1).

- A disease-causing **agent** must be present. An agent may be biological, such as a bacteria or virus, chemical, such as medications or pesticides, or physical, such as radiation or heat.
- A **reservoir** where the agent can survive must be present. This reservoir must contain the proper nutrients to keep the agent alive.
- A **portal of exit** from the reservoir to the susceptible host must be available. This can occur through body secretions such as saliva, blood, and urine.

portal of exit the route by which an agent moves from the reservoir to the susceptible host; may be through body secretions such as saliva, blood, and urine.

mode of transmission the way in which the susceptible host is moved between the portal of exit and the portal of entry.

FIGURE 19-1

■ A **mode of transmission** between the portal of exit and the portal of entry to the susceptible host must exist.

■ A **portal of entry**, the route by which the agent enters the host, must be available. This may be through breaks in the skin, inhalation of contaminants, and through insect bites.

■ A **susceptible host** must be present for the agent to be transferred. The host is usually vulnerable to disease due to lack of resistance.

Nosocomial infections, which are now called *hospital-acquired infections*, are infections that were not present at the time of hospital admission or part of the patient's original condition. They result from a procedure or form of treatment the patient

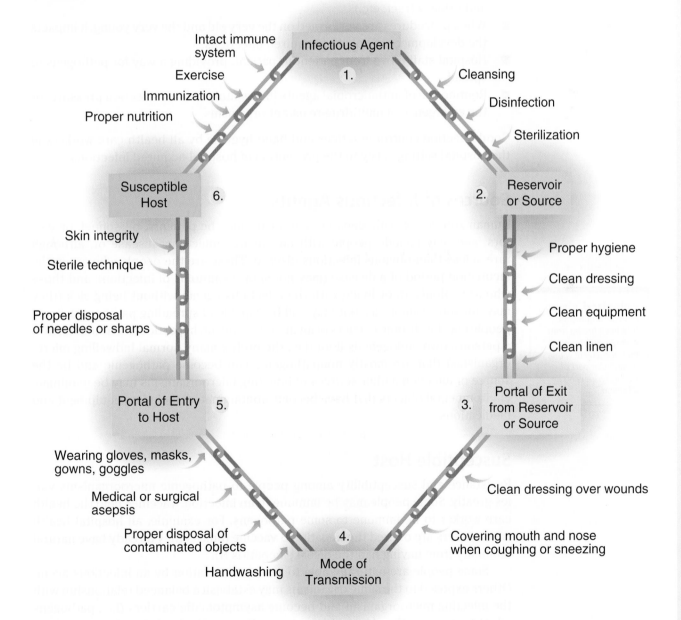

FIGURE 19-1 Chain of infection.

portal of entry the route by which the agent enters the host; may be through breaks in the skin, inhalation of contaminants, and through insect bites.

susceptible host must be present for the agent to be transferred; the host is usually vulnerable to disease due to lack of resistance.

received while in the hospital. Infections are considered hospital-acquired if they first appear after 48 hours of the patient's hospital admission, within 30 days after a surgical procedure has been performed, or within one year of a surgical procedure (for select surgeries) where an implantable device has been inserted (e.g., hip/knee replacement). In the United States, it has been estimated that as many as 2 million patients a year develop a hospital-acquired infection; one-third of these infections are considered preventable. They are even more alarming in the 21st century as antibiotic resistance has emerged.

The following are reasons for hospital-acquired infections:

- Patients in hospitals today whose immune systems are not intact may have a number of comorbities (chronic illnesses).
- The number of invasive procedures performed today on patients within the hospital may bypass the patients' normal defenses (intact skin, respiratory and urinary tract, etc.).
- When procedures are performed on the very old and the very young, it impacts the development of hospital-acquired infections.
- Hospital staff move from patient to patient, providing a way for pathogens to spread.
- Routine use of antimicrobial agents in hospitals creates selection pressure for the emergence of multidrug-resistant organisms.

Good infection control practices and hand hygiene by all health care workers in the hospital setting is key to the prevention of hospital-acquired infections.

Sources of Infectious Agents

Human sources of pathogens in health care may be patients, personnel, or visitors, and may include people with an obvious infectious disease or, although rare, a less-than-obvious infectious disease. These are the people who are in the incubation period of a disease (may not show symptoms of infection); and those who are **colonized**, or living with the infectious agents without being sick (they may not show symptoms, but may still be capable of spreading pathogens). Some people may be chronic carriers of an infectious agent. In particular circumstances, a person's own endogenous flora (i.e., the body's many normal indwelling microorganisms) that are mostly nonpathogenic can become pathogenic and be the source of infection. Other sources of infecting microorganisms may be inanimate environmental objects that have become contaminated, including equipment and medications.

colonized a group of microorganisms that have grown from a single infectious microorganism within a particular part of the body, causing an infection.

Susceptible Host

Resistance and susceptibility among people to pathogenic microorganisms varies greatly. Some people may be immune to an infection. Vaccines help the health care worker to be immune to some pathogens. For example, all hospital health care workers are offered the hepatitis B vaccine (unless they already have natural immunity from having had the disease hepatitis B).

Some people are naturally able to resist colonization by an infectious agent. Others exposed to the same organisms may establish a balanced relationship with the infecting microorganism and become asymptomatic carriers (i.e., pathogens adapt to grow on the skin and mucous surfaces of the host, forming part of the normal flora without making the person sick). Still others may develop a clinical disease.

Host factors may make people more at risk for infection. For example, one's age affects one's ability to fight off infection. Children are known to be more susceptible, and babies born prematurely are especially vulnerable. The elderly are also less able to fight off infections. Other conditions that disrupt the body's ability to fight infection include underlying diseases like diabetes and cancer, and particular treatments including the use of antimicrobials, corticosteroid therapy, and other immunosuppressive agents, as well as radiation therapy.

Procedures performed for diagnosis and treatment of disease often place the patient at higher risk and can contribute to infection. For instance, the patient is at risk for infection when there are breaks in the skin or other natural body defenses that occur during surgical operations, anesthesia, and when indwelling catheters are used.

Modes of Transmission

Microorganisms are spread five ways, or routes, and the same microorganism may be transmitted in more than one way.

Contact transmission

contact transmission a mode of transmission for microorganisms; divided into two subgroups: direct-contact transmission and indirect-contact transmission.

direct-contact transmission infection through body surface-to-body surface contact with an infected person.

indirect-contact transmission infection through contact with a contaminated object.

Contact transmission, the most important and frequent mode of transmission of infections, is divided into two subgroups: direct-contact transmission and indirect-contact transmission. **Direct-contact transmission** involves direct body surface-to-body surface contact and physical transfer of microorganisms between a susceptible host and an infected or colonized person, such as occurs when nursing personnel bathe a patient or when physicians perform invasive procedures on patients who require direct personal contact. Direct-contact transmission can also occur between two patients, with one serving as the source of the infectious microorganisms and the other as a susceptible host.

Indirect-contact transmission involves contact of a susceptible host with a contaminated intermediate object, usually inanimate, such as contaminated instruments, needles, or dressings, or contaminated, improperly washed hands, and gloves that are not changed between patients. With the advent of multidrug-resistant organisms, many of which can live on patient-care equipment for several days, environmental cleaning practices play an important role in the prevention of transmission of transmissible organisms through indirect contact.

Droplet transmission

droplet transmission infection through contact with microscopic liquid particles coming from an infected person.

Droplet transmission, theoretically, is a form of contact transmission. However, because the mechanism of transfer of the pathogen to the host is quite distinct from either direct- or indirect-contact transmission, the Centers for Disease Control and Prevention (CDC) considers droplet transmission a separate route of transmission. Droplets are generated from the source patient, primarily during coughing, sneezing, and during certain procedures such as suctioning and bronchodilator treatments. Transmission occurs when droplets containing microorganisms generated from the infected person are propelled a short distance through the air and deposited on the host's conjunctivae (eye surface), nasal mucosa, or mouth. Because droplets do not remain suspended in the air, special air handling and ventilation are not required to prevent droplet transmission. Droplet transmission must not be confused with airborne transmission.

Airborne transmission

Airborne transmission occurs by dissemination of either **airborne droplet nuclei** (small-particle residue—five microns or smaller in size—of evaporated droplets, containing microorganisms that remain suspended in the air for long periods of time) or dust particles containing the infectious agent. Microorganisms carried in this manner can be widely dispersed by air currents and may become inhaled by a susceptible host within the same room or over a longer distance from the source patient, depending on environmental factors. Therefore, special air handling and ventilation are required to prevent airborne transmission. Microorganisms transmitted by airborne transmission include mycobacterium tuberculosis, varicella (chickenpox) virus, and zoonotic diseases (diseases transferred from animal to people) such as SARS (severe acute respiratory syndrome) and avian influenza (bird flu).

Vehicle transmission

Common **vehicle transmission** applies to contaminated items such as food (salmonellosis), water (cholera, *E. coli*), medications, devices, and equipment.

Vector-borne transmission

Vector-borne transmission occurs when vectors such as mosquitoes (malaria, West Nile encephalitis), flies, rats, ticks (Lyme disease), or other vermin transmit microorganisms. This route of transmission is less significant in hospitals in the United States than in other regions of the world, but it certainly does exist.

airborne transmission infection by contact with airborne particles that contain infectious organisms.

airborne droplet nuclei small-particle residue—five microns or smaller in size—of evaporated droplets, containing microorganisms that remain suspended in the air for long periods of time.

vehicle transmission infection through contact with contaminated food or water.

vector-borne transmission infection through contact with infection-carrying insects or animals.

Control of Infections

Infection control and prevention programs have three principal goals:

1. Protect and provide a safe environment for the patient.
2. Protect the health care worker, visitors, and others in the health care environment from possible exposure to a communicable disease.
3. Accomplish the previous two goals in a cost-effective manner, whenever possible.

Because host and agent factors are more difficult to control, interruption of the transfer of microorganisms in health care facilities is the primary goal of infection control and prevention programs. The greatest opportunity for health care workers to prevent infections comes from eliminating the transmission of pathogenic organisms.

The Principles of Aseptic Techniques

To protect the patient and to prevent contamination, the basic principles of **asepsis** and the practices of aseptic techniques need to be understood.

asepsis free from germs, sterile.

- Microorganisms (germs) are capable of causing illness in humans.
- Microorganisms that are harmful to humans can be transmitted by direct or indirect contact.

■ Interrupting the transmission of microorganisms from reservoirs (i.e., infected people, whether patients, other staff members, or visitors and the environment) to susceptible hosts (other patients, health care workers, visitors) can prevent illness.

Aseptic techniques (clean practices) are used to reduce the number of microorganisms or to eliminate their transmission from one person or environment to another. The practices of aseptic technique include hand hygiene to reduce the number of skin microorganisms, the use of barriers such as gloves and gowns to avoid skin and clothing contact with contaminated surfaces, and environmental controls, ranging from and including routine environmental cleaning and disinfection to the use of controlled airflow hoods.

Standard Precautions

standard precaution
universal precautions developed by the Occupational Safety and Health Administration (OSHA) for infection control safety measures, designed to protect health care workers and patients from infections.

For many years, universal precautions and procedures for universal precautions developed by the Occupational Safety and Health Administration (OSHA) referred to infection control safety measures designed to protect health care workers from infections. The CDC (Centers for Disease Control and Prevention), responsible for both health care workers and patients, expanded universal precautions to protect both health care workers and patients and used the term **standard precautions**. Today, a facility may use either term or a combination of the two to name the infection control and prevention principle practices needed for all exposures to blood and body fluids and to equipment potentially contaminated by blood and body fluids.

Since people harboring infectious agents may not look sick, health care personnel must use precautions during the care of all patients, and for all contact with patients, clients, residents, and inmates, regardless of the diagnosis or presumed infection status. Standard precautions apply to any contact with blood, all body fluids, secretions, and excretions except sweat—regardless of whether or not they contain visible blood—nonintact skin (e.g., open cuts, wounds, surgical sites), and mucous membranes (e.g., surface of the eye, inside of the nose and mouth).

Personal Protective Equipment (PPE)

personal protective equipment (PPE)
protective gear worn by health care workers, made up of barriers used to prevent skin and mucous membrane exposure when contact with blood or other potentially infectious material is anticipated.

Personal protective equipment (PPE) is made up of barriers used to prevent skin and mucous membrane exposure when contact with blood or other potentially infectious material is anticipated. PPE includes impermeable gowns or aprons, disposable non-sterile gloves, masks, masks with eye shields, goggles, resuscitation bags, mouthpieces or other ventilation devices used for patient resuscitation, specimen transport bags, and red regulated medical waste garbage bags (Figure 19-2). Health care workers use PPE when anticipating contact with blood, body fluids, secretions, and excretions, nonintact skin, and mucous membranes.

Health care workers must wear protective gloves (most facilities today use latex-free gloves as a result of the increased sensitivity by many health care workers to latex) when it can be reasonably anticipated that there may be hand contact with blood or body fluids, other potentially infectious material, mucous membranes, or nonintact skin and when handling or touching contaminated items or surfaces. For example, gloves must be worn during venipuncture or other vascular access procedures. Gloves must be changed in between the care and contact with each patient, client, resident, inmate, and so forth. Protective gloves are to be removed before touching noncontaminated items (e.g., telephones, doorknobs).

Health care workers must wear gowns, gloves, and masks with eye shields for procedures that could involve splashing or spattering of blood or other body fluids

FIGURE 19-2

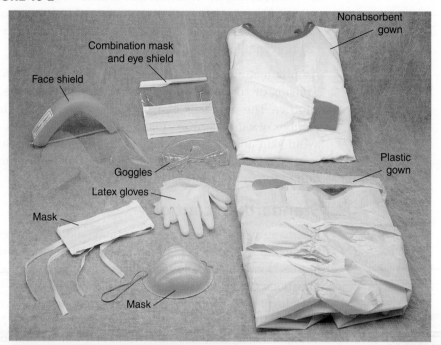

FIGURE 19-2 Personal protective equipment (PPE).

or other potentially infective materials that may be transmitted to one's eyes, nose, or mouth.

The following procedures must be observed with PPE:

■ Wash hands immediately, or as soon as feasibly possible, after removal of gloves or other PPE.

■ Remove PPE after it becomes contaminated and before leaving the work area.

■ Remove PPE either before leaving a contaminated area (e.g., a lab) or right after leaving (e.g., a TB [mycobacterium tuberculosis] airborne isolation room).

■ Remove immediately, or as soon as feasible, any garment contaminated by blood or body fluids in such a way as to avoid contact with the outer surface.

Prevention of Needlestick and Other Sharps Injuries

Precautions must be taken to prevent injuries caused by needles, scalpels, and other sharp instruments or devices during and after use. To prevent needlestick injuries, needles should *not* be recapped, purposely bent or broken by hand, removed from disposable syringes, or otherwise manipulated by hand. In the event a needle must be recapped, a "one-hand scoop" method must be employed. After use, disposable syringes and needles and all other sharp items, both used and unused, should be discarded in appropriate puncture-proof sharps biohazard containers (Figure 19-3). In today's health care system, there are a number of safety devices for using needles. For example, needles that retract into the syringe (or a sheath that will cover the needle) after the injection is given avoid the possibility of the health care worker being stuck.

Hand Hygiene

Hands and other skin surfaces must be washed immediately and thoroughly if contaminated with blood or other body fluids. Hand washing significantly reduces

FIGURE 19-3

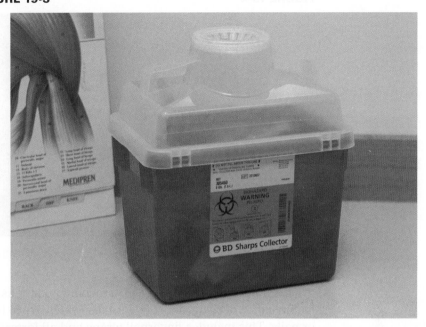

FIGURE 19-3 Sharps containers are used to dispose of needles or any other object capable of penetrating the skin.

the transmission of pathogens in hospitals and is considered the most important infection control and prevention measure that the health care worker can perform. Health care workers must wash their hands frequently. Hands must be washed before putting on gloves and immediately after gloves are removed, between patient contacts, and when otherwise indicated to avoid transfer of microorganisms to other patients or environments.

To properly wash hands, wet the hands with warm water and then add soap. Use friction to generate lather and wash hands (Figure 19-4). Use a vigorous 10- to 15-second rub to remove transient microorganisms (wash longer for more heavy contamination or after a possible exposure to **bloodborne pathogens** and other potentially infectious material). Follow with a thorough rinsing with warm water. In certain work areas a counted scrub is used for hand washing (e.g., operating room, neonatal intensive care). Health care workers need to wash hands before beginning work, before and after giving treatments or handling used equipment, before eating, and before and after using the bathroom.

Waterless alcohol-based hand hygiene products are now available in most health care facilities for hand washing procedures. Health care workers appreciate these products since they are easy to use, and because they contain emollients, they do not dry the skin. Especially important when sinks are not available, dispensers for waterless hand cleaners can be located anywhere hand washing might be needed. In some instances the health care worker may carry the hand hygiene product with them to use as needed. Soap and water must still be used when the hands are visibly soiled, since the alcohol will not disinfect the hands through the soil. Waterless products are used for routine hand washing procedures, but do not replace counted or timed scrubs. Waterless alcohol-based hand rubs are not to be used when caring for a patient with *Clostridium difficile*. The actual action of washing with an antimicrobial soap and warm water is needed to remove *C. difficile* from one's hands.

bloodborne pathogens microorganisms that are transmitted through exposure to contaminated blood products.

FIGURE 19-4

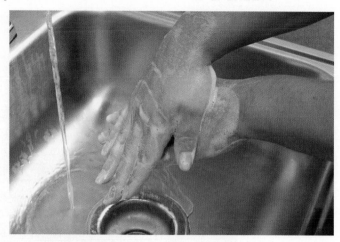

FIGURE 19-4 Hand hygiene is the single most important method of infection control.

An important aspect of the CDC recommendations for good hand hygiene is the maintenance of clean, short fingernails, which are to be free of artificial extenders or nails. This includes fingernail wraps and all forms of acrylic nails. Fashionable fingers and health care may be a recipe for infected nails, and nail beds have been found through extensive scientific studies to harbor a higher bacterial count.

Cleaning and Decontamination of Surfaces and Spills

Environmental contamination is an effective method of disease transmission for microorganisms and particularly for the hepatitis B virus (HBV). The CDC states that HBV can survive for at least one week in dried blood on environmental surfaces. Cleaning of contaminated work surfaces after completion of procedures or after spills is required to ensure that employees are not inadvertently exposed to blood or other potentially infectious material remaining on a surface from previous procedures or from a spill. All cleaning should be done with infection-control committee/institutional-approved disinfectants.

Specific procedures are used for spills of blood or other potentially infectious material. If the pharmacy technician encounters a spill, he or she should call for help from the professional staff.

Biohazard symbols (Figure 19-5) or red bags are used to warn employees who may have contact with items of the potential hazard posed by their contents.

FIGURE 19-5

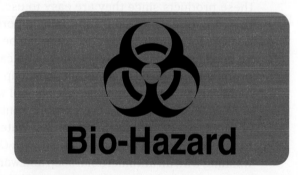

FIGURE 19-5 Biohazard symbol.

The storage of food, as well as eating, drinking, smoking, applying cosmetics or lip balm, and handling contact lenses, is prohibited in patient care areas and in other work areas where there is the likelihood of occupational exposure.

Blood and other potentially infectious materials must be handled carefully in order to minimize the potential for splashing and spraying.

Engineering and Workplace Controls

Engineering controls reduce the risk of employee exposures either by removing, eliminating, or isolating hazards.

Regulated medical waste (RMW) handling

Most hospital waste is not any more infective than residential waste. Consistent with most current state and local regulations, RMW is defined as sharps, culture/stocks, human pathological waste, animal research waste, and human blood or blood products. State regulations for proper handling and disposal of these wastes may vary and need to be checked on a state-by-state basis.

Containers with free-flowing blood or blood products, or discarded material saturated or dripping with blood (e.g., dressings, blood transfusion bags, or tubings), should be considered RMW.

Materials that produce free-flowing fluid when compressed or squeezed are considered RMW. All other hospital-related items are to be disposed of as regular waste. RMW is placed in closable containers constructed to hold all contents and prevent leakage. The containers are appropriately labeled as a biohazard or color-coded, and closed prior to removal to prevent spillage or protrusion of contents during handling.

Because pharmaceuticals are considered chemicals, the Environmental Protection Agency (EPA), the American Hospital Association, and the Joint Commission have been working together to set guidelines for the disposal of certain hazardous pharmaceuticals that must be disposed of appropriately. This is a result of the Resource Conservation and Recovery Act (RCRA) enacted by Congress in 1976. This regulation is now being enforced, and health care facilities must incorporate the proper disposal program for these select pharmaceutical agents within their medical waste program. Pharmaceutical hazardous waste has been divided into three categories by the Resource Conservation and Recovery Act: the P-List, the U-List, and the D-List. P-List wastes are considered acutely hazardous and are the most dangerous chemicals for acute exposure if they present as the sole active ingredient of a product. Examples are arsenic and epinephrine. U-List wastes are considered toxic and involve the majority of chemotherapy agents. Items in the D-List are considered hazardous waste as a result of their ability to ignite and their toxicity, corrosiveness, and reactivity. All health professional organizations must identify, segregate, document, properly store, manifest, transport, and dispose of RCRA hazardous waste according to specific procedures. Each health care facility will have a very specific plan to address this issue.

Sharps disposal containers

Leakproof, puncture-resistant sharps disposal containers labeled with a biohazard label are located in all patient rooms, all patient care areas, and all other areas where contaminated sharps might be encountered. All sharps must be discarded into such containers as soon as possible.

Safety devices and proper work practices

Needlestick-prevention devices with engineered safety features are part of the comprehensive program to reduce the risk of bloodborne pathogen exposures. Safer medical devices used to prevent percutaneous injuries before, during, or after use, through safer design, are becoming increasingly available on the market and are being evaluated throughout the United States in response to a recent OSHA rule. Examples of safer devices include shielded-needle devices, blunt needles, needleless IV connectors, and IV access devices.

Proper work practices, such as reducing hand-to-hand instrument passing in the operating room and no-hands procedures in handling contaminated sharps (including broken glassware picked up using mechanical means, such as a brush and dustpan), reduce the risk of bloodborne pathogen exposure. Examples of engineered devices that are used as part of proper work practices include mechanical pipetting devices, centrifuge safety cups, splashguards, and biological safety cabinets.

Hospital Isolation Precautions

Isolation precautions are used in hospitals for patients known or suspected to be infected with highly transmissible microorganisms, for which additional precautions beyond universal-standard precautions are needed to interrupt the transmission of disease. The particular isolation precautions used are based on the way the infectious disease or microorganism is transmitted. These precautions might also be used in other parts of the health care system where the infectious disease is diagnosed prior to admission to the hospital.

Hospitals modify isolation systems to meet the needs of the patient population served and to meet federal, state, or local regulations. Each hospital isolation system, however, must preserve the principles of infection prevention and control and include precautions to interrupt the spread of infection by all routes (contact, airborne, droplet) likely to be encountered. Most hospitals use standard precautions (the use of good hand washing practices and the use of PPE when contamination is anticipated) and transmission-based precautions.

Communicable diseases and conditions require different types of transmission-based precautions (isolation). In most hospitals, a color-coded transmission-based precaution-isolation sign (or card) is placed outside of the patient's room to alert health care workers and visitors to the procedures required to prevent transmission of the disease or condition the patient is harboring. The isolation sign lists the requirements of the isolation (e.g., whether masks or gowns are required). Before entering any hospital room, be sure to check for these signs.

Pharmacy personnel, when in direct contact with patients, must be aware and trained in transmission-based isolation precautions. Those not trained in hospital isolation precautions are considered visitors and need to follow the instructions printed on the sign outside the patient's door: "Report to the Nurses' Station Before Entering the Room." The nurse will instruct visitors on what precautions are required to prevent transmission.

There are three types of transmission-based precautions: airborne precautions, droplet precautions, and contact precautions. They may be combined for diseases that have multiple routes of transmission. When used either singly or in combination, they are to be used in addition to standard precautions (good hand washing and the use of PPE).

Standard precautions are designed to reduce the risk of transmission of microorganisms from both recognized and unrecognized sources of infection in hospitals. Since people harboring infectious agents may not look sick, health care personnel must use precautions during the care of all patients and for all contact with patients, clients, residents, and inmates, regardless of the diagnosis or presumed infection status.

Airborne precautions

Airborne precautions require the use of a private room with a special air-handling system that creates negative air pressure and discharges room air to the outdoors or out through a high-efficiency filter before the air is circulated to other areas in the hospital (Figure 19-6). Those entering the room are required to wear National Institute of Occupational Safety and Health (NIOSH)-approved respirators, unless they are immune to the disease.

Airborne precautions are used for patients diagnosed with or suspected of having measles, varicella (chickenpox), suspected or diagnosed pulmonary

FIGURE 19-6

AIRBORNE PRECAUTIONS
(In addition to Standard Precautions)

VISITORS: Report to nurse before entering

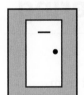

Patient Placement
Private room that has:
    Monitored negative air pressure,
    6 to12 air changes per hour,
    Discharge of air outdoors or HEPA filtration if recirculated.
Keep room door closed and patient in room.

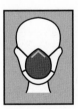

Respiratory Protection
Wear an **N95 respirator** when entering the room of a patient with known or suspected infectious pulmonary **tuberculosis**.
Susceptible persons should not enter the room of patients known or suspected to have **measles** (rubeola) or **varicella** (chickenpox) if other immune caregivers are available. If susceptible persons must enter, they should wear an **N95 respirator**.(Respirator or surgical mask not required if immune to measles and varicella.)

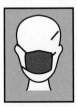

Patient Transport
Limit transport of patient from room to essential purposes only.
Use **surgical mask** on patient during transport.

FIGURE 19-6 Airborne precautions (From Brevis Corporation, 225 West 2855 South, Salt Lake City, UT 84115. Copyright © 1996, Brevis Corporation).

tuberculosis, and other possible airborne diseases. The door to the room used for airborne precautions must remain closed to maintain negative air pressure in the room in relation to surrounding areas and to contain microorganisms that remain suspended in the air for long periods of time to prevent them from being widely dispersed by air currents.

Droplet precautions

Droplet precautions require the use of a private room, or that the patient be placed in a room with a patient who has active infection or colonization with the same microorganism but with no other infection (Figure 19-7). This is called **cohorting**. Surgical masks with or without eye protection are used when entering the room or when within a certain distance of the patient.

Droplet precautions are used for patients diagnosed or suspected to have some types of meningitis, serious bacterial respiratory infections such as pertussis (whooping cough), influenza (flu), streptococcal pharyngitis, pneumonia or scarlet fever in infants and young children, and serious viral infections. Trans-

> **cohorting** a patient is placed in a room with a patient who has active infection or colonization with the same microorganism but with no other infection.

FIGURE 19-7

DROPLET PRECAUTIONS
(In addition to Standard Precautions)

VISITORS: Report to nurse before entering

Patient Placement
Private room, if possible. Cohort or maintain spatial separation of **3 feet** from other patients or visitors if private room is not available.

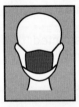

Mask
Wear mask when working within **3 feet** of patient (or upon entering room).

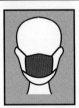

Patient Transport
Limit transport of patient to essential purposes only.
Use **surgical mask** on patient during transport.

FIGURE 19-7 Droplet precautions (From Brevis Corporation, 225 West 2855 South, Salt Lake City, UT 84115. Copyright © 1996, Brevis Corporation).

mission occurs when droplets are propelled a short distance through the air, but because droplets do not remain suspended in the air, special air handling and ventilation are not required to prevent droplet transmission. Droplet transmission must not be confused with airborne transmission.

Contact precautions

Contact precautions require the use of a private room, or that the patient be placed in a room with a patient who has active infection or colonization with the same microorganism, but with no other infection (cohorting) (Figure 19-8). Gloves are used when entering the room. Depending on what the patient is on contact precautions for, gowns may be indicated. Check the isolation sign on the door. When possible, patient care equipment (e.g., blood pressure machines, stethoscopes) should be dedicated to a single patient or cleaned and disinfected before use on another patient.

Contact precautions are used for patients known or suspected of having illnesses easily transmitted by direct patient contact or by contact with items in the patient's environment, including gastrointestinal, respiratory, skin or wound infections, or colonization with multidrug-resistant bacteria judged by the institution to be significant.

Preventing Infections in Health Care Workers

Following the AIDS epidemic that began in the early 1980s, and in response to the threat of other serious on-the-job infections, federal and state legislatures have written into law the requirement for institutions to give all their health care workers infection control and prevention education, which is to encompass safe infection control practices as well as preventative measures the health care worker is required to take within the institutional environment, and what to do if the health care worker has been exposed to a communicable disease. In the past number of years, the health care industry has been charged with the task to evaluate all occupational exposures and to adopt safety practices and devices to prevent health care worker injuries and exposures to bloodborne pathogens and airborne infectious diseases. Some possible bloodborne infectious diseases are hepatitis B, hepatitis C, and HIV (human immunodeficiency virus), which causes AIDS. Some airborne infectious diseases are pulmonary TB and varicella (chickenpox).

Hepatitis B Vaccination

Employees found to be nonimmune to hepatitis B must be encouraged to receive the hepatitis B vaccination, which must be available at no charge to the employee. Nonimmune employees choosing to decline the hepatitis B vaccination must sign a declination form. The employee may rescind a declination at any time.

Infection Control Education

All health care facilities are required to have infection control programs that establish infection control and prevention standards of care. Hospital staffs are required to review these infection control policies and procedures, some of which are specific to a department (such as the pharmacy), and others that relate to all members of the health care team on a yearly basis.

CONTACT PRECAUTIONS

(In addition to Standard Precautions)

VISITORS: Report to nurse before entering

Patient Placement
Private room, if possible. Cohort if private room is not available.

Gloves
Wear gloves when entering patient room.
Change gloves after having contact with infective material that may contain high concentrations of microorganisms (**fecal** material and **wound drainage**).
Remove gloves before leaving patient room.

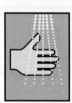

Wash
Wash hands with an **antimicrobial** agent immediately after glove removal. After glove removal and handwashing, ensure that hands do not touch potentially contaminated environmental surfaces or items in the patient's room to avoid transfer of microorganisms to other patients or environments. If hands are not visibly soiled, use an alcohol-based hand rub for routinely decontaminating hands.

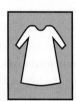

Gown
Wear gown when **entering** patient room if you anticipate that your clothing will have substantial contact with the patient, environmental surfaces, or items in the patient's room, or if the patient is **incontinent**, or has **diarrhea**, an **ileostomy**, a **colostomy**, or **wound drainage** not contained by a dressing. **Remove** gown before leaving the patient's environment and ensure that clothing does not contact potentially contaminated environmental surfaces to avoid transfer of microorganisms to other patients or environments.

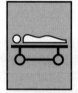

Patient Transport
Limit transport of patient to essential purposes only. During transport, ensure that precautions are maintained to minimize the risk of transmission of microorganisms to other patients and contamination of environmental surfaces and equipment.

Patient-Care Equipment
Dedicate the use of noncritical patient-care equipment to a single patient. If common equipment is used, clean and disinfect between patients.

FIGURE 19-8 Contact precautions (From Brevis Corporation, 225 West 2855 South, Salt Lake City, UT 84115. Copyright © 1996, Brevis Corporation).

Pharmacy personnel are not at high risk for occupational exposure to infectious diseases unless they are involved in direct patient care and have contact with body fluids or patients with an airborne communicable disease. In some situations, the pharmacist might assist the medical team (e.g., during cardiac arrest response) and could possibly have contact with body fluids or a patient with an airborne disease. Other situations with less potential for pharmacy staff occupational exposure might nonetheless be harmful if basic infection control principles are not followed. For instance, during the delivery and distribution of pharmaceuticals to patient care areas, there could be an unexpected encounter with patients, patient linens, or with soiled patient care equipment. Health care worker duties requiring contact with blood or body fluids, or with equipment that is contaminated with blood and other potentially infectious materials such as body fluids, create the most risk for exposure to serious infections.

To protect themselves and others from infection, all health care workers use universal-standard precautions whenever they are in a health care environment. The details of these precautions are mandated by the U.S. Occupational Safety and Health Administration (OSHA) and the Public Employee Safety and Health Administration (PESH) and are based on recommendations from the Centers for Disease Control and Prevention (CDC).

Through the Bloodborne Pathogen Standard (law), OSHA and PESH ordered that all health care facilities have in place **exposure control plans** to protect workers from exposure to infectious diseases. These plans must include infection control training for health care workers at risk for occupational exposure to blood and other potentially infectious material, because these may contain bloodborne pathogens or patients that are harboring an airborne pathogen. The tuberculosis control plan is required to be reviewed because some health care workers may be at risk for exposure to this disease.

The bloodborne pathogens of most concern in health care include but are not limited to the hepatitis B virus (HBV), which causes hepatitis B infection; the human immunodeficiency virus (HIV), which causes acquired immunodeficiency syndrome (AIDS); and the hepatitis C virus (HCV), which causes hepatitis C infection. Other bloodborne pathogens include microorganisms that are considered less of a risk to health care workers from exposures, but can potentially cause diseases like syphilis, malaria, and viral hemorrhagic fever.

Not all tasks within the health care setting carry the same chance of contact with blood, potentially infectious body fluids, or an airborne communicable disease. Tasks that carry a high risk of exposure require that the health care worker wear appropriate clothing (PPE), including cover gowns, gloves, masks, and protective eye wear. OSHA requires that the health care facility must provide all protective equipment free of charge to their employees.

Pulmonary Tuberculosis Testing

All new employees in hospitals and other health care facilities must have a baseline evaluation for evidence of tuberculosis infection, consisting of a two-stage **tuberculin skin test (TST)**, unless they have a history of positive TSTs. Health care workers with negative TSTs must be re-tested at periodic intervals; annually in most cases, every six months or more frequently for employees in work areas that are at high risk for tuberculosis. Health care workers with positive TSTs are evaluated to rule out active disease and must receive counseling regarding current recommended treatments and the symptoms of tuberculosis disease (including

exposure control plan guidelines to follow in the event of an exposure to an infectious disease, including infection control training.

tuberculin skin test (TST) a test performed to identify exposure to the tuberculosis bacillus.

coughs and fevers that last two weeks or longer, night sweats, weight loss, blood in sputum). People with positive TSTs but without active disease have TB infection and may require treatment.

TB infection is not the same as having pulmonary TB disease. Pulmonary TB infection is a condition in which living tuberculosis organisms are present in a person without causing continuing destruction of tissue. The healthy immune system usually keeps the infection in check, but prophylactic treatment with INH (isoniazid) is needed to kill the mycobacterium tuberculosis organism. If not treated and the immune system fails, TB disease may develop. Pulmonary TB disease is a condition in which living tuberculosis organisms produce progressive destruction of tissue. Pulmonary TB disease is contagious. TB infection is not contagious.

Multidrug-resistant (MDR) TB

Some strains of TB have developed resistance to the drugs used to treat tuberculosis disease. The main reason that MDR strains of TB have developed is that TB patients have not followed their prescribed drug treatment. The drugs used to treat TB usually alleviate the symptoms within two to three weeks; however, they do not eliminate the underlying infection unless they are taken for at least six months. When patients do not adhere to their prescribed drug regimen, the bacteria can become resistant to the drugs being used. Symptoms can return and the patient can transmit these resistant organisms to others, including health care workers. Employees exposed to pulmonary tuberculosis in the workplace will be evaluated for evidence of infection as a result of the exposure through a post-exposure evaluation.

Occupational Exposures

Infectious body substances that carry a risk for bloodborne pathogen transmission include blood, bloody fluid, semen, vaginal secretions, and synovial, pleural, peritoneal, pericardial, cerebrospinal, or amniotic fluid. Exposures that may place a health care worker at risk for bloodborne pathogen infections include a percutaneous injury (e.g., a needlestick or cut with a sharp object); contact of mucous membrane, conjunctivae, or nonintact skin (e.g., when the exposed skin is chapped, abraded, or afflicted with dermatitis) with blood, tissue, or other body fluids; and contact with intact skin when the duration of contact is prolonged (i.e., several minutes or more) or involves an extensive area with blood, tissue, or other body fluids.

What to Do If Exposed

Clean the affected area *immediately*. Wash with soap and water.

- For needlesticks, cuts, or skin contact, wash the area with soap and running water for several minutes. Do not vigorously disrupt the skin, and do not use bleach or other strong chemicals, since these can increase chances of infection through skin damage.
- For eye contact, flush the eyes with copious amounts of running water for several minutes.

Notify the area supervisor *immediately*. Complete an employee accident form. Report to the emergency department or to the employee health service as directed by the hospital *immediately*. Smaller hospitals and other institutions may make arrangements with area hospital emergency departments for their staff to be seen for occupational exposures.

Post-exposure prophylaxis (PEP) is recommended for individuals exposed to potentially infectious body substances within one to two hours of a reported event, ideally within one hour. Health care workers must not delay seeking evaluation and treatment. (CDC-specific antiretroviral recommendations may vary from your state's department of health recommendations.)

The risk of hepatitis B virus infection following a needlestick with infected blood appears to be approximately 6 percent to 30 percent. The risk of hepatitis C infection following a needlestick with infected blood appears to be approximately 3 percent. The risk of HIV infection following a needlestick with infected blood appears to be 0.3 percent to 0.5 percent.

Post-exposure services must be available 24 hours a day, every day, in a designated center to any employee who sustains an occupational exposure. All expenses for medical evaluations and procedures, vaccines, and post-exposure prophylaxis must be at no cost to the employee.

Post-Bloodborne Pathogen Exposure Evaluation and Follow-Up

Health care workers need to be tested for hepatitis B, hepatitis C, and HIV and referred for follow-up care. Laws may vary by state, but usually the health care worker will be asked to consent to HIV testing. If consent is given, the source individual's blood will be tested as soon as feasible, and after consent is obtained in accordance with state and local laws relating to this matter. If the health care worker has never been infected with hepatitis B or has not been vaccinated against hepatitis B, the vaccine will be offered along with hyperimmune gamma globulin (HBIG), if indicated.

The source (patient) will be requested to sign an informed consent authorizing disclosure of his or her HIV status information to the exposed worker or to undergo consented HIV testing with disclosure of the test results to the exposed worker. Follow-up care is offered to the health care worker or person exposed, either through the employee health services or by a physician.

Health Care Worker Work Restrictions

Health care workers with infections can infect patients and other health care workers. Personnel with open draining lesions like abscesses or wounds must remain away from their jobs in the hospital and other health care settings and are to return only after cleared for work by the employee health service. Employees with herpetic lesions (herpes infections) should not care for patients in high-risk categories, including nursery, oncology, and ICU, until cleared by employee health. Health care workers should not work with rashes (especially if susceptible to varicella/chickenpox and after known exposure to chickenpox) or conjunctivitis until they have seen or spoken with their physician or employee health clinic.

Contamination of Pharmaceuticals

Contamination of pharmaceutical preparations has led to epidemics. Pharmacy personnel are required to know how to prevent contamination in the first place and must be prepared to participate in curtailing disease when contamination does occur. For example, if the possibility of an incident has occurred, the pharmacy staff will be a key part of a multidisciplinary team that will perform a complete investigation. Other important members of the team will be the infection control professional, the director of medical services, the nursing services representative, and other team members who may glean insight into all the medications that are involved, whether the medications were intrinsically contaminated (which occurs during the manufacturing process) or extrinsically contaminated (which occurs subsequent to manufacturing, during the admixture process or while the infusate was in use), and to whom the contaminated medications were administered. The pharmacy technician will be involved in aiding in the coordination process for all recalls that occur in cases of manufacturer contamination.

Intravenous Products

Preparation of intravenous products in areas outside of the pharmacy (in areas not providing a class 100 environment—for example, preparation of IVs outside a laminar air flow hood) may lead to contamination. Intravenous (IV) solution contamination rarely occurs, but when it does, bloodstream infections can cause bacteremia or fungemia, resulting in patients becoming critically ill and possibly developing septic shock. Also, intravenous solution contamination has the potential to result in outbreaks and possibly an epidemic because of the likely wide distribution and use of the contaminated solutions. Solutions intrinsically contaminated during production have caused widespread outbreaks of bloodstream infections in different facilities, extending at times to different states, which may escalate to epidemic proportions, increasing patient mortality and morbidity. Extrinsic contamination is a constant threat during the admixture process or while the infusate is in use. The threat of extrinsic contamination is always possible when aseptic technique is improperly used. Recommendations for the prevention of contamination of intravenous infusions include the following:

- Compound all admixtures in the pharmacy. The Centers for Disease Control and Prevention (CDC) and the Intravenous Nursing Society Standards of Practice both recommend that all parenteral fluids be prepared in the pharmacy using a laminar air flow hood.
- Prepare sterile products using facilities and equipment recommended by the American Society of Health-System Pharmacists (ASHP) and the standards implemented by the United States Pharmacopoeia (USP) Chapter 797.
- The sterile product preparation area is to have directly adjacent to it a hand washing facility with hot and cold running water and a facility-approved antimicrobial soap. The ASHP recommends personnel preparing sterile products wear clothing covers or gowns that generate low numbers of particles, and masks and coverings for head and facial hair. All hair, whether on your head, face, or arms, holds particles that may contaminate the sterile product during preparation. It is important to ensure this safety practice is utilized at all times during the preparation process.

■ All sterile products should be prepared in a class 100 environment with the use of a vertical or horizontal laminar air flow hood. The area is to be separate from other areas, with limited personnel traffic. Particle-generating items such as cardboard boxes are not to be stored in the sterile preparation room. Opening cardboard boxes generates dissemination of possible contaminated particles into the air, which in turn can contaminate stored pharmaceutical products. Solutions and/or medications should be removed from the boxes prior to storage within the pharmacy area. It is important to note that the pharmacy technician is typically the first person within the pharmacy to visualize IV solutions and medications that enter the pharmacy. This professional should carefully inspect solutions and medications for defects, expiration dates, and product integrity. For example, if the pharmacy technician notes that IV solutions appear cloudy or there are abnormal particles within the solution, the technician must remove the product and alert the pharmacist immediately.

Use the following aseptic techniques to prevent contamination of pharmaceuticals:

■ Perform hand and forearm hygiene before preparing sterile products. Use an antimicrobial or detergent soap with warm running water, or use a waterless alcohol skin hygiene product if no organic matter is present on your hands or forearms, as directed by the latest CDC hand hygiene guidelines.
■ Abstain from eating, drinking, and smoking in the preparation area.
■ Wipe or spray the rubber stoppers of containers with a 70-percent alcohol preparation before accessing the container.
■ Disinfect the entire surface of ampoules, vials, and container closures, including automated devices used for compounding sterile products, before placing them in the laminar airflow hood, as recommended by the ASHP.
■ Avoid touching sterile supplies, which may result in contamination of the product.

Contaminated multi-dose vials (MDVs) are excellent vehicles for the transmission of bacteria into the patient and the possible development of an infection. Although contamination of in-use vials is rare according to several well-controlled studies, epidemics have been traced to their use. In the past, most hospitals established policies to discard MDVs after a set period of time, usually 28 days, although some hospitals continue to use the manufacturer's expiration date on the vial.

Recommendations for the prevention of contamination of MDVs include the following:

■ When MDVs are used, the vial is dated once opened, and CDC recommendations call for the refrigeration of the vial after opening *ONLY if recommended by the manufacturer.*
■ Each time a vial is accessed, the rubber diaphragm of the vial must be cleaned carefully with an alcohol wipe, allowing the alcohol to dry (this is key to ensure the effectiveness of the antiseptic) before inserting a sterile needle into the vial; and avoid hand contamination of the device before penetrating the rubber diaphragm.
■ Discard the MDV when empty, when suspected or visible contamination (e.g., cloudiness) is present, or when the manufacturer's stated expiration date has been reached.

Inadequate quality control practices may lead to contamination of pharmaceuticals. The pharmacy is responsible for the storage of all pharmaceuticals, for monitoring for expiration dates (rotation of stock may be indicated for items that do not move quickly), and for monitoring the temperature of refrigerators and freezers used to store pharmaceuticals in all locations.

Recommendations for the prevention of contamination include the following:

- Sterile products should be examined for leaks and cracks and for turbidity or particulate matter that could indicate contamination. Keep in mind the growth of microorganisms, even in high numbers, may not be evident.
- Labeling all admixed parenterals according to ASHP recommendations provides for patient safety, and the use of control or lot numbers for batch-prepared items should assist with recalls, if needed.
- Admixed parenterals may be stored in the refrigerator for up to one week, providing that refrigeration begins immediately after preparation and is continuous, unless stability of ingredients dictates a shorter storage time. According to the ASHP, some admixed parenterals may be stored longer, depending on the sterile product preparation procedures used and the storage temperature.

Multidrug-Resistant Organisms

multidrug-resistant organism (MRDO) microorganisms, predominantly bacteria, that are resistant to one or more classes of antimicrobial agents (antibiotics).

Microorganisms, predominantly bacteria, that are resistant to one or more classes of antimicrobial agents (antibiotics) are known as **multidrug-resistant organisms (MDROs)**. Over the past 20 years, MDROs have steadily impacted the direct care of patients. In most instances, patients with MDROs have clinical symptoms similar to infections caused by susceptible microorganisms; however, options for treating patients with infections caused by MDROs are often extremely limited. For example, at one point we had only one antibiotic that would treat methicillin-resistant staphylococcus aureus (MRSA), which is an invasive skin bacterium that can cause a raging infection. Today, we have a number of MDROs within the health care system. Patients who are colonized with these organisms can transmit them to other patients and cause an infection to occur. Many of these organisms are transmitted from person to person and from inanimate object to person if cleaning practices are not adequate. Once again, good hand hygiene practices are the key to the prevention of transmission of these pathogenic organisms.

The role of the pharmacy in infection control and prevention extends beyond assuring the integrity of pharmaceuticals. The dramatic increase in the last several decades of the loss of activity of standard antibiotics to common bacteria has led to an incredible challenge. There is a demand for a pharmacy leadership role in the selection, use, and control of antibiotics as hospitals and other health care facilities deal with infections caused by bacteria that are resistant to multiple antibiotics. Working together with physicians, microbiologists, and infection control professionals, pharmacists participate in programs that limit unnecessary antibiotic use and seek to prevent the spread of multidrug-resistant microorganisms. These programs attempt to influence practitioner antimicrobial prescribing practices and the antibiotic habits of the public.

Summary

The prevention and control of infection is a high priority in all health institutions. The pharmacy is an integral part of the health care system. The pharmacist and pharmacy technician are key players on the health care team. This chapter identifies areas of concern and methods to be employed to prevent and control the spread of infection in institutions where people with infections are routinely treated.

Two areas of major concern that are addressed is preventing contamination of pharmaceuticals and ensuring sterility of all injectable medications.

TEST YOUR KNOWLEDGE

Multiple Choice

1. Some of the general causes of contamination of IV fluids during preparation include
    a. not cleaning the rubber stopper of the medication vial with alcohol prior to entry with needle and syringe.
    b. touching the sterile ports of IV fluids with sterile gloves.
    c. preparing parenteral nutrition solutions under the laminar air flow hood.
    d. examining fluids for turbidity.

2. Good hand washing practices are
    a. used by pharmacy personnel mainly while handling sterile medications and solutions.
    b. important in health care mostly when caring for patients in isolation rooms.
    c. used by medical personnel primarily to protect themselves from infections.
    d. considered the single most important infection control measure practiced by health care workers.

3. The principles of asepsis include the idea that
    a. microorganisms can be completely eliminated from humans.
    b. pathogens can be transmitted by direct or indirect contact.
    c. pathogens do not cause infection in health care workers.
    d. microorganisms cannot be spread in clean hospitals.

4. Aseptic techniques
    a. are used to reduce the transmission of germs.
    b. are not used routinely by pharmacy personnel.
    c. are needed only when working with items that are obviously soiled.
    d. decrease the number of bloodborne pathogens in blood and body fluids.

5. Pharmacy personnel
    a. are at great risk for infection at work.
    b. face no threat of infection on the job.
    c. are not included in infection control education programs because they do not have direct contact with patients.
    d. need to know how to protect themselves from contact with blood or body fluids, from airborne diseases, and from contaminated equipment.

6. For an infection to develop,
    a. organisms have to be transmitted from people who have obvious infections.

b. microorganisms are transmitted from an infected or contaminated source to a susceptible host (person).
c. the health care workers have to be very young or very old.
d. pathogens have to be contacted by hand.

7. In hospitals, microorganisms are most frequently spread
   a. by mosquitoes and flies.
   b. by contaminated food and water.
   c. by contact with contaminated people or objects.
   d. by droplets.

8. Standard precautions are used
   a. by doctors when shaking hands with patients and visitors.
   b. by some health care workers in the laboratory.
   c. by health care workers when they anticipate possible contamination with a patient's blood, body fluids, and/or wounds.
   d. by health care workers when they have contact with a patient who is sweating profusely.

9. Hospitalized patients are placed on isolation precautions
   a. to prevent the spread of microorganisms that are highly transmissible or resistant to multiple antibiotics.
   b. to alert hospital staff to the special precautions required to prevent infection from the disease or condition being isolated.
   c. to alert pharmacy personnel and other visitors there is a need to check with the nursing staff for special instructions before entering the room.
   d. all of the above.

10. An occupational exposure that might place a pharmacy worker at risk for exposure to a bloodborne pathogen includes
    a. a needlestick from a needle that was used to inject medication into IV solution.
    b. a needlestick from a needle that was used to draw blood from a vein.
    c. a needlestick from an unused needle.
    d. a finger skin cut from paper in the pharmacy.

11. In the event of possible or actual exposure to a patient's blood or body fluids,
    a. wash the area with bleach and call for help.
    b. cover the area thoroughly with a dressing.
    c. wash skin area immediately with soap and water, or flush the eyes with copious amounts of running water for several minutes.
    d. report to your supervisor during your next scheduled evaluation session.

12. Pulmonary tuberculosis
    a. might be spread to or from a pharmacy worker; therefore, all pharmacy workers in hospitals must be screened.
    b. does not exist in pharmacy personnel; therefore, screening is not required.
    c. is spread by people with tuberculosis infection as evidenced only by a positive tuberculin skin test.
    d. is a disease of third-world countries and not a problem in the United States.

13. Health care workers can infect others
    a. if they work while they have an open, draining wound or abscess.
    b. if they have never had chickenpox and come to work with a rash.
    c. if they have pinkeye or conjunctivitis.
    d. all of the above.

Matching

Match the disease with the type of pathogen causing that disease.

1. _____ athlete's foot   a. bacteria
2. _____ malaria   b. virus
3. _____ Lyme disease   c. fungi
4. _____ hepatitis   d. protozoa
5. _____ pneumonia   e. rickettsia

Fill in the Blank

1. The single most important infection control measure practiced by health care workers is _____.
2. The _____ must contain the proper nutrients to keep the agent alive.
3. _____ transmission occurs as a result of coughing and sneezing.
4. Gloves, gowns, and masks are all examples of _____.
5. Placing patients with the same active infection in the same room for treatments is called _____.

References

American Society of Hospital Pharmacists. (2000). *ASHP technical assistance bulletin on quality assurance for pharmacy-prepared sterile products.* Best Practices for Health System Pharmacy Positions and Guidance Documents of ASHP.

DeCastro, M. A. (2000). Aseptic technique. In *APIC text of infection control and epidemiology* (p. 27). Washington, DC: Association for Professionals in Infection Control and Epidemiology.

Department of Health and Human Services. (2006). *Management of multidrug-resistant organisms in healthcare settings, 2006.* Jane D. Siegel, MD; Emily Rhinehart, RN, MPH, CIC; Marguerite Jackson, PhD; Linda Chiarello, RN, MS; the Healthcare Infection Control Practices Advisory Committee, Centers for Disease Control and Prevention.

Department of Labor, Occupational Safety and Health Administration. Occupational exposure to bloodborne pathogens: Needlesticks and other sharps injuries. *Final Rule*, 29 C.F.R. § 1910. 1030(b) (2001).

Hospital Infection Control Practices Advisory Committee. (1996). Recommendations for isolation precautions in hospitals. *American Journal of Infection Control*, 24, 24–52.

Hospital Infection Control Practices Advisory Committee. (1996). Recommendations for the prevention of nosocomial intravascular device related infections. *American Journal of Infection Control*, 24, 262–293.

Hospital Infection Control Practices Advisory Committee. (1998). Guidelines for infection control in health care personnel. *American Journal of Infection Control*, 26, 289–454.

Intravenous Nurses Society. (1998). Intravenous nursing standards of practice. *Journal of Intravenous Nursing*, 21, S1–S95.

Montgomery, P. A., & Cornish, L. A. (2000). Pharmacy. In *APIC text of infection control and epidemiology* (p. 68). Washington, DC: Association for Professionals in Infection Control and Epidemiology: A Consensus Panel Report. *Infection Control and Epidemiology*, 19, 114–124.

Montgomery, P. A., & Cornish, L. A. (2004). Pharmacy: Diagnostic and therapeutic services. *APIC text of infection control and epidemiology*, 68, 1–8. Washington, DC: Association for Professionals in Infection Control and Epidemiology.

Saljoughian, M. (2004). Disposal of hazardous pharmaceutical waste. *U.S. Pharmacist*. HS-22-HS-24.

Siegel, J. D., Rhinehart, E., Jackson, M., Chiarello, L., and the Healthcare Infection Control Practices Advisory Committee. (2007). *CDC guideline for isolation precautions: Preventing transmission of infectious agents in healthcare settings, June 2007*. Available at www.cdc.gov/ncidod/dhqp/pdf/isolation2007.pdf.

USP Pharmacists' Pharmacopoeia. (2005). *Pharmaceutical compounding-sterile preparations*, Chapter 797 (1st ed.). United States Pharmacopeial Convention: Rockville, MD.

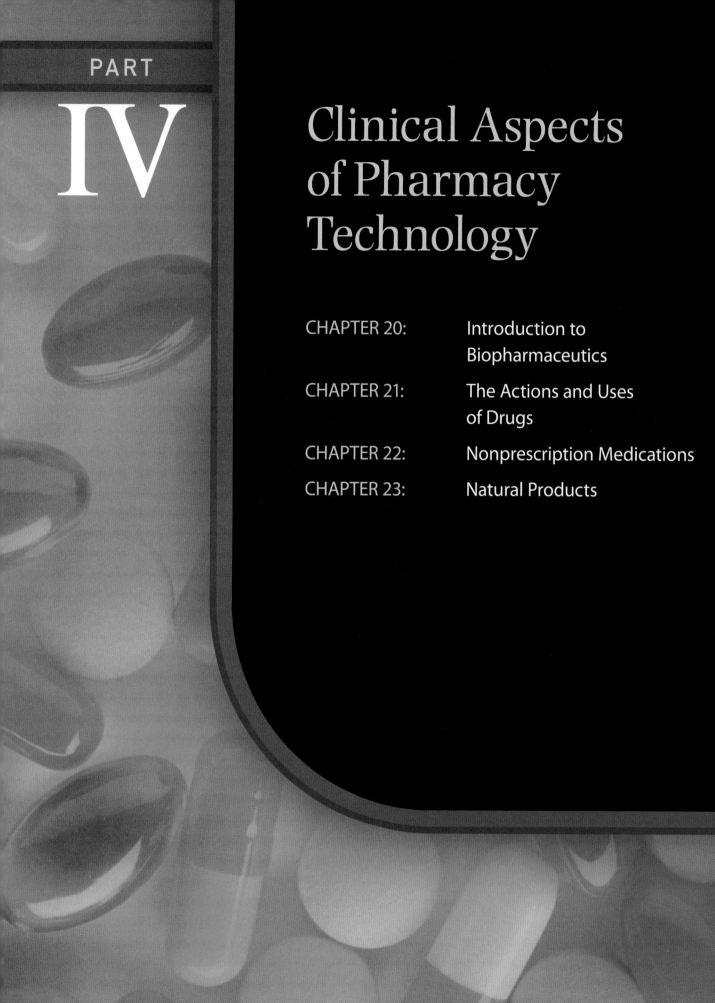

PART IV

Clinical Aspects of Pharmacy Technology

Introduction to Biopharmaceutics

Competencies

Upon completion of this chapter, the reader should be able to

1. Describe key factors that can affect the absorption of a drug.
2. Define bioavailability, and calculate it given the appropriate information.
3. Describe the processes of drug distribution, metabolism, and elimination.
4. List factors that could decrease the bioavailability of a drug administered orally.
5. Define the three parameters obtained from drug plasma concentration-time data to assess bioequivalence.
6. Identify a current reference for obtaining information on bioequivalence of drug products, and use this reference to determine whether two products may be legally substituted.

Key Terms

absorption
area under the plasma concentration-time curve (AUC)
bioavailability
bioequivalence
C_{max}
distribution
elimination
elimination half life
first-pass metabolism
metabolism
T_{max}

Introduction

Biopharmaceutics focuses on the interrelationship between the rate and extent of systemic drug **absorption** (method for drugs to enter the body's circulation) and the physiochemical properties of the drug molecule, the drug dosage form, and the route of administration of the dosage form. **Bioavailability** is the extent of drug absorption, and it is defined as the fraction of an administered dose that ultimately reaches the systemic or whole body circulation. The rate of drug absorption is evaluated by the magnitude or height of the maximum drug concentration (C_{max}) and by how long it takes to reach that maximum concentration (T_{max}).

Many factors can affect the rate and extent of drug absorption from a particular dosage form and, consequently, the therapeutic effect of the drug. These factors include the route of administration, and various anatomical and physiological factors.

Routes of Administration

Drugs are given by many different routes of administration. These routes can be divided into two categories: intravascular and extravascular administration. *Intravascular administration* refers to the direct administration into the vasculature or bloodstream by an intravenous or intra-arterial route. *Extravascular administration* includes all routes of administration in which the drug is not delivered directly to the bloodstream. These routes include oral, sublingual, buccal, intramuscular, subcutaneous, transdermal or percutaneous, pulmonary or inhalation, rectal, and intranasal. Any drug administered extravascularly must first be absorbed from its site of administration to subsequently enter the bloodstream.

Many factors must be considered when determining the best route of administration for a particular drug in an individual patient. These factors range from the physiochemical properties of the drug, anticipated patient adherence, severity of the disease state, concurrent disease states, and cost. There are numerous benefits of oral administration, including ease of administration, patient acceptance, cost, and the ability to formulate modified release dosage forms. Therefore, the most common route of administration is oral, and consequently, a complete understanding of factors affecting absorption from oral dosage forms is very important.

Factors Affecting Drug Absorption from an Extravascular Route

A drug administered by an extravascular route must overcome a number of barriers before it can reach the bloodstream. These barriers can affect both the amount of drug reaching the bloodstream and the rate at which the drug reaches the bloodstream. These barriers include drug release from the dosage form, dissolution of the drug in the surrounding fluid, and diffusion of the drug into the bloodstream. A simple diagram of this process for an oral tablet is presented in Figure 20-1.

Drug release from the dosage form

A solid drug product, such as a tablet, must disintegrate into smaller particles so the drug can be released from the formulation. Other dosage forms can release

FIGURE 20-1

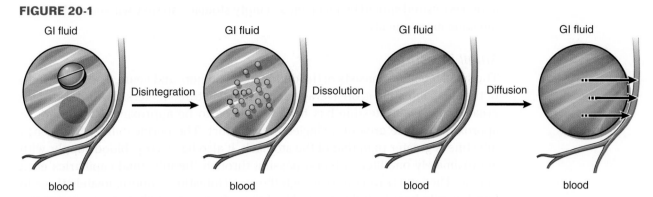

FIGURE 20-1 Extravascular drug absorption.

the drug without disintegrating. These include depot injections, implants, patches, creams, and ointments. The rate and extent that the drug is released from the dosage form directly influences the rate and extent of drug absorption into the bloodstream.

Dissolution

Unless the drug is already in solution when it is released from the dosage form, it must dissolve in the aqueous fluid surrounding it before diffusion can occur. In general, compared to drugs with good solubility in the surrounding biological fluid, a drug with poor solubility will be absorbed more slowly or incompletely.

Diffusion

Once the drug is in solution, it is able to diffuse across biological membranes. However, particular substances in gastrointestinal fluid, including some drugs, may then bind or adsorb the drug and prevent its diffusion. To prevent this type of interaction, the administration of certain combinations of drugs must be separated by several hours (e.g., levothyroxine and cholestyramine). For an oral dosage form, the drug must diffuse across the gastrointestinal epithelium. The lipid nature of biological membranes, including the gastrointestinal epithelium, results in their being more permeable to lipid-soluble substances.

Anatomic and Physiologic Considerations

Since orally administered drugs must diffuse across the epithelium of the gastrointestinal tract, the anatomic and physiologic features of the gastrointestinal tract are very important in determining how much of a drug diffuses. The amount of drug that will diffuse across the epithelium of the gastrointestinal tract is dependent on various factors including the permeability of the epithelium, the surface area, the amount of time the drug is in the area of the epithelium, the blood supply, and the pH and nature of the gastrointestinal contents.

Stomach

The stomach has a relatively small surface area, so diffusion is usually very limited in the stomach. Parietal cells in the stomach secrete hydrochloric acid that yields a very acidic environment with a fasting pH of 2 to 6 and decreasing to 1 to 2 in the presence of food. Food, especially fatty food, inhibits the emptying of the gastric contents into the small intestine. Therefore, most drugs in which a rapid onset of action is desired should be taken on an empty stomach so they will reach the small intestine more quickly.

Small intestine

The small intestine consists of the duodenum, jejunum, and ileum. The total length of the small intestine is on average approximately three meters. The total surface area of the small intestine has been estimated to be approximately 200 m^2, or approximately the area of a singles tennis court. The permeability of the small intestine is greater than that of the stomach. It also has a large blood supply, with approximately one liter of blood passing through the intestinal capillaries each minute. The total travel time through the small intestine is approximately three to four hours in healthy individuals. All of these factors contribute to the enormous absorptive capacity of the small intestine. Therefore, the principal site of absorption for most orally administered drugs is the small intestine.

Duodenum

The duodenum is the first section of the small intestine. Gastric contents are released into the duodenum through the pyloric sphincter. Bicarbonate from the pancreas buffers the contents coming from the stomach to a pH of 4 to 6. The anatomical structure of the duodenum includes villi and microvilli. These are small finger-like processes that project from the surface of the epithelium, yielding a very large surface area. Due in part to this large surface area, the duodenum is the primary site of diffusion for many drugs into the blood.

Jejunum

The jejunum is the center section of the small intestine. Although there is a gradual decrease in the diameter of small intestine and the number of villi and microvilli along its length, the jejunum still has a large surface area. The normal pH of the jejunum is in the range of 5 to 7. Due to these continuing favorable conditions, a significant amount of drug diffusion still occurs in the jejunum.

Ileum

The ileum is the terminal section of the small intestine. The diameter and number of villi and microvilli continue to decrease, but the ileum still has a relatively large surface area. The normal pH of ileum is in the range of 7 to 8. The blood supply to the ileum is much less than the blood supply to the duodenum and jejunum. Drug absorption continues to occur in the ileum, but not the extent that occurs in the duodenum and jejunum.

Large intestine

The large intestine is, on average, slightly more than one meter in length and consists of the cecum, colon, and rectum. The contents of the small intestine are released into the cecum through the ileocecal valve. Due to a lack of villi and microvilli, the large intestine has a much smaller surface area than the small intestine. The contents of the large intestine are also more viscous and begin to take on a semisolid to solid form. These factors limit the capacity for the diffusion of drugs in the large intestine. The pH of the large intestine can vary widely from 4 to 8. The rectum and anal canal are a straight, muscular tube that begins at the terminal colon and extends to the anus. Drug absorption by rectal administration can occur in the rectum via the hemorrhoidal veins.

FIGURE 20-2

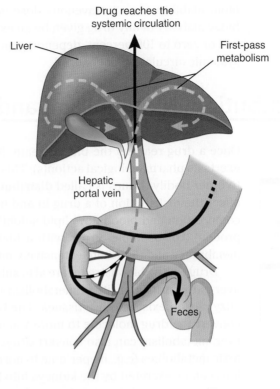

FIGURE 20-2 First-pass metabolism.

First-pass metabolism in the liver

Once an orally administered drug diffuses across the gastrointestinal epithelium into the blood of the hepatic portal vein, the drug is delivered directly to the liver before it can pass into the rest of the body (Figure 20-2). The liver then has the opportunity to metabolize the drug before it reaches the systemic or whole body circulation. This initial **metabolism** is known as **first-pass metabolism** because it occurs during the first pass of the drug through the liver. First-pass metabolism can significantly reduce the total amount of an orally administered drug reaching the systemic circulation, even if the drug diffuses completely from the gastrointestinal tract into the blood. A drug with a very large first-pass effect cannot be administered orally because not enough of the drug will make it into the systemic circulation to achieve its desired therapeutic effect (e.g., nitroglycerin). The drug would have to be administered by routes not subject to first-pass metabolism (e.g., sublingually, transdermally, intravenously).

metabolism the process by which an organism converts food to energy needed for anabolism.

first-pass metabolism occurs when a drug is rapidly metabolized in the liver after oral administration with minimum bioavailability.

Bioavailability

The amount of drug in the dosage form that ultimately clears all these barriers and reaches the systemic circulation unchanged is considered to be bioavailable. The bioavailability (F) of a dosage form can be defined by the following equation:

$$F = \frac{\text{amount of drug reaching the systemic circulation unchanged}}{\text{amount of drug in the administered dosage form}}$$

Since intravenous doses are administered directly into systemic circulation, the bioavailability of an intravenous dose is always 1 or 100 percent. However, the bioavailability of any drug given by an extravascular route can range from zero to one or zero to 100 percent, depending on the amount of the dose that reaches the systemic circulation unchanged.

Drug Distribution, Metabolism, and Elimination

Once a drug reaches the bloodstream, it must then move to the site(s) where it exerts its pharmacological action(s). This movement of drug from the bloodstream to other bodily tissues is called **distribution**. Several characteristics of the tissue affect the distribution of a drug in and out of the tissue (e.g., regional pH, tissue composition and blood flow, lipid solubility of the drug, extent of drug bound to protein). For example, drugs with a high lipid solubility easily cross biological membranes and distribute extensively into adipose or fat tissue.

distribution the movement of a drug from the bloodstream to other bodily tissues.

Drugs in the bloodstream are also subject to metabolism and **elimination**. The liver is the principal site of metabolism in the body, although drug-metabolizing enzymes do exist in other tissues. The typical purpose of drug metabolism is to convert the drug molecule to more water-soluble and inactive metabolites. However, metabolism can also convert drugs to active (e.g., codeine to morphine) or toxic metabolites (e.g., meperidine to normeperidine). Finally, the drug or metabolites can be excreted by the kidneys into the urine and eliminated from the body.

elimination the removal of waste material from the body.

The amount of time it takes to eliminate one-half of the total amount of drug in the blood is the **elimination half-life**. For example, if the concentration in the blood is 10 mg/L and the half-life is 6 hours, then the concentrations presented in Table 20-1 would result if no additional doses were administered. After five half-lives, the drug is clinically considered to be completely eliminated from the body, although a small residual amount would remain.

elimination half-life the amount of time it takes to eliminate one-half of the total amount of drug in the blood.

The half-life of a drug usually is also related to its duration of activity and therefore the allowable length of time between doses. Drugs with short elimination half-lives must be dosed more frequently to maintain adequate amount of drug in the body to achieve the desired therapeutic effect. Alternatively, a modified-release formulation designed to slowly release the drug from the dosage form can be developed for drugs with short half-lives. The drug can then be given less frequently, which increases the consistency and accuracy with which a patient follows the directions for taking the medication. Patient adherence with four-times-

TABLE 20-1 Half-Life and Drug Concentration

TOTAL TIME AFTER MEASURED CONCENTRATION	NUMBER OF HALF-LIVES ELAPSED AFTER MEASURED CONCENTRATION	EXPECTED DRUG CONCENTRATION (mg/L)
0	0	10.0
6	1	5.0
12	2	2.5
18	3	1.2
24	4	0.6
30	5	0.3

The expected drug concentrations from a single dose of a drug with a half-life of 6 hours and a measured drug concentration of 10 mg/L.

a-day regimens has been shown to average about 40 percent, whereas patients receiving once daily and twice-daily regimens have average adherence rates of approximately 70 percent.

Bioavailability Studies

area under the plasma concentration-time curve (AUC) plasma drug concentration can be determined by calculating the rate and extent of systemic absorption, as visualized by the plasma concentration-time curve.

bioequivalence the comparison of the bioavailability of different drug products with the same active ingredient.

Bioavailability studies are generally conducted to determine both the rate and the extent (i.e., absolute bioavailability) to which a drug is absorbed from the dosage form into the systemic circulation. There are three measures of the rate and extent of drug absorption: C_{max} (maximum plasma concentration achieved), T_{max} (time of the maximum plasma concentration), and **AUC (area under the plasma concentration-time curve)**. Information of the rate and extent of systemic absorption from a dosage form can be visualized graphically by the concentration-time profile (Figure 20-3).

During drug product development, bioavailability studies are routinely employed to compare different formulations of the same drug product. The formulation with the most desirable rate and extent of absorption can then be pursued. The desired rate and extent of absorption will depend on the therapeutic application of the drug in the dosage form. For example, it would be desirable for a dosage form of drug used to treat acute pain to provide a fast rate of release and absorption of the drug to quickly relieve the pain. In contrast, a drug needed to control a patient's blood pressure around-the-clock would be appropriate for manufacture as a controlled or slow-release product.

Bioequivalence studies are bioavailability studies specifically comparing two or more formulations of the same dose of the same drug in the same dosage form. The purpose of bioequivalence studies is to determine if the concentration-time profiles produced by test formulations are similar to an innovator's product that is or soon will be off-patent. If a test formulation is statistically found to be bioequivalent in terms of C_{max}, T_{max}, and AUC to the innovator's or reference's formulation, then it is considered to be bioequivalent. Since the innovator's product has already undergone extensive safety and efficacy testing to be approved by the Food and Drug Administration (FDA), it is assumed that the bioequivalent formulation will be

FIGURE 20-3

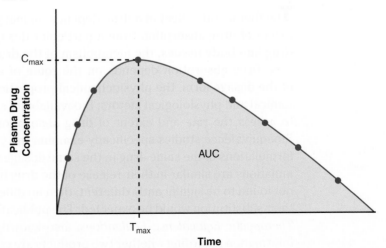

FIGURE 20-3 AUC (area under the plasma concentration-time curve).

unlikely to result in any clinically significant differences in therapeutic responses or adverse events. Bioequivalence studies are one of the requirements for pharmaceutical companies trying to gain FDA-approved generic status for their formulation of off-patent products.

Generic Substitution

To reduce drug costs, most private and public third-party formularies require the substitution of a trade name product with an appropriate generic product, when available. It is important for pharmacists and pharmacy technicians to know where to obtain accurate and current information on the therapeutic equivalence of drug products so that they may choose an appropriate generic product. The publication *Approved Drug Products with Therapeutic Equivalence Evaluations*, also known as the Orange Book, contains a list of all drug products approved by the FDA on the basis of safety and efficacy. This publication also contains therapeutic equivalence codes that provide the user with information regarding whether two products are considered equivalent and thus may be substituted. The Orange Book may be accessed electronically at the following Web site: www.fda.gov/cder/ob, and detailed information on using this reference is available on the same Web site in the preface section.

To use the Orange Book to identify a substitutable generic product, you may search the Electronic Orange Book using the "Proprietary Name" search to determine the ingredient(s). Then use the "Active Ingredient" Search to obtain a list of approved products grouped by dosage form and route of administration. For each group there is a reference listed drug (RLD) to which potential generic products are compared. If there are approved generic products from another manufacturer, the RLD will be "No" and all of the products within the group will have a therapeutic equivalence code (TE code). These TE codes are two-letter designations and can be divided into two general groups. Those that the FDA considers therapeutically equivalent, and that may be substituted, have a TE code that begins with the letter *A* (e.g., AB), and those that are not considered equivalent are designated with the first letter *B*.

Summary

The therapeutic effect of a drug depends on many factors, including the rate and extent of drug absorption from a particular dosage form, the distribution of the drug into body tissues, the metabolism of the drug, and the rate of drug elimination. Drug absorption depends on the route of administration, the formulation of the dosage form, the physiochemical properties of the drug, and various anatomical and physiological factors. Bioavailability studies are commonly employed to assess the rate and extent of drug absorption from different dosage forms. Bioequivalence studies specifically examine the C_{max}, T_{max}, and AUCs of different formulations of the same drug in the same dosage form to determine if the two formulations are similar in their release of the drug from the dosage form. If they are not found to be significantly different, then no differences in clinical outcome from their substitution would be expected. The publication *Approved Drug Products with Therapeutic Equivalence Evaluations*, also known as the Orange Book, contains information regarding whether two products are considered equivalent by the FDA and thus may be substituted.

TEST YOUR KNOWLEDGE

Multiple Choice

1. Bioequivalence studies assess the similarity of plasma concentration-time profiles by comparing
    I.   AUC.
    II. C_{max}.
    III. T_{max}.
    a. I only
    b. I and II only
    c. II and III only
    d. I, II, and III

2. Which of the following therapeutic equivalence (TE) codes indicate(s) a product appropriate for generic substitution?
    I.   AB
    II. AT
    III. BC
    a. I only
    b. III only
    c. I and II only
    d. I, II, and III

3. The bioavailability of a drug administered intravenously is
    a. 0 percent.
    b. 25 percent.
    c. 50 percent.
    d. 100 percent.

4. The elimination half-life of a drug is
    a. the time required to completely eliminate the drug from the body.
    b. the time required to eliminate one-half of the drug in the body.
    c. the time required to absorb one-half of the drug from the dosage form.
    d. the time required to completely absorb the drug from the dosage form.

5. If 1,000 mg of a drug is administered in an oral tablet and 400 mg of the drug is absorbed into the systemic circulation, then the absolute bioavailability (F) is
    a. 20 percent.
    b. 40 percent.
    c. 60 percent.
    d. 80 percent.

6. The bioavailability of an oral tablet could be decreased due to
    I.   incomplete dissolution.
    II. incomplete diffusion.
    III. first-pass metabolism.
    a. I only
    b. I and II only
    c. II and III only
    d. I, II, and III

7. Bioavailability is defined as
   a. the amount of an administered dose that reaches the systemic circulation.
   b. the fraction of an administered dose that fails to reach the systemic circulation.
   c. the amount of an administered dose that fails to reach the systemic circulation.
   d. the fraction of an administered dose that reaches the systemic circulation.

8. Which of the following is/are extravascular route(s) of administration?
   I.   oral
   II. subcutaneous
   III. intravenous
       a. I only
       b. III only
       c. I and II only
       d. I, II, and III

9. Which one of the following represents the correct order of events an oral dosage form must go through for the drug to reach the bloodstream?
   a. disintegration, dissolution, diffusion
   b. dissolution, disintegration, diffusion
   c. disintegration, diffusion, dissolution
   d. diffusion, dissolution, disintegration

10. The principal site of absorption for most orally administered drugs is the
    a. liver.
    b. stomach.
    c. small intestine.
    d. large intestine.

Matching

Please select the appropriate term and match it with the correct description.

1. _____ Movement of the drug from the blood to other body tissues.

2. _____ The purpose of this process is to convert the drug molecule to more water-soluble and inactive metabolites.

3. _____ Method for drugs to enter the body's circulation.

4. _____ This term refers to two drugs that have comparable concentration-time profiles when administered by the same route.

5. _____ One of the three measures of the rate and extent of drug absorption, with C_{max} (maximum plasma concentration achieved) and T_{max} (time of the maximum plasma concentration).

a. absorption

b. area under the plasma concentration-time curve (AUC)

c. bioavailability

d. bioequivalence

e. distribution

f. elimination

g. half-life

h. metabolism

Fill In The Blank

1. _____ is the fraction of an administered dose that ultimately reaches the systemic or whole body circulation.

2. A _____ drug product must disintegrate into smaller particles so the drug can be released from the formulation.

3. The liver has the opportunity to metabolize the drug before it reaches the systemic or whole body circulation; this is called the _____.

4. This movement of drug from the bloodstream to other bodily tissues is called _____.

5. _____ studies are bioavailability studies specifically comparing two or more formulations of the same dose of the same drug in the same dosage form.

References

Allen, L., Popovich, N., & Ansel, H. (2005). *Pharmaceutical dosage forms and drug delivery systems* (8th ed.). Baltimore: Lippincott Williams & Wilkins.

Burton, M., Shaw, L., Schentag, J., & Evans, W. (2006). *Applied pharmacokinetics & pharmacodynamics: Principles of therapeutic drug monitoring* (4th ed.). Baltimore: Lippincott Williams & Wilkins.

Dipiro, J., Spruill, W., Wade, W., Blouin, R., & Pruemer, J. (2005). *Concepts in clinical pharmacokinetics* (4th ed.). Bethesda, MD: ASHP.

Seeley, R., Stephens, T., & Tate P. (2007). *Anatomy and physiology* (8th ed.). New York: McGraw-Hill.

Shargel, L., Wu-Pong, S., & Yu, A. (2004). *Applied biopharmaceutics and pharmacokinetics* (5th ed.). New York: McGraw-Hill.

The Actions and Uses of Drugs

Competencies

Upon completion of this chapter, the reader should be able to

1. Describe the advantages and disadvantages of the various routes of drug administration.
2. Recognize the standard abbreviations for the various routes of administration.
3. Describe the major factors that affect variability in drug response.
4. Describe the role of drug therapy in some common disease states.
5. Know the therapeutic category for commonly prescribed drugs.
6. Match the generic and brand names of commonly prescribed medications.

Key Terms

adherence
extravascular
intravascular
pharmacogenetic polymorphism
prodrug

Introduction

Drugs are prescribed to treat a wide variety of medical conditions; therefore, the knowledge of the action and use of individual drugs is critical. Responses to the actions of drugs are varied, and the many factors contributing to a drug's actions will be addressed here. This chapter also describes the use of drugs through the major therapeutic classes of drugs and categorizes drugs with both their trade and generic names.

Factors Affecting Drug Response

Once drug therapy is initiated in a patient, many factors will affect the outcome of the drug therapy. All of these factors combined can result in large patient variability, which is the difference in drug response from patient to patient. The route of administration is one factor that can significantly affect drug response. Each route offers advantages and disadvantages that must be taken into consideration. There are also many patient-specific factors that affect drug response, including patient adherence with administration directions, drug-food interactions, drug-drug interactions, drug-disease interactions, and the age, weight, and genetics of patients.

Route of Administration

Drug dosage forms are given by various routes of administration. Although the pharmacological effect of the same drug administered by different routes should be similar, the route can affect both the speed at which the desired effect is attained and the intensity of the effect. These differences between the various routes of administration are covered in detail in Chapter 20.

Intravenous

intravascular
injection into a blood vessel.

extravascular
outside of the blood vessels or lymphatic vascular channel.

Directly injecting a sterile drug into a vein is known as the *intravenous* (or **intravascular**) route of administration, which is abbreviated as "IV" on a prescription. Advantages to intravenous administration of drugs include a more rapid onset of drug action—which can be extremely valuable in emergency situations—and allowing the use of drugs that may not be suitable for **extravascular** administration (outside the body vessels) due to poor absorption into the bloodstream or significant first-pass metabolism. Several disadvantages to intravenous administration include possible pain, irritation, and increased risk of infection at the injection site and in the bloodstream. Pantoprazole can be administered via the intravenous route as a treatment for increased stomach acid production.

Intra-arterial

Drugs are occasionally injected into the arterial side of the bloodstream. This route is usually reserved for delivery of some anticancer drugs and diagnostic agents to a particular tissue or organ for localized effects. Otherwise, it offers the advantages and disadvantages of intravenous administration. Cisplatin is an example of a drug that can be administered via the intra-arterial route to treat various types of cancer.

Oral

For oral administration, the drug dosage form is placed into the mouth and swallowed; it is abbreviated as "po" on a prescription. This route is the most common, convenient, and economical route for delivery of many drugs. In addition, dosage forms can be designed to offer sustained or prolonged action of the drug, which decreases the frequency with which the drug must be taken. Disadvantages include limited absorption of some drugs, destruction of some drugs by digestive enzymes or the acidic pH of the stomach, and significant metabolism of some drugs during first-pass metabolism. When a drug is taken orally, it must pass through the liver before it can reach the systemic bloodstream. Therefore, the liver has the first chance to metabolize the drug before it reaches the rest of the body. Ibuprofen is often taken orally for pain relief and fever reduction.

Buccal, sublingual, and translingual

Buccal, sublingual, and *translingual* routes represent the drug dosage form being placed into the mouth without being swallowed. For buccal administration, the dosage form is placed between the cheek and gum. For sublingual administration, the dosage form is placed under the tongue to dissolve and is abbreviated as "SL" on a prescription. For translingual administration, the drug is sprayed directly onto the tongue or mouth tissue. These routes of administration offer several advantages, including rapid absorption and, therefore, rapid onset of drug action. The direct absorption into the bloodstream prevents the drug from encountering the acidic environment of the stomach and first-pass metabolism. One disadvantage is that unless properly instructed, patients may swallow the medication before it is completely absorbed. Nicotine gum is used for quick absorption through the cheek into the bloodstream. Nitroglycerin preparations are often administered sublingually and translingually for rapid relief of anginal chest pain, but if the dosage form is swallowed, nitroglycerin will undergo a very large first-pass metabolism and be ineffective.

Intramuscular

Intramuscular administration means a sterile drug is directly injected into a skeletal muscle; it is abbreviated as "IM" on a prescription. Common sites include the deltoid (shoulder) and gluteus maximus (buttocks). Absorption of the drug occurs as the drug diffuses from the site of injection into surrounding muscle fibers and into the blood vessels in those fibers. The rate of absorption into the bloodstream depends on the blood flow to the muscle. For example, the deltoid has a higher blood flow than the gluteus maximus; therefore, absorption is normally quicker from the deltoid muscle. The rate of absorption is also dependent on the formulation of the injection. For example, aqueous or water-based injections are generally more rapidly absorbed than oil-based ones. Advantages include the potential for a sustained release while bypassing gastrointestinal absorption problems and first-pass metabolism. As with intravenous administration, disadvantages include pain, irritation, and risk of infection at the injection site. Tetanus vaccinations are administered as intramuscular injections.

Subcutaneous

Subcutaneous administration means the injection of a sterile drug just beneath the surface of the skin, and is abbreviated as "subc," "subq," "SC," or "SQ" on a prescription. This route can only be used for drugs that are not irritating to the tissue and can be given in a small volume. The rate of absorption varies with blood flow to the area of the injection and formulation of the product. Advantages include the potential for a sustained release while bypassing gastrointestinal absorption problems and first-pass metabolism. Disadvantages may include pain and irritation at the injection site. Insulin is injected under the skin, or subcutaneously.

Topical and transdermal

Topical and *transdermal administration* involves applying a drug directly on the surface of the skin and is abbreviated as "top." on a prescription. Topical administration is used for local drug effects in the skin and is most commonly administered as a lotion, cream, or ointment. Triamcinolone cream is commonly used as a topical steroid cream. Transdermal administration is mainly used to deliver a drug into the bloodstream for systemic effects. However, transdermal patches can be used for local action. A transdermal patch is designed to control the release of drug and, therefore, provide a sustained absorption of the drug into the bloodstream. In addition to the potential for sustained effects, transdermal products bypass any problems with gastrointestinal absorption and first-pass metabolism. A selegiline patch has recently been made available for transdermal use, used as an adjunct in the treatment of Parkinson's patients.

Inhalation

Inhalation administration delivers a sterile drug directly into the lungs. This route is mostly used for local effects in the lungs, but is sometimes used for absorption of a drug into the bloodstream for systemic effects. The advantages of this route include a rapid onset of activity and avoidance of gastrointestinal absorption problems and first-pass metabolism. In addition, there are few-to-no systemic side effects when this route is used for local effects. Albuterol is often used via inhalation for the treatment of asthma and chronic obstructive pulmonary disease (COPD). There could be a slight increase in heart rate (systemic), but the key local effect is the bronchodilation.

Rectal

Rectal administration means insertion of a drug suppository directly into the rectum and is abbreviated as "rect." or "PR" on a prescription. This route is used for either local effects in the rectum or for absorption of drug into the bloodstream for systemic effects. This route is an inexpensive alternative to the oral route for unconscious or vomiting patients when a systemic effect is desired. Advantages include a relatively low cost while bypassing gastrointestinal absorption problems and first-pass metabolism. The disadvantages of this route can include variable absorption and patients' dislike of inserting dosage forms into the rectum. The administration of prochlorperazine (Compazine®) suppositories for the management of nausea and vomiting is a good example of the effective use of the rectal route of administration.

Vaginal

Vaginal administration involves the insertion of a drug directly into the vagina. This route is primarily used for local vaginal disorders, but some drugs can be absorbed into the bloodstream. Many vaginal preparations are antifungal agents in the form of creams, gels, ointments, and suppositories. Metronidazole is used as a vaginal cream and gel to treat vaginal bacterial infections.

Intranasal

Intranasal administration means administering a drug directly into the nasal cavity. This route is used for either local effects in the nasal passages or for absorption of drugs into the bloodstream for systemic effects. The advantages of this route for systemic effects are the avoidance of gastrointestinal absorption problems and first-pass metabolism. When used for local effects, such as decongestant sprays, there are minimal systemic side effects. Phenylephrine is used as a nasal decongestant and causes constriction of the nasal blood vessels, decreasing congestion while only minimally causing an increase in heart rate.

Ophthalmic and otic

Ophthalmic and *otic administration* refers to giving a sterile drug directly into the eye or ear, respectively. Both of these routes are used for local drug effects that minimize or eliminate any systemic side effects. Ciprofloxacin preparations to treat bacterial infections are available for the ears and eyes.

Patient Variability

In addition to variability in drug response due to the route of administration, many patient-specific factors can affect an individual patient's response to drug therapy. The patient-specific factors include adherence, drug-food interactions, drug-drug interactions, drug-disease interactions, age, weight, or genetics.

Adherence

adherence the act of complying with prescribed directions.

Adherence is the consistency or accuracy with which patients follow the prescribed directions for taking their medication. A general lack of adherence is a serious public health problem with major health and economic implications. Studies report adherence rates in adults range from about 8 percent to 93 percent, depending on the medication and the frequency with which the medication should be taken. If not taken properly, the best possible therapeutic effect of the drug will not be achieved.

Drug-food interactions

Drug-food interactions occur when the presence of food results in altered absorption of orally administered drugs. Drug-food interactions can be a significant source of patient variability for certain drugs and can occur by several mechanisms. Some foods, particularly those high in fat, can significantly slow the rate of stomach emptying into the small intestine, thereby extending the drug's presence in the acidic pH of the stomach. The presence of food also influences the pH of the stomach. For these reasons, certain medications must be taken either with or without food, according to the instructions of the manufacturer. One example of a drug-food interaction is the intake of foods rich in vitamin K (e.g., spinach), which can counteract the blood-thinning effects of warfarin (Coumadin).

Drug-drug interactions

Drug-drug interactions occur when a patient taking two or more drugs concurrently has an altered response to one or more of these drugs caused by the other drug(s). The effect of drug-drug interactions can be insignificant, or it can decrease the therapeutic effect or increase the incidence and severity of side effects for one or more of the drugs the patient is taking. The interactions can be due to alterations in the absorption, distribution, metabolism, and elimination of one or more of the interacting drugs or a pharmacologic interaction (i.e., additive, synergistic, or antagonistic effects).

Absorption. Altered drug absorption due to the interaction of two or more drugs can occur by several mechanisms. The rate and extent of absorption of drugs depends on many factors that can be altered by the presence of other drugs. Drugs administered to elevate the pH in the stomach can affect the absorption of certain drugs. Absorption can also be altered by the binding of two or more drugs in the gastrointestinal tract, thereby preventing the drug's absorption. Finally, drugs that alter stomach emptying rate or gastrointestinal motility can affect the absorption of certain drugs by affecting the amount of time the drug takes to be absorbed. For example, there can be a delay in onset of the analgesic effect of acetaminophen or aspirin when taken with a meal due to a delay in gastric emptying.

Distribution. Altered drug distribution due to the interaction of two or more drugs normally occurs due to changes in plasma protein binding of drugs. Some drugs are highly bound to proteins in the blood. Interacting drugs that are also highly bound to these same proteins can competitively displace the other drug from its protein binding sites. This displacement leads to more unbound drug in the bloodstream, which is free to diffuse out of the bloodstream into other tissue, which is the process of distribution. The net effect of this interaction is an increase in the distribution of the drug into tissues outside of the bloodstream. In addition, more unbound drug translates to more pharmacologic activity, which can lead to increased side effects. Quinidine (Quin-Tab) alters the distribution of digoxin (Lanoxin), so more digoxin distributes into the bloodstream and can result in higher than normal digoxin concentrations.

Metabolism. Altered drug metabolism due to the interaction of two or more drugs can occur by two primary mechanisms: enzyme induction and inhibition. Most drugs are metabolized to some extent by various enzymes, including the cytochrome P450 system in the liver and other parts of the body. These enzymes can have increased or decreased activity due to the presence of one or more drugs, as well as non-drug substances. These increases and decreases in metabolism due to other drugs are known as *enzyme induction* and *enzyme inhibition*, and the drugs causing these changes in activity are known as *inducers* and *inhibitors*. Enzyme induction can lead to lower blood concentrations of drugs metabolized by that enzyme, which can result in a decreased or lack of therapeutic effect. Enzyme inhibition can lead to higher blood concentrations of drugs metabolized by that enzyme, which can result in an increased incidence of side effects. For example, fluconazole (Diflucan) inhibits the metabolism of phenytoin, which can lead to higher than normal concentrations of phenytoin.

Elimination. Altered drug elimination due to the interaction of two or more drugs can occur by several mechanisms. The kidney is the primary organ for drug elimination, and it is involved in both the elimination of the administered drug (i.e., parent drug) and its metabolites. Interacting drugs may increase or decrease the elimination of certain drugs by the kidneys. As with altered metabolism, these changes in elimination can lead to decreased drug concentrations in the blood and a corresponding decrease or lack of therapeutic effect, or increased drug concentrations and a corresponding increased incidence of side effects.

Additive, synergistic, and antagonistic pharmacologic interactions. Two or more drugs can combine to exert their individual pharmacological effects in an additive manner. Two or more drugs can also combine to exert their pharmacological effects in a manner resulting in an overall effect that is more than what would result from a simple additive effect, analogous to "one plus one equals three." This type of interaction is known as a *synergistic interaction*. An *antagonist interaction* results when one or more drugs inhibit the pharmacological effect of another drug. These interactions can be beneficial and used in the treatment of a patient's medical condition. But these interactions can also decrease the effectiveness of the patient's drug therapy if they are not recognized. All drug interactions should be carefully considered since the result can be dangerous. For example, the combination of sildenafil (Viagra) and nitrates (e.g., isosorbide dinitrate, isosorbide mononitrate, and nitroglycerin) can cause a severe and potentially deadly drop in blood pressure.

Drug-disease interactions

Drug-disease interactions occur when a patient's disease state results in altered drug response. Therefore, the overall health of the patient can significantly affect the response to drug therapy. The liver is the primary location for drug metabolism, so diseases such as hepatitis and alcoholic liver disease can result in decreased drug metabolism (e.g., procainamide). The kidney is the primary organ of drug elimination, so diseases such as acute and chronic renal failure can result in decreased drug elimination (e.g., gentamicin). Both of these examples would lead to higher concentrations of drugs in the blood, which can increase side effects and the drug's effectiveness.

Age and weight

Weight progressively increases from birth through adolescence, increases more slowly through adulthood, and then gradually declines in the elderly. Body water, muscle mass, and organ mass are all related to body weight. In addition, many bodily functions, including organ blood flow and organ function, are related to body weight. Some individuals may be considerably underweight or overweight compared to normal individuals. All these factors can lead to the requirement of greatly different doses to achieve the desired therapeutic response, depending on an individual patient's age and weight. For example, elderly patients are normally started on lower than normal doses of many medications.

pharmaco-genetic polymorphism
a genetic variation accounting for changes in severely decreased drug metabolism, or when a normal dose is given, toxic concentrations can result.

Genetics

Genetic variation can account for large variability in drug response. Genetic variation in drug-metabolizing enzymes usually results in severely decreased drug metabolism. These genetic variations are known as **pharmacogenetic polymorphisms**, and they have been identified in the cytochrome P450 system and other drug-metabolizing enzymes. The changes in drug metabolism due to pharmacogenetic polymorphisms can be very dramatic and can result in toxic concentrations of drugs when normal doses of the medications are taken.

prodrug a class of drugs; the pharmacological action of which results from their biotransformation in the body.

Pharmacogenetic polymorphisms can also result in a lack of therapeutic effect if the administered drug is a **prodrug**, meaning it requires metabolic conversion in the body to an active compound. Codeine is a good example of a prodrug that requires conversion to morphine by cytochrome P450 2D6 to exert its analgesic activity. However, 8 percent to 14 percent of Caucasians have pharmacogenetic polymorphisms of this particular enzyme and, therefore, cannot convert codeine to the active analgesic, morphine. Unmetabolized codeine results in a lack of pain relief and may cause nausea and vomiting.

Common Disorders and Associated Drug Therapies

This section provides information on drugs and their therapeutic category. It is divided into bone and joint disorders, cardiovascular disorders, endocrinologic disorders, gastrointestinal disorders, gynecologic and obstetric disorders, infectious diseases, neurologic disorders, psychiatric disorders, and respiratory disorders.

The list of medications is not all-inclusive, but attention has been placed on the most-prescribed drugs in each category. Some prescription drugs are available without a prescription, but are usually in lower strengths as compared to their prescription counterparts. These over-the-counter (OTC) products will be marked with an asterisk (*).

Bone and Joint Disorders

Bone and joint disorders including osteoporosis, osteoarthritis, and pain can often be effectively treated with medication. What once was assumed to be simply associated with getting older can now be treated and increase patients' quality of life.

Osteoporosis

Osteoporosis is a condition of diminished bone density. Many factors can contribute to osteoporosis, but the result is bone mass being lost faster than it is being formed. This decrease in bone density leads to an increased risk of fractures. Osteoporosis is most common in elderly women, but also occurs in men. Treatment and prevention of osteoporosis includes bisphosphonates, calcium supplements, estrogens, and vitamin D therapy. A list of drugs used to treat osteoporosis can be found in Table 21-1.

Osteoarthritis and pain

Almost 50 percent of individuals over age 65 are afflicted with osteoarthritis. Osteoarthritis is marked by a degeneration of cartilage, primarily in weight-bearing joints. The lack of cushioning between articulating bones results in inflammation, mild to moderate pain, and limited range of motion. Appropriate pain management is vital when treating osteoarthritis. It is best to begin therapy with an agent that will have the fewest side effects. These usually include aspirin, acetaminophen, and nonsteroidal anti-inflammatory drugs. Narcotic analgesics are rarely used in osteoarthritis, but are usually reserved for moderate to severe pain from other causes. Analgesics are often taken orally, while there are some available as transdermal and injectable products. Anesthetics can also be used for acute and chronic pain. These agents can be injected or applied topically and work by blocking painful nerve impulses. Pain medications used in the treatment of osteoarthritis are found in Table 21-2.

TABLE 21-1 Drugs Used to Treat Osteoporosis

GENERIC NAME	COMMON BRAND NAME(S)
Bisphosphonates	
alendronate and combinations	Fosamax, Fosamax Plus D
ibandronate	Boniva
risedronate and combinations	Actonel, Actonel with Calcium
Estrogens	
conjugated estrogens	Premarin
esterified estrogens	Estratab, Menest
mircronized estradiol	Estrace
transdermal estrogen	Climara, Estraderm, Vivelle
Miscellaneous agents	
calcitonin	Miacalcin
calcium*	Tums, Viactiv, Oscal, Citracal
raloxifene	Evista
vitamin D*	Various

*Over-the-counter product

TABLE 21-2 Pain Medication

GENERIC NAME	COMMON BRAND NAME(S)
Analgesics (non-narcotic)	
acetaminophen*	Tylenol
acetylsalicylic acid*	Aspirin
celebrex	Celecoxib
diclofenac	Voltaren
ketoprofen*	Orudis KT
ibuprofen*	Advil, Motrin
indomethacin	Indocin
nambumetone	Relafen
naproxen*	Naprosyn
naproxen sodium	Aleve, Anaprox
Analgesics (narcotic)	
codeine (and combinations)	Tylenol with Codeine #3
fentanyl	Duragesic
hydrocodone combinations	Lorcet, Lortab, Vicodin
hydromorphone	Dilaudid
meperidine	Demerol
methadone	Dolophine
morphine	MS Contin, MS IR
oxycodone (and combinations)	OxyIR, Percocet, Tylox, Percodan
oxycodone	OxyContin
propoxyphene (and combinations)	Darvon, Darvocet-N 100
pentazocine	Talwin, Talwin NX
tramadol (and combination with acetaminophen)	Ultram, Ultracet

*Over-the-counter product

(Continued)

TABLE 21-2 Pain Medication (continued)

GENERIC NAME	COMMON BRAND NAME(S)
Anesthetics	
bupivacaine	Marcaine
dibucaine	Nupercaine
halothane	Fluothane
lidocaine	Xylocaine
procaine	Novocain
propofol	Diprivan
thiopental	Pentothal
tetracaine	Pontocaine

Cardiovascular Disorders

Cardiovascular disorders are the number one cause of death in the United States, according to the National Vital Statistics Report published by the Centers for Disease Control and Prevention. These disorders include arrhythmias, coronary artery disease, hyperlipidemia, and hypertension.

Arrhythmias

An arrhythmia is a disruption in the heart's normal beating or rhythmic pattern. This abnormal electrical conduction can occur in different areas of the heart. Some common examples of arrhythmias are sinus bradycardia, sinus or ventricular tachycardia, atrial fibrillation, and ventricular fibrillation. Antiarrhythmic drugs are used to treat these arrhythmias (Table 21-3) and are classified into four types based on their electrophysiological properties.

TABLE 21-3 Classifications of Antiarrhythmic Drugs

GENERIC NAME	COMMON BRAND NAME(S)
Type 1A	
disopyramide	Norpace
procainamide	Procanbid, Pronestyl
quinidine	Quin-Tab, Quinaglute, Quinidex
Type 1B	
lidocaine	Xylocaine
mexiletine	Mexitil
tocainide	Tonocard
Type 1C	
flecainide	Tambocor
propafenone	Rythmol
Type 2	
beta-adrenergic blockers	(see Table 21-6)
Type 3	
amiodarone	Cordarone, Pacerone
bretylium	Bretylate
dofetilide	Tikosyn
sotalol	Betapace, Betapace AF

TABLE 21-3 Classifications of Antiarrhythmic Drugs (continued)

GENERIC NAME	COMMON BRAND NAME(S)
Type 4	
diltiazem	Cardizem, Dilacor XR, Tiazac
verapamil	Calan, Covera, Isoptin, Verelan
Miscellaneous agents	
adenosine	Adenocard
digoxin	Lanoxin

Coronary artery disease

Coronary artery disease (CAD) develops as atherosclerotic plaques form on the inner walls of cardiac vessels. There are modifiable and nonmodifiable risk factors involved in the development of CAD. Angina pectoris is a common condition that is associated with coronary artery disease. When the vessels of the heart become blocked with plaque or fatty material, the oxygen demand of the body may not be able to be met. Vasodilators, calcium channel blockers, and beta-adrenergic blockers are often used in the treatment of angina pectoris. A thrombus, or clot, can also form in vessels and block blood flow through those vessels. Antithrombotic agents can prevent platelet aggregation and reduce the likelihood of clot formation. Thrombolytic agents are used to dissolve previously formed clots. A list of agents used in the treatment of coronary artery disease can be found in Table 21-4.

TABLE 21-4 Agents Used in Coronary Artery Disease

GENERIC NAME	COMMON BRAND NAME(S)
Antithrombotic agents	
argatroban	Argatroban
dalteparin	Fragmin
enoxaparin	Lovenox
fondaparinux	Arixtra
heparin	Hep-Lock
Coumadin thrombolytic agents	
alteplase	Activase
streptokinase	Streptase
urokinase	Abbokinase
Calcium channel blockers	
amlodipine	Norvasc
diltiazem	Cardizem, Dilacor, Tiazac
felodipine	Plendil
nifedipine	Adalat CC, Procardia XL
verapamil	Calan, Covera, Isoptin, Verelan
Nitrates	
isosorbide dinitrate	Isordil
isosorbide mononitrate	Imdur
nitroglycerin	Nitrostat, Nitro-Bid

Hyperlipidemia

Hyperlipidemia is an abnormally high concentration of lipids, or cholesterol, in the blood. Cholesterol is synthesized in the liver and is contained in many foods. The human body can use cholesterol as an energy source or store it. Cholesterol and triglycerides are two major lipids found in the body. A total cholesterol level of less than 200 mg/dL is desirable. Hyperlipidemia increases patients' chances of developing coronary artery disease (CAD) and peripheral vascular disease (PVD). Several classes of drugs with different mechanisms of action are used to treat hyperlipidemia. Bile acid resins bind with bile acid to inhibit cholesterol absorption and storage. Fibrates cause an increase in enzymes, which results in an increase in cholesterol metabolism. HMG-CoA reductase is an important enzyme that catalyzes in vivo cholesterol synthesis. HMG-CoA reductase inhibitors target this enzyme and inhibit its activity. Drugs used to lower cholesterol are listed in Table 21-5.

Hypertension

Hypertension, or high blood pressure, is a constant elevation in the systolic or diastolic blood pressure. Blood pressure is considered to be high when the systolic pressure is greater than 140 mmHg and the diastolic pressure is greater than 90 mmHg.

Numerous mechanisms cause elevations in blood pressure. Drugs with different mechanisms of action can be utilized to reduce blood pressure effectively in individual patients. Alpha-adrenergic blockers hinder the nerve conduction to the

TABLE 21-5 Drugs Used to Treat Hyperlipidemia

GENERIC NAME	COMMON BRAND NAME(S)
Bile acid resins	
cholestyramine	Questran, Questran Light
colestipol	Colestid
colesevelam	Welchol
Fibrates	
fenofibrate	Tricor
gemfibrozil	Lopid
HMG-CoA Reductase inhibitors	
atorvastatin	Lipitor
lovastatin	Mevacor
pravastatin	Pravachol
rosuvastatin	Crestor
simvastatin	Zocor
Miscellaneous agents	
amlodipine and atorvastatin	Caduet
ezetimibe	Zetia
niacin*	Niaspan

*Over-the-counter product

heart and block nerve impulses that would make the heart beat faster. Angiotensin-converting enzyme inhibitors (ACE inhibitors) and angiotensin II receptor blockers (ARBs) work against the body's own mechanisms for raising blood pressure. Beta-adrenergic blockers regulate the heart rate. Calcium channel blockers weaken muscle contractions and decrease the workload placed on the heart. Diuretics lower blood pressure by lowering the volume of the vasculature, and vasodilators relax the walls of blood vessels. All of these agents are commonly used in treating hypertension (Table 21-6).

TABLE 21-6 Drugs Used to Treat Hypertension

GENERIC NAME	COMMON BRAND NAME(S)
Alpha-adrenergic blockers	
doxazosin	Cardura
prazosin	Minipress
terazosin	Hytrin
Angiotensin-converting enzyme inhibitors	
benazepril	Lotensin
captopril	Capoten
enalapril	Vasotec
fosinopril	Monopril
lisinopril	Prinivil, Zestril
quinapril	Accupril
ramipril	Altace
Angiotensin II receptor blockers	
candesartan	Atacand
irbesartan	Avapro
losartan	Cozaar
telmisartan	Micardis
valsartan	Diovan
Beta-adrenergic blockers	
atenolol	Tenormin
bisoprolol	Ziac
carvedilol	Coreg, Coreg CR
labetalol	Normodyne, Trandate
metoprolol	Lopressor, Toprol XL
nadolol	Corgard
propranolol	Inderal, Inderal LA
Calcium channel blockers	
amlodipine	Norvasc
diltiazem	Cardizem, Dilacor, Tiazac
felodipine	Plendil
nifedipine	Adalat CC, Procardia XL
verapamil	Calan, Covera, Isoptin, Verelan

(Continued)

TABLE 21-6 Drugs Used to Treat Hypertension (continued)

GENERIC NAME	COMMON BRAND NAME(S)
Diuretics	
bumetanide	Bumex
furosemide	Lasix
hydrochlorothiazide	Esidrix, HydroDIURIL, Oretic
spironolactone	Aldactone
triamterene and hydrochlorothiazide	Dyazide, Maxzide
Renin inhibitor	
aliskiren	Tekturna
Vasodilators	
hydralazine	Apresoline
minoxidil	Loniten
sodium nitroprusside	Nitropress
Miscellaneous agents	
clonidine	Catapres, Catapres-TTS
methyldopa	Aldomet
potassium chloride	K-Dur, Klor-Con, Micro-K, Slow-K

Endocrine Disorders

Common endocrine disorders include diabetes and thyroid disorders. These disorders are the result of inappropriate hormone release. Drug therapy can help control these disorders and improve the patients' quality of life.

Diabetes mellitus

Diabetes mellitus is the body's inability to either produce or efficiently use insulin, resulting in high blood sugar, or hyperglycemia. Type I diabetes is characterized by the inability to produce insulin. Type II diabetes differs in that the body cannot efficiently utilize the insulin that it makes. Type I diabetics are usually diagnosed during adolescence, while Type II diabetes usually manifests later in adulthood. The goal of therapy in diabetes mellitus is to maintain blood sugar levels within 80 to 120 mg/dL. Insulin is used more often by Type I diabetics as compared to Type II diabetics. However, both populations can utilize oral hypoglycemic agents to control blood glucose concentrations. Drugs used to treat diabetes are listed in Table 21-7.

Thyroid disorders

The thyroid gland plays a crucial role in growth, body development, and metabolism. Thyroid disorders involve either producing excess thyroid hormone or failing to produce an adequate amount.

Hyperthyroidism is an increase in production of thyroid hormone. *Hypothyroidism* is a decrease in thyroid hormone production. Treatment consists of suppressing thyroid hormone production in hyperthyroidism, or supplying an exogenous source of thyroid hormone for hypothyroidism. Drugs used for this purpose are listed in Table 21-8.

TABLE 21-7   Drugs Used to Treat Diabetes Mellitus

GENERIC NAME	COMMON BRAND NAME(S)
Insulin preparations	
intermediate-acting insulin	Humulin N, NPH-N, Novolin N
lente	Humulin L, Novolin L
long-acting insulin	Humulin U, Lantus, Levemir
rapid-acting insulin	Humalog, NovoLog, Apidra
NPH-regular combinations	Humulin 70/30, Novolin 70/30
short-acting insulin	Humulin R, Novolin R
Oral hypoglycemic agents	
acarbose	Precose
chlorpropamide	Diabinese
glimeperide	Amaryl
glipizide	Glucotrol, Glucotrol XL
glyburide	DiaBeta, Glynase, Micronase
metformin	Glucophage, Glucophage XR
nateglinide	Starlix
pioglitazone	Actos
repaglinide	Prandin
rosiglitazone	Avandia
sitagliptin	Januvia
Combination oral agents	
glyburide and metformin	Glucovance
rosiglitazone and glimeperide	Avandaryl
rosiglitazone and metformin	Avandamet
sitagliptin and metformin	Janumet

TABLE 21-8   Drugs Used to Treat Thyroid Disorders

GENERIC NAME	COMMON BRAND NAME(S)
Hyperthyroidism agents	
methimazole	Tapazole
propylthiouracil	Propyl-Thyracil
Hypothyroidism agents	
levothyroxine	Levothroid, Levoxyl, Synthroid
liothyronine	Cytomel
liotrix	Thyrolar
thyroid USP	Armour Thyroid

Gastrointestinal Disorders

Common gastrointestinal disorders include diarrhea, constipation, and gastro-esophageal reflux disease.

Diarrhea and constipation

Diarrhea is an abnormally frequent occurrence of watery or semisolid stools. Diarrhea can be caused by disease, drugs, infection, and toxins. This increased frequency of watery defecation can lead to dehydration. Treatment consists of agents that can absorb the excess water or slow down the intestinal motility. Constipation is a decrease in stool frequency. This decreased frequency could be caused by certain medications. It is also often directly related to dietary fiber consumption. Common treatments of constipation are aimed at softening stools, increasing motility, and increasing bulk or volume of feces. Medications used to treat diarrhea and constipation are listed in Table 21-9.

Gastroesophageal reflux disease

Gastroesophageal reflux disease (GERD) is a condition where gastric acid and other stomach contents come back up into the esophagus, causing pain and irritation. Common foods such as chocolate, coffee, and carbonated beverages can worsen GERD. Certain medications can also worsen gastroesophageal reflux disease. Treatment usually consists of over-the-counter antacids and histamine receptor (H2) blockers, or prescription proton pump inhibitors (Table 21-10).

Gynecologic and Obstetric Disorders

Contraception and hormone replacement therapy are common treatments for gynecological patients. Contraception is simply the prevention of pregnancy or conception. There are various methods of contraception, but this section will focus on oral contraception. Oral contraception involves the manipulation of estrogen and its role in normal physiology. Most oral contraceptives contain a form of estrogen and a progestin component. Hormone replacement therapy usually begins during menopause to decrease associated symptoms. Drugs used as contraceptives and for hormone replacement are listed in Table 21-11.

TABLE 21-9 Drugs Used to Treat Diarrhea and Constipation

GENERIC NAME	COMMON BRAND NAME(S)
Absorbing agents for diarrhea	
polycarbophil*	Fiberall, Fibercon
Antimotility agents	
diphenoxylate	Lomotil
loperamide*	Imodium
Laxative and cathartic agents for constipation	
bisacodyl*	Dulcolax
docusate*	Colace
glycerin*	various
lactulose	Chronulac
mineral oil*	various
polyethylene glycol	GoLYTELY, MiraLax,* NuLYTELY
psyllium*	Metamucil
saline*	various
senna and combinations*	Senokot, Senokot S
*Over-the-counter product	

TABLE 21-10   Drugs Used to Treat GERD

GENERIC NAME	COMMON BRAND NAME(S)
Antacids	
aluminum-containing*	Alterna GEL
calcium-containing*	Rolaids, Tums
magnesium/aluminum combinations*	Gaviscon, Maalox, Mylanta
sodium bicarbonate*	various
Histamine receptor (H2) blockers	
cimetidine*	Tagamet
famotidine*	Pepcid
nizatidine*	Axid
ranitidine*	Zantac
Proton pump inhibitors	
esomeprazole	Nexium
lansoprazole	Prevacid, Prevacid Solutab
omeprazole*	Prilosec, Prilosec OTC
pantoprazole	Protonix
rabeprazole	Aciphex
Miscellaneous agents	
metoclopramide	Reglan
misoprostol	Cytotec
sucralfate	Carafate

*Over-the-counter product

TABLE 21-11   Drugs Used for Contraception and Hormone Replacement

GENERIC NAME	COMMON BRAND NAME(S)
Estrogens	
conjugated estrogens	Premarin
conjugated estrogens with medroxyprogesterone	Premphase, Prempro
esterified estrogens	Estratab, Menest
micronized estradiol	Estrace
transdermal estrogen	Climara, Estraderm, Vivelle
Progestins	
medroxyprogesterone	Provera
norethindrone	Aygestin, Micronor, Nor-QD
norgestrel	Ovrette
progesterone	Prometrium
Combined oral contraceptives	
ethinyl estradiol and desogestrel	Desogen, Mircette
ethinyl estradiol and levonorgestrel	Lybrel, Quasense, Seasonale
ethinyl estradiol and norethindrone	Estrostep, Ortho-Novum, Ovcon
ethinyl estradiol and norgestimate	Ortho-Cyclen, Ortho Tri-Cyclen, Ortho Tri-Cyclen
ethinyl estradiol and norgestrel	Ovral, Lo/Ovral, Low-Ogestrel-28

Infectious Diseases

Infectious diseases can be bacterial, fungal, or viral. Antibiotics used to treat bacterial infections are classified as either bacteriostatic or bacteriocidal. Bacteriostatic drugs inhibit the growth of an infecting organism, and bacteriocidal drugs kill the infecting organism. Antibiotics also work by various mechanisms of action. Penicillins and cephalosporins disrupt the cell wall of the organism. Aminoglycosides, fluoroquinolones, macrolides, and tetracyclines move into the cell to inhibit RNA and protein synthesis. Antifungal agents are used to treat both topical and systemic fungal infections. Antiviral agents are reserved for the treatment of viral infections. Antibiotics used to treat infections are found in Table 21-12.

TABLE 21-12 Drugs Used to Treat Infections

GENERIC NAME	COMMON BRAND NAME(S)
Aminoglycosides	
amikacin	Amikin
gentamicin	Garamycin
neomycin	Mycifradin
streptomycin	various
tobramycin	Nebcin
Antifungal agents	
amphotericin B	Abelcet, Fungizone
clotrimazole*	Mycelex, Lotrimin
fluconazole	Diflucan
itraconazole	Sporanox
ketoconazole*	Nizoral
miconazole*	Monistat
nystatin	Mycostatin
voriconazole	Vfend
Antiviral agents	
acyclovir	Zovirax
amantadine	Symmetrel
didanosine	Videx
famciclovir	Famvir
ribavirin	Virazole
rimantadine	Flumadine
stavudine	Zerit
valacyclovir	Valtrex
zidovudine	Retrovir
Cephalosporins	
cefaclor	Ceclor
cefadroxil	Duricef
cefpodoxime	Vantin
cefprozil	Cefzil
ceftazidime	Fortaz
ceftriaxone	Rocephin
cephalexin	Keflex

TABLE 21-12 Drugs Used to Treat Infections (continued)

GENERIC NAME	COMMON BRAND NAME(S)
Fluroquinolones	
ciprofloxacin	Cipro, Cipro XR
gatifloxacin	Tequin
moxifloxacin	Avelox
Macrolides	
azithromycin	Zithromax, Z-Pack
clarithromycin	Biaxin, Biaxin XL
erythromycin	E.E.S., Ery-Tab
Penicillins	
amoxicillin	Amoxil, Trimox
amoxicillin/clavulanate	Augmentin
ampicillin	Principen
ampicillin/sulbactam	Unasyn
penicillin G	various
piperacillin	Pipracil
piperacillin/tazobactam	Zosyn
ticarcillin	Ticar
Penicillin-related agents	
aztreonam	Azactam
imipenem/cilastin	Primaxin
meropenem	Merrem IV
Tetracyclines	
doxycyline	Vibramycin
minocycline	Minocin
tetracycline	Sumycin
Miscellaneous anti-infectives	
isoniazid	INH
metronidazole	Flagyl, Flagyl ER
nitrofurantoin	Macrobid, Macrodantin
rifampin	Rifadin
sulfamethoxazole/trimethoprim	Bactrim, Septra

Neurologic Disorders

Neurologic disorders are disorders that affect the nervous system. Common neurologic disorders that are often treated with prescription medications are epilepsy and numerous psychiatric disorders.

Epilepsy

Epilepsy is a term that encompasses various symptoms that can range from some alteration in consciousness to uncontrollable convulsions or seizures that result from altered brain function. Decreasing the frequency of these attacks or seizures

TABLE 21-13 Drugs Used to Treat Epilepsy

GENERIC NAME	COMMON BRAND NAME(S)
Anticonvulsant agents	
carbamazepine	Tegretol
clonazepam	Klonopin
fosphenytoin	Cerebyx
gabapentin	Neurontin
lamotrigine	Lamictal
phenobarbital	Luminal
phenytoin	Dilantin
topiramate	Topamax
valproic acid	Depakote
zonisamide	Zonegran

greatly increases the quality of life in epileptics. Drugs used to treat epilepsy are found in Table 21-13.

Psychiatric disorders

Psychiatric disorders range from depression, anxiety, and sleep disorders to more severe illnesses. Depression is an overwhelming feeling of sadness or guilt. There are numerous options for treating depression. Serotonin reuptake inhibitors are often used to treat depression. Anxiety disorders are characterized by abnormal restlessness and worry. Anxiety is commonly treated with benzodiazepines. With disruptions in mood, a lack of restful sleep often follows. Hypnotics are used to induce sleep in patients. Drugs used to treat psychiatric disorders can be found in Table 21-14.

Respiratory Disorders

Asthma and chronic obstructive pulmonary disease are two common respiratory disorders. Asthma is a condition that is characterized by inflammation of the airways. Wheezing, chest tightness, and coughing occur frequently with asthma. Environmental factors, exercise, and certain drugs can all be triggers of asthmatic episodes.

Chronic obstructive pulmonary disease (COPD) has two main causes: chronic bronchitis and emphysema. COPD has an inflammatory component along with airway obstruction. Treatments of asthma and COPD are similar. Bronchodilators are used to relax the bronchial smooth muscle and assist in breathing. Mast cell stabilizers and steroids are used to treat the inflammatory components of asthma and COPD. Drugs used to treat asthma and COPD are listed in Table 21-15.

Colds, inflammation, and allergic reactions

Antihistamines block the activity of histamine that is released during colds, inflammation, and allergic reactions. Histamine receptors are found throughout the body, but this section will mainly be focusing on the H-1 receptor. Antihistamines block this receptor, which helps prevent the watering, redness, and swelling that is characteristic of a histamine reaction. Decongestants are often added to cold preparations to help alleviate a stuffy nose. Decongestants cause a constriction of

TABLE 21-14   Drugs Used to Treat Psychiatric Disorders

GENERIC NAME	COMMON BRAND NAME(S)
Antianxiety agents	
alprazolam	Xanax
buspirone	BuSpar
clonazepam	Klonopin
diazepam	Valium
hydroxyzine	Atarax, Vistaril
imipramine	Tofranil
lorazepam	Ativan
oxazepam	Serax
velafaxine	Effexor, Effexor XR
Antidepressants	
amitriptyline	Elavil
bupropion	Wellbutrin SR, Wellbutrin XL
citalopram	Celexa
duloxetine	Cymbalta
escitalopram	Lexapro
fluoxetine	Prozac
mirtazapine	Remeron
nortryptiline	Pamelor
paroxetine	Paxil, Paxil CR
sertraline	Zoloft
trazadone	Desyrel
Hypnotic agents	
flurazepam	Dalmane
midazolam	Versed
ramelteon*	Rozerem
temazepam	Restoril
triazolam	Halcion
zaleplon	Sonata
zolpidem	Ambien

*Only agent in class that is not a controlled substance

TABLE 21-15   Drugs Used to Treat Asthma and COPD

GENERIC NAME	COMMON BRAND NAME(S)
Anticholinergic agents	
ipratropium	Atrovent, Atrovent HFA
tiotropium	Spiriva Handihaler
Beta-2 adrenergic agonists	
albuterol	Proventil HFA, Ventolin HFA
epinephrine*	Primatene Mist
levalbuterol	Xopenex, Xopenex HFA
metaproterenol	Alupent
pirbuterol	Maxair
salmeterol	Serevent
terbutaline	Brethine

(Continued)

TABLE 21-15 Drugs Used to Treat Asthma and COPD (continued)

GENERIC NAME	COMMON BRAND NAME(S)
Leukotriene antagonists	
montelukast	Singulair
zafirlukast	Accolate
Mast cell stabilizing agents	
cromolyn*	Intal, Nasalcrom*
nedocromil	Tilade
Steroids	
beclomethasone	Beclovent, Beconase, Vancenase, Vanceril
budesonide	Pulmicort
flunisolide	AeroBid
fluticasone	Flovent, Flonase
prednisone	Deltasone, Orasone
triamcinalone	Azmacort
*Over-the-counter product	

blood vessels and allow for better breathing through the nose. It is important to note that individuals who have high blood pressure should contact their pharmacist or physician before using any products containing decongestants. Drugs used as antihistamines and decongestants are listed in Table 21-16.

TABLE 21-16 Antihistamines and Decongestants

GENERIC NAME	COMMON BRAND NAME(S)
Antihistamines	
brompheniramine combinations*	Dimetapp
cetirizine	Zyrtec*
chlorpheniramine*	Chlor-Trimeton
desloratadine	Clarinex
diphenhydramine	Benadryl
fexofenadine	Allegra
loratidine*	Alavert, Claritin
meclizine*	Antivert, Bonine
promethazine	Phenergan
Decongestants	
ephedrine*	Ephadron Nasal, Vatronol
phenylephrine*	Neosynephrine
pseudoephedrine*	Sudafed
Steroids	
Budesonide	Entocort, Rhinacort AQ
Fluticasone	Flonase, Veramyst
Mometasone	Nasonex
Triamcinolone	Nasacort AQ
*Over-the-counter product	

Summary

This chapter first noted the advantages and disadvantages of the various extra-vascular and intravascular modes of drug administration. Drug action is also affected by patient characteristics, such as adherence with directions for taking the drug, interactions of drugs with food and other drugs, and patient pathology, as well as age, weight, and genetic predispositions. The second major part of the chapter dealt with common disorders and the major therapeutic classes of drugs in use today to treat those disorders. The generic and trade names of the drugs in each category have been included. Both the actions and the uses of drugs have been described and noted to provide the pharmacy technician with a sound basis for understanding the basics of drug therapy.

TEST YOUR KNOWLEDGE

Multiple Choice

1. Which of the following route(s) of administration avoid first-pass metabolism?
    I.   oral
    II. sublingual
    III. intravenous
        a. I only
        b. III only
        c. I and II only
        d. II and III only

2. Which one of the following routes of administration is best when a rapid onset of systemic drug action is required in an emergency situation?
    a. transdermal
    b. rectal
    c. intravenous
    d. oral

3. Induction of drug-metabolizing enzymes is mostly likely to cause
    a. increased drug concentrations and increased side effects.
    b. increased drug concentrations and decreased therapeutic effects.
    c. decreased drug concentrations and increased side effects.
    d. decreased drug concentrations and decreased therapeutic effects.

4. Which of the following drugs is a beta-adrenergic blocker?
    a. albuterol
    b. captopril
    c. metoprolol
    d. fluconazole

5. Which of the following drugs is used to treat pain?
    a. diltiazem
    b. hydrocodone
    c. minoxidil
    d. atorvastatin

6. Albuterol, Spiriva, and Flovent HFA are common treatments for
   a. coronary artery disease.
   b. respiratory disorders.
   c. hypertension.
   d. bacterial infections.

Matching

Match the abbreviation with its meaning.

1.	_____ prn	a.	intramuscular
2.	_____ o.u.	b.	subcutaneous
3.	_____ IM	c.	both eyes
4.	_____ OS	d.	left eye
5.	_____ SC, SQ	e.	as needed

Match the generic name with the brand name.

1.	_____ digoxin	a.	Lasix
2.	_____ acetaminophen	b.	Zoloft
3.	_____ warfarin	c.	Norvasc
4.	_____ sertralin	d.	Coumadin
5.	_____ furosemide	e.	Ambien
6.	_____ amlodipine	f.	Lanoxin
7.	_____ zolpidem	g.	Tylenol

Fill In The Blank

1. _____ administration means a sterile drug is directly injected into a skeletal muscle.

2. Two or more drugs can combine to exert their individual pharmacological effects in a/an _____ manner.

3. _____ is the consistency or accuracy with which patients follow the prescribed directions for taking their medication.

4. _____ is an abnormally high concentration of lipids, or cholesterol, in the blood.

5. A/An _____ is a disruption in the heart's normal beating or rhythmic pattern.

References

Brunton, L., Lazo, J., & Parker, K. (Eds.). (2006). *Goodman & Gilman's The pharmacological basis of therapeutics* (11th ed.) New York: McGraw-Hill.

DiPiro, J., Spruill, W., Wade, W., Blouin, R., & Pruemer, J. (2005). *Concepts in clinical pharmacokinetics* (4th ed.). Bethesda, MD: ASHP.

DiPiro, J., Talbert, R., Yee, G., et al. (Eds.). (2005). *Pharmacotherapy: A pathophysiologic approach* (6th ed.). New York: McGraw-Hill.

Shargel, L., Wu-Pong, S., & Yu, A. (2004). *Applied biopharmaceutics and pharmacokinetics* (5th ed.). New York: McGraw-Hill.

22

Nonprescription Medications

Competencies

Upon completion of this chapter, the reader should be able to

1. Define the term over-the-counter medication, and provide other common terms used to identify these agents.
2. Describe the various dosage formulations available as over-the-counter medications.
3. List the various therapeutic categories most commonly used for the purpose of self-care by patients.
4. Identify a specific nonprescription medication and recognize which therapeutic category it belongs to.
5. List common indications, adverse effects, and drug-disease interactions of select nonprescription medications.

Key Terms

allergies
analgesic
antacids
antihistamines
antitussives
cold
constipation
diarrhea
expectorant
gastroesophageal reflux disease (GERD)
nonprescription medications
over-the-counter medications (OTCs)
peptic ulcer disease (PUD)

Introduction

nonprescription medications
drugs available for patients suffering from conditions that are considered self-treatable.

over-the-counter medications (OTCs) drugs that can be sold without a prescription.

Those practicing in a pharmacy environment must be familiar with agents that may be purchased by the consumer without a prescription from their health care provider. These **nonprescription medications**, also known as **over-the-counter medications (OTCs)**, are available for patients suffering from conditions that are considered self-treatable. Patients commonly come into the pharmacy seeking these medications to provide relief from various symptoms. Not only are they seeking relief, but often they have been exposed to direct-to-consumer advertising, which may result in them asking the pharmacy personnel for specific brand-name products. The product they come in asking for may not necessarily be the best one for their condition. The pharmacist has the responsibility to offer consultation on the best product option, depending on the patient's symptoms, other disease states, and medications.

An advantage to nonprescription medications is that they do not require patients to see their physician in order to gain access to them. This alleviates a substantial burden on the health care community, and because the pharmacy is so accessible, it allows opportunities for the pharmacist to provide direct patient care. It also allows individuals more control over their own personal health needs.

The disadvantage to nonprescription medications is that without their physician's guidance, patients may misdiagnose their condition, and a far more serious condition may remain unrecognized. This can lead to inadequate treatment. For this reason, one of the roles of the pharmacist is to appropriately triage patients, either recommending self-treatment with nonprescription medications as appropriate or directing the patient to see a physician if the pharmacist thinks a more serious condition may be present.

In addition, OTCs have pharmacological activity. Thus, they have the potential to cause significant side effects and interact adversely with other medications a patient may be taking. Certain nonprescription medications may not be safe for those patients with specific disease states; therefore, it is important for the pharmacist and pharmacy technician to be aware of the OTCs a patient is taking to allow the pharmacist to effectively counsel a patient. For the reasons just stated, nonprescription medications are not benign, and all considerations used by the pharmacist when evaluating prescription medications should be employed when a patient purchases an OTC medication.

A technician can be of great assistance to the pharmacist in identifying patients who may require additional counseling by the pharmacist. When patients come into the pharmacy to purchase a nonprescription medication or to fill a prescription, the pharmacy technician may ask the patient about his or her nonprescription medication use so that it can be placed in the patient's profile. Information that a pharmacy technician obtains during a casual conversation with the patient should be communicated to the pharmacist and will aid in identifying potential problems that may have otherwise gone unrecognized. In order to be able to do this effectively, a technician should be familiar with the numerous available OTC products. This chapter will highlight the most common therapeutic agents that patients may purchase without a prescription.

Dosage Forms

OTCs are available in many different formulations, similar to prescription drugs. The most widely used agents are available as oral dosage forms and include capsules, tablets, suspensions, solutions, and effervescent tablets. It is important for patients to shake a suspension well, while solutions do not require this step. Effervescent tablets, such as Alka-Seltzer, need to be dissolved in water or another compatible liquid prior to ingesting. These agents also tend to have an increased amount of sodium, which becomes important in those patients who are on salt-restricted diets for disease states such as hypertension or heart failure. If an alternative dosage form is available, the pharmacist should make a recommendation that the patient take that rather than the effervescent tablet. Sugar-free and alcohol-free formulations are also more appropriate for certain patients.

Topical agents include creams, ointments, and lotions. Other dosage forms include eardrops, eyedrops, suppositories, enemas, and shampoos. These dosage forms should never be taken by mouth since they are intended for external use only.

Nonprescription medications may contain multiple active ingredients. This is often the case with cough, cold, flu, and allergy products. The patient may end up taking a drug for which there is no indication, increasing the risk of side effects. If the patient's symptoms are known by the pharmacist, this scenario may be avoided. An additional important point to note about nonprescription product formulations is that the active ingredients in a brand may change. Sometimes this is done while keeping the same brand name, so it is always important to look at the active ingredients specified on the product label.

Pain

analgesic an agent that relieves pain without causing loss of consciousness (e.g., codeine).

Agents used to treat a patient's pain are known as **analgesics**. A patient may have pain for various reasons, and it may manifest as headaches, muscle pain, or bone or joint pain. Pain is often categorized as either *acute* or *chronic*. Acute pain is due to a recent, sudden occurrence such as an injury, medical procedure, or accident, while chronic pain is usually the result of an underlying disease state such as cancer, rheumatoid arthritis, or multiple sclerosis. In general, nonprescription analgesics are most appropriately utilized in patients suffering from acute pain or as adjunctive agents in those with chronic pain. They are effective for mild to moderate pain. The pharmacist should direct the patient to see his or her physician for a complete evaluation if the pain has not resolved within 10 days of taking an OTC analgesic. Some analgesics are also commonly used as antipyretics to decrease a patient's fever. The pharmacist should direct the patient to see his or her physician for a complete fever workup if the fever has not subsided within three days of taking an OTC antipyretic.

Internal analgesics are those that can be taken by mouth (po) and include salicylates (e.g., aspirin), acetaminophen, and nonsteroidal anti-inflammatory drugs (NSAIDs). See Table 22-1 for examples of agents that are available without a prescription. OTC NSAIDs include ibuprofen, ketoprofen, and naproxen. The doses of OTC NSAIDs are considerably less than their prescription counterparts.

Common side effects of salicylates include bleeding and gastrointestinal irritation. These agents should be avoided in pregnant patients. Children and adolescents are at increased risk of developing Reye's syndrome, a fatal illness, especially if they have the flu or chickenpox. Therefore, salicylates are generally avoided in this population. An important drug interaction to consider with the salicylates is that they may cause increased risk of bleeding in those patients also taking warfarin. This interaction is also seen in patients taking NSAIDs and, to a lesser degree, acetaminophen.

Like salicylates, NSAIDs also cause significant stomach upset, dyspepsia, and heartburn. To help prevent stomach upset, the pharmacist should instruct patients to take these agents with food, milk, or antacids. The NSAIDs should be avoided in those patients who are allergic to aspirin or have asthma, ulcers, renal impairment, or heart failure.

Acetaminophen is also widely used for pain and is well tolerated, but may be damaging to the liver in higher doses, especially in those who are malnourished or drink heavily. Acetaminophen is available in several different dosage formulations and strengths for both the adult and pediatric populations. These include drops, syrups, suspensions, suppositories, chewable tablets, caplets, tablets, and gelcaps.

Combination products are available for the consumer to purchase as well. The most common combination products include caffeine, which may increase the analgesic activity of the primary ingredient. They may also contain combinations of two of the agents just discussed.

Topical OTCs are available and are applied externally to the affected area of pain. External analgesics, including topical NSAIDs, are of questionable efficacy. They may decrease pain, itching, and burning. Counterirritants produce mild pain

TABLE 22-1 Nonprescription Analgesic Agents

THERAPEUTIC CATEGORY	GENERIC NAME	BRAND NAME	FORMULATION
Salicylates	aspirin	Anacin, Ascriptin, Bayer, Bufferin, Ecotrin	tablets, caplets
	magnesium salicylate	Doan's, Momentum	caplets
	choline salicylate	Arthropan	liquid
Nonsteroidal anti-inflammatory drugs	ibuprofen	Advil, Motrin, Nuprin	tablets, chewtabs, caplets, capsules, geltabs, drops, suspension, liquid
	ketoprofen	Actron, Orudis KT	caplets, tablets
	naproxen sodium	Aleve	caplets, tablets
Other	acetaminophen	Tylenol, Tempra	effervescent tablet, tablets, chewtabs, caplets, capsules, geltabs, drops, suspension, liquid, susuppositories
Counterirritants	menthol	Absorbine Jr., BenGay, Flexall, Therapeutic Mineral Ice	topical liquid, gel, cream
	capsaicin	Capzasin, Zostrix	topical lotion, gel, cream
	trolamine salicylate	Aspercreme, Aspergel, Myoflex	cream, lotion

and inflammation at a site close to the affected area and decrease the severity of the patient's pain. This masks the patient's pain to make it more tolerable. Camphor, menthol, capsaicin, and trolamine salicylate are the most commonly used counterirritants. See Table 22-1 for available formulations. The pharmacist should warn users not to apply counterirritants to wounded skin or in the eyes. Bandages should not be placed over these products. Patients should be made aware that these agents might cause a burning sensation when applied and are never to be ingested.

Cold and Allergy

cold a self-limiting viral infection of the respiratory tract.

antitussive a drug used for the relief of cough.

antihistamine reduces runny nose and sneezing.

allergy a disorder in which the body becomes hypersensitive to a particular antigen (called an *allergen*).

A **cold** is a self-limiting viral infection of the respiratory tract. The main goal in patients suffering from a cold is to alleviate their symptoms, because a cold cannot be cured by the administration of antibiotics. Decongestants are used for patients' nasal stuffiness, analgesics are used for fever and pain, and **antitussives** are used for coughs. **Antihistamines** can also be utilized to help control a runny nose and sneezing. Many combination products are available, because many patients experience one or more cold symptoms. Multiple medications used separately can be quite confusing and cumbersome for the patient, and the likelihood of mistakes is much higher.

Allergies are characterized by sneezing, itchy and watery eyes, and an itchy, runny nose. The person with allergies may also experience increased fatigue, irritability, and worsening moods. These symptoms are triggered by an allergen, such as mold, pollen, cigarette smoke, dust, or pet dander. The symptoms of allergies are treated with antihistamines, intranasal cromolyn, and topical decongestants.

OTC decongestants are available as eye drops, nasal sprays/drops/inhalers, and various oral formulations. Eye drops contain naphazoline, oxymetazoline, phenylephrine, and tetrahydrozoline, and are utilized most often in those patients suffering from allergies. Intranasal formulations contain ephedrine, epinephrine, naphazoline, phenylephrine, tetrahydrozoline, xylometazoline, oxymetazoline, desoxyephedrine, and propylhexedrine. The oral decongestants, including pseudoephedrine and phenylephrine, are absorbed into the bloodstream and can result in cardiovascular and central nervous system stimulation. This results in increased blood pressure, palpitations, high heart rate, restlessness, tremors, anxiety, insomnia, and fear. The oral decongestants may worsen hypertension, hyperthyroidism, diabetes, coronary heart disease, ischemic heart disease, and benign prostatic hypertrophy. In general, patients with these conditions should avoid the oral decongestant agents.

As of September 2006, federal regulations mandated that pseudoephedrine be stored behind the pharmacy counter or in locked cabinets because of its abuse potential. It has been used to synthesize methamphetamine; therefore, its distribution needs to be limited. Purchasers must provide photo identification and sign a log for each purchase of pseudoephedrine. The pharmacy must keep records of the name, address, signature, product purchased, quantity purchased, and the date and time of the purchase. These records must be retained for two years and do not apply to the purchase of single-dose packages that contain less than 60 milligrams. A single individual cannot purchase more than 3.6 grams per day or 9 grams per month. Pharmacies must also submit a statement notifying the Attorney General that all pharmacy staff members have been trained on these regulations.

As a result of this mandate, many manufacturers have reformulated their pseudoephedrine products to contain phenylephrine instead, which can remain OTC and cannot be used to synthesize methamphetamine. Some still make their pseudoephedrine products in addition to the reformulated products.

Antitussives are those agents that are approved to suppress a patient's cold-related cough. The generic names of the nonprescription antitussives are codeine and dextromethorphan. Some states sell OTC codeine with certain restrictions, while others do not allow the sale of codeine as a nonprescription medication. Common side effects of codeine include nausea, vomiting, sedation, dizziness, and constipation. Codeine should not be used in those who have respiratory problems or a history of addiction.

> **expectorant** a substance that promotes the ejection of mucus or an exudate from the lungs, bronchi, and trachea.

Dextromethorphan is well tolerated and does not cause sedation or respiratory depression, or have addictive properties. Guaifenesin is an **expectorant** that loosens thick secretions to make a cough more productive and, therefore, should only be used in those patients suffering from a nonproductive cough. There is a popular nonprescription combination product that contains both guaifenesin and dextromethorphan. This product is irrational because it contains an agent that suppresses the cough and one that causes the cough to be more productive.

Antihistamines are also used to control symptoms of the common cold and allergies. Some OTC antihistamines can cause sedation, but some cause it to a greater degree than others. The first generation antihistamines are the sedating antihistamines and include brompheniramine, chlorpheniramine, clemastine fumarate, diphenhydramine, and doxylamine. Of these, brompheniramine and chlorpheniramine are the least sedating. First-generation antihistamines can cause dry mouth, blurred vision, decreased urination, constipation, and an increased heart rate. They may also impair a patient's ability to perform tasks, such as those required for driving or working. The pharmacist should instruct patients with glaucoma or benign prostatic hypertrophy to avoid these antihistamines. Non-sedating or second generation antihistamines were traditionally only available by prescription; however, because of its favorable safety profile, loratidine was recently made available OTC. Loratidine needs to be used with caution in patients with liver or kidney disease and should be used at recommended doses, because going above the recommended dose makes the drug more likely to be sedating.

Cromolyn is used to treat the symptoms of allergies and is available as an intranasal spray. The pharmacist should inform the patient that it may take three to seven days to begin to take effect and up to a month for maximum benefit. The most common side effects include sneezing and nasal burning and stinging, primarily due to its administration. See Table 22-2 for a list of commonly used nonprescription cold and allergy products.

Constipation

> **constipation** difficult, incomplete, or infrequent bowel evacuation.

A decrease in the frequency of stool to below that of the patient's normal frequency is known as **constipation**. Constipated patients may experience abdominal discomfort, lower back pain, difficult passage of stool, bloating, and flatulence. Constipation is usually the result of inadequate exercise and the inadequate intake of water or fiber. Nonprescription treatment options that facilitate the elimination of stool include bulk laxatives, saline laxatives, hyperosmotic laxatives, and stool softeners.

TABLE 22-2 Nonprescription Agents for Cold and Allergy

THERAPEUTIC CATEGORY	GENERIC NAME	BRAND NAME	FORMULATION
Topical nasal decongestants	oxymetazoline	Afrin 12-hour, Dristan 12-hour, Neosynephrine 12-hour, Vicks Sinex 12-hour	nasal spray, pump, drops
	phenylephrine	Afrin, Dristan, Little Noses, Neosynephrine, Vicks Sinex	nasal spray, drops
	xylometazoline	Otrivin	nasal spray, drops
	naphzoline	Privine	nasal spray
Oral decongestants	phenylephrine	Sudafed PE	tablets, caplets
	pseudoephedrine*	Sudafed	tablets, capsules
Antitussives	dextromethorphan	Benylin, Robitussin, Sucrets, Vicks	liquid, lozenges
Antihistamines	diphenhydramine	Aler-Dryl, Benadryl	caplets, tablets, liquid
	chlorpheniramine	Chlor-Trimeton	tablets
	brompheniramine	Dimetapp, Dimetane	tablets, elixir
	loratidine	Alavert, Claritin, Tavist ND	tablets, orally disintegrating tablets

*Found behind the pharmacy counter (see text)

Bulk-forming laxatives are used for fiber replacement therapy and are usually mixed with a liquid and taken by mouth. These include methylcellulose, polycarbophil, psyllium, and malt soup extract and are the safest of the laxatives. Bulk laxatives can be utilized for both prevention and treatment of constipation. These agents take as long as three days to work; therefore, patients who take these should not expect a bowel movement until then. The pharmacist must also instruct the patient to drink sufficient water with these agents to avoid blockage. They should also take the medications two hours prior to or two hours after taking other medications by mouth, because they can interact with medications such as digoxin, warfarin, and salicylates.

Saline laxatives may be used to treat more severe constipation and should be used with caution in those who are dehydrated because these agents pull a significant amount of water into the intestine to soften the stool. There are magnesium and sodium-containing saline laxatives available. The sodium-containing laxatives should be avoided in those patients on a low-salt diet, such as patients with hypertension or heart failure. Sodium-containing laxatives are most commonly used as enemas. Also, many sodium-containing laxatives contain phosphate; therefore, they should not be used in patients with kidney impairment. Patients with kidney impairment must also avoid magnesium-containing laxatives. The oral saline laxative will take effect in 30 minutes to three hours, while the enemas will take two to five minutes to work.

Hyperosmotic laxatives include glycerin and sorbitol. They can be given rectally in the form of suppositories and enemas, which may cause mild discomfort for the patient. The laxative effects usually occur within 15 to 60 minutes.

Stool softeners allow for easier and less painful passage of the stool by softening it. Docusate is the only available OTC softener. It is available as sodium or calcium salt and takes 12 to 72 hours to take effect. Docusate is well tolerated and has minimal side effects.

TABLE 22-3 Nonprescription Agents for Constipation

THERAPEUTIC CATEGORY	GENERIC NAME	BRAND NAME	FORMULATION
Bulk-forming laxatives	polycarbophil	FiberCon, Mitrolan	tablets
	methylcellulose	Citrucel	powder
	psyllium	Konsyl, Metamucil, Perdiem	powder, granules
	malt soup extract	Maltsupex	liquid
Saline laxatives	magnesium citrate	Citroma	liquid
	sodium phosphate	Fleet	enema
	magnesium hydroxide	Milk of Magnesia	suspension
Hyperosmotic laxatives	glycerin	Fleet Babylax, Fleet suppositories	liquid, suppositories
Stool softeners	docusate sodium	Colace, Ex-Lax	liquid, gelcaps, capsules
Lubricant laxative	mineral oil	Fleet, Kondremul	oil, enema
Stimulant laxatives	bisacodyl	Correctol, Dulcolax, Fleet	tablets, caplets, suppositories
	senna	Ex-Lax, Correctol, Senokot	tablets, herbal tea, syrup
	castor oil	Neoloid, Purge	oil

Mineral oil is the only available lubricant laxative and is available as an enema or an oil that is taken by mouth. Mineral oil takes about six to eight hours to work. It should not be used as a first-line laxative because of its many adverse effects and interactions. Patients may aspirate the mineral oil; therefore, the pharmacist should warn the patient to remain upright when taking it and to take it at least 30 minutes prior to going to bed. Because mineral oil prevents the absorption of the fat-soluble vitamins, it should be taken two hours prior to or two hours after a meal.

Stimulant laxatives are available as liquids, tablets, granules, or suppositories. These laxatives force the bowel to expel its contents within 6 to 12 hours. Taking stimulants for an extended period of time may result in damage to the intestines. Senna, cascara, and casanthranol are known as the *anthraquinones*. These agents turn urine a pink to red or brown to black color. It is important to warn the patient about this effect. Diphenylmethanes include bisacodyl, which is the only bowel stimulant available as a suppository as well as a tablet. Castor oil is also a stimulant laxative. In most cases the stimulant laxative should be combined with a stool softener. The stimulant alone may not soften the stool adequately, leading to pain and discomfort when the stool is passed. See Table 22-3 for a list of commonly used nonprescription products for constipation.

Diarrhea

diarrhea increased frequency of stool that is loose and watery.

An increased frequency of stools with loose and watery consistency is known as **diarrhea**, which can be the result of diet, infection, or medications. A pharmacist should always instruct parents or guardians of pediatric patients that have had persistent diarrhea or have a fever associated with their diarrhea to consult with a physician. Children under three years old are more prone to the effects of fluid losses and should consult with their pediatrician. Dehydration and electrolyte abnormalities can manifest from just two days of diarrhea depending upon the severity; therefore, these patients should see a physician. They may require the administration of intravenous fluids to correct the abnormalities. Patients with a fever may have an infectious cause of diarrhea and should be put on appropriate therapy, such as antibiotics, rather than OTC products. Patients with infectious diarrhea should generally avoid OTC antidiarrheal agents because they inhibit the removal of the pathogen by slowing the gastrointestinal transit time, which could result in longer duration or increased severity of diarrhea. The nonprescription agents used to treat diarrhea include polycarbophil, attapulgite, bismuth subsalicylate, kaolin, loperamide, lactobacillus, activated charcoal, and oral rehydration solutions.

Calcium polycarbophil is a bulk laxative that was discussed earlier in the constipation section. It can be utilized for both constipation and diarrhea. It absorbs up to 60 times its weight in water to help "bulk up" the consistency of the stool. The pharmacist must inform patients that they should maintain adequate fluid intake and to chew the tablets before swallowing them. Patients who are on tetracycline should stagger their dose to minimize the effect of calcium binding to the tetracycline. Adsorbents include attapulgite, kaolin, pectin, and bismuth subsalicylate. These agents work by binding to toxins, bacteria, and noxious materials that can cause diarrhea. Because these agents work by binding to substances, which can result in decreased amount of drug available for activity, they should generally be given at least two hours prior to or two hours after other medications. Kaolin alone may be effective, but has not been proven to be effective when given with pectin and was therefore removed from older products containing the combination. Older kaolin-pectin combination products were reformulated to contain attapulgite, which is effective in treating diarrhea. Some attapulgite products, like Kaopectate, were later reformulated to contain bismuth subsalicylate. Bismuth subsalicylate is available as a suspension and contains salicylate. For this reason, caution should be used in the pediatric population, those who are allergic to aspirin, and in those who are taking other salicylates or anticoagulants such as warfarin. Bismuth subsalicylate may darken the tongue and stool.

Loperamide helps with the symptoms of diarrhea by slowing gastrointestinal motility and is available as caplets or a solution. Adverse effects are rare and include drowsiness, dizziness, and constipation.

Lactobacillus has not been proven effective, but may promote regrowth of normal flora in the bowel. This agent must be refrigerated and may cause flatulence. Activated charcoal is not proven to be effective and is not recommended for the treatment of diarrhea. Oral rehydration solutions may be helpful while a patient is waiting to see a physician.

Please see Table 22-4 for a list of select agents and their brand names.

TABLE 22-4   Nonprescription Agents for Diarrhea

THERAPEUTIC CATEGORY	GENERIC NAME	BRAND NAME	FORMULATION
Bulk laxative	calcium polycarbophil	Equalactin, Mitrolan	tablets
Adsorbents	attapulgite	Donnagel	tablets, capsules,
	bismuth subsalicylate	Pepto-Bismol, Kaopectate	tablets, capsules, liquids
Motility agent	loperamide	Imodium AD	caplets, liquid

Acid/Peptic Disorders

This section will emphasize the common gastrointestinal disorders that can be controlled with OTC medications. These include **gastroesophageal reflux disease (GERD)** and **peptic ulcer disease (PUD)**. PUD is ulceration of the stomach or duodenal lining. Patients must be seen by a physician and diagnosed with PUD before the pharmacist can aid in the selection of a nonprescription medication. Nonprescription medications used for patients with PUD are used as adjunctive agents in addition to prescription medications. Antacids can be used for pain relief, and bismuth subsalicylate can be used as part of a regimen including prescription medications to treat *H. pylori*, an infectious cause of PUD.

GERD, also called heartburn, is a process that causes a burning sensation in the chest area. This burning is the result of reflux of the acidic contents of the stomach up into the esophagus. The reflux causes irritation to the lining of the esophagus that can lead to discomfort and ulceration. Dietary and lifestyle modifications are key to the management of a patient suffering from heartburn. These measures include elevating the head of the bed, eating smaller meals, eating meals at least three hours before bedtime, and avoiding trigger foods such as mints, chocolates, citrus juices, spicy foods, foods with tomatoes, and coffee. It may also be helpful to lose weight, quit smoking, and avoid alcoholic beverages. Agents for heartburn that are available without a prescription include antacids, alginic acid, histamine$_2$ receptor antagonists, and more recently omeprazole (a proton pump inhibitor). In general, patients should not have symptoms of gastric distress for longer than a two-week period; if they have, the pharmacist should advise the patient to see their physician.

Antacids neutralize the acid in the stomach to produce minimal irritation to the lining of the gastrointestinal tract. Calcium carbonate, sodium bicarbonate, aluminum hydroxide, aluminum phosphate, magnesium hydroxide, and magnesium chloride are the antacids available over the counter. Suspensions usually allow for quicker dissolution over tablet formulations; therefore, suspensions usually have a quicker onset of action. Calcium carbonate and aluminum hydroxide dissolve more slowly than sodium bicarbonate and magnesium hydroxide and take about 10 to 30 minutes to see an effect. Magnesium-containing antacids can cause diarrhea, while aluminum-containing antacids may cause constipation. For this reason, combination products are available to negate the effects of either agent. Magnesium can accumulate to cause central nervous system depression in patients with renal failure; therefore, the pharmacist should recommend an alternative antacid for these patients. Aluminum and sodium bicarbonate antacids should also be avoided in patients with renal impairments due to accumulation. Alginic acid has been combined with sodium bicarbonate. This combination forms a viscous solution that floats on the acidic contents of the stomach, and instead of acid refluxing into the esophagus, the viscous solution is refluxed, which decreases irritation and symptoms. Antacids interact with many medications, and the pharmacist should be aware of these in order to counsel the patient.

Histamine$_2$ receptor antagonists (H$_2$RAs) are available in prescription and nonprescription strength. The nonprescription strength is available in a lower dosage form. The H$_2$RAs that are available over the counter are cimetidine, famotidine, nizatidine, and ranitidine. These agents decrease gastric acid secretion, which decreases damage done to the gastrointestinal mucosa. The nonprescription strength of these agents is not adequate to heal gastrointestinal ulcers due to

TABLE 22-5   Nonprescription Agents for Acid/Peptic Disorders

THERAPEUTIC CATEGORY	GENERIC NAME	BRAND NAME	FORMULATION
Antacids	magnesium hydroxide	Mag-Ox, Phillips' Milk of Magnesia, Uro-Mag	tablets, suspension, capsules, chewtabs
	aluminum hydroxide	ALternaGEL, Alu-Cap, Alu-Tab, Amphojel, Basaljel	tablets, suspension, capsules, liquid
	aluminum/magnesium hydroxide	Maalox, Riopan, Mylanta	suspension
	calcium carbonate	Amitone, Chooz, Tums	chewtabs, liquid
	calcium/magnesium	Rolaids, Mylanta	chewtabs
	aluminum/magnesium/alginate	Gaviscon	tablets, suspension, chewtabs
H₂ receptor antagonists	cimetidine	Tagamet	tablets
	famotidine	Pepcid	tablets
	nizatidine	Axid	tablets
	ranitidine	Zantac	tablets
Proton pump inhibitors	omeprazole	Prilosec OTC	tablets

GERD and PUD. The patient should be notified that these agents may not result in relief of symptoms for one to two hours; therefore, they should be taken one hour before a meal rather than at the time of symptoms. Common side effects from non-prescription doses of H₂RAs include headache, dizziness, constipation, nausea, and vomiting. Significant drug-drug interactions may occur with the H₂RAs. Cimetidine is associated with the most drug interactions of the drugs in this category.

Proton pump inhibitors (PPIs) prevent acid production and are also available with or without a prescription. Currently, omeprazole is the only PPI available without a prescription version. It is a 20 milligram delayed-release tablet. The patient should be notified that omeprazole will not provide immediate relief and that relief of symptoms may not occur for one to four days. Significant drug-drug interactions may occur with omeprazole, and patients taking certain medications should consult their doctor prior to taking omeprazole. Patients should not take this drug for more than a 14-day course or more than one course every 4 months, unless directed by their physician. Table 22-5 lists common agents for use in acid/peptic disorders.

Summary

It is imperative that those working in a pharmacy environment be familiar with over-the-counter agents sold to patients. These products have significant interactions and adverse effects and should be treated much like prescription medications. The technician can aid the pharmacist in identifying those patients who may require further pharmacist counseling on nonprescription products. Knowledge of over-the-counter agents can help the technician do this effectively and with greater confidence. This chapter covers some of the most common problems that are self-treated with over-the-counter drugs.

TEST YOUR KNOWLEDGE

Multiple Choice

1. All of the following are true statements regarding nonprescription medications *except*
   a. OTCs are available for conditions that are considered to be self-treatable.
   b. OTCs allow the patient more control over health care needs.
   c. OTCs have pharmacological activity.
   d. OTCs do not have the potential to cause adverse reactions.

2. Which of the following products is an option for the patient with hypertension?
   a. Alka-Seltzer
   b. Fibercon
   c. Sudafed
   d. Fleet's Enema

3. All of the following are examples of NSAIDs *except*
   a. naproxen.
   b. ketoprofen.
   c. acetaminophen.
   d. ibuprofen.

4. Which of the following should be shaken well prior to administration?
   a. solution
   b. suspension
   c. elixir
   d. lotion

5. All of the following are topical dosage forms *except*
   a. Doan's.
   b. Capzasin.
   c. Mineral Ice.
   d. Icy Hot.

6. Dextromethorphan belongs to which of the following therapeutic categories?
   a. decongestant
   b. antitussive
   c. antihistamine
   d. expectorant

7. Which of the following antihistamines is *not* available OTC?
   a. diphenhydramine
   b. chlorpheniramine
   c. fexofenadine
   d. brompheniramine

8. In most cases, senna should be given with which of the following nonprescription agents to decrease pain and discomfort of constipation?
   a. Citroma
   b. Colace

    c. Maltsupex
    d. Milk of Magnesia

9. Which of the following can be used for the treatment of both constipation and diarrhea?
    a. polycarbophil
    b. docusate
    c. loperamide
    d. senna

10. Which of the following agents can be safely used in a patient with renal impairment?
    a. Alu-Tab
    b. Tums
    c. Milk of Magnesia
    d. Amphogel

Matching

Match the drug category with what it is used to treat.

1. _____ analgesic
2. _____ antacid
3. _____ antitussive
4. _____ antihistamine
5. _____ laxative

a. cough
b. excess stomach acid
c. pain
d. runny nose and sneezing
e. constipation

Fill In The Blank

1. Tablets, suspensions, and solutions are examples of _____ dosage forms.
2. _____ agents include creams, ointments, and lotions.
3. A _____ is a self-limiting viral infection of the respiratory tract.
4. _____ are characterized by sneezing, itchy, and watery eyes, and an itchy, runny nose.
5. _____ is defined as a decrease in the frequency of stool to below that of the patient's normal frequency.

References

Berardi, R. R., Kroon, L. A., McDermott, J. H., et al. (Eds.) (2006). *Handbook of nonprescription drugs* (15th ed.). Washington, DC: American Pharmaceutical Association.

McEvoy, G. K. (Ed.). (2007). AHFS Drug Information. Bethesda, MD: American Society of Health-System Pharmacists, Inc.

Pray, W. S. (2006). *Nonprescription product therapeutics* (2nd ed.). Philadelphia: Lippincott Williams & Wilkins.

Natural Products

Competencies

Upon completion of this chapter, the reader should be able to

1. Describe what makes a product an herbal (or botanical) versus a drug.

2. Describe how herbals are regulated by the Food and Drug Administration (FDA) in the United States.

3. Explain the preparation and administration routes of most herbals.

4. Explain the potential for possibly dangerous interactions between herbals and standard drug therapy.

5. Be able to find reliable sources of current information on herbal safety and effectiveness.

6. List some common traditional uses of the major herbals.

Key Terms

dietary supplement
GRAS list
Herb Contraindications and Drug Interactions
herbal
hypersensitivity reaction
metabolite
secondary plant metabolite

Introduction

By definition, a *drug* is "any substance or mixture of substances intended for the cure, mitigation, diagnosis, or prevention of disease." This definition comes mainly from the Pure Food Act of 1906, which formed the basis of what is now the Food and Drug Administration. Regulation of drugs in the United States is discussed elsewhere in this text and summarized in a subsequent section in this chapter.

When most people talk about "natural products," they are referring to herbal preparations. An **herbal** substance is defined in the 1994 Dietary Supplement and Health Education Act (DSHEA) as a **dietary supplement**, not a drug. The DSHEA definition of a dietary supplement is any "product that contains a vitamin; mineral; amino acid; an herb or other botanical; a dietary substance for use by man to supplement the diet by increasing total daily intake; or a concentrate metabolite constituent, extract, or combinations of these ingredients."

Because they are not drugs, herbals and other dietary supplements cannot claim to cure, prevent, treat, or diagnose disease. They can claim to have a health action such as promoting healthy digestion. However, it is important to recognize that as a dietary supplement, herbal products are not evaluated by the FDA for either safety or effectiveness in the same manner that prescription drugs are evaluated. The reasons for this situation are discussed later in this chapter. In addition, the regulatory oversight that we have come to expect from the FDA with regard to drug manufacture has not necessarily been followed for the production of herbal products. On June 25, 2007, the FDA released revised regulations that set forth Good Manufacturing Practices (GMP) guidelines for dietary supplements. These guidelines came into force in June 2008 for large manufacturers (500 or more employees) and will be phased in for small companies through June 2010.

Those changes not withstanding, lack of assurance as to safety, quality, and effectiveness often places the pharmacist in a difficult position when asked for recommendations about herbal products. One of the goals of this chapter is to provide some guidelines for the review of herbal preparations and sources of reliable safety information.

> **herbal** a plant with therapeutic properties that can be used for nutritional or medical purposes.
>
> **dietary supplement** any product containing a vitamin, mineral, amino acid, or herb that is intended to supplement the diet by increasing overall intake of a particular substance.

History of Herbal Preparations

From colonial times until well into the 1900s, one of the primary roles of the pharmacy was the compounding or mixing of medicines. Pharmacists were not alone in this function. Unlike today, numerous physicians also compounded and dispensed medicines. Also unlike today, patients did not have to go to a physician to get a prescription to buy medicines. Indeed, as late as the 1920s, less than 25 percent of all medicines and drugs purchased in drugstores were bought using prescriptions.

Most of the early medicines compounded were based upon plant materials. One important example of such a medicine is digitalis, which was used to treat congestive heart failure. The active ingredients were usually harvested from the purple foxglove (*Digitalis purpurea*) or from the white foxglove (*Digitalis lanata*). In fact, the medicine derived its name from the genus name of the plants from which it was harvested. This medication was popularized by William Withering, a British physician, who published a monograph in 1785 on the use of extract of foxglove and the beneficial effects of digitalis on dropsy (the old name for congestive heart failure). Withering's treatise was one of the first published scientific studies of an herbal compound. Although crude digitalis extract is no longer used in the United States, digoxin and digitoxin (members of the cardiac glycoside drug class), which are the main components of the extract, are currently available.

To aid pharmacists in preparing compounds in a more consistent manner, several national publications arose. The United States Pharmacopoeia (USP), started in 1820, and the National Formulary (NF), started in 1888 by the American Pharmaceutical Association, are two publications that have taken on the status of being official compendiums that set national standards. The USP describes standards for drug identity, strength, quality, purity, packaging, and labeling. The NF sets standards for excipients, botanicals, and other similar products. The NF was purchased by the USP in 1975, combining the two publications under one cover entitled the USP-NF.

Early on, these publications had numerous monographs on the preparation of botanical products. At its peak, the USP published over 600 monographs on botanicals. By 1900 that number had decreased to about 169 monographs. Between 1900 and 1990, the increasing use of synthetic organic drugs resulted in a further reduction in attention to plant-derived medicines. Thus, in the latter quarter of the 20th century, the USP-NF had few monographs on botanicals. Fortunately, that situation is changing, and the USP-NF has reenergized its efforts to review botanicals and herbal products and publish appropriate monographs.

Historical Review of Drug Regulations

At this point, a brief history of drug regulation in the United States is useful. Prior to the early 1900s, there were few enforceable laws pertaining to medicines or what we would now call drugs. In 1906 the Pure Food Act was passed by Congress and signed into law. The legislation was enacted largely due to public concern over adulteration of foods as described by authors such as Upton Sinclair. Sinclair's book *The Jungle* described horrific practices at some meat packing plants and sparked public outrage demanding regulatory oversight over the production of food and medicines.

Although the title of the 1906 Pure Food Act suggests that it was about purity and food safety, in reality the law focused on making sure only that foods and drugs were truthfully and accurately labeled. The 1906 law had several important impacts on pharmacy. The law defined what constituted a drug and prohibited adulterated or misbranded drugs; however, it did not require that a drug be proven safe or effective. The 1906 law also converted the USP and NF from private publications into the official standards for the manufacture and compounding of drugs. And finally, the law essentially triggered the creation of what has become the Food and Drug Administration (FDA).

To enforce the provisions of the 1906 legislation, the Department of Agriculture's Division of Chemistry, headed by Harvey W. Wiley, was enlarged and renamed the Bureau of Chemistry. The Bureau of Chemistry was charged with assaying and checking the accuracy of content labels. By 1927, the regulatory aspects of the Bureau of Chemistry had become so large that they were moved to a new agency named the Food, Drug, and Insecticide Administration. In 1931 the name was shortened to the Food and Drug Administration (FDA).

As described above, the 1906 act was primarily concerned with truth in labeling. The Bureau of Chemistry could only act if a drug was misbranded or adulterated. There were no requirements that a drug be proven effective or even safe before being sold to the public. Then in 1937, the "elixir of sulfanilamide" tragedy occurred. A pharmaceutical company mixed sulfanilamide with diethylene glycol because it dissolved well and had a reasonable taste. Unfortunately, diethylene glycol, like ethylene glycol (the main component in automobile antifreeze), is poisonous to humans, causing potentially fatal central nervous system (CNS) and kidney (renal) damage. More than 100 of the patients who ingested the mixture died due to renal failure. Because there was no requirement that drugs be proven safe prior to sale, the FDA could only charge the pharmaceutical company with misbranding because the name of the drug used the term *elixir* in its name. Elixir is used to indicate an alcohol solution, and there was no alcohol in the mixture. A fine of slightly more than $26,000 was levied on the company, but no other action could be taken.

Once again, public outrage led to enactment of new legislation. In 1938 the Federal Food, Drug, and Cosmetic Act was signed into law. This legislation focused on demonstration of drug safety. The law spelled out procedures for how applications for new drug approval had to occur. For the first time medical devices were included in FDA regulations. Perhaps most importantly, the regulations gave special treatment to prescriptions written by physicians, veterinary doctors, and dentists. They distinguished between prescription and over-the-counter (OTC) drugs, which led to the prescription-only method of drug acquisition common today. The 1938 Federal Food, Drug, and Cosmetic Act is the foundation of drug regulation as it exists in the United States.

However, the 1938 legislation still did not require a drug to be effective. This was corrected by the Drug Amendments of 1962 (often called the Kefauver-Harris Amendments) that required that all drugs marketed after 1962 in the United States be proven both safe and effective. Although already in committee in Congress, enactment of this legislation was spurred by the thalidomide tragedy. Although never approved for sale in the United States, use of thalidomide in pregnant women often led to phocomelia, a birth defect in which the child is born missing one or more limbs. While nothing in the 1962 Drug Amendments would have specifically prevented clinical testing of thalidomide in the United States, it did encourage the mentality that the FDA should decide what drugs would be allowed on the market and then tightly regulate how they should be used.

To determine which drugs were effective, the FDA worked with the National Academy of Sciences' National Research Council to organize a drug efficacy study. This study examined the effectiveness of some 4,000 drugs that contained about 300 different chemicals. A final report was made in 1969. This report established much of how we think about prescription drugs in pharmacy today.

The drugs that could be purchased without a physician's prescription, the over-the-counter (OTC) drugs, were not examined (to any great extent) in the drug efficacy study. To deal with this, the FDA set up 17 panels in 1972 to evaluate the effectiveness of the active ingredients of OTC drugs. However, lack of sufficient data and resources to evaluate many of the OTCs led to a less than satisfactory result. The panels only examined ingredients if they were asked to do so and then only evaluated evidence presented to them. In 1990, when the final OTC study was released to the public, the safety and efficacy of many herbals was still in question.

A few botanicals, such as senna leaves (which act as a laxative), were found to be safe and effective and classified as Category I (safe and effective). Almost 150 herbals were classified as Category II (unsafe or ineffective). However, more than a hundred herbals were classed as Category III (insufficient evidence to evaluate). Note that a Category III designation does not mean that an herbal is not safe or effective. Category III means only that there has been no decision because of lack of supporting evidence. For those looking for more direction on the use of herbals in medical practice, this was a disappointing outcome. This classification system certainly did not provide pharmacy with much guidance in dealing with herbals.

Regulation of Herbals in the United States

GRAS list a list of food additives generally recognized as safe by the Food and Drug Administration.

One approach to address the concerns over herbals was to use the **GRAS list**. A number of herbals are listed on the 1958 list of GRAS (generally recognized as safe) food additives. However, as the name indicates, this list is directed primarily at food and flavoring agents and not at therapeutic actions. Thus, little reliable information was available to the pharmacy to evaluate safety and effectiveness of herbals as compared to prescription drugs.

Finally, in 1994 the Dietary Supplement Health and Education Act (DSHEA) was signed into law. This law treats herbals as dietary supplements, not drugs, and allows them to make claims with regard to general health promotion but not treatment of disease claims (like drugs). Much like the 1906 Pure Food Act, DSHEA focuses on the labeling of herbals (as well as other dietary supplements), spelling out what constitutes a misbranded or adulterated botanical (herbal).

According to DSHEA, an herbal must (1) be labeled as a dietary supplement, (2) identify all ingredients by name, (3) list the quantity of each ingredient, (4) identify the plant and the plant part from which the ingredient is derived, (5) comply with any standards set by an official compendium (such as the USP and the NF), and (6) meet the quality, purity, and compositional specifications as established by validated assays. Failure to comply with these regulations means that an herbal is misbranded. The DSHEA also sets guidelines to prevent adulteration of dietary supplements. The DSHEA even states that a botanical or herbal must be "prepared, packed, or held" under Good Manufacturing Practices (GMP) protocols. Mandating GMP is meant to ensure quality at the manufacturing (or preparation) stage of herbal production. As noted previously, although mandated in 1994, the final guidelines for GMP standards were not published until June 25, 2007 (FDA 21 CFR Part 111). The regulations will be phased into practice between June 2008 (for manufacturers with 500 or more employees) and June 2010 (for small companies). The expectation is that these GMP guidelines will result in enhanced quality assurance and safer herbal products. A summary review of the FDA's final GMP guidelines for dietary supplements has recently been published in the journal of the American Botanical Council.

However, to follow GMP during manufacture or preparation requires absolute standards that do not presently exist for many herbals. The new GMP guidelines require only that the methods be "scientifically valid" while allowing the manufacturers to establish their own specifications for identity, purity, potency, and relative composition. Furthermore, the DSHEA regulations say that the FDA may not "impose standards for which there is no currently and generally available analytical methodology."

For example, in the preparation of St. John's wort (an herbal often used for depression), which of the many components of the plant should be used by a manufacturer to standardize its manufacturing process? Two major components in St. John's wort are hypericin and hyperforin. Currently, many companies use hypericin levels as their assay standard for preparation of St. John's wort extract. However, there is no direct evidence that hypericin is the active ingredient in St. John's wort. Indeed, recent evidence suggests that if St. John's wort is effective in depression, the active ingredient may be hyperforin, not hypericin. Until the exact efficacious ingredient(s) have been determined for a particular herbal, exact potency (and therefore dosage) will be problematic.

In summary, as the brief history of the regulation of herbals presented here indicates, herbals have a unique status in the United States. Manufacturers can only market them with health claims and may not make any claims as to their use in treating disease (i.e., disease claims). However, millions of consumers (and patients) are purchasing these preparations to treat disease. While health care professionals at many levels are concerned about the safety and effectiveness of these preparations, current limitations on the FDA make it unlikely that this agency will be able to readily address these concerns in the near future. This leaves the pharmacy in the difficult position of trying to counsel the consumer (patient) without adequate information. Certainly, the easiest, most conservative advice would be to not purchase or use herbals unless under the directions of a physician. However, without specific warnings (e.g., "Use of this preparation has caused liver failure in patients with your condition!"), the "Do not use" advice is likely to be ignored. Annual sales of dietary supplements are estimated to be in the $19 billion-plus range. More and more people are turning to herbals as part of their health care. Thus, the rest of this chapter is directed toward helping pharmacy technicians understand and obtain up-to-date, useful information on herbals.

Chemical Structure of Herbals

secondary plant metabolite derived from primary plant metabolites.

metabolite a chemical synthesized within cells as part of a metabolic pathway.

Although the term *herbal* has been applied to any plant substance used for health purposes, most herbals are **secondary plant metabolites**. The term **metabolite** refers to a chemical synthesized within cells as part of a metabolic pathway. Primary plant metabolites are compounds that are essential for basic plant cell function and life. Primary metabolites fall into five general classes: proteins, nucleic acids, carbohydrates (sugars), simple organic acids, and lipids (fats). Secondary metabolites are derived from the primary metabolites, but have their own specialized pathways of synthesis. Secondary metabolites may be important for the success and health of the plant, but they are not as essential to basic plant cell survival as primary metabolites.

The functions of secondary metabolites in plants are quite varied. It is important to recognize that plants face many of the same environmental challenges that humans do, except they cannot change their location in response to these challenges. Thus, some secondary metabolites evolved to help conserve moisture for the plant (e.g., the suberins and waxes); some evolved to help ward off herbaceous animals (predators) as a form of chemical self-defense (e.g., various plant toxins such as nicotine); and some evolved to fight fungal, bacterial, and viral infections in plants. It is this last group of substances that is of particular interest to modern medicine and pharmacy because some of these compounds can also be used to fight infections in humans.

For simplicity, secondary plant metabolites can be divided into three major groups or classes of compounds: the terpenoids, the alkaloids, and the phenylpropanoids (including the flavonoids) and allied phenolics. Of these, the terpenoids are by far the most numerous in occurrence with more than 25,000 identified chemically. By comparison, there have been about 12,000 alkaloids identified and approximately 8,000 plant phenolics characterized. The chemical characteristics of secondary plant metabolites have been reviewed and summarized in numerous texts such as those of Dewick (*Medicinal Natural Products*), Dey and Harborne (*Plant Biochemistry*), and Buchanan, Gruissem, and Jones (*Biochemistry & Molecular Biology of Plants*). Although these secondary metabolites have been extensively characterized chemically, only a fraction of them have been tested for possible medicinal benefits.

Preparation and Routes of Administration of Herbals

Up until the mid-20th century, much of the work in the pharmacy was focused on preparation and compounding of plant material into herbal medicines. Today, however, most herbal preparations will enter the pharmacy already packaged. One reason for this is because few pharmacists are currently trained in pharmacognosy. Pharmacognosy is the science of selecting and preparing plant materials for medical use (see text by Robbers, Speedie, and Tyler). It should be emphasized that the selection and harvesting of plant material for herbal preparation should only be performed by trained and experienced professionals. There is significant risk of plant misidentification and subsequent toxicologic misadventure. Use of published identification standards is recommended (for example, see Applequist).

A second reason is economic; that is, it is cheaper to purchase the material ready to sell rather than to have to prepare and package it. This is certainly the case with many OTC preparations. However, compounding of an herbal product may be the only way to get it into a form usable to a patient. Even with prepackaged materials, there is still the matter of product safety, which is more complicated for herbals, as discussed in the next section.

Many retail herbal preparations are supplied as tablets, capsules, lozenges, liquids, or tinctures to be taken orally (po). Some herbals are supplied in a dry form to be taken po as a powder or made into a tea or similar drink. A number of herbals are for external skin or topical use only and are supplied as a gel, cream, or ointment. It is difficult to obtain herbal products that meet the microbiological and particulate safety standards needed for injection of product in the human body. Thus, for safety reasons, *herbal products should not be given by injection*; that is, by intravenous (IV), intramuscular (IM), or intra-arterial routes.

Safety of Herbals

Advocates for herbals often state that they are safer than modern drugs because they have been used by humans for a long time. In some instances, herbals have been used as a food or dietary supplement for generations. In general, most herbals are safe at low to moderate dosages. However, a number of issues must still be considered by the pharmacist. The most important of these issues are (1) the potential of a hypersensitivity (i.e., allergic) response to an herbal, (2) that the product actually contains the herbal claimed, (3) potential contamination of the herbal product with toxic material, and (4) the potential for herbal-drug interaction.

Hypersensitivity (Allergic) Reactions

hypersensitivity
reaction the reac-
tion that occurs after a
person is exposed to
a compound and has
generated antibodies
against the compound.

Just as with any newly administered drug or food, attention must be paid to the possibility of a hypersensitivity reaction to a component of the herbal product by the patient. A **hypersensitivity reaction** occurs when a patient has been exposed to a compound previously and has made antibodies against the compound. When the patient takes the compound again, a *hyper* or larger than normal immune response occurs, and the patient's own antibodies or immune cells begin to cause problems. Examples of hypersensitivity reactions are a pollen allergy or a food allergy, such as to peanuts. Hypersensitivity reactions can range in intensity from an immediate allergic reaction (such as anaphylactic shock) that can lead to death, to the skin rashes common in delayed hypersensitivity. Unfortunately, there is no easy way to predict which patients will have a hypersensitivity response to a particular food, compound, or drug. With herbal products, the concern about potential allergic responses is heightened because of the complex chemical nature of herbals. An herbal product may contain dozens to hundreds of compounds that might react with the immune system. On the other hand, immune tolerance can be induced by a number of food components, and certain herbals may be better tolerated because of a cross-tolerance effect.

In summary, given the potential severity and unpredictability of hypersensitivity reactions, the patient should be counseled to be on the lookout for the signs and symptoms of hypersensitivity, not just the first time an herbal is taken but also with each subsequent use. The pharmacy personnel should also be on the lookout for such reactions. *If there is an indication that the patient is having an allergic response to an herbal product, use of the product should be immediately discontinued, and appropriate medical treatment should be sought at once.*

Content and Concentration of the Herbal Product

The concern that the product may not contain the herbal listed on the label or may have varying concentrations of the herbal is still a significant problem. Several analytical testing laboratories have examined herbal products from a number of manufacturers or producers and found a wide disparity in the contents of the product. An important next step in the herbal industry will have to be the standardization of various products. With the new GMP guidelines published, manufacturers must establish and maintain records of identity, purity, strength, and relative composition of components in their product, starting in 2008. There is no requirement that an expiration date be placed on an herbal product. However, if a date is provided, the manufacturer must maintain records that support the choice of date (i.e., shelf life of the product). Quality assurance for the new GMP regulations requires that each manufacturer test subsets of each batch of finished herbal product in a manner consistent with currently accepted statistical sampling methods. The resultant data must be maintained for at least one year after the product expiration date (if one is used) or for two years beyond the date of distribution of the last of the batch of herbal product. The new regulations and the increased involvement of the FDA should clarify some of the issues about quality and content in herbals.

However, as previously pointed out, absolute nationally recognized standards for many herbals do not exist at this time. In many cases, no single active ingredient has been identified. This leaves the question of content of an herbal open-ended. In the end, a pharmacy (or parent organization such as retail chain or hospital) must investigate to determine how well an herbal manufacturer is meeting the required

GMP standards. In addition to the FDA's involvement, several other organizations are offering verification programs to assist the pharmacy in this regard.

Potential Contamination of the Herbal Product

In addition to the question of how much of the desired herbal may be in the finished product, there is the concern of undesired plant material or heavy metal or other toxic contaminant levels. Particularly if an herb is harvested from a wild or uncultivated field, there is a significant possibility of undesired plant contamination.

This issue has taken on a heightened concern with the reported incidents of toxic contamination on the increase. In one case in Europe, an herbal product for weight reduction was found to be adulterated with the plant contaminant aristolochic acid. This compound has been reported to be nephrotoxic in laboratory animals. In an investigation reported in 2000, this compound was also associated with the development of urothelial carcinoma in a number of Belgian consumers of the weight-reduction herbal.

In another case, an herbal product was found to be contaminated with *Digitalis lanata* (white foxglove). The contamination was discovered when a consumer of the herbal was admitted to the hospital with digitalis poisoning. After an investigation by the FDA, the manufacturer voluntarily removed the product from the market. Although the manufacturer responded appropriately to protect the public safety, it should be noted that this contamination was only discovered after consumers had been exposed to the risk. Similar incidents have been reported with regard to heavy metal contamination such as lead, mercury, and cadmium of glucosamine products derived from mollusks. The only solution to such situations is extensive screening and testing for toxic contaminants by the manufacturer or producer of an herbal. Unfortunately, many small manufacturers do not currently have the expertise or equipment for such screening. This issue has been a major problem in determining the safe use of herbals.

The new GMP regulations require manufacturers to list if there are any contaminants in their finished herbal products and to determine the identity of any such contaminants. However, the FDA regulations do not specify upper limits for any contaminants. This suggests that there may be a range of responses to this particular section of the guidelines. Therefore, it will probably take some time before the FDA clarifies this aspect of the regulations to the satisfaction of health care providers.

Meanwhile, there are several third-party organizations that can assay and report on potential contaminants in herbal products. Some of these are trade associated organizations or for-profit companies. From a scientific viewpoint, an independent not-for-profit organization with the requisite testing experience and facilities is preferable. One such organization is the National Sanitation Foundation International or NSF International (not to be confused with the National Science Foundation). This is a nonprofit organization that began operation in 1944, focusing initially on water purity and then branching out into public health. NSF International is used by the American Herbal Pharmacopoeia.

The United States Pharmacopoeia (USP) also has a verification and testing program. In 2002 the USP launched an initiative entitled the Dietary Supplement Verification Program (DSVP), in which manufacturers voluntarily submit their products to USP testing. Any product passing USP testing will be awarded the DSVP verification mark. The goals of the DSVP are to assure consumers and health care professionals that a dietary supplement product contains the ingredients listed on the label at the declared concentrations, the product meets requirements (as listed in the USP-NF) on potential contaminants, and that the product has been manufactured in compliance with GMPs proposed by the FDA and USP. Although manufacturer enrollment is voluntary, this program has examined and verified more than 200 product lines to date. For pharmacists, the USP standard is perhaps the most trusted one in practice. Details of the verification program and an up-to-date list of verified companies can be found on the USP Web site (www.usp.org).

Potential Herbal-Drug Interactions

Just as with drug-drug interactions, the concomitant usage of herbal preparations with prescription drugs may lead to significant herbal-drug interactions with adverse outcomes. Herbals and orally administered drugs are absorbed across the GI tract, metabolized by the liver, and excreted by the kidneys. Therefore, it is not surprising that the presence of herbals may alter the absorption, metabolism, or excretion of drugs. For example, use of St. John's wort has been reported to decrease the absorption of digoxin and indinavar (an antiviral) and to increase the metabolism of warfarin, cyclosporine, and oral contraceptives. Each of these interactions would decrease the amount of prescription drug concentrations in patients, potentially resulting in subtherapeutic doses. In short, patients might be undertreated even though they were receiving the correct dosage of a prescription drug. The difficulty of predicting such interactions with herbals is greatly complicated because they are not single compounds. There is no evidence, for example, that the effects of St. John's wort as just described are due to a single constituent.

A useful resource on herbal-drug interactions for the pharmacy is the text *Herb Contraindications and Drug Interactions* by Francis Brinker. Additional information can be found on the Natural Medicines Comprehensive Database Web site (www.naturaldatabase.com) under the "Natural Product/Drug Interaction Checker." In addition to being accessible via the Internet, this database may be downloaded to a personal digital assistant or PDA, making it handy during patient counseling and information review.

Herb Contra-indications and Drug Interactions a useful resource by Francis Brinker on herbal-drug interactions for the pharmacy.

Therapeutic Value of Herbals

Most of the discussion so far has focused on the issues of safety under the premise of "first do no harm." Of course, the real reason for using herbals is their potential therapeutic value. Unfortunately, there is no easy answer to the question "Do herbals have therapeutic effects?" While some herbals may logically be expected to be very useful in treatment (after all, most of our early medications were derived from botanicals), clinical trials have been lackluster in demonstrating or in definitively ruling out efficacy. Numerous reasons exist for this state of affairs, including poor clinical trial design, poor execution, and clear bias. Moreover, the source of many herbals used in some trials has come under significant scrutiny. A well-designed and well-executed clinical trial is to no avail if the product tested does not actually contain the herbal compound under investigation. Thus, the source of the herbal (which has not been extensively considered or documented in most trials) is paramount to a sound study. For all of these reasons, the effectiveness of herbals in treatment remains to be worked out on a case-by-case basis.

Where to Get More Information on Herbals

Concerns over safety and efficacy clearly underscore the need for information on herbals that is updated in a timely manner and made rapidly available to the pharmacy. Until recently, it has been hard to obtain such information in the United States. Now, however, some very useful sources are available.

1. The United States Pharmacopoeia (USP) is a mainstay of pharmacy in the United States. The USP-NF publications essentially set the standard of practice in pharmacy. As such, USP monographs on particular herbals will be central to any pharmacy's information database. From 1995 to 2005, the USP reinvigorated its efforts to publish up-to-date information on botanicals and herbals in its dietary supplements section. At this time, the USP has more than 80 monographs on botanicals/herbals. Starting in 2008, all dietary supplement monographs will be published in one volume. Furthermore, as of November 2007, the USP has announced 11 new proposed monographs on dietary supplements with the following breakdown: six turmeric-related monographs, three soy isoflavone monographs, and two amino acid formulations (*Pharmacopeial Forum* 33(6)). These monographs are in addition to others announced in July 2007 on decaffeinated green tea extract and powdered bilberry extract. Updates as to the progress of these monographs can be found on the USP Web site (www.usp.org).

2. *The ABC Clinical Guide to Herbs*, edited by Mark Blumenthal, is a handy compendium of relevant facts on various herbals and summaries of published clinical trials. Although there are numerous similar publications available, none has the range of information as well as the clinical data. Additionally, rapid updates on clinical information as well as a searchable database are available via the ABC Web site (www.herbalgram.org) for members of the American Botanical Council. As a single reference on herbals in the pharmacy, this text is a valuable resource. The ABC Web site also contains a wealth of information, but you must pay a fee to access some resources.

3. The Natural Medicines Comprehensive Database (www.naturaldatabase .com) is also a fee-based Web site. However, it also has many useful features, including access to clinical trial information and updates.

4. The USP Dietary Supplement Verification Program (DSVP) sets a high standard for herbals in the United States and assures the pharmacy of the safety of a product. Manufacturers voluntarily submit their products to USP testing. Updates and details about the DSVP can be found at the USP Web site (www.usp.org). This program has verified more than 200 product lines to date.

5. One of the provisions of the DSHEA of 1994 was the formation of an Office of Dietary Supplements (ODS) at the National Institutes of Health (NIH). The mission of the ODS is to "strengthen knowledge and understanding of dietary supplements by evaluating scientific information, stimulating and supporting research, disseminating research results, and educating the public. . . ." The ODS has created and maintains two large databases on herbals: IBIDS (the International Bibliographic Information on Dietary Supplements) and CARDS (Computer Access to Research on Dietary Supplements). CARDS covers all federally-funded research projects, such as

those from the NIH from 1999 on. IBIDS covers all "published, international, scientific literature on dietary supplements" and includes almost 700,000 entries. Both databases can be accessed free of charge at the ODS Web site (ods.od.nih.gov).

6. Another very useful Web site is the National Center for Complementary and Alternative Medicine (nccam.nih.gov). This site contains information on current clinical trials and drug interactions between herbals and drugs.

7. MedWatch (www.fda.gov/medwatch/) contains information from the FDA Safety Information and Adverse Event Reporting Program. This site is not focused exclusively on herbals or dietary supplements, but adverse events, drug interactions, and important safety announcements are reported here. This is a very useful site for the pharmacy.

8. The publication in English of the *German Commission E Monographs on Herbals* provides an excellent reference based on the accepted medicinal uses of herbals in Europe. The text is entitled *Herbal Medicine: Expanded Commission E Monographs*, and is available in hardback and as a CD-ROM. The text's European perspective on the use of herbals in medicine is quite useful in providing another viewpoint for making clinical decisions.

Some Traditional Uses of Herbals

The following list contains some common herbal products and their traditional or common uses. Please note that this section is not an endorsement of clinical efficacy of any particular herbal, nor is this meant to be an exhaustive list of all herbals used. Rather, these are merely examples of typical herbal products.

Common Name: Angelica
Botanical Name: *Angelica archangelica* (divided into many different species)
Typical Uses: To relieve symptoms of flatulence (i.e., GI gas), as a diuretic (i.e., to increase urine flow), and a diaphoretic (i.e., sweat producer). Also used as a flavoring agent in several liqueurs and in gin (along with juniper berries).

FIGURE 23-1

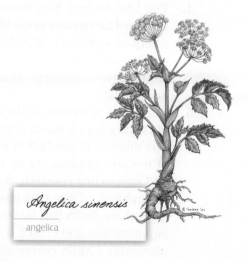

Angelica sinensis

angelica

FIGURE 23-1 Angelica

Common Name: Black Cohosh (black snakeroot)
Botanical Name: *Cimicifuga racemosa*
Typical Uses: To relieve symptoms of menopause and various menstrual
    problems.

FIGURE 23-2

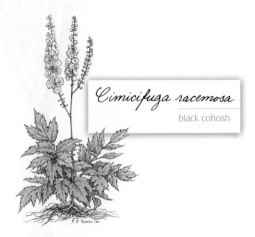

FIGURE 23-2 Black Cohosh

Common Name: Feverfew
Botanical Name: *Tanacetum parthenium*
Typical Uses: To relieve symptoms of migraine headaches, arthritis, and men-
    strual problems.

FIGURE 23-3

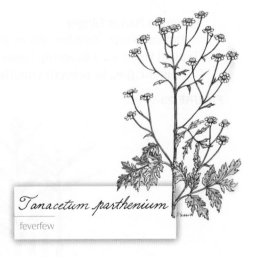

FIGURE 23-3 Feverfew

Common Name: Garlic
Botanical Name: *Allium sativum*
Typical Uses: As a flavoring agent in salads, soups, and other foods; as a cholesterol-lowering agent.

FIGURE 23-4

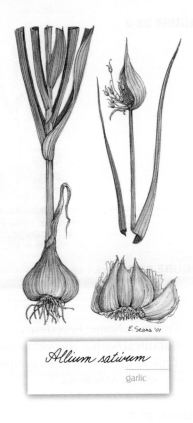

FIGURE 23-4 Garlic

Common Name: Ginger
Botanical Name: *Zingiber officinale* Roscoe
Typical Uses: As a flavoring agent in foods; as a digestive aid; and as an anti-emetic (i.e., to prevent vomiting).

FIGURE 23-5

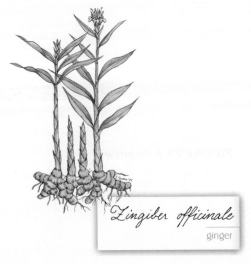

FIGURE 23-5 Ginger

Common Name: Ginkgo
Botanical Name: *Ginkgo biloba*
Typical Uses: As an antiasthmatic, bronchodilator, and to treat memory loss or headache.

FIGURE 23-6

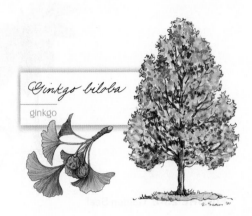

FIGURE 23-6 Ginkgo

Common Name: Ginseng
Botanical Name: *Panax ginseng* (Asian ginseng) or *Panax quinquefolius* (American ginseng)
Typical Uses: As an "adaptogen" to increase resistance to environmental stress and to promote immune response.

FIGURE 23-7

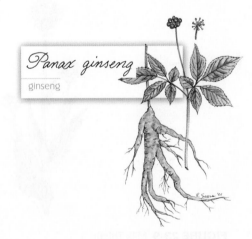

FIGURE 23-7 Ginseng

Common Name: Golden Seal
Botanical Name: *Hydrastis canadensis*
Typical Uses: As a bitter tonic for gastric and urogenital disorders.

FIGURE 23-8

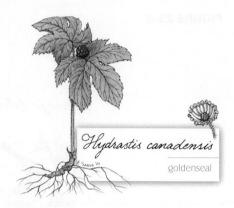

FIGURE 23-8 Golden Seal

Common Name: Milk Thistle
Botanical Name: *Silybum marianum*
Typical Uses: As an antihepatotoxic agent (i.e., liver protectant), especially against poisoning from *Amanita* sp. mushrooms, which contain compounds such as phallotoxins.

FIGURE 23-9

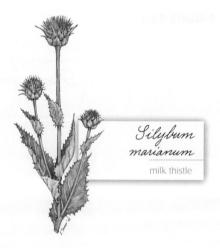

FIGURE 23-9 Milk Thistle

Common Name: Purple Coneflower or Echinacea
Botanical Name: *Echinacea purpurea*
Typical Uses: As an anti-infective, antiseptic, and immunostimulant agent.

FIGURE 23-10

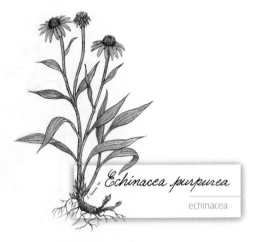

FIGURE 23-10 Purple Coneflower (Echinacea)

Common Name: Saw Palmetto
Botanical Name: *Serenoa repens*
Typical Uses: To relieve the symptoms of benign prostatic hypertrophy (i.e., noncancerous enlarged prostate gland).

FIGURE 23-11

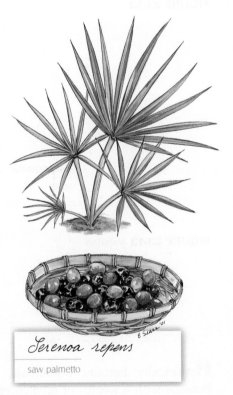

FIGURE 23-11 Saw Palmetto

Common Name: St. John's wort
Botanical Name: *Hypericum calycinum* (divided into many different species)
Typical Uses: To relieve the symptoms of depression.

FIGURE 23-12

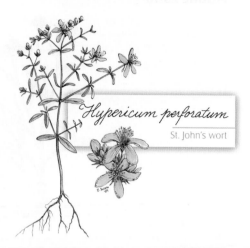

FIGURE 23-12 St. John's wort

Common Name: Valerian
Botanical Name: *Valeriana officinalis*
Typical Uses: To relieve the symptoms of restlessness, sleep disturbances, or nervousness.

FIGURE 23-13

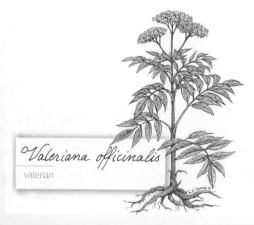

FIGURE 23-13 Valerian

Summary

Historically, herbals, botanicals, and natural plant products have provided humans with a wealth of medicines. Herbals are currently regulated as dietary supplements and not as drugs under the 1994 Dietary Supplement Health and Education Act (DSHEA). According to DSHEA, herbals may not claim to cure, mitigate, diagnose, or prevent disease. However, herbals have been and continue to be used by many consumers to prevent or self-treat disease. While some herbal preparations may be useful, the effectiveness (efficacy) and safety of many herbals has yet to be demonstrated. Fortunately, new regulatory initiatives and programs are beginning to address the safety concerns over herbals. Moreover, reliable, professional health care information is becoming increasingly available on the Internet, allowing rapid access for the pharmacist. This chapter reviews the regulatory history of herbal products in the United States, the major classes of secondary plant metabolites that make up most herbals, and the sites where professional herbal information is freely available.

TEST YOUR KNOWLEDGE

Multiple Choice

1. Which of the following is the best regulatory definition of an herbal?
   a. plant material that smells nice
   b. any substance or mixture of substances intended for the cure, mitigation, diagnosis, or prevention of disease
   c. a dietary supplement that contains an herb or other botanical for use to supplement the diet and to promote health
   d. all of the above

2. Which of the following prohibited misbranded or adulterated drugs, but did not require that a drug be safe or effective before being sold?
   a. 1906 Pure Food Act
   b. 1938 Federal Food, Drug, and Cosmetic Act
   c. 1962 Kefauver-Harris Drug Amendments
   d. 1994 Dietary Supplement Health and Education Act

3. Chemically, most herbal products would be described as
   a. proteins.
   b. primary metabolites.
   c. nucleic acids.
   d. secondary metabolites.

4. To be compliant with DSHEA, an herbal must be
   a. labeled as a dietary supplement.
   b. identify all ingredients by name and list the quantity of each ingredient.
   c. identify the plant by genus and species and the plant part from which the ingredient is derived.
   d. all of the above.

5. Herbal remedies are never administered as a
   a. tablet.
   b. lozenge.
   c. injection.
   d. topical ointment.

6. Which of the following is not an important safety concern with the use of herbal products?
   a. the potential of a hypersensitivity (allergic) response to the herbal
   b. the potential that the product does not contain the herbal declared on the label
   c. the potential that the herbal product is contaminated with toxic material
   d. the potential that the herbal product does not taste very good

7. Which of the following is the Web site for the Dietary Supplement Verification Program and the updates on the United States Pharmacopoeia-National Formulary monographs on herbals?
   a. ods.od.gov
   b. www.usp.org
   c. www.fda.gov/medwatch
   d. nccam.nih.gov

8. Which of the following is traditionally taken by individuals as an herbal treatment for depression?
   a. saw palmetto (*Serenoa repens*)
   b. milk thistle (*Silybum marianum*)
   c. St. John's wort (*Hypericum calycinum*)
   d. purple coneflower or echinacea (*Echinacea purpurea*)

9. Which of the following is traditionally taken by individuals to help prevent illness such as colds?
   a. saw palmetto (*Serenoa repens*)
   b. milk thistle (*Silybum marianum*)
   c. St. John's wort (*Hypericum calycinum*)
   d. purple coneflower or echinacea (*Echinacea purpurea*)

Matching

Match the herbal with its use.

1. _____ cholesterol-lowering agent   a. ginger
2. _____ bronchodilator   b. ginseng
3. _____ anti-emetic   c. garlic
4. _____ stimulates immune system   d. valerian
5. _____ used for insomnia   e. ginkgo

References

Applequist, W. (2006). *The identification of medicinal plants: A handbook of botanicals in commerce.* St. Louis, MO: Missouri Botanical Garden Press.

Blumenthal, M., et al. (Eds.). (2003). *The ABC clinical guide to herbs.* New York: Thieme Medical Publishers.

Blumenthal, M., Goldberg, A., & Brinckman, J. (Eds.). (2000). *Herbal medicine: Expanded commission E monographs.* Newton, MA: Integrative Medicine Communications.

Brinker, F. (2001). *Herb contraindications and drug interactions* (3rd ed.). Sandy, OR: Eclectic Medical Publications.

Buchanan, R. B., Gruissem, W., & Jones, R. L. (2000). *Biochemistry & molecular biology of plants*. Rockville, MD: American Society of Plant Physiologists.

Cavaliere, C., & Blumenthal, M. (2007). Review of FDA's final GMPs for dietary supplements. *HerbalGram: The Journal of the American Botanical Council*, 76: 58–91.

Dewick, P. M. (1998). *Medicinal natural products: A biosynthetic approach*. New York: John Wiley & Sons.

Dey, P. M., & Harborne, J. B. (Eds.). (1997). *Plant biochemistry*. San Diego: Academic Press.

Goldman, P. (2001). Herbal medicines today and the roots of modern pharmacology. *Annals of Internal Medicine*, 135, 594–600.

Harkey, M. R., Henderson, G. L., Gershwin, M. E., Stern, J. S., & Hackman, R. M. (2001). Variability in commercial ginseng products: An analysis of 25 preparations. *American Journal of Clinical Nutrition*, 73, 1101–1106.

Israelsen, L. D. (1998). Botanicals and DHSEA: A health professional's guide. *Quarterly Review of Natural Medicine*, Fall, 251–257.

Linde, K., Ramirez, G., Mulrow, C. D., Pauls, A., Weidenhammer, W., & Melchart, D. (1996). St. John's wort for depression—An overview and meta-analysis of randomized clinical trials. *British Medical Journal*, 313, 253–258.

Nortier, J. L., Martinez, M. C., Schmeiser, H. H., Arlt, V. M., Bieler, C. A., Petein, M., et al. (2000). Urothelial carcinoma associated with the use of a Chinese herb (*Aristolochia fanchi*). *New England Journal of Medicine*, 342, 1686–1692.

Robbers, J. E., Speedie, M. K., & Tyler, V. E. (1996). *Pharmacognosy and pharmacobiotechnology*. Baltimore, MD: Lippincott Williams & Wilkins.

Slifman, N. R., Obermeyer, W. R., Aloi, B. K., Mussler, S. M., Correll, W. A., Cichowicz, S. M., et al. (1998). Contamination of botanical dietary supplements by *Digitalis lanata*. *New England Journal of Medicine*, 339, 806–811.

Srinivasan, V. S., & Kucera, P. (1998). Botanicals in the USP-NF. *Pharmacopeial Forum*, 24, 6623–6626.

Temin, P. (1980). *Taking your medicine: Drug regulation in the United States*. Cambridge, MA: Harvard University Press.

Web Sites

American Botanical Council (fee required)
www.herbalgram.org

MedWatch (FDA Safety Information and Adverse Event Reporting Program)
www.fda.gov/medwatch

The National Center for Complementary and Alternative Medicine
nccam.nih.gov

Natural Medicines Comprehensive Database (fee required)
www.naturaldatabase.com

NIH Office of Dietary Supplements (with the IBIDS [International Bibliographic Information on Dietary Supplements] and CARDS [Computer Access to Research on Dietary Supplements] databases)
ods.od.nih.gov

The United States Pharmacopoeia (USP-NF) and the Dietary Supplement Verification Program (DSVP)
www.usp.org

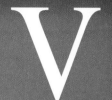

PART

V

Administrative Aspects of Pharmacy Technology

The Policy and Procedure Manual

Competencies

Upon completion of this chapter, the reader should be able to

1. Define and differentiate a *policy* and a *procedure*.
2. Give five reasons to justify the need for a policy and procedure manual.
3. Explain the rationale for inclusion of job descriptions in the policy and procedure manual.
4. Give examples of the sections that may be included in a pharmacy policy and procedure manual.
5. List five topics that could be included in each of the following pharmacy areas: administration, distribution, and clinical.
6. Describe the rationale for the use of a policy and procedure manual for new pharmacy employees.

Key Terms

policy
procedure

Introduction

policy a defined course to guide and determine present and future decisions; established by an organization or employer who guides the employee to act in a manner consistent with management philosophy.

In every organization rules or policies are developed to accomplish the objectives of the organization. There are also specific ways in which these policies are to be carried out. These ways of carrying out policies are called *procedures*.

A **policy** is an overall plan embracing general goals and objectives of what is to be done. A **procedure** is a particular way of accomplishing the objectives set forth in the policy—a series of steps and ways of doing things. In other words, a policy is a decision by an organization or a department to do something; a procedure is a step-by-step method used to accomplish that policy.

Need for Policies and Procedures

procedures guidelines on the preferred way to perform a certain function; particular actions to be taken to carry out a policy.

When new employees begin work in a pharmacy, there are literally hundreds of things to learn. Not only must the newcomers learn the work, but they must also learn about lunch hours, benefits, hours of operation, the chain of command, what scope of services is provided by the department, and so on. By reading a manual in which policies and procedures are described, new employees should be able to learn a considerable amount about their respective jobs. So the first reason for having a policy and procedure manual is to use it in the training of new employees.

If written policies and procedures did not exist, employees would have to be trained and instructed verbally by other employees. As everyone may not be a good teacher or able to explain things fully or correctly, having information in writing ensures it is presented in a clear and consistent manner. Therefore, the second reason to have a written policy and procedure manual is to prevent errors from verbal communication.

People handle different situations in different ways. In a pharmacy, however, it is important to ensure that the same accurate and consistent results occur and that people and situations are treated the same way every time. Thus, a set way for doings things is established and set forth in a policy and procedure manual. Another reason for having a policy and procedure manual is consistency—to ensure that the same policy is followed in a particular situation all the time.

The pharmacy department uses a large number and variety of drugs and supplies. Although many drugs are expensive, labor and supplies used in compounding, packaging, and labeling in a pharmacy can also comprise a considerable component of the cost of bringing drugs to patients. If procedures are performed in an efficient and economical manner, waste of both materials and manpower can be minimized, thus reducing the cost of providing services.

A good manager is responsible for assuring that the work is done and that employees are aware of how well they are performing their jobs. One way this may be accomplished is through periodic evaluations of personnel job performance (i.e., how well an employee is following procedures). Effective evaluations can be accomplished only if there are written policies, procedures, and job descriptions against which job performance can be measured (Figure 24-1). Policy and procedure manuals are often used to evaluate job performance.

Because of potential harm to patients, pharmacy departments take considerable care to ensure that medications are purchased, stocked, packaged, compounded, labeled, dispensed, administered, and charted accurately. Despite this care, adverse outcomes do occur, resulting in lawsuits. Unfortunately, these are not uncommon and it is sometimes necessary to determine how a specific procedure should have been performed. Policy and procedure manuals, therefore, often serve as legal documents in the event of a lawsuit to protect the individual and the institution.

FIGURE 24-1

MEDICAL CENTER
JOB DESCRIPTION – PERFORMANCE APPRAISAL

EMPLOYEE NAME:	EMPLOYEE NUMBER:

DATE OF HIRE:	DATE IN POSITION:

EVALUATION DATE:	EVALUATION PERIOD:

☐ INTRODUCTORY   ☐ ANNUAL

JOB TITLE: Pharmacy Technician   **JOB CODE: TECH04**
DEPARTMENT: Pharmacy   **REPORTS TO: Senior Pharmacist**

JOB SUMMARY: Assist the pharmacist in the day to day activities of the hospital pharmacy with emphasis on cassette filling, label filling, and drug distribution. Adheres to the medical center/department policies and procedures and Joint Commission/regulatory agency requirements. Demonstrates and promotes service excellence at all times.

MINIMUM QUALIFICATIONS:

Education: High school diploma or equivalent

Experience/skills: Technician certification preferred.

Licensure:

Risk Exposure;
Hazard Assessment:
Physical Demands:
Mental Demands:

PERFORMANCE RATING SCALE:

Exceeds – Performance consistently exceeds performance standard. (Comments preferred.)
Meets – Performance consistently meets performance standards.
Needs Improvement – Performance inconsistently meets performance standards. **(Comments required.)**
Does Not Meet – Performance consistently does not meet performance standards. **(Comments required.)**
Not Applicable/Unable to Evaluate – Performance could not be evaluated to date for standard.

Validation methods used in evaluating performance are as follows, but not limited to, direct observation, written tests, skills checklist, attendance records, incident reports, patient comments/letters and medical record reviews.

Approval Signatures	
Department Head:	Date:
Human Resources:	Date:

FIGURE 24-1 Technician job description-performance appraisal form.

FIGURE 24-1 (Continued)

PERFORMANCE STANDARD	EX	MTS	NI	DNM	UE	COMMENTS
*Standard #1. Demonstrates the ability to assist in inpatient drug distribution activities.	☐	☐	☐	☐	☐	
A. Fills/exchanges patient's cassettes accurately and efficiently.	☐	☐	☐	☐	☐	
B. Fills prescription labels accurately and efficiently.	☐	☐	☐	☐	☐	
C. Delivers medications to patient care areas in a timely manner.	☐	☐	☐	☐	☐	
D. Assists pharmacists with phone/window in a courteous, professional manner.	☐	☐	☐	☐	☐	
*Standard #2. Demonstrates the ability to perform IV Room activities.	☐	☐	☐	☐	☐	
A. Accurately prepares add-a-vial stock and adheres to logging procedures.	☐	☐	☐	☐	☐	
B. Sets up TPN pump/prepares TPN fluids.	☐	☐	☐	☐	☐	
C. Maintains inventory by ordering medications and restocking solutions.	☐	☐	☐	☐	☐	
D. Accurately labels premixed intravenous admixtures/piggybacks.	☐	☐	☐	☐	☐	
Standard #3. Able to assist in daily maintenance activities.	☐	☐	☐	☐	☐	
A. Generates and processes fill lists, transfer/discharge lists, reports, etc.	☐	☐	☐	☐	☐	
B. Maintains floor stock/Pyxis.	☐	☐	☐	☐	☐	
C. Pre-packs medications as per policy and procedure.	☐	☐	☐	☐	☐	
D. Files daily orders/controlled substance sheets.	☐	☐	☐	☐	☐	
Standard #4. Demonstrates the knowledge and skills necessary to provide care and/or services to patients/guests of specific age groups as designated.	☐	☐	☐	☐	☐	*Attach age specific competency, if applicable.*
A. Neonate/Infant (Birth–1 yr)	☐	☐	☐	☐	☐	
B. Child (1–11 yrs)	☐	☐	☐	☐	☐	
C. Adolescent (12–17 yrs)	☐	☐	☐	☐	☐	
D. Adult (18–65 yrs)	☐	☐	☐	☐	☐	
E. Older Adult (65+ yrs)	☐	☐	☐	☐	☐	
F. All Ages	☐	☐	☐	☐	☐	
Standard #5. Fosters change initiatives to ensure continued improvement of service quality and performance improvement.	☐	☐	☐	☐	☐	

* ADA Essential Functions

FIGURE 24-1 (Continued)

PERFORMANCE STANDARD	RATING SCALE					COMMENTS
	EX	MTS	NI	DNM	UE	
A. Facilitates change initiatives in a manner that promotes continued performance improvement.	☐	☐	☐	☐	☐	
B. Willingly contributes talents and skills to achieve individual, departmental, and hospital goals and objectives.	☐	☐	☐	☐	☐	
C. Attends meetings and participates on committees as directed.	☐	☐	☐	☐	☐	
D. Performs activities that foster a culture of safety within the department and organization.	☐	☐	☐	☐	☐	
E. Identifies safety/risk reduction strategies and communicates these to department director.	☐	☐	☐	☐	☐	
Standard #6. Incorporates Medical Center's service excellence standards by identifying patient/guest expectations and working to exceed them. Promotes positive "Guest Services" throughout the organization by demonstrating care, compassion, and respect to patients, physicians, guests, and staff.	☐	☐	☐	☐	☐	
A. Anticipates, understands, and meets the needs of the guest. Is supportive and gives help before asked. Is consistently courteous to all guests in all forms of communication including in person, on the telephone, and in writing.	☐	☐	☐	☐	☐	
B. Demonstrates compassion, empathy, concern, and a respectful behavior toward guests. Exhibits an "always caring" attitude.	☐	☐	☐	☐	☐	
C. Promotes positive co-worker, team building relationships, within the department and between departments. Works collaboratively and is respectful of others. Takes individual responsibility for living and energizing the Medical Center Service Excellence Standards.	☐	☐	☐	☐	☐	

FIGURE 24-1 (Continued)

PERFORMANCE STANDARD	RATING SCALE					COMMENTS
	EX	MTS	NI	DNM	UE	
Standard #7. Incorporates Hospital's Corporate Compliance Program into the work environment by adhering to the "Standards of Conduct" outlined in the Compliance Assurance Program Handbook.	☐	☐	☐	☐	☐	
A. Conducts himself/herself in a professional and ethical manner when acting on behalf of the Medical Center. Is honest and truthful in all of his/her dealings with other employees or organizations that do business with the Hospital.	☐	☐	☐	☐	☐	
B. Participates in Corporate Compliance Program by receiving formal in-service education, obtaining a copy of the Compliance Assurance Program Handbook, and attesting to abide by the Standards of Conduct outlined in the handbook.	☐	☐	☐	☐	☐	
C. Understands the disciplinary policies for violations of the Corporate Compliance Program.	☐	☐	☐	☐	☐	
D. Understands the manner in which a violation of the Corporate Compliance Program can be reported.	☐	☐	☐	☐	☐	
Standard #8. Complies with general policies and procedures of the organization/department including:	☐	☐	☐	☐	☐	
A. Is knowledgeable of and exemplifies the beliefs, mission, and vision of Health Services at the Medical Center.	☐	☐	☐	☐	☐	
B. Maintains confidentiality of patients, employees, department, and hospital information including computer passwords.	☐	☐	☐	☐	☐	
C. Follows emergency/disaster preparedness protocols.	☐	☐	☐	☐	☐	
D. Maintains safe work environment; follows fire/safety prevention protocols.	☐	☐	☐	☐	☐	

FIGURE 24-1 (Continued)

PERFORMANCE STANDARD	RATING SCALE					COMMENTS
	EX	MTS	NI	DNM	UE	
E. Complies with departmental and organizational in-service education program requirements.	☐	☐	☐	☐	☐	
F. Complies with dress, appearance, and uniform requirements.	☐	☐	☐	☐	☐	
G. Follows infection control practices and procedures.	☐	☐	☐	☐	☐	
H. Complies with Human Resources attendance/punctuality policy.	☐	☐	☐	☐	☐	
I. Adheres to Joint Commission and other regulatory requirements.	☐	☐	☐	☐	☐	
Standard #9. Provides support and leadership within the department.	☐	☐	☐	☐	☐	
A. Resolves problems regarding department operations and assists in resolving co-worker problems/issues.	☐	☐	☐	☐	☐	
B. Promotes and communicates commitment, values, and ethics within the department.	☐	☐	☐	☐	☐	
C. Provides assistance to co-workers in meeting the goals and objectives of the department.	☐	☐	☐	☐	☐	
D. Promotes continued development and morale among co-workers.	☐	☐	☐	☐	☐	
E. Fosters effective employee communications, teamwork, and participates in department staff meetings.	☐	☐	☐	☐	☐	
Standard #10. Works to enhance professional growth and development.	☐	☐	☐	☐	☐	
A. Participates in educational programs, in-service meetings, workshops, conferences, and committees.	☐	☐	☐	☐	☐	
B. Keeps abreast of current literature and professional trends.	☐	☐	☐	☐	☐	
C. Participates in professional organizations.	☐	☐	☐	☐	☐	
Standard #11. Performs related duties as necessary.	☐	☐	☐	☐	☐	
A. With appropriate training, accepts additional related duties as needed.	☐	☐	☐	☐	☐	

Responsibilities may be added, changed, or deleted at any time at the discretion of the Department Head or Administration formally or informally, either verbally or in writing.

It must be recognized that pharmacies and hospitals are highly regulated establishments. They are governed by laws, rules, regulations, standards, and guidelines that must be followed. Many of these federal, state, and local regulating agencies require written policies and procedures.

In summary, policy and procedure manuals exist for the following reasons:

- To train new employees or retrain existing employees.
- To prevent errors due to verbal communication.
- To ensure consistency of policy and job performance.
- To minimize the waste of human resources and materials.
- To evaluate job performance.
- To serve as legal documents in the event of a lawsuit.
- To comply with regulatory and accreditation agencies' requirements.

Composing a Policy and Procedure Manual

Let us now examine what information can be found in a pharmacy department's manual.

Format

To avoid confusion and for the sake of consistency, a similar format to follow for all policies and procedures is best. Some institutions use special preprinted forms on which to write their policies and procedures. Most institutions, however, follow some kind of standard format that sets forth the basic information required. Let us examine some of the items that should be part of every policy and procedure manual.

Title

First, every policy and procedure should have a title. This tells the reader what subject is covered in the policy and procedure. This title is also used in a table of contents or an index.

Date

Every policy and procedure should be dated. Initially, a date of implementation indicates when the policy and procedure went into effect. Often, however, it is necessary to change, update, expand, or modify an existing policy or procedure. Therefore, additional dates indicate when the policy or procedure was revised. Many institutions use just the original and latest revision dates. For example:

Approved and Implemented: 9-19-05
Revised: 10-25-07

Signatures

Policies and procedures should also contain the signatures of those who wrote or approved the policy where the policy and procedure is most frequently carried out. These signature(s) are valuable because they indicate who is responsible for generating the policy and procedure and document the agreement of the administrative personnel on the highest level.

Design

It has been suggested that a useful policy and procedure manual must answer the following questions regarding a specific activity. Figure 24-2 is an example of a format used in a community hospital

What must be done?

Who should do it?

How should it be done?

When should it be done?

FIGURE 24-2

HOSPITAL

PHARMACY POLICY AND PROCEDURE MANUAL

	Manual Code:	Inpatient – 60
Subject:	Verbal Orders for Treatment	

Effective Date: 5/85	**Revised Date:** 9/08	**Supersedes:** 9/92

POLICY

All orders for treatment shall be in writing. A verbal order shall be considered to be in writing if dictated to a nurse functioning within her sphere of competence and signed by the responsible practitioner. A pharmacist can accept a verbal order dictated by a physician to correct and/or clarify an already existing medication order on the Order Sheet.

PROCEDURE

Orders to clarify an existing medication order will be placed on the Physician Order Sheet. All orders dictated over the telephone shall be signed by the nurse or pharmacist to whom dictated with the name of practitioner per his/her own name.* The responsible practitioner shall authenticate such orders within 24 hours and failure to do so shall be brought to the attention of the Executive Committee for appropriate action.

A verbal order shall be considered to be in writing if dictated to a pharmacist for outpatient prescriptions acceptable over the telephone. All prescriptions dictated and accepted over the telephone shall be signed by the pharmacist to whom dictated with the name of the practitioner per his/her own name.

* **All orders dictated over the telephone shall be "received" by 2 pharmacists (one pharmacist to whom dictated, and one pharmacist confirming the verbal order)**

FIGURE 24-2 Sample format of a policy and procedure manual.

The Approval Process

In most hospitals the Pharmacy and Therapeutics Committee serves as the liaison between the medical staff and the department of pharmacy services. The Joint Commission requires that the Pharmacy and Therapeutics Committee annually review and approve the policies and procedures of the pharmacy department. Although some pharmacy departments indicate the approval of the Pharmacy and Therapeutics Committee on each policy and procedure itself, most pharmacy departments use a cover page at the beginning of the manual indicating all approvals. Figure 24-3 is an example of a cover page for the approval of the policy and procedure manual.

A number of hospitals and other health care institutions have a subcommittee of the Pharmacy and Therapeutics Committee that deals specifically with medication procedures, which also may also serve as a pharmacy-nursing liaison committee. Many policies and procedures dealing with medication distribution, control, administration, and documentation are developed jointly by the nursing and pharmacy department members of this committee.

FIGURE 24-3

MEDICAL CENTER
DEPARTMENT OF PHARMACY

POLICY AND PROCEDURE MANUAL

THE POLICIES AND PROCEDURES OF THE DEPARTMENT OF PHARMACY
HAVE BEEN APPROVED BY THE MEDICAL STAFF OF THE HOSPITAL
THROUGH THE PHARMACY AND THERAPEUTICS COMMITTEE

Jack Royale
President & Chief Executive Officer

Elizabeth Prime
Director of Clinical Services

Alex Zimmerman, Chairman
Pharmacy & Therapeutics Committee

Alison Zaza
Pharmacy & Therapeutics Committee

FIGURE 24-3 Cover approval page for the policy and procedure manual.

Contents of a Policy and Procedure Manual

The format and contents of a policy and procedure manual will vary from hospital to hospital. The most common methods for organizing policy and procedure manuals fall into two main groups. The first method has policies and procedures placed in a book in alphabetical order by title; for example, Abbreviations, Absenteeism, Adverse Drug Reactions, Alcohol Dispensing and Control, Ambulatory Care, and Aseptic Technique. A second common method of organizing a manual is to group policies and procedures into three or more categories with separate sections for each category.

An example of this format follows:

Section I: Organization—This section contains information on the hospital and pharmacy department itself, organizational charts for both the hospital and the department, services offered, pharmacy department participation on hospital committees (e.g., Pharmacy and Therapeutics Committee, the Infection Control Committee), security/confidentiality, and so forth.

Section II: Personnel—This section may contain job descriptions/performance appraisals; orientation, staffing, and scheduling information; personnel policies; educational benefits, and so forth.

Section III: Administrative Policies—This section contains policies and procedures on the department's hours of operation, purchasing policies and procedures, inventory control, interdepartmental requisitions, control and accountability of controlled drugs, performance improvement (PI) activities, material safety data sheets (MSDS), administrative reports, annual reports, in-service education, and so forth.

Section IV: Distribution Services—These policies and procedures involve the compounding, labeling, packaging, dispensing, and control of medications; formulary operation; automatic stop orders; intravenous admixture services, including parenteral nutrition and antineoplastic therapy; outpatient pharmacy services; non-sterile compounding and manufacturing, and so forth.

Section V: Clinical Pharmacy Services—This section includes the clinical pharmacy services provided by the department, which may include drug therapy monitoring, pharmacokinetic consultation services, drug information services, investigational drugs, in-service education, discharge counseling, and so forth.

Section VI: Facilities and Equipment—These policies and procedures pertain to the use and maintenance of the department's physical facilities and equipment, their maintenance and repair, service contracts, and the like.

This format of grouping policies and procedures into categories with separate sections for each category requires a comprehensive table of contents or index for each section so that any policy and procedure can be easily and readily located.

No matter which system a department uses to organize its policy and procedure manual, there is no one "right way." Some prefer not to include job descriptions in their manuals. Some have separate sections for inpatient and outpatient operations. The key factor of a good manual is that it meets the needs of the department and that it is a useful reference for the staff.

Distribution

A policy and procedure manual is a dynamic entity since it is constantly changing. Policies and procedures are being revised, added, or deleted on a continuing basis. Therefore, the more copies of a manual that are available, the more difficult it is to keep each copy current. A copy of the policy and procedure manual, however, should be readily available to every employee so that it may be used as a reference in handling both new and repeat situations, and a number of copies should be available for the orientation of new employees.

In hospitals that have hospital-wide computerized information systems, it is now possible to place the policy and procedure manual on the system's computer network. This permits access to the policy and procedure manual from any terminal in the hospital and makes updating the policy and procedure manual quick and easy since the network file can be easily modified. Individuals can also generate a hard copy of any policy and procedure as needed.

Summary

Each policy and procedure manual is unique for a particular pharmacy. It addresses the mission, goals, and objectives of the pharmacy; it incorporates the contemporary professional standards of practice as well as current legal and quasi-legal regulations of the profession; and it provides the basis for a cooperative professional environment where there is a strong sense of direction for the pharmacy staff.

Comprehensive and current policy and procedure manuals are necessary, useful tools in the proper running of any well-managed organization. They should be viewed as meaningful, helpful guides in providing efficient and consistent service to the patients and staff whom the pharmacy department serves.

TEST YOUR KNOWLEDGE

Multiple Choice

1. A policy is
   a. a series of steps to follow.
   b. a memorandum to accomplish in a definite order.
   c. a traditional way of doing a task.
   d. all of the above.

2. A procedure is
   a. a step-by-step method used to carry out a task.
   b. a verbal communication.
   c. a decision to do something.
   d. all of the above.

3. New employees must become familiar with
   a. their job description.
   b. the hours of work.
   c. policies and procedures.
   d. all of the above.

4. Policy and procedure manuals are used to
   a. train and inform new employees.
   b. prevent errors from verbal communications.
   c. ensure that the same policies are followed in the same situations.
   d. all of the above.

5. Which of the following is not true regarding policy and procedure manuals?
   a. Many regulating agencies require written policies and procedures.
   b. Any change requires approval of the chief operating officer of the institution.
   c. They minimize waste of manpower, time, and materials by providing direction in repetitive tasks.
   d. They provide a new employee with valuable information about his or her new job.

Matching

1. _____ operational manual
2. _____ policy
3. _____ memo
4. _____ policy and procedure manual
5. _____ procedure

a. guidelines that contain goals and methods of carrying out the goals
b. a particular way of acting
c. a directive in message form
d. overall plan of general goals
e. internal workings of the pharmacy department

Fill In The Blank

1. A definite course or method of action is a _____.

2. A particular way of accomplishing something is a _____.

3. Every policy and procedure should be _____.

4. In most hospitals, the _____ serves as the liaison between the medical staff and the department of pharmacy services.

5. The policy and procedures manual may be organized _____ or _____.

References

American Society of Health-System Pharmacists. *Best practices for hospital and health-system pharmacy, 2007–2008*. Bethesda, MD.

Brown, T. R. (Ed.). (2006). *Handbook of institutional pharmacy practice* (4th ed.). Bethesda, MD: American Society of Health-System Pharmacists.

Materials Management of Pharmaceuticals

Competencies

Upon completion of this chapter, the reader should be able to

1. List the functions involved in the drug procurement process in the institutional pharmacy.

2. Explain the major methods used to distribute drugs in the hospital.

3. Describe the function of the Pharmacy and Therapeutics Committee in drug selection.

4. Enumerate the seven basic principles essential for group purchasing.

5. List the records and reports required to be maintained in the materials management section.

6. State the information that must be included in a pharmacy purchase order.

7. Describe checkpoints to be observed when a drug order is received in the hospital.

8. List the environmental considerations required in the storage of drugs, and define temperature requirements.

9. Calculate an inventory turnover rate, and state the desirable turnover level range.

10. Describe acquisition alternatives when manufacturer's back orders or distributor shortages impose a supply dilemma.

11. List the benefits associated with the use of a bar-coded medication system.

Key Terms

bioengineered therapies
group purchasing organizations (GPOs)
just in time (JIT)
materials management
prime vendor
therapeutic equivalent
turnover rate

Introduction

This chapter will address the methods used to select, acquire, and organize a drug inventory for institutional use; describe the various systems of drug distribution and control; recognize the impact of cost-containment strategies used by pharmacy personnel; and describe the scope of activities qualified pharmacy technicians can assume.

Health care costs at both the federal and state levels have increased more rapidly than any other category of products or services used in our society. Private insurance companies and government agencies have been overwhelmed with requests for payment of expensive charges for state-of-the-art diagnostic procedures and sophisticated treatments and therapies. The costs associated with pharmaceuticals continue to increase at astronomical rates due to a constant flow of costly new **bioengineered therapies** (e.g., Epoetin alfa, various insulin preparations, etc.), resulting from advances in research and sophisticated marketing programs. Bioengineered therapies (or biotechnology) refers to the use of genetically modified living organisms in the production of pharmaceutical products having beneficial uses. As a result of increased costs for health care services and a decrease in resources to pay for them, assessing cost containment in all aspects of pharmacy service has become essential for pharmacy department managers.

The objective of this chapter is to identify and describe the methods used by pharmacy personnel to deliver the appropriate drug to the right patient, at the right time, and at the most reasonable cost (i.e., to identify pharmacy services that are both effective and affordable).

bioengineered therapies the process used in the manufacture of therapeutic agents through recombinant DNA (deoxyribonucleic acid) technology.

Materials Management

Controlling the costs associated with a complete pharmacy service includes not only the acquisition cost of drugs, but also the total cost of "managing" materials. An institutional pharmacy **materials management** program includes the following:

materials management the division of a hospital pharmacy responsible for the procurement, control, storage, and distribution of drugs and pharmaceutical products.

- *Procurement*—drug selection, source selection, cost analysis, group purchasing, prime-vendor relationships, purchasing procedures, recordkeeping, receiving control.
- *Drug storage and inventory control*—storage conditions, security requirements, proper rotation of inventory, computerized inventory control.
- *Repackaging and labeling considerations*—unit-dose and extemporaneous packaging, labeling requirements.
- *Distribution systems*—unit-dose, floor stock, compounded prescriptions, intravenous admixtures, emergency drugs.
- *Recapture and disposal*—unused medication, returns and reuse, environmental considerations.

In a hospital, the overall responsibility for the materials management of pharmaceuticals lies with the director of the pharmacy department. The Pharmacy and Therapeutics Committee approves all drugs and therapeutic agents that are to be available in the institution. This committee is chaired by a physician appointed by the medical board, and the secretary is the director of pharmacy services. The committee consists of representatives from the medical staff, the pharmacy, nursing and dietary departments, quality assurance, and the hospital administration. Having the clinical and technical knowledge of pharmacists, physicians, and nurses is essential when making decisions regarding which drug products should be included in the formulary to ensure adequate and appropriate therapy.

The director of pharmacy delegates certain aspects of the pharmacy materials management program to trained pharmacy personnel to deliver effective and efficient pharmacy services. The official list of drugs available is known as the *hospital formulary* and is reviewed and modified on an ongoing basis as required.

Procurement

The procurement of medications is the responsibility of the pharmacy department. The following section will outline the steps involved in the process and the responsibilities of the pharmacy technician.

Drug selection

The drug selection process may begin with a physician's request for a new drug. All requests for the addition of a drug to a hospital formulary must be reviewed and approved by the Pharmacy and Therapeutics Committee. The pharmacist processes the request and prepares an objective review of the medication. The pharmacist will then add the request to the Pharmacy and Therapeutics Committee agenda. If the drug required is similar to other drugs on the formulary, it is important to determine if the benefits justify admission to the formulary. Guidelines for the evaluation of drugs are provided by the ASHP Guidelines on Formulary System Management.

The pharmacy department's objective review includes cost analysis information, which is an important factor in this age of cost containment. The Pharmacy and Therapeutics Committee considers how much a drug costs per dose, per day, or even per treatment cycle. The decision regarding whether to add a new drug to the formulary is not based solely on whether it is a better therapeutic agent, but whether the perceived benefit is worth the additional cost (cost-benefit analysis). The pharmacy department's research and presentation can have a profound effect on whether a new drug is added to the hospital formulary.

The most cost-effective materials management programs are the result of combining the required expertise and specialty knowledge of a pharmacist with the materials management and systems expertise of a trained pharmacy technician. The pharmacist selects the brands or acceptable generic equivalents. The trained pharmacy technician may monitor inventory levels, input purchase order and receiving information into a computer system or manual recordkeeping system, and organize inventory. Under supervision of the pharmacist, the technician will fill and deliver floor stock orders, repackage medication for unit-dose distribution, and may inspect medication storage areas for proper environmental conditions. The degree of supervision by a pharmacist will vary, depending on the ability of the technician and the policy of the pharmacy department. The pharmacist responsible for materials management supervises the entire process.

Source selection

Another aspect of procurement deals with source selection. One aspect of source selection deals with the concept of generic drugs versus brand-name drugs. The pharmacist determines if the generic product is a **therapeutic equivalent** of the brand-name product and then makes the source selection.

therapeutic equivalent a drug product that, when administered in the same amount, will provide the same therapeutic effect and pharmacokinetic characteristics as another drug to which it is compared.

The Food and Drug Administration regulates the manufacturing of generic drug products to make every effort to ensure therapeutic efficacy. To minimize therapeutic inadequacies, the pharmacist carefully considers the reputation of the generic drug manufacturer and reviews drug analysis data and information. Although cost savings associated with the use of generic drugs have proven to be of great value, selection is made based on quality assurance of the product. Therapeutic equivalence is sometimes difficult to ascertain. However, the reputation of the generic manufacturer and an ongoing surveillance of the professional literature assist the pharmacist in determining if the amount of savings realized by purchasing a generic drug is cost-justified. Guidelines are provided by the ASHP Guidelines for Selecting Pharmaceutical Manufacturers and Suppliers.

Cost analysis

Procurement also includes cost considerations. Drug product cost analysis is an essential step in assessing cost-containment strategies. Information regarding acquisition cost of the product is readily available, and a price comparison of therapeutically equivalent drugs can be studied. Non-acquisition costs may include costs related to storage, time required to prepare products for patient use, and even packaging considerations. Non-acquisition costs include those related to getting the medication to the patient, not simply getting the drug to the pharmacy.

Group purchasing and prime vendor relationships

Group purchasing and prime vendor relationships are two important strategies utilized in an attempt to control the purchase price of drugs. **Group purchasing organizations (GPOs)** are a cooperative of many hospitals that decide to pool their purchasing resources to gain competitive pricing. In general, as a result of group purchasing, the unit cost of a drug is lowered as the projected quantity of the drug to be purchased is increased. Simply stated, group purchasing allows each participating hospital the benefit of quantity discounts as a result of pooling the projected quantities of each hospital and negotiating one contract that applies to all participating members. In addition to contracting, GPOs also work with their members to help initiate drug utilization programs to reduce costs. The seven basic principles essential for effective group purchasing are as follows:

> **group purchasing organizations (GPOs)** a group of hospitals or pharmacists that buys drugs directly from the manufacturer.

1. Most hospitals should have generic formularies allowing across-the-board evaluation opportunities to all vendors.
2. All group members should be committed to buy from the awarded agreement.
3. The group should normally award each item to only one supplier.
4. A pharmacy committee should be established to ensure thorough product quality and vendor review. The pharmacy committee, when it addresses issues for the entire group, can direct the group to many years of successful agreements.
5. The management of individual hospitals should support group programs, especially pharmacy purchasing.
6. The group director should maintain open communication with vendors through newsletters, cooperation in dealing with compliance issues, and approval of regular visits.
7. The group should be willing and able to consider the addition of new products to the bid.

prime vendor a drug wholesaler who contracts directly with hospital pharmacies for the purpose of their high volume pharmaceuticals.

A **prime vendor** relationship is with a distributor of pharmaceuticals who warehouses all drugs from various drug manufacturers. The hospital procures the drugs from its prime vendor wholesaler at the contract price negotiated with the drug manufacturers. A prime vendor relationship allows the pharmacy to reduce the size of inventory. This reduction frees dollars to pay other outstanding debts or to pay bills on time, minimizing the amount of costly premiums associated with late payments. A drug wholesaler can make same-day deliveries, six days per week. Some manufacturers maintain their own direct shipment service as well as a wholesaler distribution program, whereas others distribute exclusively through wholesalers, thereby eliminating the need for their own distribution facilities.

Purchasing procedures

Most wholesalers sell products at established contract prices plus an additional handling fee that can vary from 2 percent to −2 percent, depending on the payment terms and dollar value established with the hospital. The shorter the payment period, the lower the wholesaler markup will be. If the hospital minimizes the markup charge by maintaining an efficient accounts payable schedule, the cost benefits realized from reducing the pharmacy inventory will far outweigh the additional costs associated with the wholesaler's fee. The following questions will assist the pharmacy technician to understand the intricacies of purchasing pharmaceuticals:

1. Is a single-brand purchasing policy in effect for the pharmacy department?
2. Has the Pharmacy and Therapeutics Committee approved a written therapeutic substitution policy?
3. Is competitive bidding used for high-cost items? For high-volume items?
4. Is either of these methods used to set prices: guarantee of bid prices or price ceiling set for the term of the contract?
5. Are the following considered when evaluating bids: prompt payment discount, terms of payment, nonperformance penalties, delivery time limitations, returned and damaged goods policy, and services?
6. Are contracts negotiated when appropriate?
7. Are contracts renegotiated on a regular basis (e.g., annually)?
8. Is group purchasing used when advantageous?
9. If group purchasing is used, are prices guaranteed, and is there a mechanism for determining that group prices are competitive?
10. Are primary wholesalers or wholesale contracts used for specific drugs when appropriate?
11. Are the wholesaler costs equal to or less than the costs of purchasing the same drugs directly? (Consider all factors such as increased investment revenues, decreased number of purchase orders, reduced inventory value, and receiving costs.)
12. Have inventories been adequately reduced?
13. Have ordering and receiving costs been adequately reduced?
14. Do outages that require payment of premium prices occur frequently?
15. Are there frequent outages?
16. Are volume discounts evaluated for net savings before purchase (i.e., gross savings minus increased carrying cost)?

Impact of drug shortages. The unavailability of drugs has increased in frequency and severity over the past few years for many reasons. One major factor is the overwhelming economic pressure that affects all aspects of the health care industry. Hospitals receive less reimbursement from insurers, and distributors and manufacturers compete for lower margin business affected by aggressive contracts from group purchasing organizations (GPOs). Unfortunately, there are strong indications that all parties in the supply chain are too aggressive in attempting to reduce costs and meet business objectives.

Drug shortages may cause treatment delays and a need for alternative therapeutic approaches, which sometimes result in less desirable treatment outcomes. There are many frustrations associated with drug shortages, such as determining the cause of a drug shortage and the expected duration, locating an alternative source of the product or a generic substitution, selecting therapeutic alternatives, managing increased costs, and coping with strained relationships. Alternative agents may also increase the potential for medication errors leading to adverse reactions. Some of the contributing factors include poor communication throughout the supply chain, aggressive inventory practices, manufacturer issues, inaccurate product use projections, and the FDA's regulatory influence.

In an ideal world, providers of health care would be able to consistently anticipate and order the appropriate quantity of drugs in a timely manner so that manufacturers could produce sufficient quantities and distributors could deliver the drugs just prior to the time they are needed. The reason for a **just-in-time (JIT)** inventory strategy is to minimize tying up large sums of money for long periods of time and, in addition, to reduce the cost associated with inventory management. Hospitals, distributors, and manufacturers all implement a JIT strategy, which leaves very little room for error. Using JIT strategies, manufacturers maintain approximately 30 days of raw material and product, distributors maintain approximately 43 days of product, and hospital pharmacies average between 10 and 16 inventory turns per year.

A pharmacy technician working as an inventory manager must consistently monitor the utilization trends of critical drugs and expensive products and communicate changes in utilization to the distributor every day. Distributors, in turn, need to frequently monitor the quantities being ordered and modify the quantities ordered from the manufacturer. Manufacturers should adjust production quantities as the demand for products change, but unfortunately, this is not always done.

There are many factors that influence the production of drug products. Some of these factors include industry consolidation, complex manufacturing processes, raw material shortages, FDA certification problems, profitability, and obligation to shareholders. Sometimes production shortages occur when manufacturers underestimate the demand for product as a result of poor planning, shifts in clinical practice, new indications, and new treatment guidelines. Marketing strategies, unexpected withdrawals, contracting changes, or halting production when annual quotas are met can also be factors. An interesting and difficult-to-anticipate phenomenon is when one drug shortage causes a rapid increase in the use of another product, which causes a secondary shortage.

The impact that drug shortages have on the hospital pharmacy can be devastating and may include increases in drug expenditures as a result of purchasing non-contracted drugs, which may adversely affect bundled product contracts. There are sometimes costs associated with getting manufacturers to drop-ship emergency allocations of product that are no longer available from the distribu-

just in time (JIT)
an inventory strategy to minimize inventory levels, thus minimizing tying up large sums of money.

tors. There is also a tendency to overstock an item when it has been backordered or difficult to obtain.

In order to be prepared, a hospital pharmacy buyer should take a proactive approach and establish contingency procedures. An excellent source of information on this topic can be found in the ASHP Guidelines on Managing Drug Product Shortages.

Recordkeeping

The pharmacy department must also establish and maintain adequate records to meet government regulations, standards of practice requirements, accreditation standards, hospital policies, and management information requirements. These records include budget reports, productivity and workload documents, purchase orders, inventories, receiving and dispensing reports, and controlled substances and alcohol records. The pharmacy's materials manager should be intimately involved with the development and maintenance of many of these documents.

The purchase order. The purchase order document should be prepared at the time the order is placed by telephone, mail, computer, or fax. The information included on the purchase order includes the following:

- The name and address of the hospital.
- The shipping address.
- The date the order was placed.
- The vendor's name and address.
- The purchase order number.
- The ordering department's name and location.
- The expected date of delivery.
- Shipping terms (e.g., FOB, Net 30).
- The account number or billing designation.
- A description of items ordered.
- The quantity of items ordered.
- The unit price.
- The extended price.
- The total price of the order.
- The buyer's name and phone number.

Receiving control

Accepting the responsibility for receiving drugs for the pharmacy department is another important role that can be filled by the pharmacy technician. When receiving deliveries, the pharmacy technician should follow these basic rules:

- Check the shipping address to be sure the package received was intended for delivery to the pharmacy department.
- Check the outside of the package for visible signs of damage to the carton or the contents. Note any damage on the receiving document before you sign for the delivery.
- Look for any shipping documents attached to the outside of the package, and determine if special handling is required (e.g., store in freezer, controlled substance).
- Carefully open the package, and check each item for breakage.
- Check each item for expiration date, and make note of any short-dated material for immediate use or return.

■ Verify the order received against a copy of the purchase order. Make a notation of any variation. Refer to the shipping document or packing slip to determine if items are backordered or out of stock.

■ Refer any order discrepancies to the supervising pharmacist.

Complete accountability of drugs from receiving to patient administration requires a tightly controlled, coordinated effort on the part of all pharmacy and nursing personnel.

All drugs should be delivered directly to the pharmacy department or a secured pharmacy receiving area to prevent diversion of drug orders. Controlled substances and tax-free alcohol require special handling and must be closely supervised by a licensed pharmacist to minimize loss or adulteration. All controlled drugs and tax-free alcohol are accounted for in a perpetual inventory. Every individual dose must be accounted for from procurement, receipt, storage, and dispensing to administration. Records for controlled drug inventory management must be maintained for two years. Some states may require these records to be maintained for five years.

Drug Storage and Inventory Control

The next step in the material management process is the safe storage of drugs that have been ordered and received.

Storage

After drugs have been selected, ordered, and received, they must be properly stored. Appropriate storage requires environmental considerations, security issues, and safety requirements.

The inventory may be divided into an active drug inventory and a backup storeroom inventory for large, bulky items that require more space. The inventory may also be divided by how the drugs will be used. For example, parenteral medication for intravenous (IV) administration may be stored in the IV admixture room only (Figure 25-1).

FIGURE 25-1

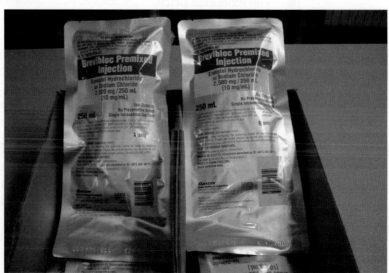

FIGURE 25-1 Organization of inventory allows a pharmacy to maintain stock and work efficiently.

Environmental considerations. Environmental considerations include proper temperature, ventilation, humidity, light, and sanitation. Standards have been developed and are referenced in various statutes as a basis for determining appropriate storage requirements since they affect strength, quality, purity, packaging, and labeling of drugs and related articles. These important standards are contained in a combined publication that is recognized as the official compendium, the United States Pharmacopoeia (USP) and the National Formulary (NF).

For example, the USP defines *controlled room temperature* as the acceptable temperature when a variation is not specified. In addition, specific requirements are stated in some drug monographs where it is considered that storage at a lower or higher temperature may produce undesirable results. Printing specific storage conditions in product literature and on drug packaging and drug labels to ensure proper storage and product integrity is required. The conditions are defined by the following terms:

- *Cold*—any temperature not exceeding 8°C (45°F). A refrigerator is a cold place in which the temperature is maintained thermostatically between 2° and 8°C (36° and 46°F). A freezer is a cold place in which the temperature is maintained thermostatically between –20° and –10°C (–4° and 14°F).
  a. *Protection from freezing*—When freezing subjects an article to loss of strength or potency or to destructive alteration of its characteristics, the container label bears an appropriate instruction to prevent the article from freezing.
- *Cool*—any temperature between 8° and 15°C (46° and 59°F). An article for which storage in a cool place is directed may alternatively be stored in a refrigerator, unless otherwise specified in the individual monograph.
- *Room temperature*—the temperature prevailing in a working area. Controlled room temperature is a temperature maintained thermostatically between 15° and 30°C (59° and 86°F).
- *Warm*—any temperature between 30° and 40°C (86° and 104°F).
- *Excessive heat*—any temperature above 40°C (104°F).

When no specific storage directions or limitations are provided in the individual monograph, it is understood that the storage conditions include protection from moisture, freezing, and excessive heat.

Additional standards regarding the preservation, packaging, storage, and labeling of drugs are described in the "General Notices and Requirements" section of the USP/NF. Those involved in any aspect of materials management of pharmaceuticals must be familiar with the official standards and definitions as they relate to the proper storage and handling of drugs. The pharmacy technician shares this obligation with all other members of the health care team involved in medication-related activities.

Security requirements

Security requirements that restrict access to drugs to "authorized personnel only" are often the result of legal requirements, hospital policy, and established standards of practice. All medications must be maintained in restricted locations so that they are only accessible to professional staff who are authorized to receive, store, prepare, dispense, distribute, or administer such products.

Legend drugs must be dispensed by a licensed pharmacist. However, a pharmacy technician under the direct supervision of a pharmacist can receive and fill floor stock orders and deliver the medication to a drug storage location. Medication storage areas located on nursing units must also be secured and restricted to authorized personnel only. Controlled substances and tax-free alcohol require additional restrictions. Only a licensed pharmacist can order, receive, prepare, and dispense these drugs. However, a qualified pharmacy technician under the direct supervision of a pharmacist can assist in storing and delivering these products. Special security procedures, such as daily physical counts of pharmacy and nursing units' inventories, are essential to ensure that there is no diversion or misuse of controlled substances. Tax-free alcohol, which is most often used only by the pathology department, is controlled by performing periodic record audits and physical inventories.

Safety precautions must also be carefully considered when handling materials that have a high potential for danger. For example, when storing volatile or flammable substances, it is important to have a cool, properly ventilated location that has been specially designed to reduce fire and explosion potential. Another consideration would be to store caustic substances, such as acids, in a location that would reduce any potential for the container being dropped and broken (e.g., in a locked cabinet instead of an open shelf). Oncology drugs used to treat cancer are often cytotoxic themselves and therefore must be handled with extreme care. These drugs should be received in a sealed protective outer bag that restricts the dissemination of the drug if the container leaks or is broken. They should also be stored in a secure area that has limited access and a restricted traffic flow. When the potential exists for exposure to chemotherapy, all personnel involved must wear protective clothing and equipment while following a hazardous materials cleanup procedure. All exposed materials must be properly disposed of in chemohazardous waste containers.

Proper rotation of inventory

Segregating inventory by drug category also helps to prevent errors that could increase the potential for harm. For example, the standards of the Joint Commission require that internal and external medications must be stored separately to reduce the potential for someone dispensing or administering an external product for internal use. Rotating inventory and checking expiration dates on products when drugs are received helps to reduce the potential for dispensing or administering expired drugs and also maximizes the utilization of inventory before drugs become outdated.

Computerized inventory control

Many of these functions can be better controlled with the use of computer programs dedicated to monitor the purchasing, receiving, and dispensing functions on an ongoing basis. Perpetual inventory systems are now being utilized to indicate when predetermined reorder points are reached. Most dedicated pharmacy systems can generate management reports that allow the materials manager to review drug use. For example, the monthly usage rate of each drug can be monitored and utilization can be tracked to determine which clinical department or patient population is using specific drugs. Computers also enable the materials manager to closely monitor budget trends and year-to-date purchases by drug category. The pharmacy technician must remember that computer systems are only as effective as the users are accurate when inputting information. Therefore, the materials management technician must have a basic understanding of how the pharmacy computer works and must be properly trained to maximize the potential benefits of inventory control programs. More detail on pharmacy computerization is discussed in Chapter 27.

Turnover rate

Determining the pharmacy's inventory **turnover rate** is a good method of measuring the overall effectiveness of the purchasing and inventory control programs. The inventory turnover rate is calculated by dividing the total dollars spent to purchase drugs for one year by the actual value of the pharmacy inventory at any point in time. The number produced by this calculation offers an indication of how many times a year the inventory may have been used or replaced. The larger the number of inventory turnovers, the stronger the indication that the inventory control program is efficient.

In the 1980s, a turnover rate of 6 percent to 7 percent was considered acceptable. In the 2000s, turnover rates of 12 percent to 15 percent were easily achievable because of more efficient methods of purchasing, such as prime-vendor programs and computerized order-entry systems. Even higher turnover rates will be achieved in the 21st century due to new materials management techniques and business strategies such as consignment of inventory programs. The following questions may further assist the pharmacy materials manager in his or her attempt to maintain adequate controls on a very large and complex inventory.

1. Has an inventory turnover rate been calculated for your hospital?
2. Is this rate optimal for the facility?
3. Is the storeroom checked at regular intervals to verify that appropriate purchasing and inventory methods are being followed?
   a. Are reorder points adjusted as needed?
   b. Is this rate optimal for the facility?
4. Are inventories controlled in dispensing areas?
   a. Are minimum and maximum inventories maintained?
   b. Is the space allotted for each product restricted?
   c. Is there a routine check for outdated drugs and excesses?
   d. Are exchange systems used when appropriate (e.g., carts, self-units, boxes)?
5. Are nursing-unit drug inventories controlled?
   a. Is an approved floor-stock list used for drug items?
   b. Are there maximum allowable quantities for each item?
   c. Are inventory dollar limits set for each nursing unit?
   d. Are units checked monthly for excesses and outdated drugs?
6. Are inventories controlled in the emergency, operating, and recovery rooms?

Repackaging and Labeling Considerations

In-house packaging and labeling are sometimes necessary when required dosage forms are not available commercially. The pharmacy technician is often directly involved in preparing unit-dose packaging that utilizes automated packaging equipment. The pharmacy technician must be adequately trained to ensure the stability of the product and appropriate labeling.

There are different types of containers to choose from depending on the product, the desired route of administration, and the method of dispensing—for example, unit-dose packaging for solid oral forms (e.g., tray-fill blister packaging, cadet foil packaging) and oral liquids (e.g., Baxa cups, oral syringes). In addition, some of the new automated dispensing technologies require packaging unique to their dispensing design (e.g., robot-ready cards, Pyxis Cubies).

Regardless of which type of packaging container is used, it should be clean, and special precautions and cleaning procedures may be necessary to ensure that extraneous matter is not introduced into or onto the drugs being packaged. It is also essential to be sure that the container does not interact physically or chemically with the drug being placed in it so as to alter the strength, quality, or purity of the article beyond the official requirements.

Some drugs may have special packaging requirements as described in the manufacturer's literature and in official monographs published in the USP/NF. The following requirements for use of specified containers may apply when in-house packaging is required:

- *Light-resistant container*—protects the contents from the effects of light by virtue of the specific properties of the material of which it is composed, including any coating applied to it. Alternatively, a clear and colorless or a translucent container may be made light resistant by means of an opaque covering, in which case the label of the container bears a statement that the opaque covering is needed until the contents are to be used or administered. When it is directed to "protect from light" in an individual monograph, preservation in a light-resistant container is required.
- *Tamper-resistant packaging*—is required for a sterile article intended for ophthalmic or otic use, except when extemporaneously compounded for immediate dispensing on prescription. The contents are sealed so that they cannot be opened without obvious destruction of the seal.
- *Tight container*—protects the contents from contamination by extraneous liquids, solids, or vapors, from loss of the article, and from efflorescence, deliquescence, or evaporation under the ordinary or customary conditions of handling, shipment, storage, and distribution.
- *Hermetic container*—is impervious to air or any other gas under the ordinary or customary conditions of handling, shipment, storage, and distribution.
- *Single-unit container*—is one that is designed to hold a quantity of drug product intended for administration as a single dose, or a single finished device intended for use promptly after the container is opened. Each single-unit container should be labeled to indicate the identity, quantity, strength, name of manufacturer, lot number, and expiration date of the drug or article.
- *Single-dose container*—is a single-unit container for articles intended for parenteral administration only. Examples of single-dose containers include prefilled syringes, cartridges, fusion-sealed containers, and closure-sealed containers when so labeled.
- *Unit-dose container*—is a single-unit container for articles intended for administration by routes other than the parenteral route as a single dose, direct from the container.

Each label must include at least the following information:

- Generic name of the product (brand name optional).
- Strength in units (e.g., mg, mL, oz).
- Drug form (e.g., tablet, capsule, suppository).
- Lot number and manufacturer's name.
- Expiration date for repackaged drug.

The expiration date used on repackaged drugs should be based on the prevailing community standard of practice or based on an evaluation of scientific information. In all cases a maximum expiration date should be adhered to as identified in law and regulation. The 17th edition of the USP states, "In the absence of stability data to the contrary, such date should not exceed (1) 25 percent of the remaining time between the date of repackaging and the expiration date on the original manufacturer's bulk container, or (2) a six-month period of time from the date the drug is repackaged, whichever is earlier."

All repackaged drugs must be carefully checked by a licensed pharmacist, and approvals must be documented in writing before repackaged drugs are put into active inventory. Documentation of the repackaging process should include the following information:

- Date of repackaging.
- Name and strength of drug.
- Quantity of drug repackaged.
- Manufacturer's name.
- Manufacturer's lot number.
- Manufacturer's expiration date.
- In-house code number.
- In-house expiration date.
- Initials of packaging technician.
- Initials of pharmacist.

Benefits associated with bar coding

In March 2003, the FDA announced that it would require bar codes on all medications in an effort to reduce the high rate of medical errors. This is an important step in automating the medication use process and reducing the amount of human interpretation in the ordering, dispensing, and administration of drugs. During a study of more than 88 million doses from April 2002 to June 2003, it was estimated that only 36 percent of the dose level drugs had bar coding. The FDA estimates that it would cost pharmaceutical companies $50 million to add bar codes to all drugs manufactured and used in the United States, and hospitals would spend over $7 billion on scanners and computer systems to support the initiative.

The Institute of the National Academy of Sciences has estimated that of the more than 98,000 people killed from medical errors each year, about 7,000 of those deaths were directly attributed to medication errors. According to Michael R. Cohen, president of the Institute for Safe Medication Practices, early studies indicate that bar coding should reduce the number of medications errors by over 50 percent.

Early indications suggest that some manufacturers will reduce the number of drugs presently available in individual dose packaging in order to avoid the increased cost associated with the new FDA requirement. This trend will result in an even greater need for providers to repackage and bar code drugs that will no longer be available in unit-dose packaging. This change will have a direct impact on the pharmacy technician's role and responsibilities. The pharmacy technician will need to become knowledgeable regarding the different types of packaging and scanning equipment available, the limitations and compatibility of bar coding systems, and the associated changes in the medication use process. For example, bar coded labels that are read by automated dispensing technology may not be compatible with a scanner used by a nurse at the patient's bedside. A bar code label placed on a unit-dose product may or may not contain an expiration date that would be helpful for inventory management purposes. Due to the current lack of standardization related to bar coding in the health care industry, pharmacy providers must carefully scrutinize the compatibility of the bar coding systems and equipment in order to ensure that the outcomes desired are achieved.

The obvious goal of the government's initiative is to have all drugs bar coded to the dose level, which in turn will make products available that can be used as part of an automated system that will reduce the incidence of medication errors. Additional benefits will be realized as a result of streamlining the entire medication use process. For instance, a physician can order a patient's medication online with less chance of a selection error or interpretation error occurring and with a faster transmission time.

A pharmacist can review the order as part of an electronic patient medication profile programmed to identify potential medication errors such as the wrong drug, wrong dose, or a drug that may not be compatible with other medication the patient is receiving. Patient profile systems can also identify drug-food allergies and possible allergic reactions as a result of known patient allergies. Drugs can also be dispensed using bar coded labels or overwrap containers compatible with automated dispensing technology either in the pharmacy or at the patient's point of care. A nurse can scan the patient's ID bracelet, her own ID badge, and the medication bar code as a final check to ensure the right medication and right dose is being administered to the right patient at the right time. If all of these checks are accepted, the medication administration documentation and the associated charge for the drug can be automatically processed as a post-administration step in the process.

The infrastructure required to accomplish these goals includes having medication with a bar coded label, bar coded patient ID bracelets, bar coded nurse badges, a wireless network, and point-of-care hardware (reader/scanner). Bar coding is the critical communication link, the common denominator used by automated systems to ensure that supply chain processes and the clinical checks and balances work in concert to support the best results. Bar coding uniquely identifies a specific product and a specific dose. The savings associated with automating the medication use process will eventually offset the cost of the technology and systems required to support a "closed loop" initiative, but the initial cost can only be justified as cost avoidance associated with reducing the incidence of medication errors and improving the quality of patient care. Pharmacy technicians will play a significant role in developing and supporting the FDA's bar coding initiative.

Distribution Systems

Drug distribution systems have changed considerably in the last 10 years. In the past it was acceptable to dispense large containers of drugs (bulk packaging) to be stored at the nursing unit for use whenever a nurse needed to administer a drug to a patient. This method, known as a *floor stock system*, does not allow the pharmacist to review drug therapy before it is administered to a patient. It is therefore potentially dangerous. Also, floor stock medication cannot be reused once it is removed from the original container because there is no way to guarantee product integrity. As a result, this method increases the potential for waste. Today the Joint Commission and most state agencies require unit-dose dispensing and pharmacy-based intravenous additive programs. (The importance of these programs is discussed in Chapter 18.)

Certain emergency drugs are still maintained as floor stock because they may be urgently needed. Emergency drugs may be stored in mobile units for quick transfer to a patient's bedside when resuscitation techniques are required. Emergency drugs are necessary for patients in emergency situations who cannot wait for drug orders to be processed and delivered by the pharmacy department. Determining when it is appropriate to circumvent a pharmacist review of drug therapy to have medication available for immediate administration is a difficult undertaking. Code Cart Committees made up of physicians, nurses, pharmacists and central sterile personnel determine the appropriate drugs and supply, as needed, to be stocked in these mobile units.

Recapture and Disposal

The final step in the material management process is the appropriate handling of medications not administered to patients and returned to the pharmacy.

Returned medications

Properly processing medication that is returned to the pharmacy department is an important role that can be fulfilled by a pharmacy technician. When unit-dose packaging is used, the pharmacy technician can check return medication for package integrity and proper dating before putting the drug back into stock. In case of a manufacturer's recall, each dose of medication can be located by lot number to ensure its removal. Records of all recall information should be maintained to ensure that a proper review of all potentially dangerous drugs has been completed. All controlled drugs returned or destroyed must be removed from perpetual inventory. Records of destruction or returned drugs must be kept for five years.

Expiration dates

All drug packages have expiration date notations that identify the date when the medication is no longer suitable for use. The expiration date will be designated in one of two ways: month and year (e.g., June 2008), which means that the packaged material, if properly stored, is good until the last day of the month; or more specifically as month, day, and year (e.g., June 15, 2008). Every hospital pharmacy must have a system whereby drugs are checked for expiration dates on a regular basis to guarantee that only properly dated drugs are available for use. Expired drugs must be segregated from active inventory to prevent a potentially dangerous dispensing error. Many pharmaceutical companies will give full credit for expired medication. It is essential for the pharmacy materials manager to determine the return policy for each company.

Environmental considerations

When disposing of partially used drugs or expired drugs that cannot be returned for credit, it is important to consider the negative impact that certain drugs may have on the environment. For example, many oncology drugs used for the treatment of cancer are carcinogenic (i.e., they have the potential to cause cancer themselves). Strict precautions must be taken and procedures followed to properly dispose of these items. Another concern is related to partially used injectable medication that may have come in contact with a patient who has a communicable disease. Once again the drug, needle, and syringe must be disposed of in a special puncture-resistant container that can be handled safely and then properly destroyed.

In 1976, the Resource Conservation and Recovery Act (RCRA) was enacted to provide a mechanism for tracking hazardous waste from generation to disposal.

These regulations are enforced by the Environmental Protection Agency. Several drugs (e.g., epinephrine) require handling, containment, and disposal as RCRA hazardous waste. Today, many pharmacy departments contract with the "reverse" distribution companies to assure that drugs that require tracking are disposed of appropriately. The inventory personnel will keep a manifest of the disposal on file. For further information, see the ASHP Guideline: Drug Distribution in Preparation and Handling (2006).

Summary

It is important for the pharmacy technician to realize that the responsibilities of materials management are comprehensive and must be carried out in an organized and consistent manner to ensure patient safety and guarantee cost-effective pharmaceutical care.

TEST YOUR KNOWLEDGE

Multiple Choice

1. An institutional pharmacy materials management program includes
   a. procurement.
   b. drug storage.
   c. inventory control.
   d. all of the above.

2. In a hospital, overall responsibility for the materials management of pharmaceuticals lies with the
   a. chairperson of the Pharmacy and Therapeutics Committee.
   b. director of pharmacy services.
   c. hospital administration.
   d. chief pharmacy technician.

3. A drug distribution system includes
   a. unit dose.
   b. floor stock.
   c. compounded prescriptions.
   d. all of the above.

4. Environmental considerations in the storage of pharmaceuticals include
   a. proper temperature and ventilation.
   b. proper humidity.
   c. proper temperature.
   d. all of the above.

5. The pharmacy department is responsible for
   a. preparing purchase orders.
   b. receiving and securing shipments of pharmaceuticals.
   c. monitoring the inventory of controlled substances and tax-free alcohol.
   d. all of the above.

6. Inventory control may include
   a. minimum and maximum reorder points maintained.
   b. return of outdated stock.
   c. drug usage report.
   d. all of the above.

7. The Food and Drug Administration's bar coding rules are estimated to reduce the number of medication errors by which of the following?
   a. 36 percent
   b. 50 percent
   c. 70 percent
   d. 90 percent

Matching

Match the following.

1. _____ cold temperature
2. _____ freezer
3. _____ room temperature
4. _____ refrigerator
5. _____ excessive heat
6. _____ warm

a. −20° to −10°C (−4° to 14°F)
b. 15° to 30°C (59° to 86°F)
c. not exceeding 8°C (46°F)
d. 30° to 40°C (86° to 104°F)
e. 2° to 8°C (36° to 46°F)
f. above 40°C (104°F)

Match the following.

1. _____ select the drug source
2. _____ prepare the drug order
3. _____ check the incoming drug products
4. _____ maintain a proper drug storage environment
5. _____ prepare formulary revision

a. pharmacist's responsibility
b. technician's responsibility

References

ASHP guidelines for drug distribution and control: Preparation and handling. (2006). *American Journal of Health-System Pharmacy*, 63: 1172–1193.

ASHP guidelines for selecting pharmaceutical manufacturers and suppliers. (1991). *American Journal of Health-System Pharmacy*, 48: 523-524.

ASHP guidelines on formulary system management. (1992). *American Journal of Health-System Pharmacy*, 49: 648–652.

ASHP guidelines on managing drug product shortages. (2001). *American Journal of Health-System Pharmacy*, 58: 1445–1450.

Joint Commission. Pharmacy services. (2007). *Comprehensive Accreditation Manual for Hospitals*. Oak Brook Terrace, IL.

Okeke, C. C., Bailey, L., Medwick, T., & Grady, L. T. (2000). Revised USP standards for product dating, packaging, and temperature monitoring. *American Journal of Health-System Pharmacy.* 57(15): 1441–1445.

United States Pharmacopoeia. (2007). General notices and requirements: Preservation, packaging, storage, and labeling. *The United States Pharmacopoeia XXX/The National Formulary XXV*, 10–13.

The Pharmacy Formulary System

Competencies

Upon completion of this chapter, the reader should be able to

1. Outline the five core attributes of the formulary system.
2. Explain the impact of a formulary in pharmacy practice in relation to managed care organizations and pharmacy benefit managers.
3. List the steps in the process for adding a new drug to the formulary.
4. List three surveillance activities fostered by the formulary system.
5. Describe how using new technologies will improve formulary compliance.
6. Illustrate why it is important to revise the formulary regularly.

Key Terms

National Formulary

Introduction

Throughout much of the history of pharmacy, the term formulary has referred basically to a listing of drugs. The spectrum of sophistication of a formulary can range from a simple list for use in a small institution to an elaborate compendium of detailed standards, which may in fact carry some official weight as a legally recognized standard. In some cases an institution's formulary is actually a complete reference manual for the policies and procedures, guidelines for use, and criteria for evaluation of the medications approved for use at that particular institution. Formularies can be used for many purposes. Perhaps the most historically significant of the ancient formularies is the Ebers Papyrus (c. 1500 B.C.), a listing of complex prescriptions and cures from ancient Egypt. Formularies have documented the state-of-the-art therapeutic knowledge of the cultures that compiled them.

Not all formularies are from the Old World. Some very complete ones, usually described as *codices*, are attributed to Central American native civilizations. In fact, some of the drugs, such as digitalis and cocaine, appeared in these formularies many years before they were "discovered" by Western or Oriental medicine. The most revered formulary in the United States is the **National Formulary**. Many pharmacists are familiar with the initials *NF* following drug names. The National Formulary has since been incorporated into the United States Pharmacopoeia (USP) as the official compendium of drug standards in the United States. Formularies, then, are a continuation of a worldwide, centuries-old pharmacy tradition.

In their modern form, formularies are usually associated with hospitals or other organized medical care settings, but increasingly larger organizations, such as pharmacy benefit managers (PBMs), managed care organizations (MCOs), and other payer-based entities have established their own formularies for their beneficiaries or member population. In most instances, these formularies are identified as Preferred Drug List or PDL. The implementation of Medicare Part D brought formularies to the forefront of the general public.

The utility and effectiveness of formularies, despite their ancient heritage and pervasiveness, are not without controversy. Some agencies and organizations seem to depend on them increasingly more. For example, the Veterans Affairs system has adopted a "national" formulary (not to be confused with the official compendium, *National Formulary*) and uses it to optimize therapy and as a tool to negotiate price savings. The Center for Medicare and Medicaid Services (CMS) developed specific guidelines and requirements requiring all prescription drug plans (PDPs) to abide by their guidelines for developing formularies. Formularies are tools, and like any tool, how one uses it determines the overall judgment of its value. As part of this tradition, certain attributes come to mind when using the term *formulary*. It is interesting that some ancient concepts embodied in formularies are now being used to expand the role of the pharmacy profession for technician practitioners as well as for pharmacists.

> **National Formulary** a database of drugs of established usefulness not found in the U.S. Pharmacopoeia.

The Formulary System

The formulary system describes how formularies are derived and how the drug-use process can be guided, controlled, and accounted for when a particular formulary is in effect. The core attributes of a formulary and formulary system include the following:

- Formularies represent a selective list of the drugs available for beneficiaries.
- Formularies are either considered open or closed. A closed formulary excludes drugs from various therapeutic classes, and an open formulary includes all drugs, placing them on various benefit tiers.
- A formulary is developed through the consensus of the Pharmacy and Therapeutics Committee (P&T Committee) (Appendix B). The committee reviews each therapeutic class, looking for any superiority within a class, placing emphasis on the most effective therapeutic agents to be used in the practice.
- Formularies should contain additional information about the drugs and their use, such as dose regulations, tables comparing similar drugs within a related class, common drug interactions, suggestions for patient information, and so forth.
- The formulary system defines policies and procedures along with coverage criteria concerning drug use, and it defines the scope of the formulary.
- Formularies must be continuously reviewed and revised.

Consensus is important for the formulary to be effective. The members of the P&T Committee should be selected with this in mind and should represent a cross section of disciplines from the medical and pharmacy community.

Today, MCOs (managed care organizations) and PBMs (pharmacy benefit managers) utilize the clinical pharmacy department as a lead role. The clinical pharmacy department develops the white paper (described below) and clinical review documents. There are several strategies to gain consensus:

1. Additions to the formulary should be requested in a formal fashion through the use of a request form. This form can channel the thoughts of the requester by including some questions such as "Are there similar drugs on the formulary?" or "What are the advantages of this drug?"
2. Requests can be forwarded to the chairman or secretary (usually the Director of Pharmacy) of the P&T Committee.
3. The P&T Committee should prepare a "white paper" report on the advantages, disadvantages, and therapeutic impact. Generally, the financial impact may be part of a request to add a drug to the formulary.
4. The actions of the committee and their reasons for including or not including a drug should be published as soon as possible after the meeting. If actions were not to include a drug, it is particularly important to specify the reasons why.

Formularies must be inclusive. The formulary should be selective and represent the best drugs available for the population subject to the formulary. The factors contributing to the best drugs for a formulary can vary over a wide range: for example, indication, adverse events, factors affecting patient compliance, ease of administration, special storage or security requirements, the inherent safety profile, and cost of the medication.

There are many therapeutic reasons supporting a selective formulary; the elimination of unnecessary and potentially confusing duplications is one. A second reason deals with economics. Watching carefully how the money is spent is now much more important for all institutions, hospitals, and insurance companies. The advent of high-tech drugs such as colony-stimulating factors, monoclonal antibodies, drugs produced by recombinant technology, genetically engineered drugs, and biotech drugs can precipitate an economic crisis for the hospital or MCO if the potential economic impacts of these agents are treated in a cavalier fashion and not monitored. The pharmacy budget as a percentage of total drug spending has increased dramatically in the past few years. All indications are that this trend will continue indefinitely because of the many new, high-tech, and innovative agents in the pipeline. It should be noted, however, that many new drugs coming to the market are in fact very similar to those drugs already available. These drugs perhaps do not contribute added therapeutic value, but in many cases increase the cost of therapy for a particular disease state. A formulary provides the opportunity to provide optimal drug coverage while providing some economic containment through the availability of manufacturer discounts.

Application of Formulary in the Community

Formularies are utilized in many settings. They are an important component in all hospital systems and are now extremely prevalent in the community setting. A majority of health insurance plans utilize pharmacy benefit managers (PBMs) to administer coverage of drugs for their subscribers. This includes the Medicare prescription drug plan known as Medicare Part D. The predominant formulary seen in the marketplace today is an open formulary. An open formulary, also known as a *preferred drug list*, provides subscribers with access to quality, appropriate, clinical drug therapy at various cost-share levels.

To help manage the formulary, many PBMs and insurance companies utilize a tiered formulary. The tier placement of medication affects the copayment the member pays for the medication. Many plans work with a two or three tier plan, with Tier 1 being generic medications, Tier 2 the preferred medications, and Tier 3—the highest copayment tier—reserved for non-formulary or non-preferred medications. The goal is for physicians to prescribe cost-effective tier medications for their members, because studies show member compliance is generally better when their cost share is less.

Prior authorization (PA) is another way insurance companies and Medicare Part D plans control costs. Requiring a PA generally means a member must try a specific medication or class of medications before a more expensive medication may be prescribed. In addition, the use of prior authorizations may ensure the member has a specific diagnosis before a specific medication may be used. An example of this would be oral chemotherapy medications. Many PBMs have a prior authorization for these medications, based on the type of cancer, to ensure the medication is used according to the manufacturer's specific indications.

A third way to monitor appropriate use of medications is through *quantity limits*. This is limiting the amount of medication a member can get in a given time period to ensure the member is compliant with therapy.

Medicare Part D is of major importance due to the growing number of senior citizens in the United States. There is much confusion due to the large number of programs and the larger number of formularies. Many of the insurance companies offer a Medicare Part D plan, and these plans may offer two or three formularies with different deductibles and copayment tiers. In addition, each plan has a different formulary with varying tier placements of medications. The same medications may not be covered by all formularies. In addition, different plans offer different PA and limits on the same medications. This may cause disruption of therapy in senior citizens who are stable on medications if they are forced to change medications due to their Medicare Part D plan. The formulary information is available to senior citizens, pharmacists, and pharmacy technicians on the CMS Web site; however, this still has not eliminated all of the confusion.

The following information from the CMS Web site concerns Medicare Part D-covered drug definitions:

- Drugs included in a Part D plan's formulary, or treated as being included in a Part D plan's formulary, as a result of a covered determination or appeal.
- Drugs categorized as "less than effective" (LTE) are not included. Such drugs are identified by having a DESI (Drug Efficacy Study Implementation) indicator code of either 5 or 6.
- These are the excluded drugs:
  - Agents used for anorexia, weight loss, or weight gain.
  - Agents used to promote fertility.
  - Agents used for cosmetic purposes or hair growth.
  - Agents used for the symptomatic relief of coughs and colds.
  - Prescription vitamins and mineral products, *except* prenatal vitamins and fluoride preparations.
  - Nonprescription drugs.
  - Barbiturates.
  - Benzodiazepines.
  - Agents used for the treatment of sexual or erectile dysfunction.

Like hospital-based formularies, community-based formularies provide clinical programs that require certain trials and failures of preferred drugs prior to coverage of non-preferred drugs. It is important to understand the procedures to request coverage for non-preferred drugs.

Complications can arise when trying to be selective and trying to reach a consensus at the same time. Little doubt remains that as pressure increases to become more selective, consensus will also become important and possibly more difficult to achieve.

The information a formulary contains, aside from the listing of the available drugs, can often be a decisive factor in determining its effectiveness and quality over another formulary. Reviewing formularies from pharmacy benefit managers would indicate a remarkable similarity in the drugs they contain. Although the additional information they convey is different, even in this aspect, uniformity seems to be more common. Additional information, for example, may list certain policies about drug use in a single place. Sample protocols for drug use can be listed. (Think of a protocol as a recipe for how to use a specific drug.) Often, charts comparing the features or costs of an important drug class are included.

The formulary system defines the policies of drug use and can be effective in several aspects. For example, the system not only has the responsibility to select drugs and to foster rational drug therapy, but can also function in an educational role as a means of quality assurance. The educational role of the P&T Committee is carried out through the formulary system. Traditionally, education was in the form of written communications. Today's education involves more direct in-service programs sponsored or conducted by the P&T Committee.

Some surveillance activities fostered by the system have an education and quality assurance aspect. For example, monitoring non-formulary drugs can provide staff members with certain trends that would otherwise go unnoticed. Many monitoring activities or drug utilization evaluations (DUEs) that fall into this category are discussed elsewhere.

An exciting outgrowth of the formulary system linked to computer technology is the ability to track adverse drug reactions (ADRs). Sophisticated database management programs often allow a more rapid identification of trends that might not otherwise be obvious and thus result in interventions to avoid such reactions. Recent literature provided data that quantify the cost of ADRs—and the number is remarkable! For example, an overall average of the additional cost involved in ADRs is $2,000 per incident, but the range may vary from $6,700 per case for "bleeding" to $9,000 for "induced fever." These observations support the view that there is more to the relationship of formulary management, drug therapy, and cost than may be at first apparent.

The traditional application of the formulary system could be described as occurring in two dimensions: (1) mostly in writing, and (2) often after the fact. However, the growing trend is to apply sophisticated computer techniques to how information is used. As a result, many of the formulary system's procedures and protocols can move away from the "scripture-like" status of written documents to a prospective and often interactive status. For example, in some computer applications, the program can alert the pharmacist to a drug's formulary status and to any restrictions that apply and document special criteria for use—all while the order is being entered. Pharmacists are encouraged to discuss available formulary alternatives with prescribing physicians. As electronic prescribing becomes prevalent in society, physicians will prescreen their patient's plan formularies and prescribe within the patient's plan guidelines. You will no doubt hear more about the implications of such technology before too long, as more systems with these capabilities are installed in physician's offices.

New ways to improve the medication use process are becoming the focus of medical safety efforts. Often referred to as *computerized physician order entry (CPOE)* or, more precisely, *computer-assisted provider order entry (CAPOE)*, these systems are extremely complex, very expensive, and require major changes in the organizational culture, affecting all aspects of the medication use process from drug selection to administration and monitoring. While such technologies are promoted as the ultimate answer to medical safety, they are not an easy or inexpensive answer. The principles of the formulary system design discussed in this chapter will continue to play an important role in the success or failure of CAPOE system development and implementation.

Electronic medical records are also being initiated in many states. This involves the physician's office keeping the complete patient medical record on a computer. This allows the physician to submit prescriptions electronically, directly to the pharmacy. The system checks for possible drug interactions, correct dosing, available generic medication, duplications, and formulary tier substitutions before the prescription is transmitted. It will also alert the physician if a prior authorization is required by the patient's insurance company, saving a telephone call later from the pharmacy or patient when the pharmacy claim is denied. In some cases, this technology also allows for direct faxing to the pharmacy if the physician's office system is not set up for the electronic prescribing (e-prescribing) as just described.

Revision to the formulary is an important function because its effectiveness depends on how current the formulary is. Keeping a formulary current is a difficult task. New drugs are being introduced at a faster rate than in previous years, making formulary revision a constant activity.

Formularies are usually published once a year, even though they may be revised after each P&T Committee action. Changes that occur between official revisions can be communicated in several ways. Communication may be done via newsletters sent to physicians and pharmacy providers, or the P&T Committee may release a special publication when changes are made. The information contained in classic formularies is printed and published in book form. Formularies are revised continuously, and the logistics of assuring that all previous copies are updated can be overwhelming. Typically, new editions of the formulary are published on a regular basis, and this too can get extremely expensive. More recently, there is a trend toward using modern electronic means to disseminate formularies, and a vast array of drug information has revolutionized health care practice. Literally thousands of articles on the use of Web-based (Internet and Intranet) media and a bewildering variety of personal digital assistants (PDAs) or pocket PCs have been published, and commercial information services are competing for attention in this dynamic market.

Summary

Formularies and the formulary system are ancient concepts that have been adapted to the dynamic environment of modern medical care. When sound therapeutic management principles are applied in a practical, scientific manner, they can also become very effective tools for clinical safety and quality of care.

TEST YOUR KNOWLEDGE

Multiple Choice

1. An institution's _____ is actually a complete reference manual for the policies and procedures, guidelines for use, and criteria for evaluation of the medications approved for use at that particular institution.
    a. policy and procedures manual
    b. formulary
    c. compendium
    d. risk management plan

2. A formulary consisting of tiered benefits is considered
    a. regulated.
    b. closed.
    c. open.
    d. static.

3. The committee that develops the formulary is the
    a. Pharmacy and Therapeutics Committee.
    b. U.S. Pharmacopoeia.
    c. Veterans Affairs system.
    d. Pharmacy Benefits Managers.

4. The Pharmacy and Therapeutics Committee investigates drugs for addition to the formulary and reports on their findings in
    a. the policy and procedures manual.
    b. a white paper.
    c. a business plan.
    d. a research journal.

5. Health insurance companies may utilize _____ to administer coverage of drugs to their subscribers.
   a. private pharmacists
   b. a board of directors
   c. Medicare and Medicaid officers
   d. pharmacy benefit managers

6. The portion of the Medicare plan that specifies how prescription coverage is handled is
   a. Medicare Part A.
   b. Medicare Part B.
   c. Medicare Part C.
   d. Medicare Part D.

7. How many times in a year are formularies published?
   a. once
   b. twice
   c. four (quarterly)
   d. twelve (monthly)

Fill In The Blank

1. The most revered formulary in the United States is the _____ Formulary.

2. A _____ formulary excludes drugs from various therapeutic classes.

3. Insurance companies may try to control costs through _____.

4. The use of computer technology for formularies has led to the ability to better track _____.

5. _____ is an important function.

References

Academy of Managed Care Pharmacy. *Principles in practice.* May 2005.

American Society of Health-System Pharmacists. (1996–1997). ASHP technical assistance bulletin on assessing cost-containment strategies for pharmacies in organized health-care settings. *Practice standards of ASHP, 1996–1997* (p. 147). Bethesda, MD.

American Society of Health-System Pharmacists. (1997). ASHP statement of the pharmacy and therapeutics committee. *Practice standards of ASHP, 1997.* Bethesda, MD.

American Society of Health-System Pharmacists. (2003). ASHP guidelines on formulary management. *Practice standards of ASHP formulary management, 2003.* Bethesda, MD.

American Society of Health-System Pharmacists. ASHP hospital drug distribution and control. *Practice standards of ASHP, 2004–2006* (update). Bethesda, MD.

Classen, D. C., Pestotnik, S. L., & Evans, R. S. (1997, January). Adverse drug events in hospitalized patients: Excess length of stay, extra costs, and attributable mortality. *Journal of the American Medical Association,* 277 (4).

CMS Medicare Part D Manual. Chapter 6: Part D Drugs and Formulary Requirements.

Joint Commission. *Accreditation manual for hospitals.* Oak Brook Terrace, IL.

27

Computer Applications in Drug-Use Control

Competencies

Upon completion of this chapter, the reader should be able to

1. List various pharmacy activities that automation and computerization have improved.

2. Describe how computer systems interact within the pharmacy and with other systems in the health care delivery process.

3. Describe how computerization within the health care system can better patient care.

4. Explain the concept of project management relating to the implementation of a computer system.

5. Describe the role of the pharmacist and the pharmacy technician in the management of a pharmacy information system.

6. Describe the general terms used in reference to information systems and automation.

Key Terms

admission, discharge, and transfer system (ADT)
charge capture system
computerized physician order entry (CPOE)
electronic data interchange (EDI)
hospital information system (HIS)
patient accounting system

Introduction

The management of medication administration plays a critical role in the patient care process. The data stored in the pharmacy information system is not only vital to the operation of the pharmacy, but it is also extremely important to other health care professionals in the management of the patient's care. Many extremely important decisions are made each day concerning drug therapy and the adjustment of drug therapy based upon the information that is retrieved from the pharmacy information system.

Pharmacy information systems have been used successfully in hospital and retail pharmacies for many years. In recent times, automation has become more and more prevalent in pharmacy practice. These automated systems not only improve productivity, but also help in reducing errors. Today it would be hard to find a pharmacy that does not have a pharmacy information system and some level of automation. As a matter of fact, without the use of a pharmacy information system, it would be nearly impossible to comply with all state, federal, and third-party insurance companies' demands.

As medical care becomes more and more complex, both clinically and administratively, pharmacy information systems have also become more and more complex. In the past, pharmacy information systems were nothing more than a system to retrieve prescription data in order to generate a label that was needed to fill either a prescription or drug order. Now pharmacy information systems screen for drug allergies and drug interactions, perform drug reviews, perform billing functions, automatically transmit information to insurance companies, allow the user to do sophisticated database searches or queries, interface with other information systems such as laboratory computer systems, and link themselves to other devices in the pharmacy that are involved in automation.

It should also be noted that as more and more hospitals and pharmacies merge, the need for these information systems to communicate with each other (networking) becomes extremely important. Chain drugstores can now look up prescription data from any of the stores in their network or chain. The same holds true for hospitals. The sharing of information between hospitals not only helps with the efficiency of the member institutions, but it also helps disseminate vital information to members of the health care team.

This chapter reviews the evolution of information systems within the hospital pharmacy and the role that pharmacists and technicians have played in their use. Some of the basic terminology information technology specialists use when speaking of these integrated pharmacy information systems is also discussed. Finally, a look toward what the future may hold will be addressed.

Computer Terminology

Computer systems have a language all their own. Understanding of computer technologies hinges on understanding the language used. Table 27-1 summarizes computer terminology.

TABLE 27-1   Computer Terminology

Abort	The abnormal termination of a program or process through user input or program failure.
Access speed	The average amount of time it takes for a storage device (floppy disk, hard drive, or CD drive) to find a particular piece of data on a disk.
ActiveX	Microsoft-based technology built to link desktop applications to the World Wide Web. Using ActiveX development tools, software developers can create interactive Web content for their applications.
ADT	Admission/discharge and transfer.
Algorithm	A detailed sequence of actions performed to accomplish a task of some kind.
Alias	A name, usually short and easy to remember, that is translated into another name, usually long and difficult to remember.
Application	Software that one uses to perform a specific task (e.g., word processors, spreadsheets, database programs).
Backbone	Carries data to smaller lines of transmission, just as the human backbone carries signals to many smaller nerves in the body. A local backbone refers to the main network lines that connect several local area networks (LANs) together. The result is a wide area network (WAN) linked by a backbone connection.
Backup	The action of copying important data to a second location to protect against data loss through equipment failure and unforeseen events.
Bandwidth	Refers to how much data can be sent through a network or modem connection. It is usually measured in bits per second (bps).
Batch file	A type of script that contains a list of commands. These commands are executed in sequence and can be used to automate processes.
Beta software	A version of an application or software made just prior to its accepted completion. Beta testing is carried out after alpha testing and involves ironing out any of the last few bugs or issues.
Bluetooth	Wireless technology that enables communication between Bluetooth-compatible devices. It is used for short-range connections between desktop and laptop computers, PDAs (like the Palm Pilot or Handspring Visor), digital cameras, scanners, cellular phones, and printers.
Booting	The act of starting up a computer and loading the system software into memory.
Cache	A section of memory used to temporarily store files.
Client	A computer that is able to access the resources of other computers on the network.
Cookie	Data sent to a computer by a Web server that records the user's actions on a certain Web site.
CPU (central processing unit)	The brain of the computer where almost all information processing is carried out.
Crash	A sudden, unexpected system failure.
Data	Any information stored in an electronic fashion.
Default	A preset value for some option in a computer program.
DOS	Disk operating system.
Driver	A piece of software that tells the computer how to operate an external or added device, such as a printer or hard disk.
Ethernet	A common method of networking computers.
File attributes	Markers assigned to files that describe properties of the file and limit access to the file. File attributes include archive, compress, hidden, read-only, and system.
File server	A computer that controls which other computers are allowed access to its storage media.
File transfer	Transferring files electronically from one computer to another, whether the computer is in the same room or miles away.
File transfer protocol (FTP)	Protocol used to move files between two computers linked via a network.

(Continued)

TABLE 27-1 (Continued)

Firewall	A combination of hardware and software that acts as a gatekeeper. Firewalls restrict other computers from gaining access to data.
Firewire	High-speed interface used to connect peripherals.
Firmware	A software program or set of instructions programmed on a hardware device.
Gateway	Hardware or software that acts as a bridge between two networks so that data can be transferred between several computers.
Gigabyte	1,024 megabytes (MB) or 1,073,741,824 bytes.
Graphical user interface (GUI)	Allows users to click on buttons with a mouse, light pen, or touch screen instead of typing commands at the command line.
Hard drive	The main storage device in a computer's hardware.
HIS	Hospital information system.
Hyperlink	A word, phrase, or image that the user can click on to jump to a new document or a new section within the current document.
Hypertext	Text that links to other information.
IP (Internet Protocol)	A standard set of rules for sending and receiving data through the Internet.
IP address	A code, also known as an "IP number" or simply an "IP," made up of numbers separated by three dots that identifies a particular computer on the Internet. Every computer, whether it be a Web server or a personal computer, requires an IP address to connect to the Internet. IP addresses consist of four sets of numbers from 0 to 255, separated by three dots. For example "66.72.98.236" or "216.239.115.148."
Kilobyte	1,024 bytes.
Local area network (LAN)	A computer network limited to the immediate area, usually the same building or floor of a building.
MAC address (Media Access Control address)	A hardware identification number that uniquely identifies each device on a network.
Megabyte	1,024 kilobytes or 1,048,576 bytes.
MIPS	Millions of instructions per second.
Motherboard	The main circuit board of a computer. The motherboard is the part of the computer where all other components are attached.
Network	A group of computers set up to communicate with one another. A network can be as small as two computers linked together or millions of computers linked together.
Operating system	The software on the computer that allows all other software to run. It is also the software that tells the computer how to run and execute commands.
P2P	Stands for "peer to peer." In a P2P network, the "peers" are computer systems that are connected to each other via the Internet.
Peripheral	A piece of hardware that is located outside of the main computer. A printer or a monitor would be a peripheral.
Post office protocol (POP)	The protocol used by e-mail clients to retrieve messages from a mail server.
Print queue	A list of print jobs waiting to be sent to a printer.
Print server	A software program that manages print jobs and print devices.
Protocol	A specific set of communication rules. When computers communicate with each other, there needs to be a common set of rules and instructions that each computer follows.
Query	The process by which a user can ask for specific information from a database.
Queue	A set of instructions waiting to be executed.
RAID	Stands for "Redundant Array of Independent Disks." RAID is a method of storing data on multiple hard disks.
Random access memory (RAM)	The physical memory installed in a computer.
Read-only memory (ROM)	Memory that can be read, but not erased.
Router	A network device that channels information from one computer to another across a network.

(Continued)

TABLE 27-1   (Continued)

SATA (Serial Advanced Technology Attachment)	An interface used to connect ATA hard drives to a computer's motherboard.
T-1	A connection capable of carrying data at 1,544,000 bits per second.
Token ring	A technology used to allow computers on a LAN to communicate.
Uninterruptible power supply (UPS)	A device that has an internal power source (battery) that enables a computer to continue operations for a short period of time during a power outage.
Upload	To send a file to another computer.
URL (Uniform Resource Locator)	The address of a specific Web site or file on the Internet.
Wide area network (WAN)	Any Internet or network that covers an area larger than a single building or campus.
Wildcard	A character (usually *) that can stand for one or more unknown characters during a search.
Workstation	Any computer that is attached to a network.
WYSIWYG (what you see is what you get)	What is seen on the screen will be pretty close to what the finished product looks like.
Zip	A zip file (.zip) is a "zipped" or compressed file.

Components of a Pharmacy Information System

There are four basic components of a pharmacy information system: (1) computer hardware, (2) application software, (3) system network, and (4) information server.

Computer Hardware

The computer hardware refers to the physical components of the computer systems and related devices. Computer hardware can be classified as internal and external. Internal computer hardware includes things like memory chips, hard drives, and the motherboard, while external computer hardware consists of components such as monitors, keyboards, mice, printers, and so on. Computer hardware is the part of the computer system that can be physically handled.

Storage of data

All information or data that resides in the computer system is stored on the system's hardware. This information can be stored locally (i.e., on the user's desktop computer) or on a server. Storing the information on a server is the more common configuration, since doing so will make it accessible to all others on the network and will prevent the end user from entering the same data more than once. When thinking about the information commonly stored, it's easy to understand why network storage makes sense. The user wouldn't want to enter demographic information on every patient on every machine. It makes a lot more sense to have this type of information stored in one place, and let all other users obtain this information when necessary.

There are two main categories of these types of storage devices: (1) disk devices (e.g., hard drives, floppy disk drives, CD-ROM drives, tape drives), and (2) memory. Memory on a computer usually refers to random access memory (RAM) chips. The main difference between these two types of storage devices is that disk drives can store information, and this information will only be erased if the user directs the computer to do so. All information stored on RAM chips will be lost when the computer is turned off or when it is rebooted.

The speed at which computers can access the information on disk drives and RAM memory differs greatly. It takes the computer much longer to access information on disk drives than it does to access information on RAM. Typically, when a particular program is run, some of the information needed to run the program is copied to the RAM chips inside the computer. The computer now runs the program from the RAM and not the disk drives. This speeds up information processing. When the user is finished working on a particular program, information is transferred back to the disk drive for safety intermittently, at specified times determined by the application. Remember that if at any time power is lost to the RAM chips, all information on these chips will be lost.

Some devices serve more than one purpose. For example, floppy disks or memory sticks may also be used as input devices if they contain information to be used and processed by the computer user. In addition, they can be used as output devices if the user wants to store information for archival purposes.

Application Software

Application software is nothing more than the programs one uses. Application software is the software that is running on any computer system in use. It could be the pharmacy software package used to enter physician orders and prescriptions into the computer, or it could be the software used by the laboratory department or software used by the payroll department to pay the employees within the company or institution. Application software used in pharmacies is usually leased from companies that supply the same software to many different pharmacies or hospitals. Usually, the organization will pay an initial fee for the installation of the software in the pharmacy or on the hospital's network and then pay monthly maintenance fees to the software company, which ensures that the software is kept current. These monthly maintenance fees also pay for any technical support that the end user might need.

System Network

The system network, simplistically, is a collection of wiring, hardware, and software that allows all computers linked to the network the ability to share information. Network management (i.e., client-server technology) controls the security of the network as well as the transfer of all data crossing over on the network. Client-server technology determines what information is passed back and forth from computer to computer. It also determines where information will be processed and on what machine the data will be stored. An example of this would be the calculation of a drug dosage. A pharmacist using a local computer in the pharmacy would obtain the age, weight, height, sex, and all other patient information needed to calculate the correct dosage from demographic information that most likely is stored on the hospital's main information server. Once all of the necessary information or data is obtained, the process of calculating the dosage can be done on the local pharmacy computer. The results of this calculation can then either be stored on the server or on the pharmacy system, depending on the way the network is set up. Normally, information is stored locally only when that information is specific for that one department.

The important thing to remember here is that, in most cases, specific data is never stored in more than one place. It would be foolish to store everything about every patient on every computer in the network. Modern networking applications allow the local computer to run local applications that obtain specific data only when needed. Storing data on multiple computers or storage devices could lead to individual users having different data sets. Storing the data on one computer or storage device ensures that everyone in the network has access to the exact same data.

Until recently, all computers on a network were physically linked together by high-capacity copper or fiber cable. More recently, wireless networks are becoming the standard. There are many advantages to wireless networks. Probably the biggest one is that buildings no longer have to be "wired." One must remember that wiring a large building with high-speed networking cable can be very expensive, and adding new computers to the network after the building is already wired is an ongoing and expensive chore. With a wireless network, any new computer can very easily be added to the network. At the present time these wireless networks are in their infancy, but one can easily predict that within the near future, copper or fiber networks will be a thing of the past. While wireless technology is much easier and possibly less expensive to set up, there are many security issues surrounding this technology that sometimes outweighs its benefits.

Information Servers

The information server is usually a larger capacity computer that aims to serve as an online repository of information resources. Demographic information such as patient names, addresses, phone numbers, ages, and sex are all types of information that would be stored on an information server. Other computers on the network access this information according to the software running on the computer and the privileges that the operator of the computer has.

System Management

Computer systems throughout most hospitals are administered or controlled by the institution's information technology (IT) department. The IT department is broken down into many divisions, but typically most IT departments will have people assigned to the following divisions:

- *Integration*—The role of this department is to make sure that the applications the institution is running integrate with the other applications on the network.
- *Help desk*—This is a support group that helps the client use applications. It is analogous to a technical support number that the user might call with software or hardware questions at home.
- *Medical informatics*—This is a group of people that make sure state-of-the-art clinical information is present for use. This could include anything from drug information applications to video conferencing with other hospitals.
- *Networking services*—This group of people maintains the institution's network.
- *Patient information services*—These are the people who ensure proper patient information (e.g., demographic information, previous admission information, drug history information) is available to all end users.
- *Technical services*—These are support personnel that maintain the information system.

Individual departments might have someone designated as the liaison between his or her department and the IT department. This person could be anyone in the department that has more than the usual computer skills. This person works with the IT department to make sure the systems in the department are running correctly and also makes sure training is available to all staff members who use applications on the system. The liaison would also be involved in the decision-making process if and when new hardware or software is deemed necessary.

Changing primary system applications or, for that matter, making major hardware revisions usually involves a team effort and is not an easy undertaking. Data on the old system must be able to be integrated into the new application, and any new hardware must be able to perform its given tasks.

Because of the complexity of such changes, a team effort is usually needed to make these major changes in operation run smoothly. The team participates in the tasks necessary to implement the system project in accordance with a well-defined work plan. The implementation of the system follows a well-defined project management methodology. A systems administrator will handle the ongoing management of the system once it is put into production.

When large revisions in hardware or system applications are necessary, the end user's responsibility is to justify and obtain funding for the procurement and ongoing enhancements for a particular system. This individual also defends departmental initiatives for the system.

Generally, when these types of large projects are initiated, someone within the department is named the project manager. The project manager is the field boss during the implementation or upgrade of the computer system. In the pharmacy, a pharmacist or pharmacy technician best fills this job. That person should have an intimate knowledge of the operation to be automated and must understand the goals and objectives of the project. In addition, this individual should possess sufficient skills to manage the pharmacy staff, participating staff from other departments, vendors, and assigned technical personnel. The project manager develops the work plan and uses it to manage the project through to its completion.

One job of the project manager is to manage the expectations of all who are involved in the project. The project manager must manage the expectations of the department, the members of the project team, and the other members of the hospital community who will be relying on the system when it goes into production. The work plan developed by the project manager must be realistic. Project milestones and other deliverables should take into consideration all steps necessary to complete the assigned tasks in a professional manner.

The project manager becomes the principal architect in designing how the system will be used in the pharmacy and how it will interact with other systems and departments throughout the hospital. The project manager also will coordinate how the work flow of the area(s) being automated will interact with the system.

A computer system can serve as a change agent to facilitate improvements of the processes being automated. If a system project automates a manual process without materially improving that process, the benefits of the system investment may be subject to question. Through the work flow design process and the development of policies, procedures, and forms, the project team has a real opportunity to effect positive change.

A well-managed system project is supported by a team working under the direction of the project manager. The project team should consist of people containing the right mix of skills, experience, and knowledge to build the desired system. The team should consist of representatives of the areas being automated.

They should be intimately familiar with the work flow in their areas of responsibility and all relevant policies and procedures of the area. Subject to the components of the system being implemented, the project team should include information systems staff with hardware, network, or programming expertise. Additional participants should be considered from areas with which the pharmacy interfaces on a regular basis (e.g., nursing, admitting, medical staff). These additional team members can assist in incorporating into the system those features and functions that will promote increased customer satisfaction through the use of the system.

Hospital Information System Application Relationships

hospital information system (HIS) a system that integrates information from many parts of the hospital.

To begin the discussion about pharmacy computer applications, an understanding of how these applications fit within the framework of the hospital's other critical applications is important.

The basic **hospital information system (HIS)** manages the processes of patient admission, charge capture, and billing. Although this is an oversimplification, it is, in essence, the set of features and functions performed within the HIS.

Admission, Discharge, and Transfer System

admission, discharge, and transfer system (ADT) a computer program for admission/discharge and transfer that provides significant demographic and clinical information for each patient.

The admission process is, of course, a more complex process often referred to as the **admission, discharge, and transfer system (ADT)**. The ADT is the system that first acknowledges a patient's existence in the hospital to every other system. The pharmacy system depends on the ADT system to know that a patient is a current patient of the hospital. It also distinguishes whether or not the patient is an outpatient or an inpatient. The ADT provides the pharmacy system with basic demographics on each patient (e.g., name, address, telephone numbers of the patient and next of kin, medical record number, bill/account number, date of birth, sex). The ADT keeps the pharmacy system informed as to each patient's location in the hospital. It also constantly updates the pharmacy system when patients are transferred or discharged. With this information, the pharmacy will know the room and bed location of each patient, where to send medication orders, where to send reports concerning patients, and if the patient has been discharged and is no longer entitled to filled orders.

In addition, the ADT provides other systems with critical information necessary to manage other processes within the hospital. Insurance information is collected here to facilitate the billing process. The ADT can also be used to help the hospital collect other valuable information such as whether the patient has a living will or durable power of attorney, who referred the patient to the hospital, and the name of the patient's physician.

The Charge Capture System

charge capture system a component of the hospital information system whereby every time an order is entered on a patient, a charge is being captured for billing purposes, and a statistic is being captured for management monitoring purposes.

The next component of the HIS is the **charge capture system**. A modern HIS system is referred to as the *order entry system*. Every time an order is entered on a patient, a charge is being captured for billing purposes, and a statistic is being captured for management monitoring purposes. Depending on the nature of an order, some charges are not computed until a test's results are delivered or the order is completed. In the case of physical therapy, an order for such a service is typically not finalized until after the physical therapist can assess the patient's condition and determine the amount of therapy required.

Medical records own a piece of the HIS. At discharge, the medical records department codes the chart with procedure and diagnostic information. This information is required for regulatory and billing purposes. A link between this coded information, charge information, and admitting information forms the basis of the billing and accounting functions performed relative to the services rendered to each patient.

Patient Accounting System

patient accounting system a component of the hospital information system; allows the hospital to bill and collect for its services.

The **patient accounting system** forms the last piece of the HIS, which is the final piece into which all previously collected information flows, and allows the hospital to bill and collect for its services. Components of this system include charge capture, accounts receivable, collection system, and cash receipts system. This system, and its relationship to the other components of the patient flow cycle, forms the basis for compliance with regulatory reporting standards of state, federal, and other accrediting organizations.

Ancillary Systems

The pharmacy system is one of many ancillary departmental systems. Other departments have specialized systems that support their operations, such as radiology, clinical pathology, surgical pathology, food and nutritional services, the operating room, and other procedure areas and specialty labs. These systems relate to the HIS system in the same manner as the pharmacy system.

The relationships of systems in many hospitals allow ancillary systems to communicate with one another to support patient care needs. For example, if a lab result indicates the need for an adjustment of a patient's medication, then such a result can be triggered to automatically place a notification in the pharmacy system for a pharmacist to review. Because a dietitian may have a similar need to manage patients' nutritional intake, certain lab values can also be automatically sent to the food and nutritional services system.

Services provided by the ancillary departments are captured within the ancillary systems. Each order entered is processed to interact with the inventory that the department manages. Issuing an item results in a reduction of the inventory on hand. The item that has been ordered and issued to the patient, with the patient's identifying information, is communicated back to the hospital's billing system so that the hospital can bill correctly for the item. To the extent that test results would accompany this communication from the ancillary system (in the case of radiology or laboratory systems), the result would be placed in a portion of the hospital's information system where it can be retrieved by caregivers who have a need to access such information. Many HIS environments support order entry via the HIS. These orders can be transmitted directly to each ancillary system via an automated interface. Order entry interfaces and their implications in the pharmacy will be addressed later in this chapter.

Business Systems

Several other systems support the day-to-day activities of a hospital. For the purposes of this chapter, they are classified as *business systems*.

The finance department requires a number of systems to support its operations: payroll systems, accounts payable systems, general ledger and budgeting systems, and cost-accounting systems. For the most part, the functions performed by these systems are self-evident by their names. It is also important to understand that the pharmacy interacts with each of these systems on paper or, in an automated sense, as it relates to the business processes of the pharmacy.

The hospital's payroll system is the vehicle that will pay the employees of the pharmacy as well as other employees within the institution. Hours have to be collected for input at the end of each pay period. Adjustments in vacation time, sick time, and staffing shift differential pay (for evening and night shift staff) need to be collected and submitted by the pharmacy's management in a timely manner so that payroll can pay all employees.

The accounts payable system processes the pharmacy's bills for payment, as it does for every other department of the hospital. This system requires that the pharmacy verify all purchases of supplies, products, or services on invoices prior to processing payment. Accounts payable systems are often linked to materials management systems to facilitate the link between purchasing and receiving and accounting for the payment of purchases.

The general ledger and budget systems allow the pharmacy to submit its budget for the coming year and track its actual expenditures against the approved budget.

Although only one system may reside in the pharmacy, it must interact with the vast majority of other computer systems in the hospital to conduct its day-to-day business.

The Hospital Pharmacy Application

Pharmacy information systems are designed to support the specific needs of pharmacy operations. These systems support activities that fall into several broad categories: inventory management, purchasing, and clinical support.

Inventory Management

A good place to start is the maintenance of the pharmacy's inventory. The level or quantity of an item in inventory triggers the need to order more product. What this means is that when the quantity on hand of a particular item reaches a certain predefined level or quantity (sometimes called the par level), some sort of notification must be sent out so that the materials management people or the purchasing component of the system knows that the item needs to be reordered.

When shipments are received, they must be checked against the purchasing documentation and then logged into inventory. Many pharmacy systems employ bar code scanners, which speed up the process of item identification and input into the system. When an order received is incomplete, the pharmacy system will track open order or back order situations. When the inventory level dips to a critical low, it will notify the purchasing component of the system and the key system user that follow-up is necessary.

As patient medication orders are filled, stock levels are automatically reduced in the inventory system. As stock items are taken to create new products (e.g., IV admixtures), the inventory system also reduces the inventory by the quantity of the item used. The term *perpetual inventory* is best understood as the quantity count of items in stock, based on the computer's calculations of purchases, less medications dispensed, plus the inventory item count at the last physical inventory. Its accuracy is dependent on several variables, including compatibility of the unit of issue with the unit of purchase, the accurate reporting of inventory shrinkage (e.g., items removed from stock due to expiration), and the accuracy of reporting of every item added to and removed from stock. It is up to the pharmacist or pharmacy technician to maintain the definitions in the inventory system in a manner so that the system can correctly perform the necessary calculations. Periodic physical counts of the inventory in stock must be performed and the results compared with the system inventory. This procedure will ensure the integrity of the information in the system and will alert the pharmacy as to any shrinkage of inventory that requires follow-up.

Purchasing/Receiving

When drugs, supplies, or other items in inventory require restocking, or new items must be purchased, the purchasing system is the vehicle that serves to facilitate the process. The purchasing system enables the management of orders placed, tracks open orders and back orders, and possesses the capability to electronically communicate new purchases to suppliers.

Whether the order for restocking is computed electronically (i.e., calculated by the system) or an item is entered for purchasing, most modern systems will be able to create a purchase requisition. Subject to the nature of the item(s) to be purchased, the system provides analysis tools to assist in analyzing supplier pricing. Once the supplier for each item is identified, requisitions are converted into purchase orders. Each purchase order contains those items to be acquired from one supplier and contains all agreed terms and conditions of the purchase.

When a purchase order is generated by the system and signed by an authorized signatory, it becomes a legally binding agreement when accepted by the supplier. Most suppliers will ship an order based only on receiving a purchase order number. Pharmacy computer systems are usually capable of generating purchase orders and transmitting them to suppliers electronically. In these instances, both the pharmacy (hospital) and the supplier are usually bound by certain terms and conditions as if a purchase order was duly signed by the purchaser and accepted by the supplier.

An electronically transmitted purchase order employs a technology referred to as **electronic data interchange (EDI)**. EDI technology is commonly used for ordering merchandise, transferring funds (e.g., electronic payroll deposits), and billing. Upon receipt of merchandise ordered, pharmacy personnel must count the items received and compare them with the items, quantities, and pricing ordered. Although the process can occur directly online on a computer terminal, it typically is more expeditious to check the order against the vendor's packing list and then check the packing list against the order and the invoice. If there is any discrepancy in the shipment against the order, the system will facilitate correcting the error. It is important to understand that the system will not correct the error, but merely provide the pharmacist or technician sufficient information to follow up on the discrepancy. When ordered merchandise is acknowledged to the system as received, the inventory on hand is updated.

electronic data interchange (EDI) commonly used to order merchandise, transfer funds, and billing.

Clinical Support

The production side of pharmacy operation relates to the receipt of medication orders for patient care, the processing of the orders, and the tracking of patients' medication history. The features and functions of pharmacy information systems and the relationship they bear to a hospital's order entry system vary widely.

Most physicians generate medication orders in their own handwriting. The issues surrounding physicians entering orders directly into a system are complex and will be discussed briefly later in this chapter. In most hospitals today, physician orders are keyed into systems in the pharmacy. Fax machines, pneumatic tubes, and couriers or transporters are all being used to transmit orders from nursing units to the pharmacy. In some instances, physicians are entering orders directly into the HIS, which is interfaced to the pharmacy system or order entry.

Upon entry of the medication order, some systems will immediately identify existing medication orders, laboratory test results, or allergies that may be incompatible with the order just placed. Other systems have a functionality that will suggest to the user that certain laboratory tests should be ordered with the medication order and other open orders should be discontinued based on the current literature. Still other features include suggesting more cost-effective medications than the one ordered. In such instances, the system is not designed to terminate the order, but merely to suggest to the pharmacist that the physician who wrote the order should be contacted to verify that the order is as intended.

The pharmacy system will generally receive relevant information on every patient from the HIS to facilitate the processing of appropriate doses. Date of birth, sex, height, weight, medical record number, and admitting (or billing) number of the patient are critical pieces of information. These data, coupled with the history of medications already ordered and dispensed to the patient, laboratory results, vital signs, diet orders and restrictions, and knowledge of procedures that have been ordered or scheduled, provide the system and the pharmacist with critical information to assist in managing the patient toward a speedy recovery.

When orders are entered, the system queues up the orders for a regular production cycle. Pharmacists and technicians prepare medication doses in accordance with schedules prepared by the system. The system also generates the appropriate labels for the medication to be administered. When robotics are being utilized, pharmacy information systems can electronically pass the order to the robot.

As the orders are packaged for shipping to the patient units, the inventory system is automatically adjusted to reflect a reduction in stock. In addition, each patient's medication administration record is updated to reflect the order and the medications dispensed. Medication lot numbers are also tracked to facilitate patient identification in the event of a manufacturer's recall.

Orders issued are communicated to other systems such as the hospital patient accounting (or billing) system, cost-accounting system, utilization review system, or other systems with authorized access.

For a pharmacist to fill a patient's medication order, the pharmacist must determine that the order was written by a physician and that the medication, dosage, and frequency of its administration are in accordance with the physician's order. The two accepted mechanisms to accomplish this process are (1) the pharmacist visually inspects the physician's written order and then enters it into the system, or (2) the physician enters the order directly into the system and uses a secret password that only he or she would know. Medication orders transcribed by a unit secretary or other personnel may result in many errors and should not be considered reliable. Most of the HIS implementations to date have not been successful in inducing the medical staff to enter medication or other orders directly into the computer without transcription, but in the near future this will change.

Soon most hospitals will incorporate some sort of **computerized physician order entry (CPOE)** process. CPOE is the process of electronic entry of physician

computerized physician order entry (CPOE) a drug order entered into a hospital-wide computer system transmitted to the pharmacy.

orders for the treatment of their patients. These orders are communicated over a computer network to the medical staff (nurses, therapists, or other physicians) or to the departments (pharmacy, laboratory, or radiology) responsible for fulfilling the order. CPOE decreases delay in order completion, reduces errors related to handwriting or transcription, allows order entry at point-of-care or off-site locations, provides error-checking for duplicate or incorrect doses or tests, and simplifies inventory and posting of charges.

Most available clinical pharmacy information comes from third-party vendors that link their products with pharmacy software. The vendors' core business is the maintenance of current information concerning medications, general pharmacology, drug-drug and drug-food interactions, and other related health care information in the form of numerous computerized database products.

The Future of Pharmacy Information Systems

The future of pharmacy information systems appears to be heading in two distinct directions. The first is the integration of the data and information-driven systems with robotics for drug dispensing. The second is the improvement of voice recognition technology to attract more physicians to enter their own orders directly into a system.

In a truly integrated environment, the management of patient medications is closely tied with laboratory results and diet. Abnormal laboratory test results can trigger alerts to clinical decision makers, which can result in a change to the patient's medications or diet. As physician order entry occurs, integrated systems can provide educational reminders or a series of cost-effective options for physicians and other clinical decision makers to consider. When orders inconsistent with the patient's treatment plan are about to be entered, the system can also alert the system user to the potential problem.

An order system linked to a robotics system can then complete the automation loop by processing and filling the orders without human involvement from the moment the order is entered. Pharmacy personnel must manage these robotic systems. Inventory levels within the robot must be periodically checked. The restocking of the robot's inventory levels also must be manually supervised.

True integration allows the hospital to operate as a whole. Information concerning all services provided to a patient can interact against a common data repository, which will form the true source for all patient information. These repositories will not only hold patient data, but also diagnostic images such as X-rays and lab slides. Clinical data repositories will form the basis of online, computerized patient records. This record will contain information concerning the most recent patient encounter and all information concerning a patient's medical history throughout a patient's life.

Voice recognition is a vehicle that holds much promise for bringing more physicians into the world of automated order entry. Consider the fact that the effort required to write an order is much easier than the effort involved in signing onto a system, flipping through order entry screens, identifying medications from the formulary, and validating the entry. Many physicians are reluctant to undertake this responsibility. Once perfected, voice recognition will provide a vehicle that will require little training and actually ease the effort for physicians.

Although the technologies described in this section do exist today, they are not widely used or are in early stages of development or release. By looking at what they are being designed to accomplish, they create a clear vision of what the near future will look like.

Summary

Early forms of automation dealt with speeding the processing of information so that productivity gains could be reached. As computers and technology have become more sophisticated, speeding the ability to access information has allowed decision makers to make more intelligent decisions. This is true for the pharmacy, as well.

This chapter was written with the goal of letting the reader understand that the role of the pharmacist and pharmacy technician is a critical one in the implementation and management of systems in a hospital pharmacy operation. A systems consultant can certainly play a role in managing a system, but the consultant ultimately leaves the project when it is completed. The pharmacists and pharmacy technicians are the individuals who will be responsible for the care and feeding of the system after the consultants leave, and they are the ones responsible for linking the features and functions of a system with the operational needs of the workplace. Lastly, it will be the pharmacists and the pharmacy technicians who will play a major role in the evolution of these systems.

Society has grown more dependent on automation over the years. Successful pharmacy professionals will be those who understand what automation can contribute, are able to harness its power, and are able to align its power with the tactical and strategic requirements of the business of pharmacy and hospital management.

TEST YOUR KNOWLEDGE

Multiple Choice

1. The software that provides desirable features and functions is the
   a. operating system software.
   b. files.
   c. application software.
   d. data.

2. Under a software lease, a user
   a. pays an installation fee.
   b. pays a monthly maintenance fee.
   c. receives technical support.
   d. all of the above.

3. A benefit of using a server for file storage is *not*
   a. to facilitate sharing common files.
   b. to store computer programs.
   c. to facilitate communication between different computer systems.
   d. to provide improved access security.

4. Which of the following describes Inventory Management Software?
   a. it can automatically order inventory when needed from the wholesaler
   b. it can incorporate bar code technology to aid in inventory control
   c. it is very costly and not actually used in many hospitals
   d. a and b
   e. all of the above

5. The information server
   a. is no longer used in most pharmacies since smaller PC-type terminals are now used.
   b. is always housed a far distance from the hospital or pharmacy.
   c. takes up too much room to be housed in a normal hospital setting.
   d. can be used by other computers to obtain information such as patient demographics.

6. The system network is
   a. a collection of wiring, hardware, and software that allows all computers that are linked to the network to share information.
   b. a place where the IT department is usually housed.
   c. a technical instruction manual.
   d. a tool used to communicate with other people in the organization.

Matching

1. _____ ADT
2. _____ Bluetooth
3. _____ CPU
4. _____ DOS
5. _____ firewall
6. _____ HIS
7. _____ MIPS
8. _____ query
9. _____ RAM
10. _____ UPS

a. wireless technology that enables communication between compatible devices

b. hospital information system

c. a combination of hardware and software that acts as a gatekeeper that restricts other computers from gaining access to data

d. millions of instructions per second

e. an electronic pathway

f. the process by which a user can ask for specific information from a database

g. admission/discharge and transfer

h. the physical memory installed in a computer

i. a device that has an internal power source (battery) that enables a computer to continue operations for a short period of time during a power outage

j. central processing unit

References

Austin, C. J., & Boxerman, S. B. (2003). *Information systems for healthcare management* (6th ed.). Ann Arbor, MI: Health Administration Press.

Campbell-Kelly, M., & Aspray, W. (2005). *Computer: A history of the information machine* (2nd ed.). New York: Basic Books.

Drazen, E. L., Ritter, J. L., Schneider, M. K., & Metzger, J. (1996). *Patient care information systems: Successful design and implementation (computers in health care).* New York: Springer Verlag.

Dudeck, J., Blobel, B., Lordieck, W., & Burkle, T. (Eds.). (2000). *Studies in health technology and informatics* (Vol. 45). Amsterdam: IOS Press.

Englander, I. (2003). *The architecture of computer hardware and systems software: An information technology approach.* New York: John Wiley.

Haux, R. (Ed.). (2004). *Strategic information management in hospitals: An introduction to hospital information systems (health informatics).* New York: Springer Verlag.

Kreider, N. A., & Haselton, B. J. (1997). *The systems challenge: Getting the clinical information support you need to improve patient care.* San Francisco: Jossey-Bass.

Long, L., & Long, N. (2003). *Computers: Information technology in perspective* (11th ed.). Upper Saddle River, NJ: Prentice-Hall.

Reis, R. A. (1996). *Understanding electronic and computer technology* (3rd ed.). Chico, CA: Technical Education Press.

Turban, E., Kelly Rainer, R., & Potter, R. E. (2002). *Introduction to information technology.* New York: John Wiley.

28

Preventing and Managing Medication Errors: The Technician's Role

Competencies

Upon completion of this chapter, the reader should be able to

1. Discuss the role of the pharmacy technician in preventing medication errors.
2. Determine and state the cause of system breakdowns that result in medication errors.
3. Define the types of medication errors that occur during the ordering and dispensing process.
4. State the 11 steps necessary for proper dispensing of medications.
5. List some commonly used drugs that result in medication error-related deaths.
6. Define confirmation bias.
7. List the steps that should be taken to minimize errors when taking verbal orders.

Key Term

confirmation bias

Introduction

The Institute of Medicine (IOM) released a report in 2006 entitled "Preventing Medication Errors," indicating that medication errors are among the most common medical errors, harming at least 1.5 million people every year. The report concluded that studies indicated 400,000 preventable drug-related injuries occur each year in hospitals. Another 800,000 occur in long-term care settings, and roughly 530,000 occur just among Medicare recipients in outpatient clinics. The committee noted that these are likely underestimates.

With increasing attention to medical and medication errors by the lay media, concern has intensified in both the public and health care sectors. Health professionals acknowledge that medication errors are a growing concern because of the increased numbers of critically ill patients, the development of more potent and potentially dangerous drugs and methods of administration, and more emphasis on fiscal constraints that affect hospital staffing and workloads in all sectors. Protecting patients from inappropriate administration of medications has become an important focus for pharmacists and technicians, including those in community and institutional settings.

Technicians play a major role in modern pharmacy practice. A recent large-scale study of both new prescriptions and prescription refills found an error rate of 1.7 percent. This dispensing error rate translates into approximately 4 errors per 250 prescriptions per pharmacy per day, or an estimated 51.5 million errors during the filling of 3 billion prescriptions each year.

While most of these errors probably have minimal clinical relevance and do not adversely affect patients, many experts believe that the medication error rate in less controlled environments—such as in the ambulatory setting where a patient purchases nonprescription medications or picks up prescription medicines from a community pharmacy—is probably higher.

This chapter focuses on system enhancements and the checks and balances needed to provide the maximum degree of safety as pharmacists and technicians prepare, dispense, and control medications in both community and institutional pharmacy settings.

Background

When a medication error occurs, it is the result of deficits in one of two areas: knowledge or performance. Because no individual knows everything and because everyone has occasional lapses in performance, all people occasionally make errors. To minimize the errors associated with medications, society has devised a system whereby one practitioner—usually a physician, but increasingly non-physician primary care providers—orders medications via prescriptions, and another professional, the pharmacist, is responsible for interpreting prescriptions, filling them accurately, and providing important information to patients.

Ordering Medications

Physicians or their designees (i.e., nurse practitioners, physician assistants) initiate the drug-dispensing and administration process through the medication order or prescribing process. Because prescribers are people, errors occur because of a lack of knowledge or because of poor performance. Computerized order entry systems have been developed and implemented and will likely become commonplace in a few years. These systems may help reduce certain types of errors, such as illegible handwriting errors (although they will introduce new types of errors as prescribers make other types of mistakes). But for now, most pharmacists dispense from handwritten medication orders. Illegible, ambiguous, or incomplete handwritten prescriptions or medication orders can contribute to many errors made by nurses, pharmacists, pharmacy technicians, and other health care workers.

Illegible Handwriting

To minimize the chance of misinterpretation, physicians with poor handwriting should print prescriptions and medication orders in block letters. In the institutional setting, physicians can review orders with the nursing staff before leaving the patient care area. In addition, including the purpose of the medication as part of the prescription or medication order can help readers distinguish the drug names when legibility of handwriting is less than ideal. Many medications have similar names, but very few name pairs that are spelled similarly are used for similar purposes. Preprinted orders, dictation, and direct order entry into the computer by physicians are other solutions for poor handwriting and improper orders.

Because even skilled individuals can misread good handwriting, a system of order/prescription transcription should be in place in which several individuals interpret and transcribe an order. In many hospitals each order is read by a unit secretary and reviewed by a nurse. At the same time, an exact copy of the order is sent to the pharmacy either directly, electronically, by fax machine, or with scanning technology. In the pharmacy, pharmacists and technicians have a number of opportunities to check the order, including a double check against labels, printouts, and the drug containers. A technician often screens the order and sometimes enters it into the computer. After data entry, a label is printed and a pharmacist interprets the original order/prescription and verifies the technician's computer entry by comparing it to the label. Later, the order and label again will be read by technicians and pharmacists as doses are prepared and dispensed. In the outpatient setting, this system should include a final check when providing counseling to the patient. In no case should pharmacy technicians interpret orders on their own, since this process does not offer enough checks in the event an error is made. In addition, orders must not be filled only from computer-generated labels; rather, the original order should accompany the label to serve as another check (Figure 28-1).

Look-Alike Drug Names

Medications with similarly spelled names can easily be misread for one another. In fact, from January 2000 to March 2004, close to 32,000 reports were submitted

FIGURE 28-1

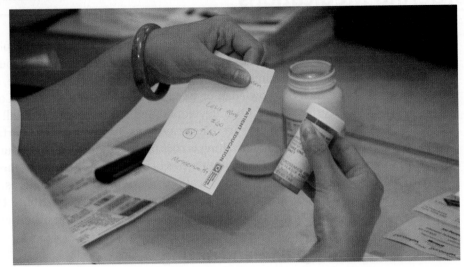

FIGURE 28-1 The pharmacist is responsible for assuring that the final product is properly labeled and matches the prescription the physician wrote.

to the USP's MedMarx Reporting System that linked errors to look-alike or sound-alike drug names. Technicians must be alert to this problem and should never guess about the prescriber's intent.

Study the handwriting in Figures 28-2 through 28-8. Would you have had difficulty reading these medication orders correctly? These are actual examples of handwritten orders in both the inpatient and outpatient setting, and each led to medication errors. The problem was not uncertainty. On the contrary, each order was misread from the start; no consideration was ever given to the alternative drug, because in each case the pharmacy staff members thought they were reading the order correctly.

FIGURE 28-2

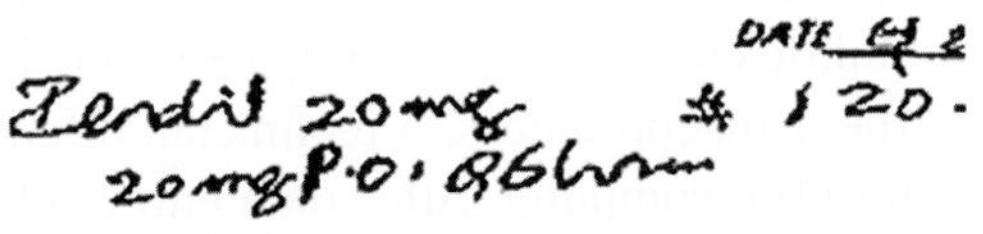

FIGURE 28-2 Prescription order for Isordil 20 mg, misread as Plendil 20 mg.

FIGURE 28-3

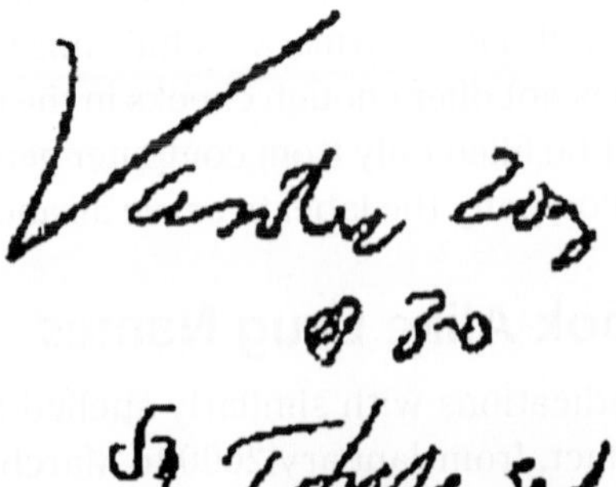

FIGURE 28-3 Order for Vantin 200 mg, misread as Vasotec 20 mg.

FIGURE 28-4

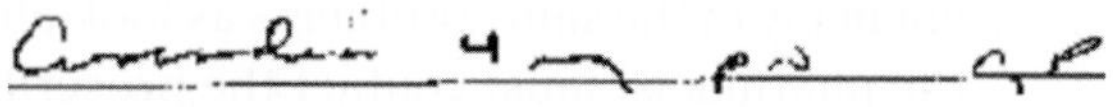

FIGURE 28-4 Order for Avandia 4 mg, misread as Coumadin 4 mg.

FIGURE 28-5

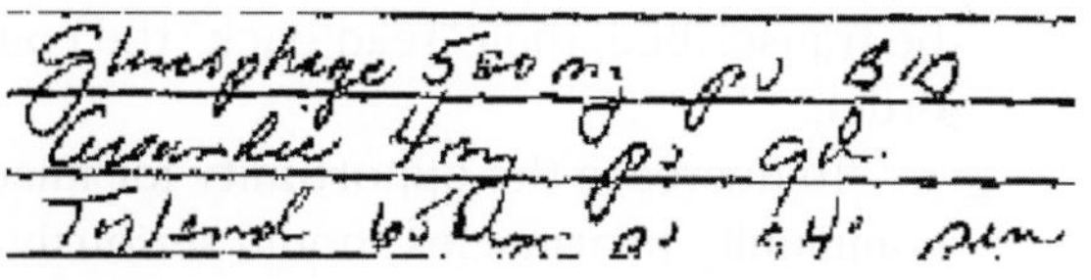

FIGURE 28-5 Order for Avandia 4 mg, misread as Coumadin 4 mg (second order).

FIGURE 28-6

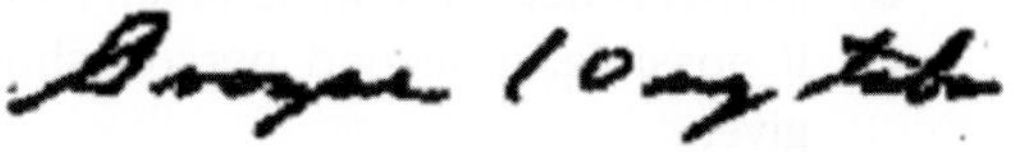

FIGURE 28-6 Order for BuSpar 10 mg, misread as Prozac 10 mg.

FIGURE 28-7

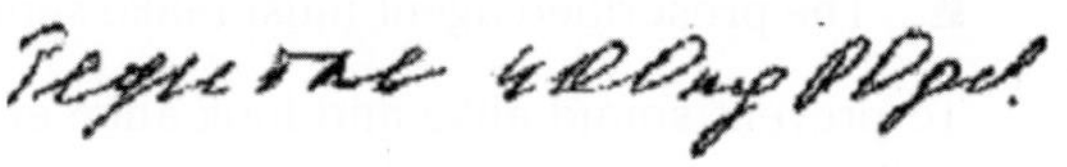

FIGURE 28-7 Order for Tequin 400 mg (misspelled with an "e"), misread as Tegretol 400 mg.

FIGURE 28-8

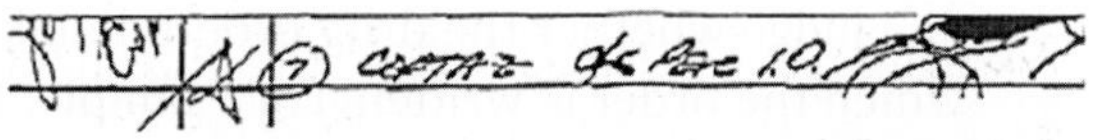

FIGURE 28-8 Ceftazidime "OK" per I.D., misread as ceftazidime "d/c" per I.D.

When pharmacists and technicians interpret prescriptions and medication orders, new drugs are a particular problem. Staff members are not as familiar with names of newly marketed drugs, and they tend to misinterpret them as older drugs. This is a good reason for health care facilities to establish policies that prohibit oral requests for medication without the pharmacy reviewing a copy of the order. Facsimile machines on each nursing unit and in the pharmacy make the process of having a pharmacist review the order easier. In the community, physicians can write both the generic and trade names legibly on the prescription, and they can add the intended purpose of the medication to further alert the pharmacy staff to the correct medication name.

Sound-Alike Drug Names

Drug orders communicated orally often are misheard, misunderstood, misinterpreted, or transcribed incorrectly. Celebrex and Cerebyx sound alike, as do Celexa and Zyprexa, Sarafem and Serophene, Lopid and Slo-bid, and thousands of other name pairs. All of these have been confused at one time or another, resulting in patients receiving incorrect medications. In many cases, serious injuries have occurred because of misinterpreted verbal orders. Sound-alike drug names present many of the same problems as look-alikes. Obviously, when uncertainties exist, the pharmacist must contact the prescriber for clarification.

The Joint Commission, a national accrediting agency for health care organizations, required in its National Patient Safety Goals that accredited organizations improve the effectiveness of communication among caregivers by implementing a process for taking verbal or telephone orders that requires a verbal order to be transcribed, then "read-back" the complete order by the person receiving the order.

To decrease the opportunity for misunderstanding, health care facilities and community pharmacies should seriously discourage verbal orders. Greater use of facsimile machines among hospital areas, medical offices, pharmacies, and nursing units will help. When verbal communication is unavoidable, strict adherence to these procedures for verbal orders can minimize errors:

- Verbal orders should be taken by a pharmacist whenever possible.
- If possible, a second person should listen while the prescription is being given.
- The order should be transcribed and read back, repeating exactly what has been understood, sometimes spelling the drug name and strength for verification (e.g., "one, five milligrams" for 15 mg).
- The prescribed agent must make sense for the patient's clinical situation.

To prevent sound-alike and look-alike errors, physicians must be encouraged to include complete directions, strengths, route of administration, and indication (purpose) for use. All of these elements can serve as identifiers. It cannot be stressed enough that even if such information is lacking on orders, by knowing a drug's purpose as well as the patient's problems, skilled health care professionals can judge whether the drug ordered makes sense for the patient in the context in which the order is written. For example, knowing that the patient has a diagnosis of diabetes would be an important clue in determining that Avandia is intended by the orders in Figures 28-4 and 28-5. Diagnostic procedures along with orders also could provide important information. This is why it is important for pharmacists to verify all orders processed by technicians. Never guess on an order. When in doubt, check with the pharmacist, who can call the physician for clarification if the intent is not completely clear. A list of sound-alike drug names can be found in Appendix C.

Ambiguous Orders

Errors can result when ambiguous orders are interpreted in a manner other than what the prescriber intended. Proper expression of doses is vital in a drug order. Technicians should be able to recognize improper expressions of doses—and the potential for error—when they see them, and they should bring them to the pharmacist's attention. When the prescriber's clarification is needed, the pharmacist must contact the prescriber. Pharmacists and technicians should avoid using improper expressions of doses as they process orders, type labels, and communicate with others. Several improperly expressed orders are analyzed and corrected in the following examples.

- *Decreased doses*—A patient with diabetes had been receiving 80 mg of prednisone daily for several months. After an office visit, the physician decided to decrease the daily dose by 5 mg, from 80 mg to 75 mg, and wrote the order

"Decrease prednisone—75 mg." The order was misinterpreted as meaning 80 mg *minus* 75 mg and was transcribed as, "Prednisone 5 mg po daily." As a result, a 5-mg dose was given, and the unintentional, sudden, large decrease in dosage caused the patient to collapse. "Decrease prednisone by 5 mg daily" would have been clearer, but the safest way would have been "Decrease prednisone by 5 mg daily. New dose is 75 mg daily."

■ *Tablet strengths*—Orders specifying both strength and number of tablets are confusing when more than one tablet strength exists. For example, "Atenolol 1/2 tablet 50 mg qd" appears clear enough; however, when you realize this product is available in both 50 mg and 100 mg tablets, it becomes clear that this order is ambiguous. What is the intended dose, 50 mg or 25 mg? Orders are clearer if the dose is specified regardless of the strengths available: "Atenolol 50 mg qd." For doses that require several tablets or capsules, the pharmacy label should note the exact number of dosage units needed. For example, the label on a 400-mg dose of Tegretol (carbamazepine), which is available in 200-mg tablets, should read "2 × 200 mg tablets = 400 mg." For a 25-mg dose of prednisone, which is available in 50 mg tablets, the label should read "1/2 tablet 25 mg." If your pharmacy prepares a computer-generated medication administration record (MAR) for the nurses, this same type of notation should be used.

■ *Liquid dosage forms*—Expressing the dose only in milliliters (or teaspoonfuls) for liquid dosage forms is confusing. For example, acetaminophen elixir is available in many strengths including 80 mg per 5 mL, 120 mg per 5 mL, and 160 mg per 5 mL. If the prescriber wrote "5 mL," the intended number of milligrams would be unclear, but "80 mg" is clear. The amount of drug by metric weight as well as the volume always should be included on the pharmacy label: "Acetaminophen elixir 80 mg/5 mL." Further, the patient dose should also be included. For a 320 mg dose the label should read "320 mg = 20 mL." The same holds true for unit-dose labels and bulk labels.

■ *Injectable medications*—For injectable drugs, the same rule applies. List the metric weight or the metric weight and volume—never the volume alone—because solution concentrations are variable. An error occurred from this problem at a hospital where hepatitis B vaccines were being administered. A preprinted doctor's order form was used to prescribe the vaccine, listing only the volume to be given. When the clinic switched to another brand of vaccine, containing a different concentration of vaccine, the same preprinted forms continued to be used, under-dosing hundreds of children until the error was discovered. This could have been avoided had the amount of vaccine been prescribed in micrograms, rather than just the volume in milliliters.

■ *Variable amounts*—A drug dose should never be ordered solely by number of tablets, capsules, ampoules, or vials because the amounts contained in these dosage forms are variable. Drug doses should be ordered with proper unit expression; for example, 20 mEq of magnesium sulfate. A patient whose doctor orders "an amp" of magnesium sulfate might get 8 mEq, 40 mEq, or 60 mEq. Under certain circumstances, the higher doses could be lethal.

■ *Zeros and decimal points*—When listing drug doses on labels or in other communications, never follow a whole number with a decimal plus a zero. For example, "Coumadin 1.0 mg" is a very dangerous way to express this dose. If the decimal point were not seen, the dose would be misinterpreted as "10 mg" and a 10-fold overdose would result. The same could happen if "Dilaudid 1.0 mg" is written. The proper way to express these orders would be "Coumadin 1

FIGURE 28-9

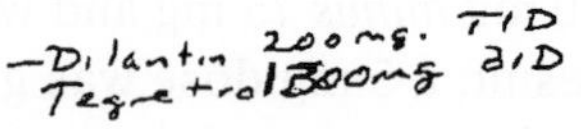

FIGURE 28-9 Order for 300 mg of TEGRETOL (carbamazepine) BID, misinterpreted as 1,300 mg BID.

mg" and "Dilaudid 1 mg," respectively. On the other hand, always place a zero *before* a decimal point when the dose is smaller than 1. For example, "Synthroid .1 mg" may be seen as "Synthroid 1 mg," especially when a poor impression of the decimal is written, such as on faxes or carbon or no-carbon-required copies. Avoid using decimal expressions at all where recognizable alternatives exist because whole numbers are easier to work with. In the above example, "Synthroid 0.1 mg" would be good, but "Synthroid 100 mcg" would be better. Use "Digoxin 125 mcg" rather than "Digoxin 0.125 mg." Use "500 mg" instead of "0.5 grams."

■ *Spacing*—Potentially serious medication errors have been reported to the Institute for Safe Medication Practices (ISMP) because a lowercase "L" was the last letter in a drug name and was misread as the number 1. For example, a prescription for 300 mg of TEGRETOL (carbamazepine) BID was misinterpreted as 1,300 mg BID (Figure 28-9). The letter "L" at the end of Tegretol had been written very close to the numerical dose of 300 mg on a prescription for the patient (e.g., Tegretol300 mg). The pharmacist was unfamiliar with the medication, and the pharmacy computer did not alert him that the dose exceeded safe limits. A similar error occurred with a prescription written for AMARYL (glimepiride) 2 mg. The "2" was written close to the "L," which led the pharmacist to misinterpret the order as Amaryl 12mg. Luckily, this error did not reach the patient (Figure 28-10).

■ *Apothecary system*—Use the metric system exclusively. You may have learned about the apothecary systems and its grains, drams, minims, and ounces, but this form of measure can be easily mistaken. For example, symbols for dram have been misread as "3" and minim misread as "55." Orders for phenobarbital 0.5 gr. (30 mg) have been mistaken for 0.5 grams (500 mg). The use of the apothecary system is no longer officially recognized by the United States Pharmacopoeia.

When typing labels, always place a space after the drug name, the dose, and the unit of measurement. It is difficult to read labels when everything runs together. Do not type "Tegretol300mg," because this can be misinterpreted as "Tegretol 1,300 mg." Instead, type "Tegretol 300 mg."

FIGURE 28-10

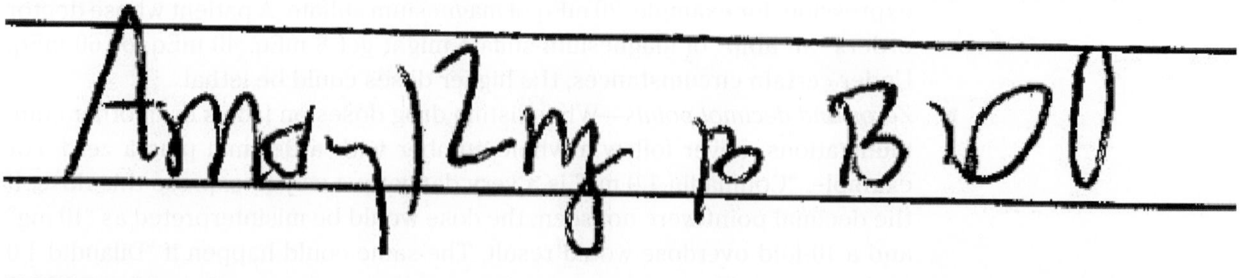

FIGURE 28-10 Is this order for Amaryl 12 mg or 2 mg?

Abbreviations to Avoid

Certain abbreviations are easily misinterpreted. Controlling dangerous abbreviations can reduce communication errors. Although many health care facilities have lists of abbreviations that are approved for use by the professional staff, it would be far safer if each hospital also developed a list of abbreviations that should *never* be used. In fact, such a negative list is easier to maintain and enforce. In addition, the Joint Commission has recommended that accredited organizations standardize abbreviations, acronyms, and symbols used throughout an organization, including a list of abbreviations, acronyms, and symbols not to use.

Table 28-1 contains several easily misinterpreted abbreviations. These should never be used in medication orders, on pharmacy labels, in newsletters or other communications that originate in the pharmacy, or in pharmacy computer systems because they may find their way to medication orders, labels, and reports.

TABLE 28-1 Misinterpretation of Abbreviations and Associated Errors

ABBREVIATION/ DOSE EXPRESSION	INTENDED MEANING	MISINTERPRETATION	CORRECTION
ʒ	dram	misunderstood or misread as "3"	use the metric system
m	minim	misunderstood or misread as "mL"	use the metric system
AU	aurio uterque (each ear)	mistaken for OU (oculu uterque—each eye)	do not use this abbreviation
D/C	discharge discontinue	premature discontinuation of medications when D/C (intended to mean "discharge") has been misinterpreted as "discontinued" when followed by a list of drugs	spell out "discharge" and "discontinue"
μg	microgram	mistaken for "mg" when handwritten	use "mcg"
o.d. or OD	once daily	misinterpreted as "right eye" (OD—oculus dexter) and results in administration of medications in the eye	use "daily"
TIW or tiw	three times a week	mistaken for "three times a day"	do not use this abbreviation
per os	orally	the "os" can be mistaken for "left eye"	use "po," "by mouth," or "orally"
Drug names			
ARA-A	vidarabine	cytarabine (ARA-C)	use the complete spelling for drug names
AZT	zidovudine	azathioprine	
CPZ	Compazine (prochlorperazine)	chlorpromazine	
HCl	hydrochloride salt	potassium chloride (the "H" can be interpreted as "K")	
HCT	hydrocortisone	hydrochlorothiazide	
HCTZ 50	hydrochlorothiazide 50 mg	hydrocortisone (seen as HCT250 mg)	
$MgSO_4$	magnesium sulfate	morphine sulfate	
MSO_4	morphine sulfate	magnesium sulfate	
MTX	methotrexate	mitoxantrone	
TAC	triamcinolone	tetracaine, adrenalin, cocaine	
$ZnSO_4$	zinc sulfate	morphine sulfate	

(Continued)

TABLE 28-1 (Continued)

ABBREVIATION/ DOSE EXPRESSION	INTENDED MEANING	MISINTERPRETATION	CORRECTION
Stemmed names			
Nitro drip	nitroglycerin infusion	sodium nitroprusside infusion	use the complete spelling for drug names
Norflox	norfloxacin	Norflex (orphenadrine)	
q.d. or QD	every day	mistaken as "q.i.d.," especially if the period after the "q" or the tail of the "q" is misunderstood as an "i"	use "daily" or "every day"
qn	nightly or at bedtime	misinterpreted as "qh" (every hour)	use "nightly"
qhs	nightly at bedtime	misread as every hour	use "nightly"
q6PM, etc.	every evening at 6 p.m.	misread as every six hours	use "6 p.m. nightly"
q.o.d. or QOD	every other day	misinterpreted as "q.d." (daily) or "q.i.d." (four times daily) if the "o" is poorly written	use "every other day"
sub q	subcutaneous	The "q" has been mistaken for "every" (e.g., one heparin dose ordered "sub q 2 hours before surgery" misunderstood as every 2 hours before surgery)	use "subcut" or write "subcutaneous"
SC	subcutaneous	mistaken for SL (sublingual)	use "subcut" or write "subcutaneous"
U or u	unit	read as a zero or a four, causing a 10-fold overdose or greater ("4U" seen as "40" or "4u" seen as "44")	unit has no acceptable abbreviation; use "unit"
IU	international unit	misread as IV (intravenous)	use "units"
cc	cubic centimeters	misread as "U" (units)	use "mL"
×3d	for three days	mistaken for "three doses"	use "for three days"
BT	bedtime	mistaken for "BID" (twice daily)	use "hs"
ss	sliding scale (insulin) or 1/2 $\overline{\text{ss}}$	mistaken for "55"	spell out "sliding scale"; use "one-half" or use "1/2 $\overline{\text{ss}}$"
> and <	greater than and less than	mistakenly used or interpreted as the opposite symbol	spell out "greater than" or "less than"
/ (slash mark)	separates two doses or indicates "per"	misunderstood as the number 1 ("25 units/10 units" read "110 units")	do not use a slash mark to separate doses; spell out "per" when that is intended
name letters and dose numbers run together (e.g., Inderal40 mg)	Inderal 40 mg	misread as Inderal 140 mg	always use a space between drug name, dose, and unit of measure
zero after decimal point (e.g., 1.0)	1 mg	misread as 10 mg if the decimal point is not seen	do not use terminal zeros for doses expressed in whole numbers
no zero before decimal dose (e.g., .5 mg)	0.5 mg	misread as 5 mg	always use zero a before a decimal when the dose is less than 1

Consider some of the abbreviations shown in Table 28-1. The abbreviation "U" for units is an example of what can go wrong; it should be on every organization's list of unacceptable abbreviations. Errors have occurred when the letter "U" was mistaken for the numerals 0, 4, 6, and 7, and even "cc," resulting in disastrous drug overdoses with insulin, heparin, penicillin, and other medications whose doses

FIGURE 28-11

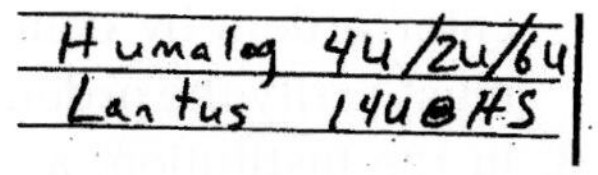

FIGURE 28-11 Erroneous order for insulin due to the use of the letter "U" for units.

are sometimes expressed in units. For example, orders written as "6U Regular Insulin" have been misinterpreted as "60 Regular Insulin," with patients receiving 60 units rather than the intended 6 units. A report sent to ISMP stated that a nurse, who was taking a patient's history, recorded his insulin dose using the letter "u" instead of the word "unit" (see Figure 28-11). The physician misread the "u" as a "4" and wrote orders for doses of 44 units, 24 units and 64 units, which is dramatically different from what the patient had been taking.

D/C is another example of an abbreviation that should not be used. It has been written to mean either discontinue or discharge, sometimes resulting in premature stoppage of patient's medications. In Figure 28-8, the "d/c" order was incorrectly interpreted as discontinuation of an antibiotic that the patient had never even received. In reality, the "d/c" is really "OK," meaning that the drug was approved for use by the infectious diseases physician.

Do not abbreviate drug names. For example, "MTX" means "methotrexate" to some health professionals, but others understand it as "mitoxantrone." "AZT" has been misunderstood as "azathioprine" (Imuran) when "zidovudine" (Retrovir) was intended. In one case, this misinterpretation led to a patient with AIDS receiving azathioprine, an immunosuppressant, instead of the intended antiretroviral agent. The patient's immune system worsened, and he developed an overwhelming infection.

Preparing and Dispensing Medications

An important safety enhancement for preventing dispensing errors is the development of a system of redundant checks from the time a prescription order is first written in the physician's office or on the nursing unit, to receipt in the pharmacy, through dispensing and administration. Such a system is suggested in this section. Obviously, the more "looks" an order receives (while efficient work flow is maintained), the better. Health professionals can review orders at several checkpoints and thereby maximize the chances of errors being discovered. Pharmacies with computerized drug distribution systems have an advantage because labels and reports can be printed so that at various steps order interpretation and order entry can be verified. Even pharmacies without computer systems should incorporate most of this suggested work flow since many of the options are available in a manual system.

Steps in Prescription Filling

The following list describes the steps a prescription goes through in the filling process:

1. The physician sees the patient; performs an assessment; determines appropriate medication, dose, and frequency; and writes the order or communicates the order verbally to nursing personnel or the pharmacy.
2. In the institution, a unit secretary reads and transcribes the order onto the medication administration record (MAR). This step is unnecessary

in hospitals where computers generate the MAR or where physicians can enter orders by computer, although the nurse and the pharmacist still must verify the order.

3. In the institution, a nurse checks the unit secretary's transcription for accuracy.

4. In both community and institutional settings, a direct copy of the order is carried or faxed to the pharmacy, or the physician's computer entry reaches the pharmacy. The pharmacy technician reads the order and enters it in the pharmacy computer system. If the technician finds a duplicate order, an incorrect dose, an allergy, or the like, it is documented and called to the attention of the pharmacist during the clinical screening in Step 5.

5. A pharmacist reviews the technician's computer entry, compares it with the original prescription (handwritten or electronic), and performs a clinical screening of the prescription with respect to the need for the drug, allergies or other contraindications, proper dose, and proper route of administration.

6. A label or a medication profile is printed. A copy of the original prescription or medication order continues to accompany the label or medication profile while the order is filled. No orders are filled solely on the basis of what appears on the label or medication profile, because the computer entry may have been in error.

7. To choose an item for dispensing, a technician reviews both the label and the medication order for possible discrepancies. If there are no discrepancies identified, the technician fills the order.

8. A pharmacist checks the technician's work, reviewing the label against the medication order copy and the dose that has been prepared. The drug is dispensed. In the community setting, the pharmacist uses the patient counseling session to further assess that the correct medication is being dispensed and that the patient has a condition treatable with the product being provided.

9. In the outpatient setting, pharmacists or technicians should ask ambulatory patients or their caregivers if they have any questions about their medications. For refills and medications patients have taken in the past, they should be informed about any changes in appearance of the product. In addition to providing patients with appropriate devices for measuring doses, such as oral syringes for administering oral solutions or suspensions, practitioners must ensure that the patient or caregiver understands how to properly use them with the medication. Demonstrate for patients how to use the device, and follow up with a return demonstration by the user.

10. In the institution, the nurse receives the drug and compares the medication and pharmacy label against the copy of the physician's order as well as the handwritten transcription made earlier in the MAR.

11. Patients in the community setting should be counseled about the common adverse effects of medications they are taking, and they should be instructed on any clinical signs to watch for and report to health professionals. In the institution, the nurse administers the dose, explaining the drug's purpose and potential adverse effects, and answers questions and concerns raised by the patient.

12. The final step in the process is the assurance of adherence to medication therapy. If the patient is taking too much medication or is not taking the

drug as frequently as prescribed, the pharmacist should speak with the patient to determine the reasons and address the variation. In addition, patients should be asked about common adverse effects and about signs of serious drug toxicities. In the institution, pharmacy personnel check unit-dose bins and MARs to make sure that nursing staff is administering the medication on the proper schedule.

Selecting Medications

The importance of reading the product label while selecting medications and filling prescriptions cannot be overemphasized. Too often the wrong drug or wrong strength is dispensed, and such errors usually stem from failure to read the label. During drug preparation and dispensing, the label should be read three times: when the product is selected, when the medication is prepared, and when either the partially used medication is disposed of (or restocked) or product preparation is complete.

Selecting the correct item from the shelf, drawer, or bin can be complicated by many factors. Similar labeling and packaging as well as look-alike names are a common trap that leads to medication errors. Restocking errors are quite common and can lead to repeated medication errors before being detected.

Automated dispensing machines have become more common on the nursing units of many hospitals. The nurse must punch a security code and a password into the dispensing device, along with the name of the patient and the name of the medication, before the machine will allow access to remove the medication. This system allows more control of items kept on the nursing unit and serves as a check for the nurse who retrieves the medication, more so than for regularly stocked floor stock items. In some cases, online communication with the hospital computer information system or pharmacy system allows a pharmacist to review medication orders before nursing access to the medication is allowed.

Automated dispensing devices create several situations that can result in errors. The machines are restocked daily, and the incorrect restocking of items (i.e., placing the wrong drug into the wrong bin) can occur. Devices that have multiple medications in each drawer and that do not require pharmacist review of orders before access have drawbacks that are identical to flaws in the old floor stock systems, in that the nurse can retrieve either the wrong item or additional items to use for other patients, and lack of pharmacist double-checking and screening of orders allows prescribing errors, wrong dosages, incorrect routes of administration, and other clinical errors to occur.

When errors occur in selection of medication by either pharmacy or nursing staff, the term **confirmation bias** is used to describe the phenomenon. When choosing an item, people see what they are looking for, and once they think they have found it, they stop looking any further. Often the health professional chooses a medication container based on a mental picture of the item. Staff members may be looking for some characteristic of the drug label, the shape and size or color of the container, or the location of the item on a shelf, in a drawer, or in a storage bin instead of reading the name of the drug itself. Consequently, they may fail to realize that they have the wrong item in hand.

A number of approaches can be used to minimize the possibility of such errors in the pharmacy and in automated dispensing machines. Physically separating drugs with look-alike labels and packaging reduces the potential for error. Some

confirmation bias a term used to describe errors that occur in selection of medication by either pharmacy or nursing staff; when choosing an item, people see what they are looking for, and once they think they have found it, they stop looking any further.

pharmacy technicians also separate drugs with similar names and overlapping strengths, especially those labeled and packaged by the same manufacturer. For example, morphine 10 mg tablets and hydromorPHONE 10 mg tablets, both from the same unit-dose packager, might pose a problem. So might chlorproMAZINE 200 mg and chlorproPAMIDE 200 mg.

Another strategy would be to change the appearance of look-alike product names on computer screens, pharmacy shelf labels and bins, and pharmacy product labels by highlighting, through boldface, color, or by the use of "tall man" letters, the parts of the names that are different (e.g., hydrOXYzine, hydrALAzine). In fact, the FDA Office of Generic Drugs requested manufacturers of 16 look-alike name pairs to voluntarily revise the appearance of their established names in order to minimize medication errors resulting from look-alike confusion. Manufacturers were encouraged to visually differentiate their established names with the use of "tall man" letters. Examples of established names involved include chlorproMAZINE and chlorproPAMIDE, vinBLAStine and vinCRIStine, and niCARdipine and NIFEdipine.

Pharmaceutical companies are aware of labeling and packaging problems, and many have responded to suggestions made by technicians and pharmacists. Health professionals can alert manufacturers about errors caused by commercial packaging and labeling problems by using the USP-ISMP Medication Error Reporting Program (MERP). Reports are forwarded to the individual pharmaceutical company and the U.S. Food and Drug Administration (FDA) and the ISMP provides follow-up when appropriate. Call 1-800-FAIL-SAF(E), go to www.ismp.org, or complete a USP-ISMP MERP report (Figure 28-12). All reports are confidential. In institutional settings and community pharmacies with several staff members, everyone should have input in deciding how and where drugs are available, how doses are prepared, who is responsible for preparing them, the appearance of the storage containers, and how they are labeled. Procedures to ensure safe medication use must be written, and the importance of adhering to the guidelines must be shared by all involved pharmacy, medical, and nursing staff members.

Selecting Auxiliary Labels

To help prevent errors, pharmacists and technicians should apply auxiliary labels in certain circumstances, especially in the community setting. For example, amoxicillin oral suspension is available in dropper bottles for pediatric use. When the suspension is used for an ear infection, some parents have been known to place the suspension in the child's ear rather than give it properly, that is, orally. An auxiliary label, "For Oral Use Only," would help prevent this error. Other such labels are "For the Ear," "For the Eye," and "For External Use Only."

However, this practice can be unsafe if the patient is unable to understand the warning. A study that appeared in the *American Journal of Health-System Pharmacy* *(AJHP)* showed that there is a high level of misunderstanding of auxiliary labels among adults with low literacy, a reading level at or below the sixth-grade level. The rate of correct interpretation of these labels ranged from 0 percent to 78.7 percent. With the exception of the label "Take with food," less than half of all patients were able to provide adequate interpretations of the warning labels' messages. In fact, none were able to correctly interpret the label "Do not take dairy products, antacids, or iron preparations within one hour of this medication." Studies have also shown that a combination of a verbal description of a warning along with visual symbols improves the overall comprehension of the warning.

FIGURE 28-12

USP MEDICATION ERRORS REPORTING PROGRAM
Presented in cooperation with the Institute for Safe Medication Practices
USP is an FDA MEDWATCH partner

Reporters should not provide any individually identifiable health information, including names of practitioners, names of patients, names of healthcare facilities, or dates of birth (age is acceptable).

Date and time of event:

Please describe the error. Include description/sequence of events, type of staff involved, and work environment (e.g., code situation, change of shift, short staffing, no 24-hr. pharmacy, floor stock). If more space is needed, please attach a separate page.

Did the error reach the patient?　❑ Yes　❑ No

Was the incorrect medication, dose, or dosage form administered to or taken by the patient?　❑ Yes　❑ No

Circle the appropriate Error Outcome Category (select one—see back for details):　A　B　C　D　E　F　G　H　I

Describe the direct result of the error on the patient (e.g., death, type of harm, additional patient monitoring).

Indicate the possible error cause(s) and contributing factor(s) (e.g., abbreviation, similar names, distractions, etc.).

Indicate the location of the error (e.g., hospital, outpatient or community pharmacy, clinic, nursing home, patient's home, etc.).

What type of staff or healthcare practitioner made the initial error?

Indicate if other practitioner(s) were also involved in the error (type of staff perpetuating error).

What type of staff or healthcare practitioner discovered the error or recognized the potential for error?

How was the error (or potential for error) discovered/intercepted?

If available, provide patient age, gender, diagnosis. Do not provide any patient identifiers.

Please complete the following for the product(s) involved. (If more space is needed for additional products, please attach a separate page.)

	Product #1	Product #2
Brand/Product Name (If Applicable)		
Generic Name		
Manufacturer		
Labeler		
Dosage Form		
Strength/Concentration		
Type and Size of Container		

Reports are most useful when relevant materials such as product label, copy of prescription/order, etc., can be reviewed.
Can these materials be provided?　❑ Yes　❑ No　　Please specify:

Suggest any recommendations to prevent recurrence of this error, or describe policies or procedures you instituted or plan to institute to prevent future similar errors.

Name and Title/Profession	( ) Telephone Number	( ) Fax Number
Facility/Address and Zip		E-mail
Address/Zip (where correspondence should be sent)		

Your name, contact information, and a copy of this report are routinely shared with the Institute for Safe Medication Practices (ISMP). Copies of reports will be sent to third parties such as the manufacturer/labeler, and to the Food and Drug Administration (FDA). You have the option of including your name on these copies.

In addition to releasing my name and contact information to ISMP, USP may release my identity to these third parties as follows (check boxes that apply):

❑ The manufacturer and/or labeler as listed above　❑ FDA　❑ Other persons requesting a copy of this report　❑ Anonymous to all third parties

Signature	Date

Return to: USP CAPS 12601 Twinbrook Parkway Rockville, MD 20852-1790	Submit via the Web at www.usp.org/mer Call Toll Free: **800-23-ERROR** (800-233-7767) or FAX: 301-816-8532	Date Received by USP	File Access Number

PSF116G

WEPDF
©USPC 2003

(Continued)

FIGURE 28-12 Form used to report medication errors or problems to the USP-ISMP Medication Error Reporting Program (Reprinted with permission of the United States Pharmacopoeia. All rights reserved. © 2002).

FIGURE 28-12 (Continued)

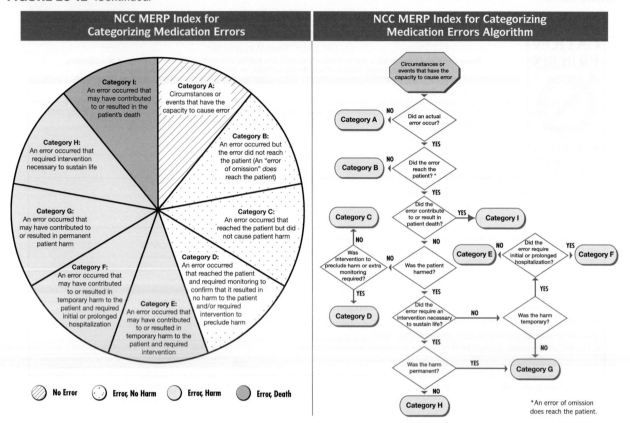

NCC MERP Index for Categorizing Medication Errors	NCC MERP Index for Categorizing Medication Errors Algorithm

 No Error   Error, No Harm   Error, Harm   Error, Death

*An error of omission does reach the patient.

© 2003 National Coordinating Council for Medication Error Reporting and Prevention

Full-size copies are available: **INDEX**—www.nccmerp.org/010612_color_index.pdf; **ALGORITHM**—www.nccmerp.org/010612_color_algo.pdf

National Coordinating Council for Medication Error Reporting and Prevention Definitions

Harm
Impairment of the physical, emotional, or psychological function or structure of the body and/or pain resulting therefrom.

Monitoring
To observe or record relevant physiological or psychological signs.

Intervention
May include change in therapy or active medical/surgical treatment.

Intervention Necessary to Sustain Life
Includes cardiovascular and respiratory support (e.g., CPR, defibrillation, intubation, etc.).

 U.S. Pharmacopeia
12601 Twinbrook Parkway
Rockville, MD 20852-1790

NO POSTAGE
NECESSARY
IF MAILED
IN THE
UNITED STATES

BUSINESS REPLY MAIL
FIRST-CLASS MAIL PERMIT NO 39 ROCKVILLE MD

POSTAGE WILL BE PAID BY ADDRESSEE:
DIANE D COUSINS RPh
THE USP CENTER FOR THE ADVANCEMENT OF PATIENT SAFETY
12601 TWINBROOK PARKWAY
ROCKVILLE MD 20897-5211

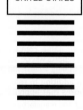
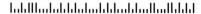

Sterile Admixture Preparation

In preparing fluids for injectable administration, the potential for grave error is increased for several reasons. First, patients who are sicker often need intravenous drugs, so the medications used have more dramatic effects on the body's function and physiology. Further, most injectable solutions are simply clear, colorless, water-based fluids, so they may look alike, regardless of what drug and how much of it is actually in the fluid.

Thus, in the sterile admixture preparation setting, the chance of dosage miscalculation or measurement error must be minimized by systems designed with procedures that require independent double checks by two staff members. The independent double check in some pharmacies might be required for all calculations or measurements, while others require it only for calculations falling into special categories, such as dosage calculations for admixture compounding for any child under 12, critical-care drug infusions requiring a dose in micrograms per kilogram per minute, insulin infusions, chemotherapy, and patient-controlled analgesia. Calculators and computer programs may improve accuracy, but they do not eliminate the need for a second person to review the calculations and solution concentrations used. Another important way to minimize calculation errors is to avoid the need for calculations. This can be accomplished by using the unit-dose system exclusively through the following methods:

- Using commercially available unit-dose systems, such as premixed critical care parenteral products.
- Standardizing doses and concentrations, especially of critical-care drugs such as heparin, dobutamine, dopamine, or morphine.

Similar steps can be taken in community pharmacies that provide sterile admixtures to physician's offices, home care programs and patients, long-term care facilities, and other clients.

The use of standard dosage charts on the floors and standard formulations in the pharmacy minimizes the possibility of error and makes calculations much easier for everyone. For example, in critical care units, physicians need order only the amount of drug they want infused and list any titration parameters. No one has to perform any calculations because dosage charts can be readily available, for choosing appropriate flow rates by patient weight and dose ordered.

Standard concentrations for frequently prepared formulations should be recorded and be readily accessible for reference in the admixture preparation area in the pharmacy. Of course, all calculations must be double-checked and documented by the pharmacist. Diluents as well as active drugs must be checked. The stock container of each additive with its accompanying syringe should be lined up in the order it appears on the container label to facilitate the checking procedure. The final edge of the plunger piston should be aligned with the calibration marks on the syringe barrel, indicating the amount used.

In many hospitals, automated compounders are being used for admixing both large- and small-volume parenterals. Automated equipment has been known to fail occasionally. Also, some accidents have occurred in which solutions were placed on the wrong additive channel. In either case, the result could be a serious medication error. Therefore, it is important that the pharmacy have an ongoing quality assurance program for the use of automated compounding equipment. This program should include double checks and documentation of solution placement within the compounder, final weighing or refractometer testing of the solution to assure that proper concentrations have been compounded, and ongoing sampling of electrolyte concentrations. Pharmacists that prepare special parenteral solutions in batches (e.g., total parenteral nutrition base solutions, cardioplegic solutions) should have additional quality assurance procedures in place, including sterility testing and quarantine until confirmation.

Effective Medication Error Prevention and Monitoring Systems

All drug-dispensing procedures should be examined regularly, and the cause of system breakdowns must be discovered so that prevention measures can be designed. Pharmacy technicians need to communicate clearly to their pharmacist supervisors what it takes to do the job correctly in terms of personnel, training programs, facilities design, equipment, drug procedures and supplies, computer systems, and quality assurance programs.

Multidisciplinary educational programs should be developed for health care personnel about medication error prevention. Because many errors happen when procedures are not followed, this is one area on which to focus through newsletters and in-service training. It also is important for pharmacy staff members to focus not just on their own internal errors, but to look at other pharmacies' errors and methods of prevention and to learn from these. The ISMP provides ongoing features to facilitate these reviews in publications such as *Pharmacy Today, U.S. Pharmacist, Hospital Pharmacy*, and *Pharmacy & Therapeutics*. The ISMP also publishes its own biweekly *ISMP Medication Safety Alert!* for hospitals and a monthly newsletter for community/ambulatory care practices that reports on current medication safety issues and offers recommendations for changes.

Summary

In institutions, the pharmacy department is responsible for the drug-use process throughout the facility. Pharmacists and other members of the pharmacy department should lead a multidisciplinary effort in examining where errors arise in this process. Pharmacists and pharmacy technicians should work together in designing quality assurance programs to obtain information that helps establish priorities and make changes. For example, joint reviews of the accuracy of unit-dose cart fills are of great help in detecting reasons for missing or inaccurate doses and changing the drug-dispensing system accordingly. Programs can be established to monitor the accuracy of order entry into computers in the pharmacy. Quality assurance efforts that include a review of medication error reports help to develop a better understanding of the kinds of system or behavioral defects being experienced so that necessary corrections can be identified. The medication error problem will never be completely eliminated, but pharmacists and pharmacy technicians, working together, can use their expertise to address issues of safety and thus ensure the safest environment possible.

TEST YOUR KNOWLEDGE

Multiple Choice

1. Medication errors are a growing concern in hospitals because of
    a. increased numbers of critically ill patients.
    b. development of more potent medications.
    c. increased media awareness.
    d. all of the above.

2. Medication errors are estimated to occur at a rate of
    a. one per patient per day.
    b. one per hospital per day.
    c. one per health care personnel per day.
    d. one per nursing unit per day.

3. The five "rights" of medication prescribing, dispensing, and administration for medications include all but
    a. patient.
    b. route.
    c. dose.
    d. prescriber.

4. Which of the following changes in process could minimize the chance of misinterpretation of handwritten orders?
    a. prescribers printing prescriptions and medication orders in block letters
    b. physicians reviewing orders with the nursing staff before leaving the patient care area
    c. including the purpose of the medication as part of the prescription
    d. all of the above

5. An order for a drug whose strength is a whole number should never be followed by a zero (e.g., 10.0 mg) because
    a. the patient could be under-dosed 10-fold.
    b. the patient could be overdosed 10-fold.
    c. the patient could be under-dosed 100-fold.
    d. the patient could be overdosed 100-fold.

6. Which order below is the most clearly written and least ambiguous?
    a. "Synthroid 100mcg daily"
    b. "Synthroid 1 tablet daily"
    c. "Synthroid 0.1 mg daily"
    d. "Synthroid 100 mcg daily"

7. Which order below is the most clearly written and least ambiguous?
    a. "Phenobarbital elixir 15 mg/5 mL: Give 15 mg 5 mL at bedtime."
    b. "Phenobarbital elixir: Give 5 mL at bedtime."
    c. "Phenobarbital elixir 15 mg/5 mL: Give 5.0 mL at bedtime."
    d. "Phenobarbital elixir: Give one teaspoonful at bedtime."

8. When you see an order for "AZT" written, it could stand for:
   a. Azidothymidine.
   b. Azathioprine.
   c. Aztreonam.
   d. all of the above—better check with prescriber before filling.

9. Computerized order entry enhances routine drug dispensing activities by
   a. serving as a double check of the patient's medication for physicians, nurses, and pharmacists.
   b. eliminating the pharmacist from having to check the technician's bin filling.
   c. eliminating the technician from having to restock floor stock items.
   d. none of the above.

10. Confirmation bias occurs when
    a. a physician orders medication for the wrong patient.
    b. an item is chosen once you confirm what you think you are looking for on the label.
    c. a nurse confirms the identity of a patient before administering medication.
    d. a pharmacist does a clinical screening of a patient's medication profile.

11. Medication errors can be reported to the USP-ISMP MERP by
    a. pharmacists.
    b. pharmacy technicians.
    c. the public.
    d. all of the above.

References

Cohen, M. R. (Ed.). (2007). *Medication errors* (2nd ed.). Washington, DC: American Pharmaceutical Association.

Flynn, E. A., Barker, K. N., & Carnahan, B. J. (2003). National observational study of prescription dispensing accuracy and safety in 50 pharmacies. *Journal of the American Pharmaceutical Association*, 43 (2): 191–200.

Flynn, E. A., Pearson, R. E., & Barker, K. N. (1997). Observational study of accuracy in compounding IV admixtures at five hospitals. *American Journal of Health-System Pharmacy*, 54, 904–912.

Institute for Safe Medication Practices. Misidentification of alphanumeric characters. *ISMP Medication Safety Alert! Community/Ambulatory Edition*. January 2003, page 3.

Institute for Safe Medication Practices. Stop U be 4 errors. *ISMP Medication Safety Alert!* October 21, 2004, Volume 9, Issue 21, 1.

Lesch, M. F. (2003). Comprehension and memory for warning symbols: Age-related differences and impact of training. *Journal of Safety Research*, 34 (5): 495–505.

Pennsylvania Patient Safety Authority. (2006). Improving the safety of verbal orders. *Patient Safety Advisory*, 3 (2): 1–7.

Santell, J. O., & Camp, S. (2004). Similarity of drug names, labels, or packaging creates safety issues. *U.S. Pharmacist*, 29 (7).

Wolf, M. S., Davis, T. C., et al. (2006). Misunderstanding of prescription drug warning labels among patients with low literacy. *American Journal of Health-System Pharmacy*, 63 (1): 1048–1055.

Reimbursement for Pharmacy Services

Competencies

Upon completion of this chapter, the reader should be able to

1. Describe the factors affecting product and service reimbursement for the drug product in hospitals, skilled nursing facilities, and community practice.

2. List factors affecting prescription coverage and reimbursement in community pharmacy practice.

3. Differentiate between the criteria in reimbursement issues in acute care and long-term care.

4. Explain existing and possible avenues for reimbursement for cognitive services.

5. Describe the role of the pharmacy technician in support of pharmacists seeking additional reimbursement for services.

6. Describe the role of the pharmacy technician in reimbursement for a health care provider.

Key Terms

average wholesale price (AWP)
carve-out
cognitive pharmacy services
maximum allowable cost (MAC)
per diem reimbursement
prior approval
wholesaler acquisition cost

Introduction

Reimbursement and insurance coverage for pharmacy services is a widely discussed subject by patients and their families. This issue now receives widespread coverage in the media because of the discussions of both existing and impending federal drug coverage legislation. Although it is a relatively small part of total health care expenditure, it is a highly visible one. While drug marketers present drugs as a small component of overall health care expenditure, we must remember that for a large segment of the population, it is the least reimbursed health care component and, therefore, the most costly portion of health care. The average Medicare beneficiary with hypertension and minor coronary disease may spend $8 on a monthly physician visit and $100 on medication each month. Therefore, opportunities for reimbursement must be carefully considered.

Ambulatory Care (Community Pharmacy) Reimbursement

In most instances there is little variance regarding reimbursement for medication products between Medicaid, indemnity insurance companies, and managed care coverage. Insurance carriers vary in their coverage on the medical side as well as on the pharmacy side. In general, the cost of medication is reimbursed, plus a fee for dispensing, monitoring, and recordkeeping. The parameters for cost reimbursement and the dispensing fee vary from carrier to carrier. Some agreements utilize **average wholesale price (AWP)**, others **maximum allowable cost (MAC)**, and others **wholesaler acquisition cost**. The latter may take into account contracts negotiated between the provider and the pharmaceutical industry. Most carrier contracts utilize a closed formulary, where there is a list of medications that will be reimbursed. In some cases, if the prescriber demonstrates evidence for individual patient need, medications outside the formulary will be reimbursed. This process is generally done according to a **prior approval** protocol. Clinical pharmacists who work for third-party payors usually review cases of nonformulary prescribing and grant approval to the member pharmacy to release nonformulary prescriptions. The evidence to grant prior approval for nonformulary drugs usually must indicate

- Patient intolerance of existing drug choices.
- Treatment failures.
- Diagnoses without any listed treatments on the formulary.
- New drug modalities.

Provider and patient preference for insurance coverage is in the order of indemnity, PPO, and HMO. Costs for these plans usually are in the same order, with indemnity policies being the most expensive.

Drug reimbursement coverage also varies from plan to plan. They include open formulary, closed formulary, copay and tiered copay systems. Open formulary plans reimburse all prescription medications. Closed formulary plans only reimburse a list of medications, generally low-cost alternatives. Copay plans divide the cost of coverage between the insurer and the patient, and are therefore at a lower cost. Tiered copays attempt to direct drug selection to lower-cost alternatives by attempting to make the patient demand of the prescriber lower-cost alter-

average wholesale price (AWP) the cost of drugs and pharmaceuticals purchased from a drug wholesaler.

maximum allowable cost (MAC) based on wholesaler acquisition costs.

wholesaler acquisition costs include contracts negotiated between the provider and the pharmaceutical industry.

prior approval the prescriber must demonstrate evidence for an individual patient's need for a medication outside the approved formulary for it to be reimbursed.

natives in order to reduce the copays. Many tiered copays also have lower copays for generic selection.

It must be kept in mind that for these patients, maintenance at a higher level of health care costs them less out of pocket for medications. This is true because Medicare pays a rate that includes medications in acute care and long-term care. Patients without prescription coverage cared for in acute care, long-term care, or in an emergency department will also receive their medication without expense directly attributable to drug cost. These higher levels of care are obviously more costly to the health care system, but patients have the incentive to seek higher levels of care to avoid out-of-pocket expense. A challenge for pharmaceutical care providers is to demonstrate the value of ambulatory pharmacy services in keeping patients at a lower level of care and to convince carriers to reimburse for this service to reduce the risk of admission to a higher level of care.

There were large segments of the population without ambulatory pharmacy prescription coverage prior to the advent of Medicare Part D on January 1, 2006. The largest group was Medicare fee-for-service patients without supplemental coverage who are now partially covered. Since most of these patients were elderly, they used more medications and, therefore, had the greatest out-of-pocket expense. Currently, the largest remaining groups still not covered at the ambulatory level are employed individuals with health coverage but no prescription coverage, employed persons without health coverage, and the unemployed.

These groups all have one thing in common: their out-of-pocket expense for drugs represents a higher percentage of their total health care outlay than one would anticipate by examination of the overall cost of health care.

The long awaited Medicare Part D prescription drug benefit requires enrollment in a private insurance plan for ambulatory and long-term care coverage. Monthly premiums averaged $32.20 in 2006. Each plan is unique, with its own formulary and benefit design. With standard coverage, the plan pays 75 percent of prescription costs, up to $2,250, after a deductible is met ($250 in 2006). At the ambulatory level the program has been well received by elderly patients who were previously unable, in many cases, to handle the expense of drug coverage.

There are some instances where reimbursement varies from coverage plan to plan. In terms of provider reimbursement, these differences include indemnity policies, HMO plans, and PPO plans. In indemnity policies the provider receives a set percentage of the usual and customary fees paid, based upon a board of peers. In PPO plans the provider agrees to a preset fee schedule, which provides some savings to the beneficiary and the insurance carrier, and the insurance carrier pays a set percentage to the provider. In HMO plans, there is also a preset fee schedule, but in addition there are "gatekeepers" or individuals (either the primary care physician or a medical director of the HMO) who determine access to various levels of care. These gatekeepers must approve access for the patient to a higher level of care.

Pharmacy technicians have opportunities to assist the pharmacist provider in adjudication of reimbursement claims. Much of this is in the area of accurate and concise recordkeeping. This includes

- Records of prescriptions dispensed.
- Records demonstrating pharmacist review of patient information such as patient profiles, medication history, and laboratory data.
- Charting demonstrating the performance of cognitive services.
- Charting of patient counseling and recommendations for patient self care.

Reimbursement for Ambulatory Care Parenteral Therapy

Significant opportunities exist for revenue generation through ambulatory care parenteral therapy. Payors have long understood that it is less expensive to treat patients in the ambulatory setting than to admit them for such treatments as chemotherapy and hemodialysis. Therefore, significant reimbursement for these services is available even in the Medicare population. The Centers for Medicare and Medicaid Services (CMS) has created a list of health insurance continuation programs (HICP) codes for drugs utilized in this setting. Reimbursable costs are also included in this listing, which provide for revenue generation between acquisition cost and reimbursable costs. This is in addition to the professional fee component and the facility fee. With this "fee-cost spread," facilities and freestanding practices are able to underwrite treatment of patients covered by other payors where the reimbursement is not so favorable. Formulary choices are detailed by manufacturers based upon "cost-reimbursement spread" rather than improvement in clinical outcomes. The pharmacy must uncover and present outcomes evidence to ensure that the most safe and effective drug modality is utilized. Over time, patient outcome evidence must be presented, because in addition to better patient care, evidence will demonstrate overall cost savings by maintaining patients at a lower level of care.

Reimbursement for Long-Term Care

Prior to the onset of Medicare Part D on January 1, 2006, reimbursement for long-term care was often done at a constant rate adjusted for annual increases in inflation. In many cases, rates were based on expenses generated 30 years ago when resident populations were far less acute, with lengthy hospital stays more acceptable and resident life spans much shorter. Medicare Part D changed all of that at the subacute level by "carving out" pharmacy from the *per diem* reimbursement rates and requiring long-term care residents to enroll in privately managed prescription drug plans when admitted to the facility. Reimbursement from these plans is now typically accomplished through direct provider pharmacy billings to individual resident plans. Residents who have dual eligibility (that is, both Medicaid and Medicare coverage) are automatically enrolled in Medicare Part D plans. Many of these Part D plans have experienced frequent changes in formularies as the plans struggle to maintain profitability. One aspect of the plans is "prior authorization," where physicians must verify the clinical need for specific higher cost medications that appear unnecessarily expensive over alternatives such as generic medications. Long-term care "friendly" formularies are important since each plan is unique and may exclude medications typical of the subacute environment, such as Alzheimer's medications. This requires formulary knowledge by the pharmacist and prior authorization protocols to avoid any unnecessary charges to the nursing home.

The long-term care industry continues to adjust to the new Part D requirements while lobbying for additional changes. A standard formulary seems to be on top of the list of desired changes. Additionally, the number of plans now available makes it impossible to make necessary comparisons to avoid unnecessary charges. Once again, not all plans are designed with a long-term population in mind, but rather an ambulatory customer base, and therefore they exclude typical long-term care drugs. Finally, clear standards are necessary to properly outline the requirements for prior authorizations.

At this level of care, it is incumbent upon those who are involved in drug administration decision making to evaluate choices. This includes formulary control and examination of epidemiological, microbacteriological, and outcomes evidence. Caregivers must utilize an ordered process to evaluate modalities to choose low-cost, safe, and effective modalities. The safety issue cannot be overemphasized. This is why the regulatory agencies developed a list of unnecessary drugs, which were determined to have excessive risk of adverse reactions. Although these medications are inexpensive, it is clear from the evidence that these medications had higher adverse event rates and poorer outcomes when compared to more expensive, newer drug modalities. The greater risk and poorer outcomes are more expensive to the facility in the long run and less contributory to good patient care as well.

Medicaid does allow "carve-out" reimbursement for a small number of medications. **Carve-outs** are the ability to charge for medication above the preestablished daily rate. This includes colony-stimulating factors such as erythropoietin, immune system mediators like GM-CSF, and the newer major tranquilizers. However, this list is not comprehensive, and some large classifications of high-use, high-cost modalities are omitted. Therefore, efficient pharmaceutical care will still conserve resources for new drug treatment modalities.

carve-out a Medicaid reimbursement for a small number of expensive medications paid directly to the long-term care facility above preestablished daily rates.

Reimbursement for Acute Care

Reimbursement for acute care pharmacy services has evolved over time and, for the most part, does not allow pharmacy services to generate profit. Often, pharmacy-related costs are calculated into the *per diem* **reimbursement** (i.e., reimbursement on a preset daily rate) hospital charge. Therefore, high medication cost and usage is often not reimbursable and causes funds to have to be allocated from other cost centers. This presents challenges for acute care pharmacists in terms of management of their distributive and clinical services. The value of pharmaceutical care in the acute care setting must be examined for its efficacy and its effect on direct and indirect costs. Examples of this are as follows:

***per diem* reimbursement** a payment on a preset daily rate.

- Labor costs to procure, store, and distribute medications efficiently.
- Labor costs to assess medication use and monitor its effects.
- Assessment of value of treatments to determine efficient outcomes and to demonstrate that medication is cost effective even if it is expensive.
- Assessment of risk of adverse events that can be caused by an individual drug or drug combination leading to drug-associated morbidity—inexpensive medications may be more expensive in the long run.
- Labor costs to monitor formulary adherence and conformity with clinical guidelines.
- Labor costs to research and evaluate clinical evidence in the literature to determine if the treatments utilized have the best probability of successful and cost-effective outcomes.
- Labor costs to assess and recommend treatments for individual patients.
- Labor costs to implement pharmaceutical care post-discharge to convey self-care instructions to patients to ensure that they benefit from less costly ambulatory care for as long as possible.

All of these services require labor costs that are not directly reimbursable, but need to be provided by a pharmacy service committed to involvement in the assessment and treatment of patients. The most efficient manner of provision of these services is to conserve labor costs from the procurement and distribution of pharmaceuticals to allow existing pharmacists to monitor and assess the effect of medications and modify treatments. Some of the methods for improving distributive efficiencies include

- Assigning the pharmacy technician to appropriate responsibilities in the dose preparation and distribution functions.
- Partnering with distributors to facilitate procurement and inventory maintenance.
- Utilizing current technology to distribute medication to the point of care.
- Computerizing inventory and billing functions at the point of care.
- Utilizing computer physician order entry to eliminate error risk and allow interactive prescribing with "rules engines" to provide executable orders at the time of prescribing.
- Initiating interactive medication administration recording with automated medication administrative records, which provide patient identification, proper administration times, prevention of dose duplication, prevention of administration of discontinued orders, and rules for medication administration as indicated.

Although these functions are not reimbursable at present, their efficiencies at the point of care eliminate duplicate paper entries, minimize risk, and lead to better outcomes, which positively impact the bottom line of a health care system. Utilization of these patient-care systems also provides data that the facility can use to demonstrate the value of pharmaceutical care. This information can be presented to payors such as managed care organizations. These organizations will recognize that utilization of a specific treatment may appear costly at first, but may lead to superior outcomes such as decreased length of stay, decreased need for monitoring of adverse effects, and maintenance at a lower level of care. Tangible results of this recognition include carve-outs (i.e., reimbursement for drug charges in addition to the preestablished daily rate), such as reimbursing a facility for the cost of an expensive medication outside of the typical *per diem* cost. This additional reimbursement conserves funds to pay for unreimbursed new technologies, enhanced pharmaceutical care, and capital investment in new drug-order and delivery systems outlined previously. It is necessary for pharmacy departments to continue outlining the value of medication that contributes to a care plan that benefits the patient, the health care system, and the payor. This will foster a climate where new drug technologies will be reimbursable once they develop a track record both in clinical trials and experiential use.

Reimbursement for Cognitive Services

cognitive pharmacy services the process of applying pharmaceutical knowledge to a particular patient to assure rational drug therapy.

Reimbursement for **cognitive pharmacy services** covers a wide variety of services across all levels of care:

- Prescriptive authority by the pharmacist.
- Patient assessment and treatment.
- Pharmacist intervention with prescribers and other health care providers.
- Patient education.
- Patient monitoring and reassessment of the progress of medication use.

The benefits of all of these services have to be presented in a way that demonstrates value and indicates that provision of these services will maintain patient care at a lower cost level. Reimbursement levels to the pharmacist pale in comparison to the costs incurred at the higher level of care. Examples of this include shorter inpatient length of stay. Another example is a switch of a patient to oral medication from an IV dosage form. Maintenance of a patient's anticoagulation status to decrease the adverse effect of bleeding with increased readmission rate also falls into this category. The more outcomes data presented that express this value of cost savings, the more payors will be inclined to encourage these services with reimbursement.

An obstacle for reimbursement for acute care pharmacy costs is in the retrospective-payor system. This means that costs are calculated from *retrospective* data (i.e., total costs from previous years). This causes delays in inclusion of reimbursement for new treatment modalities. If these treatments are more expensive than old ones, reimbursement will not go up for at least two years. In addition, costs do not include *unfunded mandates* (i.e., rules that health care systems have to follow without being paid for the resources needed to adhere to them). It costs money to pay individuals to perform these tasks. Sometimes additional equipment, such as computer programs, has to be purchased as well. Examples of these requirements include rules promulgated by regulatory agencies such as the Joint Commission, peer review organizations, the Department of Health, the Occupational Health and Safety Administration, and many others. Funds for new cognitive services must be derived at the expense of other cost centers or must be conserved from reduction of existing costs.

Evidence that priority has been placed on reimbursement for cognitive services can be seen at the national pharmacy organizational level. The National Community Pharmacists Association provides pharmacist training that includes patient assessment, disease state management, and methodologies for capturing reimbursement for cognitive pharmacist outpatient services.

Reimbursement is available for pharmacists as providers for Medication Management Therapy Services. This means that pharmacists are reimbursed for non-drug services, such as drug therapy management for diabetes, anticoagulation, anemia, hypertension, and renal failure. These avenues vary greatly from state to state, as this type of reimbursement requires government modification in the state's pharmacy practice acts and the state's board of pharmacy rules and regulations. The most advantageous way of developing these services appears to be by the use of collaborative practice agreements. In these cases, pharmacists join physician practices and have medication management delegated to the pharmacist. Practice is under the supervision of the physician, with protocols or guidelines used by the pharmacist approved by the physician. Often patients come to the office between physician visits and are seen by the pharmacist. The pharmacist orders lab tests and other measurements, and modifies therapy based upon patient response.

The Role of Pharmacy Technicians in Increased Reimbursement

The role of pharmacy technicians in efforts to enhance reimbursement cannot be overestimated. The aging of the population, the increased number of prescriptions dispensed, and the increased complexity of drug regimens require increased utilization of support personnel in all aspects of the drug distribution system.

Utilization of automation, as well as increased technician utilization, can free pharmacists from distributive services to allow greater participation in cognitive services. Technicians assist pharmacists in filling medication orders, compounding intravenous solutions, providing point-of-service distribution, billing for medications and cognitive services, triaging telephone calls, and assisting in procurement, inventory, and distribution of pharmaceuticals. As with all job categories, responsibilities vary from organization to organization and from individual to individual; however, technical support must be fostered to enhance advances in pharmaceutical care and reimbursement for pharmaceutical services.

Summary

Reimbursement for pharmaceutical care requires a proactive approach that demonstrates the inherent value of these services. Utilization of pharmacy technicians has been shown to both extend resources and release pharmacists to provide pharmaceutical care and provide evidence of its benefits. A stable, efficient, and reliable pharmacy technician staff is inherent in any successful, financially solvent pharmaceutical care program anywhere in the continuum of care.

TEST YOUR KNOWLEDGE

Multiple Choice

1. Which of the following statements is true regarding ambulatory medication costs?
   a. they are a major component of a typical Medicare patient's cash outlay
   b. they are not an important issue to senior citizens
   c. reimbursement is often duplicated by employee prescription benefits
   d. none of the above

2. Which of the following is *not* true regarding pharmacy reimbursement in ambulatory care?
   a. payors usually reimburse costs, plus a dispensing fee
   b. pharmacists are routinely reimbursed for non-dispensing related interventions
   c. the dispensing fee will vary, dependent on the insurance carrier
   d. reimbursement depends on formulary medications

3. Reimbursement for acute care pharmacy costs has which of the following pitfalls?
   a. costs are calculated from retrospective data, causing delays in inclusion of new treatment modalities that may be more costly than previous treatments

b.   costs do not include unfunded mandates, such as rules promulgated by regulatory agencies

c.   funds for new cognitive services must be derived at the expense of other cost centers

d.   all of the above

4.   Evidence required for prior approval for non-formulary drugs usually must include

a.   patient intolerance of existing choices.

b.   treatment failures.

c.   diagnoses without any representative treatments on the formulary.

d.   adverse reactions to the medication.

5.   Which of the following can improve efficient utilization of labor resources?

a.   dose preparation and distribution involving pharmacy technicians

b.   utilization of current technology to distribute medication

c.   computerization of inventory and billing at the point of care

d.   utilization of technicians in all aspects of the drug use process

6.   Use of computerized recording of medication administration can assist with

a.   patient identification.

b.   prevention of dose duplication.

c.   prevention of administration of discontinued orders.

d.   prevention of administration of the wrong medication.

7.   Unfunded mandates are

a.   physician responsibilities.

b.   regulatory requirements placed on health care systems without allowing an increase in reimbursement.

c.   not applicable to acute care facilities.

d.   applicable to ambulatory care.

8.   Regular performance review is useful for pharmacy technicians because

a.   it can demonstrate how technician support allows pharmacists to provide cognitive services.

b.   it can link compensation to retention and promotion of technicians.

c.   it can establish and measure goals for technician responsibilities.

d.   it establishes objective criteria by which technical staff can be evaluated.

9.   Cognitive pharmacy services include *all but one* of the following:

a.   prescriptive authority.

b.   patient education.

c.   trauma care.

d.   patient assessment and treatment.

10.   Patients' costs for prescription medications vary according to

a.   their individual indemnity insurance coverage.

b.   Medicaid applicability.

c.   Medicare Part D participation.

d.   acute care versus ambulatory care.

Matching

Match the following:

1. _____ prior authorization
2. _____ Medicaid
3. _____ Medicare Part D
4. _____ a cognitive pharmacist service

a. state funded program
b. request for non-formulary drug
c. prescription drug plan
d. patient education

References

American Society of Health-System Pharmacists. (2003). *The expanding role of the pharmacist and reimbursement.* ASHP government affairs division. ASHP Web site.

ASHP white paper on pharmacy technicians. (2003). Needed changes can no longer wait. *Journal of the American Society of Health-System Pharmacists*, 60: 37–51.

Pharmacy services: What you should know. New York State Health Facilities Association and Foundation for Quality Care Seminar, Oct. 19, 2007, Albany, New York.

Transforming pharmacy reimbursement: A roadmap for success. ASHP 2003, Summer meeting, June 4, 2003.

Accreditation of Technician Training Programs

Competencies

Upon completion of this chapter, the reader should be able to

1. State four objectives of the accreditation process for pharmacy technician training programs.
2. Articulate the primary reason for a differentiated workforce in the pharmacy profession.
3. Explain the ASHP's involvement in accrediting pharmacy technician training programs rather than in evaluating competency achievement of individual pharmacy technicians.
4. List the eight areas that comprise the Accreditation Standard for Pharmacy Technician Training Programs.
5. Outline the objectives that form the basis for pharmacy technician training programs.
6. List the organizations that have endorsed the Model Curriculum for Pharmacy Technician Training.

Key Terms

accreditation
Commission on Credentialing
outcome competencies
site survey

Introduction

The process of accreditation (recognition of a particular set of standards) for pharmacy technician training programs includes four main objectives: (1) upgrade and standardize the formal training that pharmacy technicians receive, (2) guide, assist, and recognize those health care facilities and academic institutions that wish to support the profession by operating such programs, (3) provide criteria for the prospective technician trainee in the selection of a program by identifying those institutions conducting accredited pharmacy technician training programs, and (4) provide prospective employees a basis for determining the level of competency of pharmacy technicians by identifying those technicians who have successfully completed accredited technician training programs.

The Need for a Differentiated Workforce

During the past decade, many of the American Society of Health-System Pharmacist's (ASHP's) initiatives have centered on pharmacy's movement toward becoming a full-fledged clinical profession. The ASHP has long recognized that as we continue to move in this *clinical* direction, other health care professions and the public will increasingly look to pharmacy for answers to complex questions in drug therapy. With pharmacists' continuing efforts to enhance the degree to which they better utilize their knowledge and skills by providing direct patient care services, it becomes more evident that many, if not all, of the technical tasks routinely done by pharmacists must be delegated (with appropriate guidance and supervision) to nonprofessional personnel.

Development of a differentiated workforce will provide a core of well-trained pharmacy technicians who can assist the pharmacist in the delivery of pharmaceutical care by performing routine tasks that were formerly part of the traditional role of the pharmacist. Expanded roles for pharmacy technicians who have completed ASHP-accredited pharmacy technician training programs even include the role of the clinical pharmacy technician, involvement in database management, management of automated drug distribution devices, pharmacy billing, involvement in telepharmacy, and many more innovative positions that are not offered to those without advanced pharmacy technician training.

The ASHP House of Delegates has even adopted policy to support the goal that technicians entering the pharmacy workforce have completed an accredited program of training. Furthermore, to encourage expansion of accredited pharmacy technician training programs, many state boards of pharmacies have started to require, or are investigating the mandate, that all pharmacy technicians must complete an ASHP-accredited pharmacy technician training program to be considered certified in that state or to work as a pharmacy technician in that state. More and more state boards of pharmacy are recognizing completion of an ASHP-accredited pharmacy technician training program as a key element to ensure the utmost in public safety. Pharmacy technicians are essential personnel in the pharmacy team to provide a safe medication-use process.

ASHP Initiatives

outcome competency the measurable, desired ability, knowledge, and skill achieved upon the completion of a program.

For over two decades the ASHP, in response to an obvious void, has promulgated documents that specifically address **outcome competencies** (standardized training goals) for pharmacy technicians. However, to date, these have not been uniformly recognized and accepted throughout pharmacy. While these documents are gaining a greater degree of acceptance among pharmacists, it remains clear that the job category of technician continues to be interpreted differently because no two technicians are necessarily measured by the same yardstick.

The ASHP has remained steadfast in its belief that an absolute prerequisite for the orderly development of pharmacy support personnel is uniform recognition and acceptance of a competency or performance standard. Moreover, it has agreed that such a standard provides the basic objective for supportive personnel training programs.

Early on, the ASHP recognized that a competency standard alone could not suffice for development of pharmacy technician training programs. In fact, the ASHP considered as part of its early deliberations such programs and whether competency-based training would be acceptable. The realization that the structure and process of these training programs would be of secondary importance was key to these deliberations; competency outcomes would be the primary concern. Further, it was agreed that the feasibility of developing competency-based training programs, which depend largely on the ability to evaluate competency achievement, would not be difficult.

Despite these considerations, and due in large measure to the advice of its members, the ASHP expressed uneasiness about promoting establishment of competency-based technician training programs. As a consequence, the ASHP decided to follow the more traditional pattern of evaluating each training program through the process of accreditation. It is easy to understand how the ASHP chose this avenue, since it already had a well-established accreditation process for postgraduate pharmacy residency training programs in place since 1963.

accreditation the process by which an agency or organization evaluates and recognizes a program of study or an institution as meeting predetermined qualifications.

Accreditation is defined as the process by which an agency or organization evaluates and recognizes a program of study or an institution as meeting certain predetermined qualifications or standards. It applies only to institutions and their programs of study or their services.

Obviously, to establish an accreditation program, the ASHP knew firsthand that it was necessary to develop an accreditation standard that would delineate specific facilities and process requirements in addition to competency outcome criteria. Therefore, in November 1980, the ASHP Board of Directors requested that an accreditation standard for technician training programs be developed. They also authorized implementation of an accreditation process for such programs at the earliest possible time.

An accreditation standard for pharmacy technician training programs was approved by the ASHP board in April 1982. The first program was accredited in September 1983.

Accreditation Program

Commission on Credentialing
the body appointed to formulate and recommend standards and administer programs for accreditation of pharmacy personnel training programs.

site survey the visit by representatives of the ASHP to review training programs to ascertain compliance with standards.

As noted in the ASHP regulations on accreditation of pharmacy technician training programs, the accreditation service is conducted by authority of the ASHP Board of Directors under the direction of the **Commission on Credentialing**. The commission reviews and evaluates applications and survey reports and, as delegated by the board, takes final action on all applications set forth in the regulations.

All pharmacy technician training programs applying for accreditation by the ASHP are evaluated by **site survey** against the ASHP Accreditation Standard for Pharmacy Technician Training Programs. The standard outlines specific requirements for administrative responsibility for the training program, qualifications of the training site, qualification of the pharmacy service that is used to provide trainees with practical experience, qualifications of the pharmacy director and preceptors, qualifications and selection of the applicant, the overall structure of the pharmacy technician training program, experimentation and innovative approaches to training, and issuance of the certificate of completion.

With respect to the competency-based objectives that must be developed as a fundamental component of any ASHP-accredited technician training program, individuals are encouraged to use the *Model Curriculum for Pharmacy Technician Training*, Second Edition. This is the updated version of the manual that was developed as a nationwide project to provide technician educators with a prototype for training technicians in all practice settings and geographic locations. Specifically, it provides a guide for structuring the curriculum of a technician-training program, a checklist of quality components of existing training programs, suggestions for strengthening technicians' skills in specific areas, a list of job responsibilities and tasks that technicians can assume to allow pharmacists time to provide direct patient care, and a descriptive list of tasks to assist technicians when writing job descriptions. A user's guide is included with the curriculum to help pare down the training menu to suit individual training needs. The curriculum consists of four components: (1) goal statements, objectives, and instructional objectives, (2) a curriculum map with suggested sequencing of the modules for instruction, (3) descriptors for each of the instruction modules, and (4) a tracking document that identifies where each objective and instructional objective are taught. An introduction of the technician's role in enhancing safe medication use, tech-check-tech, and assisting in immunizations are included in the curriculum. The Model Curriculum was a collaborative project undertaken by the American Association of Pharmacy Technicians, the American Pharmaceutical Association, the American Society of Health-System Pharmacists, the National Association of Chain Drug Stores, and the Pharmacy Technician Educators Council. The project was under the leadership of the American Society of Health-System Pharmacists. A free copy can be obtained by going to www.ashp.org under the Member Center—Technician section.

The ASHP accreditation standards accommodate training programs offered by hospital and health-system pharmacy departments, managed care facilities, community colleges, vocational/technical institutes, proprietary agencies, chain pharmacies, and military facilities. Currently, there are approximately 113 ASHP-accredited programs that are conducted in each of these types of training facilities. A directory of these programs is located at www.ashp.org under the Technician section.

Pharmacy technicians completing ASHP-accredited programs are provided with a wealth of opportunities to learn didactic information, hands-on laboratory training, and experiential rotations in a variety of pharmacy settings. Each program must be at least 600 hours in duration to be considered for accreditation and must include didactic, laboratory, and experiential elements. Graduates completing such programs gain a perspective of all aspects of pharmacy technician training practice, a substantial added value that cannot be acquired from undertaking just on-the-job training. Instructors and preceptors provide one-on-one instruction and guidance for the students to ensure that each trainee is appropriately trained to succeed as a pharmacy technician. Many of the students undertaking ASHP-accredited pharmacy technician training programs are offered job opportunities upon completion of their experiential training rotations at the specific site. A lot of the employers in areas where pharmacy technician training programs are available only hire graduates from ASHP-accredited training programs. Some employers provide higher entry-level salaries to those who are graduates from ASHP-accredited pharmacy technician training programs. ASHP accreditation is a nationally recognized accreditation. An employer in any state can review the ASHP Standards for Accreditation and review the different areas of practice in which a graduate has training. Employers reap the benefits of someone that is already familiar and trained in many areas of pharmacy technician practice.

Summary

Additional information about the ASHP program for accreditation of pharmacy technician training programs can be obtained at www.ashp.org under the Technician section or by contacting the Accreditation Services Division, American Society of Health-System Pharmacists, 7272 Wisconsin Avenue, Bethesda, MD 20814, (301) 657-3000, ext. 1251.

TEST YOUR KNOWLEDGE

Multiple Choice

1. The ASHP has accredited pharmacy technician training programs in
   a. colleges of pharmacy.
   b. vocational/technical schools.
   c. military institutions.
   d. all of the above.

2. Continuing accreditation of a pharmacy technician training program is dependent upon
   a. a site visit.
   b. adherence to accreditation standards.
   c. an increased number of graduates over previous years.
   d. all of the above.

3. A pharmacy technician may engage in the following activities:
   a. packaging and labeling medication doses.
   b. maintaining patient records.
   c. preparing intravenous admixtures.
   d. all of the above.

4. A differentiated workforce is needed in pharmacy because
   a. pharmacists provide direct patient care services.
   b. technicians answer complex questions in drug therapy.
   c. pharmacists must perform many technical functions.
   d. the personnel best suited for the role perform specialized functions.

References

American Society of Health-System Pharmacists (September 1980). ASHP position on long-range pharmacy manpower needs and residency training. *American Society of Health-System Pharmacists*, 37, 1220.

American Society of Health-System Pharmacists. (2001). *Model curriculum for pharmacy technician training* (2nd ed.). Bethesda, MD: American Society of Health-System Pharmacists.

ASHP accreditation standard for pharmacy technician training programs. *American Society of Health-System Pharmacists, Practice Standards of ASHP 1998–1999*. Bethesda, MD: American Society of Health-System Pharmacists.

ASHP regulations on accreditation of pharmacy technician training programs. *American Society of Health-System Pharmacists, Practice Standards of ASHP 1998–1999*. Bethesda, MD: American Society of Health-System Pharmacists.

Pharmacy Technician Certification Board

Competencies

Upon completion of this chapter, the reader should be able to

1. Describe the pharmacy technician's role in pharmacy practice.
2. Describe the importance of Pharmacy Technician Certification Board (PTCB) certification as a competency measure.
3. Describe the eligibility requirements to sit for the Pharmacy Technician Certification Examination (PTCE).
4. Discuss the advantages of taking the PTCE in a computer-based testing (CBT) format.
5. Define certification.
6. Understand the value of the NCCA (National Commission for Certifying Agencies) accreditation to a national certification program.
7. List the major stakeholders of the PTCB.

Key Terms

certification
certified pharmacy technician (CPhT)
recertification

Introduction

The role of pharmacy practice in modern health care continues to evolve. Today, the responsibility of pharmacists includes patient care services in addition to the oversight of the traditional medication dispensing and product fulfillment activities. As pharmacists increase the time they spend with patients, operational tasks, such as the order fulfillment process, may be shifted to competent certified pharmacy technicians to enhance the productivity and workflow of the pharmacy.

The Pharmacy Technician Certification Board (PTCB) provides high-quality programs and services that offer technicians an opportunity to demonstrate that they have mastered knowledge across pharmacy practice settings. The PTCB develops, maintains, promotes, and administers a certification and recertification program for pharmacy technicians. Through the PTCB program, pharmacy technicians are able to work more effectively with pharmacists to offer safe and effective patient care and service. Since its first exam in 1995, the PTCB has certified more than 300,000 pharmacy technicians through the examination and transfer process.

Certification

certification the act of certifying to a standard established by a written or printed statement.

certified pharmacy technician (CPhT) a pharmacy technician who has successfully passed the National Pharmacy Technician Certification Examination.

recertification a renewal of person's certification.

Certification is the process by which a non-governmental association or agency grants recognition to an individual who has met certain predetermined qualifications specified by that association or agency. The PTCB develops and implements policies related to national certification for pharmacy technicians.

In order to become a **certified pharmacy technician (CPhT)**, pharmacy technicians must sit for and pass the national Pharmacy Technician Certification Exam (PTCE). Once a pharmacy technician has passed the exam, he or she may use the designation of certified pharmacy technician (CPhT). To continue to hold one's certification, a CPhT is required to obtain 20 hours of continuing education (CE) within two years of original certification or previous recertification period (Table 31-1). One hour of the CE must be in pharmacy law.

Recertification is the renewal of an individual's certification. All certified pharmacy technicians must complete the recertification process in order to maintain their status as a CPhT. Individuals are encouraged to submit an online recertification application, but paper applications are also accepted. All valid applications must be received before 12 p.m. EST on the CPhT expiration date in order to be processed. Once the PTCB has approved the applicants' recertification materials,

TABLE 31-1 Web Sites Offering Continuing Education to the Pharmacy Technician

www.ptcb.org

www.pharmacytimes.com

www.uspharmacist.com

www.ashp.org

www.powerpak.com

a new wallet card and new PTCB certificate will be issued in approximately 60 days. Failure to successfully complete the recertification requirements will result in the loss of PTCB certification. There are no exceptions or extensions to the postmark deadlines.

The PTCB does offer a reinstatement program for up to one year after the recertification deadline. This allows pharmacy technicians whose certification has lapsed to regain their active certification without having to re-sit for the examination.

To be eligible to sit for the PTCE, the applicant must meet the following requirements:

- A high school diploma or GED by the application receipt deadline.
- No prior drug or pharmacy-related felony.
- No felony convictions in the last five years.

Interested individuals can register online at www.ptcb.org.

Computer-Based Testing

The PTCE transitioned from a paper and pencil exam format to a new computer-based testing (CBT) format in February 2007. The PTCB contracted with Pearson VUE, the industry's technology leader, as its CBT vendor. The PTCB will continue to draw upon the experience and expertise of their 12-year partner, Professional Examination Service (PES), for test development. The move to a CBT format demonstrates the PTCB's continued commitment to provide the nationally recognized examination in a psychometrically-sound format, with the highest levels of service and security.

The PTCE is available at more than 200 convenient Pearson Professional Centers located throughout the United States and its territories. The Pearson Professional Centers are carefully controlled testing environments, dedicated to both candidate comfort and test security. The test centers are quiet, distraction free, and designed to encourage peak performance from each testee. With well-lit parking and easy accessibility from major highways, the centers provide the best testing experience in the industry. A complete list of test center locations is available at www.ptcb.org.

Additional benefits of the new CBT format include faster pass/fail results; an increased number of testing center locations; added testing flexibility through a significant increase in testing days and times, including weekends; scheduling flexibility to allow candidates to schedule or reschedule their exams up to 48 hours prior to the testing time at no additional charge; state-of-the-art testing facilities; and increased exam security, including digital audio and video monitoring and digital photo and fingerprint identification processing designed to protect the integrity of the PTCB exam.

NCCA Accreditation

The PTCB's certification and recertification program is accredited by the National Commission for Certifying Agencies (NCCA). Accreditation to the PTCB's national Pharmacy Technician Certification program demonstrates that the program is in compliance with the NCCA Standards for the Accreditation of Certification Programs. The NCCA is the accrediting body of the National Organization for Competency Assurance (NOCA), which accredits certification programs based on the highest quality standards in professional certification. The process ensures that programs adhere to current standards of practice in the certification industry. The NCCA has developed criteria used to ensure that accredited programs provide fair, valid, and reliable assessment tools; defined levels of accountability and decision making; and continuing competency.

The PTCB joins an elite group of 72 organizations with 176 programs that have received and maintained the prestigious NCCA accreditation. The NCCA's review and acceptance of the PTCB's national Pharmacy Technician Certification program represents an independent audit by industry experts. NCCA accreditation shows pharmacy stakeholders and those certified that the PTCB's certification program has met independent professional standards. The PTCB is currently the only national certification program for pharmacy technicians that has received NCCA accreditation.

Background

The PTCB, a 501(c)6 organization (nonprofit), was established in January 1995 by the American Pharmacists Association (APhA), the American Society of Health-System Pharmacists (ASHP), the Illinois Council of Health-System Pharmacists (ICHP), and the Michigan Pharmacists Association (MPA). Together, the four organizations created one consolidated national certification program for pharmacy technicians to facilitate a national standard for quality in the certification of pharmacy technicians. In 2001, the National Association of Boards of Pharmacy (NABP) joined the PTCB's Board of Governors.

Examination Practices

The national PTCE samples pharmacy technicians' knowledge and skill base for activities performed in the work of pharmacy technicians. To ensure that the examination is psychometrically sound and legally defensible, the content framework of the examination is supported by a nationwide study, called a practice analysis, of the work pharmacy technicians perform in diverse pharmacy practice settings, including community and institutional settings.

The methods used to develop and administer the PTCE are designed to promote the validity, measurement precision, and integrity of the examination program. These methods follow certification examination testing procedures recommended in the Standards for Educational and Psychological Tests and testing guidelines published by the National Organization for Competency Assurance (NOCA) and the Council on Licensure, Enforcement, and Regulation (CLEAR). The NCCA's accreditation of the PTCB's certification program verifies its adherence to the industry's highest standards.

Practice Test

The PTCB offers an online practice test on its Web site at www.ptcb.org. This practice test gives candidates the opportunity to become familiar with the format of the test questions and provides an indication of preparedness for the actual exam. The new practice test is based on the content outline of the PTCB's national Pharmacy Technician Certification Examination (PTCE) and is the only assessment exam designed and developed by the PTCB.

Technology

The PTCB serves as a leading information resource on pharmacy technician issues and works closely with pharmacy stakeholders to keep abreast of current issues. The PTCB's Web site, www.ptcb.org, is an excellent resource for exam candidates, certified pharmacy technicians (CPhTs), and other stakeholders. Exam candidates are able to use the Web site to register for and schedule the examination. Upon passing the exam, CPhTs continue to use the Web site to access exclusive PTCB gear, obtain free continuing education credits, and complete the recertification process. The PTCB has linked its database and Web site to provide real-time information at the click of a button to its customer service call center, various state pharmacy associations and agencies, major employers of pharmacy technicians, and other online verification needs. The PTCB continues to expand the capabilities of its database and Web site to meet the information needs of its stakeholders.

Get Involved with the PTCB

Each fall the Pharmacy Technician Certification Board recruits volunteers to participate as item writers for the national PTCE. The examination items are prepared by volunteer subject matter experts including pharmacists, certified pharmacy technicians, or pharmacy technician educators. In all, more than 100 subject matter experts prepare items for the Pharmacy Technician Certification Examination. The volunteers for this group have many years of practice experience, have demonstrated the ability to logically define and categorize the array of tasks technicians perform in various practice environments, and have familiarity with pharmacy association work.

A select number of item writers are invited to participate in the PTCB's Annual Item Writing Workshop to review, refine, and edit items for the examination.

Regulation of Pharmacy Technicians

Pharmacy technicians are accountable to their supervising pharmacists, who are legally responsible, by virtue of state licensure, for the care and safety of patients served by the pharmacy. State rules and regulations as well as job-center policies and procedures may specifically define functions and responsibilities of pharmacy technicians. State boards of pharmacy provide regulatory oversight of the profession, most often from their state pharmacy practice acts. State boards of pharmacy continually evaluate and revise their practice acts to align with their mission to protect public safety. Some states have made PTCB certification a requirement for registration. Other states tie pharmacist-to-technician ratios, responsibilities, supervision, or other requirements to a technician's certification status.

The NABP encourages the acceptance of the PTCB certification program as a recognized assessment tool for pharmacy technicians. The use of the PTCB certification program has been incorporated into the NABP's Model State Pharmacy Practice Act and Model Rules. Language found in the Model Act can be used by state boards of pharmacy when writing their own pharmacy practice acts.

Future for Pharmacy Technicians

The Bureau of Labor Statistics reports that "employment of pharmacy technicians is expected to grow much faster than the average occupation through 2014." Their report also states that "cost-conscious insurers, pharmacies, and health-systems will continue to expand the role of pharmacy technicians."

Summary

The PTCB program offers technicians opportunities for competency recognition and greater job flexibility and satisfaction. Certification for pharmacy technicians encourages technicians to look beyond their present job and may also increase their likelihood of getting a better job. Certification may enhance the opportunities for promotion or merit increase in their responsibilities and wage.

The PTCB has been able to change the lives of thousands of pharmacy technicians across the United States. The successful launch of the certification program has not gone unnoticed in the credentialing and association management fields. The PTCB works diligently to meet the needs of the pharmacy profession and its stakeholders. With more than 270,000 certified pharmacy technicians since 1995, the PTCB has proven that pharmacy technicians are an integral part of the pharmacy team.

TEST YOUR KNOWLEDGE

Multiple Choice

1. In recent years, pharmacists have increased their use of pharmacy technicians due in part to which of the following?
   a. trends in pharmacy practice
   b. new pharmacy schools
   c. third-party reimbursement
   d. both a and c

2. What pharmacy practice trends have caused increased time demands on pharmacists?
   a. increased complexity of medication therapy
   b. increased prescription volumes
   c. increased demand for pharmacy services
   d. all of the above

3. What are some benefits for employers who use certified pharmacy technicians?
   a. better able to manage risk
   b. reduced technician training times and lower training costs
   c. increased employee satisfaction
   d. all of the above

4. Certification is
   a. a listing of practitioners maintained by a governmental entity, without educational, experiential, or competency-based requirements.
   b. the voluntary process by which a non-governmental entity grants a time-limited recognition and use of a credential to an individual after verifying that he or she has met predetermined and standardized criteria.
   c. the mandatory process by which a governmental agency grants time-limited permission to an individual to engage in a given occupation after verifying that he or she has met predetermined and standardized criteria.
   d. both a and b.

References

ASHP. (1996). *Model curriculum for pharmacy technician training.* Bethesda, MD: ASHP.

ASHP. (1999). *Accreditation standard for pharmacy technician training programs.* Bethesda, MD: ASHP.

4. Certification is

   a. a listing of practitioners established by a governmental entity without educational, experiential, or competency-based requirements.

   b. the voluntary process by which a non-governmental entity grants a time-limited recognition and use of a credential to an individual after verifying that he or she has met predetermined and standardized criteria.

   c. the mandatory process by which a governmental agency grants time-limited permission to an individual to engage in a given occupation after verifying that he or she has met predetermined and standardized criteria.

   d. both a and b.

References

ASHP (1998). *Model curriculum for pharmacy technician training.* Bethesda, MD: ASHP.

ASHP (1997). *Accreditation standards for pharmacy technician training programs.* Bethesda, MD: ASHP.

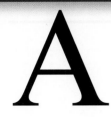

Long-Term Care

A-1: Examples of Guidelines for Automatic Stop-Order Policy in a Skilled Nursing Facility (Unless Otherwise Specified by Physician)

Drug Type

Analgesics .... 30 days
   Darvon, Darvocet

Antianemia drugs .... 30 days
   iron

Antibiotics .... 7 days
   Keflex, tetracycline

Antiemetics .... 4 days
   Compazine, Tigan

Anticoagulants .... 30 days
   Coumadin

Antihistamines .... 7 days
   Chlor-Trimeton, Seldane, Sudafed

Antineoplastics .... 30 days
   Nolvadex, Hydrea

Barbiturates .... 30 days
   phenobarbital

Cardiovascular .... 30 days
   digoxin, Vasotec, quinidine

Cathartics .... 30 days
   Pericolace, Colace, Senokot

Cold preparations .... 5 days
   Phenergan Expectorant, Robitussin

Dermatologicals .... 30 days
   Lidex, hydrocortisone, Synalar

Diuretics .... 30 days
   HCTZ, Dyazide, Aldactazide, Lasix

A-2: Medication Order Entry Flow Chart

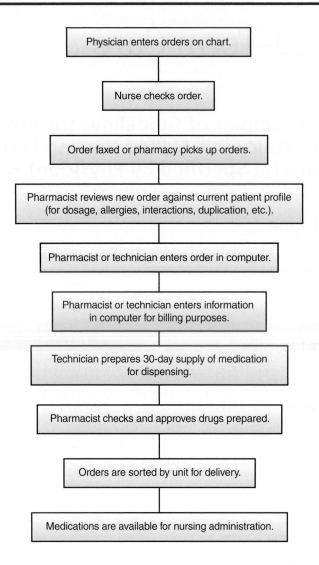

B The Hospital Formulary System

B-1: The Pharmacy and Therapeutics Committee

The Pharmacy and Therapeutics (P&T) Committee is a policy-recommending body to the medical staff and the administration of the organization on matters related to the therapeutic use of drugs. It develops policies for managing drug use and drug administration, and manages the formulary system. This committee shall be so selected as to represent different medical departments or divisions. The P&T committee should be composed of at least the following voting members: physicians, pharmacists, nurses, administrators, quality-assurance coordinators, and others as appropriate. A chairperson from among the physician representatives should be appointed. A pharmacist should be designated as secretary.

The committee shall function in both an advisory and an educational capacity.

1. It shall deal with contemporary problems in therapeutics.
2. It shall select for routine use within the institution (and its ambulatory services and clinics) therapeutic agents that represent the best available for the prophylaxis or management of disease.
3. It shall recommend the deletion of drugs from the formulary that no longer meet the needs of the hospital patients.

The department of pharmacy services shall recommend to the P&T committee quality control specifications, methods of distribution and control, and drug-utilization reviews.

Function

1. To serve as an advisory group to the medical staff, to the hospital administration, and to the department of pharmacy services on matters pertaining to drug utilization, drug-use control, and standards of practice concerning the use of drugs.
2. To evaluate clinical and scientific data regarding new drugs or agents proposed for formulary addition.
3. To establish a formulary of accepted drugs for use in the hospital and to provide for its constant revision.
4. To establish policies regarding the surveillance of investigational drugs.
5. To serve as a focal point for collecting data obtained from drug utilization reviews throughout the hospital.

B-2: Definitions and Categories of Drugs to Be Stocked in the Pharmacy

Formulary Drugs

A formulary drug is a therapeutic agent whose place in therapy is well established. It is selected by the Pharmacy and Therapeutics Committee as essential for the best patient care.

Clinical Evaluation Drugs

A clinical evaluation drug is a commercially available, non-formulary agent that is temporarily made available to a particular physician or physicians for the purpose of evaluation for formulary inclusion.

The Pharmacy and Therapeutics Committee will review these requests and if approved, the requesting physician shall complete a Clinical Evaluation Drug Request Form that will provide the following information:

- Objectives of the clinical evaluation.
- Criteria for selection of patients who will receive the drug.
- Parameters to be assessed.
- Estimated number of patients to be studied.
- Duration of study.

The requesting physician shall submit the results of the evaluation after an interim period of time (usually six months) to the Pharmacy and Therapeutics Committee.

The final report shall contain conclusions and recommendations to the Pharmacy and Therapeutics Committee concerning the drug's role relative to formulary alternatives.

Restricted Drug Guidelines

A restricted drug is a therapeutic agent, admitted to the formulary, the use of which is authorized to either specific physicians or to specific guidelines for use. The following procedures will apply:

- Drugs in the category will be dispensed only if prescribed with the approval of specific physicians, and/or if they meet specific indications for use, and/or are prescribed on specific order forms (e.g., antibiotic order form, TPN Order Sheet).

Investigational Drugs

An investigational drug is a therapeutic agent undergoing clinical investigation that is not approved by the Food and Drug Administration.

The pharmacy will be responsible for the storage, dispensing, recordkeeping, and disposition of investigational drugs. In addition, the pharmacy is charged with the responsibility for providing written drug information to the respective nursing units using these drugs.

The chief investigator will provide the following:

- Approval for the use of the investigational drugs from the Institutional Review Board.
- Provide the pharmacy with a copy of the signed patient consent form.
- Provide the pharmacy with all available pharmacologic data from the manufacturer.
- Transfer of the drug to the pharmacy.
- Indicate if the pharmacy is to have responsibility for ongoing ordering and storage of the investigational drug.

Non-formulary Drugs

A non-formulary drug is any drug other than one classified as a formulary drug, evaluation drug, restricted drug, or investigational drug. Non-formulary medications may only be prescribed by chiefs of service or attending physicians. These medications will not be dispensed without the prior submission of a Nonformulary Drug Request Form.

Upon receipt of a medication order, the pharmacist will notify the prescriber if the prescribed medication is non-formulary. The pharmacist will suggest to the prescriber alternative formulary medications in the same therapeutic class. If the prescriber still wishes to use the non-formulary medication, a Non-formulary Drug Request Form shall be completed.

B-3: Additions to the Formulary

Requests for the addition of drugs to the formulary may be initiated by an attending physician of the medical staff. A Request for Formulary Addition Form is completed and signed by the requesting physician and submitted to the secretary of the Pharmacy and Therapeutics Committee.

The Drug Information Service is responsible for preparing all drug evaluation reports. These reports review the pertinent literature concerning the requested drug and make recommendations to the committee with regard to addition of the drug based on other formulary medications, its comparable cost, adverse effects, etc.

The formulary status of a new drug may be reviewed and evaluated by the committee after a specific period of time, usually six months.

B-4: Deletions from the Formulary

Drugs may be deleted from the formulary as a result of the addition of more efficacious or safer agents, duplication of drugs in the same therapeutic category. or upon review of the annual usage.

Additions and deletions are published in a Pharmacy Newsletter, which is distributed to the medical staff.

C Common Sound-Alike Drug Names

The following is a list of common sound-alike drug names; trade names are capitalized. In parentheses next to each drug name is the pharmacological classification/use for the drug. (Reprinted from *PDR Nurse's Drug Handbook* by G. R. Spratto and A. L. Woods. Clifton Park, NY: Thomson Delmar Learning, 2004.)

Accupril (ACE inhibitor)	Accutane (antiacne drug)
acetazolamide (antiglaucoma drug)	acetohexamide (oral antidiabetic drug)
Aciphex (proton pump inhibitor)	Accupril (ACE inhibitor)
Actos (oral hypoglycemic)	Actonel (diphosphonate—bone growth regulator)
Adriamycin (antineoplastic)	Aredia (bone growth regulator)
albuterol (sympathomimetic)	atenolol (beta-blocker)
Aldomet (antihypertensive)	Aldoril (antihypertensive)
Alkeran (antineoplastic)	Leukeran (antineoplastic)
allopurinol (antigout drug)	Apresoline (antihypertensive)
alprazolam (anti-anxiety agent)	lorazepam (anti-anxiety agent)
Amaryl (oral hypoglycemic)	Reminyl (anti-Alzheimer's drug)
Ambien (sedative-hypnotic)	Amen (progestin)
amiloride (diuretic)	amlodipine (calcium channel blocker)
amiodarone (antiarrhythmic)	amrinone (inotropic agent)
amitriptyline (antidepressant)	nortriptyline (antidepressant)
Apresazide (antihypertensive)	Apresoline (antihypertensive)
Aripiprazole (antipsychotic)	lansoprazole (proton pump inhibitor)
Arlidin (peripheral vasodilator)	Aralen (antimalarial)
Artane (cholinergic blocking agent)	Altace (ACE inhibitor)
Asacol (anti-inflammatory drug)	Avelox (fluoroquinolone antibiotic)
asparaginase (antineoplastic agent)	pegaspargase (antineoplastic agent)
Atarax (antianxiety agent)	Ativan (antianxiety agent)
atenolol (beta-blocker)	timolol (beta-blocker)
Atrovent (cholinergic blocking agent)	Alupent (sympathomimetic)
Avandia (oral hypoglycemic)	Coumadin (anticoagulant)
Bacitracin (antibacterial)	Bactroban (anti-infective, topical)
Benylin (expectorant)	Ventolin (sympathomimetic)
Brevital (barbiturate)	Brevibloc (beta-adrenergic blocker)
Bumex (diuretic)	Buprenex (narcotic analgesic)
bupropion (antidepressant; smoking deterrent)	buspirone (anti-anxiety agent)
Cafergot (analgesic)	Carafate (antiulcer drug)
calciferol (vitamin D)	calcitriol (vitamin D)
carboplatin (antineoplastic agent)	cisplatin (antineoplastic agent)
Cardene (calcium channel blocker)	Cardizem (calcium channel blocker)
Cardura (antihypertensive)	Ridaura (gold-containing anti-inflammatory)
Cataflam (NSAID)	Catapres (antihypertensive)
Catapres (antihypertensive)	Combipres (antihypertensive)
cefotaxime (cephalosporin)	cefoxitin (cephalosporin)
cefuroxime (cephalosporin)	deferoxamine (iron chelator)

Celebrex (NSAID)	Cerebyx (anticonvulsant)
Celebrex (NSAID)	Celexa (antidepressant)
chlorpromazine (antipsychotic)	chlorpropamide (oral antidiabetic)
chlorpromazine (antipsychotic)	prochlorperazine (antipsychotic)
chlorpromazine (antipsychotic)	promethazine (antihistamine)
Clinoril (NSAID)	Clozaril (antipsychotic)
clomipramine (antidepressant)	clomiphene (ovarian stimulant)
clonidine (antihypertensive)	Klonopin (anticonvulsant)
Combivir (AIDS drug combination)	Combivent (combination for COPD)
Cozaar (antihypertensive)	Zocor (antihyperlipidemic)
cyclobenzaprine (skeletal muscle relaxant)	cyproheptadine (antihistamine)
cyclophosphamide (antineoplastic)	cyclosporine (immunosuppressant)
cyclosporine (immunosuppressant)	cycloserine (antineoplastic)
Cytovene (antiviral drug)	Cytosar (antineoplastic)
Cytoxan (antineoplastic)	Cytotec (prostaglandin derivative)
Dantrium (skeletal muscle relaxant)	danazol (gonadotropin inhibitor)
Darvocet-N (analgesic)	Darvon-N (analgesic)
daunorubicin (antineoplastic)	doxorubicin (antineoplastic)
desipramine (antidepressant)	diphenhydramine (antihistamine)
DiaBeta (oral hypoglycemic)	Zebeta (beta-adrenergic blocker)
digitoxin (cardiac glycoside)	digoxin (cardiac glycoside)
diphenhydramine (antihistamine)	dimenhydrinate (antihistamine)
dopamine (sympathomimetic)	dobutamine (sympathomimetic)
Edecrin (diuretic)	Eulexin (antineoplastic)
enalapril (ACE inhibitor)	Anafranil (antidepressant)
enalapril (ACE inhibitor)	Eldepryl (antiparkinson agent)
Eryc (erythromycin base)	Ery-Tab (erythromycin base)
etidronate (bone growth regulator)	etretinate (antipsoriatic)
etomidate (general anesthetic)	etidronate (bone growth regulator)
E-Vista (antihistamine)	Evista (estrogen receptor modulator)
Femara (antineoplastic)	FemHRT (estrogen-progestin combination)
Fioricet (analgesic)	Fiorinal (analgesic)
Flomax (alpha-adrenergic blocker)	Volmax (sympathomimetic)
flurbiprofen (NSAID)	fenoprofen (NSAID)
folinic acid (leucovorin calcium)	folic acid (vitamin B)
Gantrisin (sulfonamide)	Gantanol (sulfonamide)
glipizide (oral hypoglycemic)	glyburide (oral hypoglycemic)
glyburide (oral hypoglycemic)	Glucotrol (oral hypoglycemic)
Hycodan (cough preparation)	Hycomine (cough preparation)
hydrocodone (narcotic analgesic)	hydrocortisone (corticosteroid)
Hydrogesic (analgesic combination)	hydroxyzine (antihistamine)
hydromorphone (narcotic analgesic)	morphine (narcotic analgesic)
Hydropres (antihypertensive)	Diupres (antihypertensive)
Hytone (topical corticosteroid)	Vytone (topical corticosteroid)
imipramine (antidepressant)	Norpramin (antidepressant)
Inderal (beta-adrenergic blocker)	Inderide (antihypertensive)
Indocin (NSAID)	Minocin (antibiotic)
Lamictal (anticonvulsant)	Lamisil (antifungal)
Lanoxin (cardiac glycoside)	Lasix (diuretic)
Lantus (insulin glargine)	Lente insulin (insulin zinc suspension)
Lioresal (muscle relaxant)	lisinopril (ACE inhibitor)
Lithostat (lithium carbonate)	Lithobid (lithium carbonate)
Lodine (NSAID)	codeine (narcotic analgesic)
Lopid (antihyperlipidemic)	Lorabid (beta-lactam antibiotic)

lovastatin (antihyperlipidemic)	Lotensin (ACE inhibitor)
Ludiomil (alpha and beta-adrenergic blocker)	Lomotil (antidiarrheal)
Medrol (corticosteroid)	Haldol (antipsychotic)
metolazone (thiazide diuretic)	methotrexate (antineoplastic)
metoprolol (beta-adrenergic blocker)	misoprostol (prostaglandin derivative)
Monopril (ACE inhibitor)	minoxidil (antihypertensive)
nelfinavir (antiviral)	nevirapine (antiviral)
nicardipine (calcium channel blocker)	nifedipine (calcium channel blocker)
Norlutate (progestin)	Norlutin (progestin)
Noroxin (fluoroquinolone antibiotic)	Neurontin (anticonvulsant)
Norvasc (calcium channel blocker)	Navane (antipsychotic)
Norvir (antiviral)	Retrovir (antiviral)
Ocufen (NSAID)	Ocuflox (fluoroquinolone antibiotic)
Orinase (oral hypoglycemic)	Ornade (upper respiratory product)
Percocet (narcotic analgesic)	Percodan (narcotic analgesic)
paroxetine (antidepressant)	paclitaxel (antineoplastic)
penicillamine (heavy metal antagonist)	penicillin (antibiotic)
pindolol (beta-adrenergic blocker)	Parlodel (inhibitor of prolactin secretion)
Platinol (antineoplastic)	Paraplatin (antineoplastic)
Pletal (antiplatelet drug)	Plavix (antiplatelet drug)
Pravachol (antihyperlipidemic)	Prevacid (GI drug)
Pravachol (antihyperlipidemic)	propranolol (beta-adrenergic blocker)
prednisolone (corticosteroid)	prednisone (corticosteroid)
Procanbid (antiarrhythmic)	Procan SR (antiarrhythmic)
propranolol (beta-adrenergic blocker)	Propulsid (GI drug)
Provera (progestin)	Premarin (estrogen)
Prozac (antidepressant)	Proscar (androgen hormone inhibitor)
quinidine (antiarrhythmic)	clonidine (antihypertensive)
quinine (antimalarial)	quinidine (antiarrhythmic)
Regroton (antihypertensive)	Hygroton (diuretic)
Reminyl (anti-Alzheimer's drug)	Robinul (muscle relaxant)
Retrovir (antiviral)	Ritonavir (antiviral)
Rifamate (antituberculous drug)	rifampin (antituberculous drug)
rimantadine (antiviral)	flutamide (antineoplastic)
Roxicodone (oxycodone alone—analgesic)	Roxicet (oxycodone/acetaminophen analgesic)
Sarafem (for PMS)	Serophene (ovulation stimulator)
Seroquel (antipsychotic)	Serzone (antidepressant)
Serzone (antidepressant)	Seroquel (antipsychotic)
Soriatane (antipsoriasis)	Loxitane (antipsychotic)
Stadol (narcotic analgesic)	Haldol (antipsychotic)
sulfadiazine (sulfonamide)	sulfasalazine (sulfonamide)
Tegretol (anticonvulsant)	Tequin (antibacterial)
terazosin (antihypertensive)	temazepam (sedative-hypnotic)
terbinafine (antifungal agent)	terfenadine (antihistamine)
terbutaline (sympathomimetic)	tolbutamide (oral hypoglycemic)
Ticlid (antiplatelet drug)	Tequin (fluoroquinolone antibiotic)
tolazamide (oral hypoglycemic)	tolbutamide (oral hypoglycemic)
torsemide (loop diuretic)	furosemide (loop diuretic)
trifluoperazine (antipsychotic)	trihexyphenidyl (antiparkinson drug)
Trimox (amoxicillin product)	Diamox (carbonic anhydrase inhibitor)
Ultram (analgesic)	Ultrase (pancreatic enzymes)
Vancenase (corticosteroid)	Vanceril (corticosteroid)
Vasosulf (sulfonamide/decongestant)	Velosef (cephalosporin)
Versed (benzodiazepine sedative)	Vistaril (antianxiety agent)

Versed (benzodiazepine sedative)	VePesid (antineoplastic)
Xanax (antianxiety agent)	Zantac (H2 histamine blocker)
Xenical (antiobesity)	Xeloda (antineoplastic)
Xydis*	
Zebeta (beta-blocker)	DiaBeta (oral hypoglycemic)
Zinacef (cephalosporin)	Zithromax (macrolide antibiotic)
Zocor (antihyperlipidemic)	Zoloft (antidepressant)
Zofran (antiemetic)	Zantac (H2 histamine blocker)
Zosyn (penicillin antibiotic)	Zofran (antiemetic)
Zovirax (antiviral)	Zyvox (antibiotic)

*__Note__: Xydis is a technology consisting of a freeze-dried wafer that dissolves almost instantly on the tongue or contact with saliva. The name of the technology has been confused because it is written on prescriptions as if it were a drug name.

Versed (benzodiazepine sedative)	VePesid (antineoplastic)
Xanax (antianxiety agent)	Zantac (H2 histamine blocker)
Xenical (antiobesity)	Xeloda (antineoplastic)
Xylis*	
Zebeta (beta blocker)	diaBeta (oral hypoglycemic)
Zinacef (cephalosporin)	Zithromax (macrolide antibiotic)
Zocor (antihyperlipidemic)	Zoloft (antidepressant)
Zofran (antiemetic)	Zantac (H2 histamine blocker)
Zosyn (penicillin antibiotic)	Zofran (antiemetic)
Zovirax (antiviral)	Zyvox (antibiotic)

*Note: Xylis is a technology consisting of a freeze-dried wafer that dissolves almost instantly on the tongue on contact with saliva. The name of the technology has been confused because it is written on prescriptions as if it were a drug name.

absorption—the fraction of an administered drug that reaches the systemic circulation

Academy of Managed Care Pharmacy (AMCP)—a professional association of pharmacists and associates who serve patients in the managed health care system environment

accelerated care unit (ACU)—a separate unit in the hospital where patients are prepared to better care for themselves and their condition after being discharged from the hospital

accreditation—the process by which an agency or organization evaluates and recognizes a program of study or an institution as meeting predetermined qualifications

achlorhydria—the absence of hydrochloric acid in the stomach

acidosis—an acid/base imbalance causing the blood and body tissues to become excessively acidic

action plan—a concise, written document listing the objectives an employee will accomplish in a specific period of time, such as one year. The objectives are mutually agreed upon by the employee and the supervisor and should be clear, measurable, and obtainable

active transport—the movement of drug molecules against a concentration gradient (i.e., from an area of low concentration to an area of higher concentration)

acute—a severe condition, rising rapidly to a peak and then subsiding

acute illness—an illness with severe symptoms and of short duration

additive—an addition of an active ingredient to a solution that is intended for intravenous administration or irrigation

adherence—the act of complying with prescribed directions

adherence rate—an indicator of how many times out of a hundred (expressed as a percent) that a quality event occurs or fails to occur

administer—to give a patient medication, once it is checked for accuracy

administration (or route of administration)—refers to how a drug or therapy is introduced into the body. *Systemic administration* means that the drug goes throughout the body (usually carried in the bloodstream) and includes oral administration (by mouth) and intravenous administration (injection into the vein) and other routes of administration. *Local administration* means that the drug is applied or introduced into a specific area affected by disease (e.g., application directly onto the affected skin surface, called topical administration). The effects of most therapies depend upon the ability of the drug to reach the affected area, thus the route of administration and consequent distribution of a drug in the body is an important determinant of its effectiveness.

administrative section—the part of the policy and procedure manual containing the policies and procedures that pertain to the operation of the department

admission, discharge, and transfer system (ADT)—a computer program for admission/discharge and transfer that provides significant demographic and clinical information for each patient

admixture—a term used to denote one or more active ingredients in a large-volume parenteral solution

adult day care facility—provides long-term care that supplements the care an individual may be receiving at home by providing opportunities for socialization and care while the primary caregiver is at work

adverse drug reaction (ADR)—any unexpected, obvious change in a patient's condition that the physician suspects may be due to a drug

aerosol—a finely nebulized medication for inhalation therapy

agent—disease-causing; may be biological, such as a bacteria or virus, chemical, such as medications or pesticides, or physical, such as radiation or heat

AIDS—acquired immune deficiency syndrome

airborne droplet nuclei—small-particle residue—five microns or smaller in size—of evaporated droplets, containing microorganisms that remain suspended in the air for long periods of time

airborne transmission—infection by contact with airborne particles that contain infectious organisms

alkaloid—a nitrogenous basic substance found in plants or synthetic substances with structures similar to plant structures (e.g., atropine, caffeine, morphine)

alkalosis—an acid/base imbalance causing the blood and body tissues to become excessively alkaline (basic)

allergen—an agent that provokes the symptoms of an allergy

allergy—a disorder in which the body becomes hypersensitive to a particular antigen (called an *allergen*)

alligation—the relative amounts of solutions of different percentages from a mixture of a given strength

allopathy—a method of treating a disease by administering an agent that has the opposite characteristics of the disease (e.g., antipyretics to reduce fever)

almshouse—a home for the poor and indigent

alternataive medicine—herbal supplements, megavitamins, and other nontraditional remedies

ambulatory care—care provided to persons who do not require either an acute care (hospital) or chronic care (skilled nursing facility) setting; patients come in for treatment and go home the same day; they are not hospitalized

ambulatory patient—a patient who is not restricted to bed

American Association of Colleges of Pharmacy (AACP)—an organization of pharmacy colleges primarily concerned with education issues such as curricula and teaching methodologies

American Association of Pharmacy Technicians (AAPT)—a membership organization open to pharmacy technicians with access to educational services and availability of an annual meeting

American College of Apothecaries (ACA)—a small, selective association of community-based practitioners whose membership is granted only if the pharmacy and practitioners comply with specified pharmacy professional standards

American College of Clinical Pharmacy (ACCP)—a membership organization of primarily PharmD clinical practitioners and faculty members of colleges of pharmacy, with a mission to transmit the application of new knowledge in the science of pharmacotherapy

American Council for Pharmaceutical Education (ACPE)—the accrediting body for colleges of pharmacy by which high educational standards are established and monitored

American Druggist Blue Book—provides prices and other miscellaneous information about prescription drugs, over-the-counter products, cosmetics, toiletries, and other items sold in pharmacy stores

American Pharmaceutical Association (APhA)—founded in 1852, the largest association in pharmacy with more than 50,000 members

American Pharmacists Association—see American Pharmaceutical Association (APhA)

American Society of Consultant Pharmacists (ASCP)—an organization of pharmacists who provide drug therapy management services in long term care

American Society of Health-System Pharmacists (ASHP)—a national organization established in 1942; presently includes pharmacists in various institutional health care settings and contains a section for pharmacy technicians

amphetamine—a stimulant drug; also known as *uppers, bam, bennies, browns, bumblebee, butterflies*

anabolic agent—a substance that builds up tissue protein

anabolism—the body process during which proteins are synthesized and tissues are formed

analgesic—an agent that relieves pain without causing loss of consciousness (e.g., codeine)

anaphylaxis—a hypersensitivity reaction that is immediate, shock-like, and possibly fatal; a severe allergenic reaction caused by a drug or biological (or an external allergen such as a bee sting)

aneurysm—a dilation or bulging out of a blood vessel wall

anesthetic—a drug used to decrease sensation

angiotensin-converting enzyme (ACE) inhibitor—helps inhibit the renal mechanism for blood pressure elevation

anhydrous—containing no water

anionic—carrying a negative charge

antacids—an agent that neutralizes gastric acid

antagonist—a drug that opposes the action of another drug or a natural body chemical

antearea—an ISO Class 8 or better area where personnel perform hand hygiene and garbing procedures, staging of components, etc.; maintained under positive pressure in comparison to the rest of the pharmacy, but negative to the buffer area; supplied with HEPA-filtered air

anteroom—an area of the clean room that provides a clean area for hand washing and donning personnel barriers such as hair covers, gloves, gowns, or full clean-room attire

antianginal—a drug used to relieve cardiac chest pain

antiarrhythmic—an agent that restores normal heart rhythm

antibiotic—a medication that is derived from living cells or synthetic compounds and is antagonistic to other forms of life, especially bacteria; a soluble substance derived from a mold or bacterium that inhibits the growth of other organisms and is used to combat disease and infection

anticholinergic—a drug that blocks the passage of impulses through parasympathetic nerve fibers

anticoagulant—a drug that prevents or delays coagulation or clotting of blood; a "blood thinner"

antidote—a remedy for counteracting a poison

antiemetic—controls nausea and vomiting

antiflatulent—a drug that facilitates expulsion of gas from the GI tract

antigen—an agent that stimulates antibody formation

antihistamine—a drug that reduces runny nose and sneezing

antihypertensive—an agent that reduces blood pressure

antineoplastic—a substance that prevents the development or spread of tumor cells

antineoplastic agent—a chemotherapy agent or cancer drug

antipruritic—a drug that relieves itch

antipyretic—a drug that reduces fever

antiseptic—an agent that inhibits the growth of microorganisms but does not necessarily kill them

antitoxin—a specific agent neutralizing a poison or toxin

antitussive—a drug used for the relief of cough

apothecary—early American or European term for a pharmacist

apothecary system—an early English system of weights and liquid measure

apparent volume of distribution—the apparent volume of plasma that would be required to account for all the drug in the body

application software—referred to as *programs*; accepting data from the user, it calculates, stores user-specific data, and presents information according to the prescribed instructions

area under the plasma concentration-time curve (AUC)—plasma drug concentration can be determined by calculating the rate and extent of systemic absorption, as visualized by the plasma concentration-time curve

arrhythmia—an abnormal, irregular heartbeat

arteriosclerosis—a disorder characterized by thickening, loss of elasticity, and calcification of the walls of the arteries

arthritis—inflammation of joints

ascites—accumulation of fluid within the abdominal cavity

asepsis—free from germs, sterile

aseptic—a condition in which there are no living microorganisms; free from infection

aseptic processing—a method to assure that no contamination of compounded sterile products will occur during their compounding

aseptic technique—a method of preparation that will prevent contamination of a site (e.g., wound) or product (e.g., IV admixture)

assisted living facility—for individuals who are unable to remain in the home for care but who do not need the level of care provided in nursing homes

asylum—an institution for the relief or care of the destitute or afflicted and especially the insane

atherosclerosis—lipid (fat) deposits in large- and medium-size arteries

atonic—a weak tone or absence of tone

automated pharmacy systems—mechanical systems that perform operations and activities other than compounding and drug administration, relative to storage, packaging, dispensing, and distribution of medications and that collect, control, and maintain transaction information

automatic stop order—a medical decision made to discontinue the drug

autonomy—independent action

average wholesale price (AWP)—the cost of drugs and pharmaceuticals purchased from a drug wholesaler

backup systems—alternate procedures in the event the computer system should fail

bacteria—small, one-celled microorganisms that need a nourishing environment to survive

bactericide—an agent capable of killing bacteria

bacteriostat—an agent that inhibits the growth of bacteria

bar coding—a series of vertical bars and spaces of varying thicknesses and heights to represent information

beneficence—the practice of doing good; a kindly action

benign—not malignant or invasive

beta blocker—a drug that selectively blocks beta receptors in the autonomic nervous system

bile—a fluid secreted by the liver

bile salts—naturally occurring surface-active agents secreted by the gall bladder into the small intestine

bioavailability—a term used to indicate the rate and relative amount of administered drug that reaches the circulatory system intact

biodegradable—can be broken down by living organisms

bioengineered therapies—the process used in the manufacture of therapeutic agents through recombinant DNA (deoxyribonucleic acid) technology

bioequivalence—evaluates whether a second drug has the same bioavailability of the original drug regarding the active ingredient(s)

biological equivalents—those chemical equivalents that, when administered in the same amounts, will provide the same biological or physiological availability

biological fluids—includes blood, serum, plasma, lymph, etc.

biologicals—medicinal preparations made from living organisms or their products; include serums, vaccines, antigens, and antitoxins

biopharmaceutics—the branch of pharmaceutics that concerns itself with the relationship between physicochemical properties of a drug in a dosage form and the pharmacologic, toxicologic, or clinical responses observed after drug administration

biopsy—the excision of a small piece of tissue for diagnostic purposes

biotech drugs—genetically engineered therapeutic agents

biotechnology—the application of biological systems and organisms to technical and industrial processes

black plague—a worldwide epidemic of the 14th century in which some 60 million people are said to have died; descriptions indicate that it was pneumonic plague, also called *black death* or *the plague*

blending—mixing

blister packages—cardboard and plastic material that is heat-sealed to individually package medication

bloodborne pathogens—microorganisms that are transmitted through exposure to contaminated blood products

blood urea nitrogen (BUN)—an indication of kidney function

board of directors/board of trustees—the body responsible for governing the hospital in the community's best interest

body surface area (BSA)—the measurement of the height and weight of the patient to establish and estimate his or her body surface

bolus—an injection directly from the needle and syringe into a vein; also called *IV push*

botany—the science of plants, including structure, functions of parts, and classification

bradycardia—slow heart rate

brand-name drugs—drugs that are research-developed, patented, manufactured, and distributed by a drug firm

B.S. degree—bachelor of science degree; an initial entry degree originally required for admission to a state board examination to obtain a license to practice as a pharmacist

buccal—between the gum and cheek

budget—the projected costs allocated on a yearly basis for personnel, pharmaceuticals, supplies, construction, and operating expenses, among other categories

buffer—offers a resistance to pH change

buffer area—usually an ISO Class 7 area where the laminar flow hood is located; it has positive pressure to the rest of the pharmacy and is supplied with HEPA-filtered air

buffer system—used to maintain the pH of a drug solution within the range of optimum stability or when the pH of blood and body fluids are maintained virtually constant, although acid metabolites are continually being formed in the tissues or are being lost in the lungs

Bureau of Alcohol, Tobacco and Firearms (ATF)—a department of the U.S. Treasury that establishes regulatory standards for procuring, storing, dispensing, and use of tax-free alcohol for specific clinical uses

business associate—a person who, on behalf of an insured individual, performs a function or an activity involving the use or disclosure of confidential health information

calibrate—standardization of the graduations of a quantitative measuring device

calibration—a method of standardizing a measuring device

candida—a yeast organism that normally lives in the intestines, but can flourish in other parts of the body at times of immune suppression

caplet—a tablet shaped like a capsule

capsule—a soluble container enclosing medicine

carcinogen—any substance that causes cancer

cardiotonic—an agent with the effect of producing or restoring normal heart activity

carminative—a medicine that relieves stomach/intestinal gas

carve-out—a Medicaid reimbursement for a small number of expensive medications paid directly to the long-term care facility above preestablished daily rates

catabolism—the breakdown of body proteins

cataract—loss of transparency of the lens of the eye

cathartic—an agent that causes bowel evacuation

catheter—a tubular device used for the drainage or injection of fluids through a body passage; made of silicone, rubber, plastic, or other materials

cationic—carrying a positive charge

centralized dispensing system—a system of distribution in which all functions, processing, preparation, and distribution occur in a main area (e.g., the main pharmacy)

central processing unit (CPU)—the unit of the computer that accomplishes the processing or execution of given calculations or instructions

central service—an area in the hospital where general sterilization procedures are performed; serves as a storage facility for various types of supplies and equipment

certification—the act of certifying to a standard established by a written or printed statement

certified pharmacy technician (CPhT)—a pharmacy technician who has successfully passed the National Pharmacy Technician Certification Examination

chain of infection—the elements needed to take place in order for an infection to occur

chain pharmacy—a retail pharmacy owned by a corporation that consists of many stores in a particular region or nationally

charge capture system—a component of the hospital information system whereby every time an order is entered on a patient, a charge is being captured for billing purposes, and a statistic is being captured for management monitoring purposes

chelating—making a complex formation

chemical equivalents—those multiple-source drug products that contain identical amounts of the identical active ingredient in identical dosage forms

chemical sterilization—the process of completely removing or destroying all microorganisms by exposure to a chemical

chemotherapy—the treatment of an illness with medication; commonly refers to the treatment of malignancy with agents that are cytotoxic (i.e., the medication kills cells); more specifically, use of chemicals to treat cancer

cholinergic—a drug that is stimulated, activated, or transmitted by acetylcholine

chronic—of long duration or frequent recurrence

chronic illness—a disturbance in health that persists for a long time, usually showing little change or slow progression over time

Class A prescription balance—a sensitive balance scale with a range of 6 mg to 650 mg

Class 100 environment—a room or hood designed for the preparation of sterile products that indicates the environment has less than 100 particles of dust and particulates per cubic centimeter of air

clean room—a specially filtered room to create a sterile environment

clinical—involving direct observation of the patient

clinical pharmacokinetics—the branch of pharmaceutics that deals with the application of pharmacokinetics to the safe and effective therapeutic management of the individual patient

clinical pharmacy—patient-oriented pharmacy practice that is concerned with health care through rational drug use

clinical pharmacy practice—the application of knowledge about drugs and drug therapy to the care and treatment of patients

clinical section—the section of a policy and procedure manual describing patient-related activities

closed formulary—a list of reimbursable medications

C_{max}—the maximum plasma concentration of a drug to determine its bioavailability

coagulation—the blood-clotting process

cocaine—a topical anesthetic, also known as *coke, crack, snow, blow, white horse, 8-ball*

cognitive pharmacy services—the process of applying pharmaceutical knowledge to a particular patient to assure rational drug therapy

cohorting—a patient is placed in a room with a patient who has an active infection or colonization with the same microorganism but with no other infection

cold—a self-limiting viral infection of the respiratory tract

collaborative drug therapy agreement—an agreement between a physician and a pharmacist that allows the pharmacist expanded prescription authorization regarding managing drug therapy

collaborative drug therapy management (CDTM)—an agreement between a physician and a pharmacist that allows the pharmacist expanded prescription authorization regarding managing drug therapy

colonized—a group of microorganisms that have grown from a single infectious microorganism within a particular part of the body, causing an infection

colostomy—the creation of an opening into the colon through the abdominal wall

combining form—a word type that facilitates the attachment of a prefix or suffix; formed when a word root is incorporated into a medical term

Commission on Credentialing—the body appointed to formulate and recommend standards and administer programs for accreditation of pharmacy personnel training programs

community pharmacy—pharmacy service provided in community health care; sometimes called the "family drugstore" where ambulatory individuals are provided prescription and nonprescription drugs and other health-related supplies

community relations and fund development—a department that communicates with and markets hospital programs to the local community

compounded sterile preparation (CSP)—relates to the compounding of sterile preparations, including intravenous admixtures, ophthalmics, intrathecals, and so forth; prepared in a controlled, sterile environment

compounding—the preparation of a pharmaceutical that normally contains more than one ingredient, according to a prescription or formula

Comprehensive Drug Abuse and Prevention Control Act—a federal statute through which the DEA (Drug Enforcement Agency) promulgates and enforces rules and regulations controlling narcotic use

computer—a programmable electronic device used to store, process, or communicate information

computer application—a series of computer programs written for a particular function (e.g., inventory management)

computer file—a collection of like elements of information stored under a common name (e.g., Hospital Formulary)

computerized physician order entry (CPOE)—a drug order entered into a hospital-wide computer system transmitted to the pharmacy

computer network—the technology that supports the connection of multiple computers including applications, processors, printers, and microcomputers

computer server—a computer that collects and stores information for use by other computers

computer system—a combination of hardware and software working together to perform specific functions

computer terminal—a device that contains a keyboard and screen; functions as both the input and output device

congestive heart failure (CHF)—failure or diminished ability of the heart to pump an adequate blood supply to the rest of the body

confirmation bias—a term used to describe errors that occur in selection of medication by either pharmacy or nursing staff; when choosing an item, people see what they are looking for, and once they think they have found it, they stop looking any further

constipation—difficult, incomplete, or infrequent bowel evacuation

consultant pharmacist—responsible for monitoring drug usage and drug therapy of residents in nursing homes

contact transmission—a mode of transmission for microorganisms; divided into two subgroups: direct-contact transmission and indirect-contact transmission

contaminated—unclean; microorganisms are introduced into an area where they had not previously been present

continuous infusion—the administration of an intravenous drug at a constant rate over a prolonged time period

contraindicate—to indicate against; to indicate the inappropriateness of a form of treatment or a drug for a specific disease

control—any method used to eliminate or reduce the potential harm of the distributed medication

control documents—forms such as records, sheets, logs, or checklists that track conformance with established standards to reduce the likelihood of an error or negative outcome

controlled substances—drugs, controlled by the federal or state Drug Enforcement Administration, that can produce dependence or be abused (e.g., narcotics, select psychotropics, steroids)

Controlled Substances Act—a federal law regulating the manufacture, distribution, and sale of drugs that have the potential for abuse

counter balance—a double-pan balance capable of weighing relatively large quantities

counterirritant—an agent, such as mustard plaster, that is applied locally to produce an inflammatory reaction for the purpose of affecting some other part, usually adjacent to or underlying the irritated surface

covered entities—entities to which HIPAA regulations apply; namely, health plans that provide or pay the costs of medical care, health care clearinghouses that facilitate the processing of health information from another entity, and health care providers of medical or health services

CPU—central processing unit of computer hardware; the brain of the computer

crack—an illicit, pure form of cocaine, usually smoked in a pipe

cream—a water-based, semisolid external dosage form

creatinine clearance—a measure of renal function

credentialing—a process in which a formal, organized agency recognizes and documents the competencies and abilities performed by an individual or an organization

criteria—a set of statements that define quality

critical area—an ISO Class 5 area

critical site—any opening or surface that can provide a pathway between the sterile product and the environment

cyber—a cultural revolution; computerization and telecommunication that transport information through fiber optics, CD-ROMs, satellites, and the Internet

cytotoxic—a substance that causes cellular deterioration

data entry—the input function that involves recording, coding, or converting data to a form that the computer can recognize

decentralized dispensing system—a system of distribution in which all functions (processing, preparation, and distribution) occur on or near the nursing unit (e.g., satellite pharmacy)

decongestant—a drug used to open the air passages of the nose and lungs

decubitus ulcer—a bedsore

dedicated—limited to processing information for one area

deinstitutionalization—the discharge of persons with a history of long-term mental health care in a hospital back to the community

delayed-release—specifically formulated pharmaceutical dosage forms in which the active ingredient is released at a constant rate over a specific time period

density—weight per unit volume

deoxyribonucleic acid (DNA)—a double-stranded structure that is the molecular basis of heredity

departmental manual—lists those policies and procedures that affect the internal workings of the pharmacy department

diabetes mellitus—a metabolic disorder in which faulty pancreatic activity decreases carbohydrate utilization

diagnosis—the determination of the nature of a disease or symptom through physical examinations and clinical tests

diagnosis-related group (DRG)—utilized by Medicare, Medicaid, and other third-party payors to reimburse hospitals a predetermined fee for each patient based on the patient's diagnosis, irrespective of the quantity or cost of the care. Costs over this predetermined fee are not reimbursed by the government but are allocated to the hospital. The intent of implementing the DRG system was to regulate and control Medicare's health care expenditure. *See also* **prospective payment system (PPS)**

diagnostic equipment—articles or implements used to detect physical conditions that may be related to disease or biological changes; usually used at home by one patient

diarrhea—increased frequency of stool that is loose and watery

diastolic pressure—the force exerted by the blood on the blood vessels when the ventricles of the heart are in a state of rest before systole

dietary supplement—any product containing a vitamin, mineral, amino acid, or herb that is intended to supplement the diet by increasing overall intake of a particular substance

Dietary Supplement Verification Program (DSVP)—a program developed by the USP to establish standards for herbal and vitamin supplements

differentiated manpower—the distinction of responsibilities among available personnel to achieve the overall purpose of the entire group

diluent—an agent that dilutes or reconstitutes a solution or mixture

direct compounding area (DCA)—a critical compounding area meeting ISO 5 specifications

direct-contact transmission—infection through body surface-to-body surface contact with an infected person

discharge planning—a program developed to ensure continued appropriate care after the patient leaves the hospital

disease state management—a continuous, coordinated, and ongoing process that manages and improves the health status of defined patient populations over the course of an entire disease

disinfectant—a substance used to destroy pathogens; generally used on objects rather than on humans

dispensatory—a treatise on the quality and composition of medicine

dispense as written (DAW)—where the medication indicated on the prescription may not be substituted with a generic or other brand drug without the authorization of the prescriber

dispensing—the process of selecting, preparing, checking, and delivering prescribed medication and associated information; must be under the supervision of a pharmacist

dissolution—the act of dissolving

distribution—movement of a drug from the bloodstream to other bodily tissues

distributional section—the part of a policy and procedure manual that presents those policies and procedures that deal with the appropriate storage, ordering, dispensing, documentation, and disposition of drugs and supplies

diuresis—increased excretion of urine

diuretic—an agent that causes an increase in the excretion of urine

dosage—the determination and regulation of the size, frequency, and number of doses

dosage forms—the various pharmaceutical forms whereby drugs are made available (e.g., capsules, patches, injections)

dosage strength—the quantity of a drug in a given dosage form

dosage schedule—the frequency, interval, and length of time a medicine is to be given

dose—a quantity of a drug or radiation to be given at one time

droplet transmission—infection through contact with microscopic liquid particles coming from an infected person

DRG—*see* **diagnosis-related group**

drug—any substance intended to cure, prevent, or diagnose a disease or disease process

drug administration—the process by which a drug enters the body by ingestion, injection, application, inhalation, instillation, etc.

drug disposition—all processes that occur to the drug after absorption and that can be subdivided into distribution and elimination

drug distribution—the process of reversible transfer of a drug to and from the site of measurement, usually the blood

drug elimination—the irreversible loss of a drug from the site of measurement, usually subdivided into metabolism or excretion

Drug Enforcement Administration (DEA)—a federal agency established to implement the rules and regulations to enforce the Controlled Substances Act (CSA) to combat controlled substance abuse

drug formulary—a list of medicinal agents selected by the medical staff considered to be the most useful in patient care

druggist—historically, a person who compounds, dispenses, and sells drugs and medicine

drug information—information about drugs and the effects of drugs on people, the provision of which is a part of each pharmacist's practice

drug information center (DIC)—provide drug information services; usually directed by drug information specialists; purposes of a DIC vary and depend on the practice setting in which the drug information center is located; most commonly funded by or located in a hospital, academic institution, or pharmaceutical company

drug label—information placed on a drug container that includes data required by drug regulations

drug manufacturer—the company responsible for developing and producing and distributing pharmaceutical products

drug misadventures—what can go wrong in the "therapeutic adventure" of using a medication; encompasses errors in prescribing judgment, system errors in the process of bringing drug products to the ultimate users, and idiosyncratic (individual and unusual sensitivity that is not dose related) responses to medication

drug order—a course of medication therapy ordered by the physician or dental practitioner in an organized health care setting

drug recalls—the voluntary recall of a drug because of a health hazard potential

drugs of choice—the preferred or best drug therapy that can be prescribed for a specific disease state, based upon majority medical opinion

Drug Topics Red Book—a reference guide listing pharmaceuticals, medicinals, and sundries sold in drug stores, with currently available prices

drug-use control—the system of knowledge, understanding, judgments, procedures, skills, controls, and ethics that ensures optimal safety in the distribution and use of medication

drug use process—an organized, complex, and controlled system of manufacturing, purchasing, distributing, storing, prescribing, preparing, dispensing, administering, using, controlling, and monitoring of a drug's effects and outcomes to ensure that drugs are used safely and effectively

drug wholesaler—the company responsible for delivering medication, medical devices, appliances, etc. to pharmacies and retailers

dumbwaiter—an in-house elevator used to transport medications and supplies

duodenum—that area of the small intestine that is the first 25 cm after the stomach, responsible for significant drug absorption

durable medical equipment (DME)—includes health-related equipment that is used for long periods of time, is not disposable, and is rented or sold to clients for home care, such as wheelchairs, hospital beds, walkers, canes, crutches; *see also* **home medical equipment**

Durham-Humphrey Amendment—established two classes of drugs, over-the-counter and prescription, and mandated that labels of prescription drugs include the legend: "Caution: Federal Law Prohibits Dispensing without a Prescription"

elastomer—an elastometric substance

elastometric—a polymer material with elastic properties

electrocardiogram—a graphic record of the heart's action by electronic measurement

electroencephalogram—a tracing or electronic recording of brain waves

electrolytes—naturally occurring ions in the body that play an essential role in cellular function, maintaining fluid balance and establishing acid-base balance; an ionizable substance in solution (e.g., sodium, potassium chloride)

electronic balance—an electronic digital weighing balance scale that varies based on its purpose; can be used to weigh bulk quantities greater than 1 gram. Standard prescription balances are accurate up to 1 mg or smaller quantities down to 0.001 mg

electronic data interchange (EDI)—commonly used to order merchandise, transfer funds, and facilitate billing

electronic mail (e-mail)—a form of transmitting, storing, and distributing text in electronic form via a communications network

electrostatic copying machine—a photocopier

elimination—the removal of waste material from the body

elimination half life—the amount of time it takes to eliminate one-half of the total amount of drug in the blood

emboli—a blood clot; a moving or transferred blood clot

embolism—the obstruction or occlusion of a blood vessel by a transported blood clot

emergency room—a hospital unit where patients are treated for conditions that require immediate attention

emesis—the clinical term for vomiting

emetic—an agent that causes vomiting

emphysema—a lung disease caused by constriction of airway passages

employee performance evaluations—a routine, formal process by the supervisor to provide feedback on the employee's performance versus the expected performance listed in the employee's action plan

emulsifying agent—a substance used in preparing an emulsion

emulsion—a heterogeneous system of at least one immiscible liquid intimately dispersed in another in the form of droplets, stabilized by the presence of an emulsifying agent

enforcement—the process of making sure that policies and procedures, as well as laws, rules and regulations, are carefully and consistently followed

enteral nutrition—a liquid nutrient solution administered by mouth or through a feeding tube into the stomach or intestines

enteric-coated tablet—a special tablet coating that prevents the release of a drug until it enters the intestine

enterohepatic cycling—a drug is taken up by the bile, secreted into the small intestine, and may be reabsorbed back to the blood

epidemic—a disease that attacks many people in the same region at the same time

epidural—infusion therapy directly into spinal cord fluid

equivalent weight—the gram molecular weight divided by the highest valent ion in the molecule

erythrocyte—a red blood cell

estrogen—a hormone that produces secondary sex characteristics in the female

ethics—the study of precepts or principles used to assist us in making the correct choice when faced with alternative possibilities in a moral situation

etiology—the study of all of the factors that may be involved in the development of disease

excipient—an inert substance added to a drug to give form or consistency

excretion—the process whereby the undigested residue of food and the waste products of metabolism are eliminated

expectorant—a substance that promotes the ejection of mucus or an exudate from the lungs, bronchi, and trachea

expiration date—the last date of sale and/or use as determined by the manufacturer. Any sale or use after this date is unethical and may result in a levy of fines by pharmacy and or health inspectors.

exposure control plan—guidelines to follow in the event of an exposure to an infectious disease, including infection control training

extemporaneous compounding—prepared at the time it is required, with materials on hand

extended-release—drugs or capsules that are formulated in such a way as to gradually release the drug over a predetermined time period

extravascular—outside of the blood vessels or lymphatic vascular channel

facsimile equipment—a fax machine; sends orders over telephone lines

FDA—*see* Food and Drug Administration

febrile—a body temperature that is above normal

Federal Food, Drug, and Cosmetic Act (FDCA)—a federal law through which the Food and Drug Administration promulgates its rules and regulations

Federal Hazardous Substances Act—requires that hazardous household products bear cautionary labels to alert consumers of potential dangers and to inform them of measures to take to protect themselves

federal statutes—laws enacted by a legislative body that dictate the conduct of persons or organizations subject to the law

fibrillation—a rapid, ineffectual heartbeat

filtration—the process of passing a liquid through a porous substance that arrests suspended solid particles

first-pass metabolism—occurs when a drug is rapidly metabolized in the liver after oral administration with minimum bioavailability

floor stock system—medications provided to the nursing unit for administration to the patient by the nurse, who is responsible for preparation and administration

fluid extract—a liquid preparation of an herb, containing alcohol as a solvent or preservative

Food and Drug Administration (FDA)—promulgates rules, regulations, and standards; inspects drug and food facilities to ensure public safety regarding drug products

Food and Drug Administration Modernization Act of 1997 (FDAMA)—streamlined regulatory procedures, encouraged manufactures to conduct research for new uses of drugs, and encouraged drug manufacturers to perform pediatric studies of drugs

Food, Drug, and Cosmetic Act of 1938—the federal statute through which the FDA promulgates its rules and regulations

format—a standardized method of documentation for consistency

formulary—a listing of drugs of choice as determined by safety, efficacy, effectiveness, and cost, approved by the medical staff for use within the institution

franchise—authorization by a manufacturer to a distributor to sell a product

free flow—a dangerous condition in which all of the infusion is accidentally administered in a short period of time

fungi—yeasts or molds that obtain food from living organisms

galenical—a standard preparation containing one or several organic ingredients (e.g., elixir)

gargle—a substance used to rinse or medicate the mucous membrane of the throat and mouth (e.g., Listerine)

gastric—pertaining to the stomach

gastroesophageal reflux disease (GERD)—excess stomach acid that causes a burning sensation in the esophagus due to eructation of small amounts of acid into the esophagus

generic drug name—the nonproprietary (non-brand) name of a drug

generic drugs—drugs labeled by their "official" name and manufactured by a drug firm after the original patent expires

genetically engineered drugs—the exact duplication of a substance already available in the human body

geometric dilution—the addition of approximately equal amounts of the prescribed drugs when mixing in a mortar

geriatric pharmacy practice—a pharmacy practice that focuses on the medical and pharmaceutical care of the elderly

glucose tolerance test—a test for diabetes, based on the ability of the liver to store glycogen

glycoside—a compound containing a sugar molecule (e.g., digitalis)

graduate—a marked (or graduated) conical or cylindrical vessel used for measuring liquids

grain—a base unit of weight in the apothecary system

gram—a base unit of weight in the metric system

granule—a very small pill, usually gelatin-coated or sugar-coated, containing a drug to be given in a small dose

GRAS list—a list of food additives generally recognized as safe by the Food and Drug Administration

group purchasing—an arrangement where pharmaceutical companies ship larage quantities of drugs to the warehouses of hospital buying groups

group purchasing organizations (GPOs)—a group of hospitals or pharmacists that buy drugs directly from the manufacturer

habituation—an acquired tolerance for a drug

hard copy—information on a printed sheet

hardware—equipment, software, and sets of instructions that control and coordinate the activities of the hardware and direct the processing of data; refers to the actual computer system (e.g., IBM, Digital)

Hazard Communication Standard (HCS)—a regulation to ensure that the hazards in chemicals be transmitted to workers handling these hazardous substances

health care delivery—organized programs developed to provide physical, mental, and emotional health care in institutions for home-bound and ambulatory patients

Health Insurance Portability and Accountability Act (HIPAA)—an important law that requires the adoption of security and privacy standards in order to protect personal health care information

health maintenance organization (HMO)—a prepaid health insurance plan that provides comprehensive health care for subscribers, with emphasis on the prevention and early detection of disease and continuity of care. HMOs are either not-for-profit or for-profit, are designated as either an independent practice association (IPA) or a staff model, and are often owned and operated by insurance carriers. HMOs were developed as a means to control health care delivery, access, and cost

hemodialysis—a procedure by which impurities or wastes are removed from the blood

hemophilia—a hereditary blood-coagulation disorder

hemorrhage—severe bleeding

hemostat—an agent used to arrest hemorrhaging

HEN—home enteral therapy

hepatitis—inflammation of the liver

hepatitis B (HBV)—a virus transmitted through infectious bodily fluids that causes acute infection of the liver

hepatitis C (HBC)—a virus transmitted through infectious bodily fluids that causes acute and chronic infection of the liver

herb—a leafy plant used as a healing remedy or a flavoring agent

herbal—a plant with therapeutic properties that can be used for nutritional or medical purposes

Herb Contraindications and Drug Interactions—a useful resource by Francis Brinker on herbal-drug interactions for the pharmacy

heroin—an illicit drug derived from morphine; also known as *brown sugar, salt, horse*

heterogeneous—composed of parts having various and dissimilar characteristics or properties

high efficiency particulate air (HEPA) filter—used in laminar air flow hoods; they remove 99.97 percent of all particles larger than 0.3 microns in size

Hippocrates—a Greek physician, called the "Father of Medicine"

HIS—*see* **hospital information system**

HIV—human immunodeficiency virus; *see* HIV

home care—care given to patients in their own homes

home equipment management services—the selection, delivery, set up, and maintenance of equipment and the education of the patient in the use of the equipment, all performed in the home or patient's place of residence

home health agencies—providers of home health services

home health care—the provision of health care services to a patient in his or her place of residence

home health services—the provision of health care services by a health care professional in the patient's place of residence on a per-visit basis

home infusion therapy—intravenous drug therapy provided in patient's own home

home medical equipment (HME)—equipment used at home (e.g., hospital beds, crutches); *see* **durable medical equipment**

home medical services—physician services in the home

homeopathy—giving a minute quantity of a fever-producing substance; assists the body in the treatment or prevention of disease

homeostasis—a tendency toward stability in the internal body environment; a state of equilibrium

home pharmaceutical services—dispensing and delivering medications to patients who have their clinical status monitored at home

homogeneous—of uniform composition throughout

horizontal hospital integration—a situation in which a number of hospitals share administrative, clinical, and technological functions

hormone—a chemical substance, produced by cells or an organ, that has a specific regulatory effect in the body

hospice—an institution that provides a program of palliative and supportive services to terminally ill patients and their families in the form of physical, psychological, social, and spiritual care

hospital—a network of health care services for diagnosis, treatment, care of the sick, study of disease, therapy, and the training of health care professionals

hospital information system (HIS)—a system that integrates information from many parts of the hospital

human genome initiative—a program of research that studies all human genes

human immunodeficiency virus (HIV)—a virus that weakens the immune system and may progress to the development of AIDS

humor—a fluid or semifluid substance in the body; originally phlegm, blood, bile (e.g., aqueous humor is a fluid produced in the eye—not tears)

hydration therapy—replaces fluid loss

hydro-alcoholic—a mixture of water and alcohol

hydrolysis—any reaction in which water is one of the reactants

hydrophilic—"water loving"

hydrophilic drug molecules—drug molecules that are polar and water loving

hydrophobic drugs—drugs whose molecules are non-polar and lipid loving or water hating

hydrous—combined with water, forming a compound with one or more molecules of water

hygroscopic—moisture absorbing

hyperalimentation—intravenous feeding; total parenteral nutrition (TPN)

hyperglycemia—high blood glucose level

hypersensitivity—excessive response of the immune system to a sensitizing antigen

hypersensitivity reaction—the reaction that occurs after a person is exposed to a compound and has generated antibodies against the compound

hypertension—a disorder characterized by elevated blood pressure

hypertonic—having a higher osmotic pressure than a reference solution, usually referring to blood plasma or lacrimal fluid

hypnotic—a drug used to induce sleep

hypoglycemic—a drug that lowers the level of glucose in the blood; used primarily by diabetics

hypolipodemic—an agent to reduce lipids (fat) in the blood

hypometabolic—low basic metabolic rate

hypotension—low blood pressure

hypotonic—having a lesser osmotic pressure than a reference standard, usually referring to blood plasma or lacrimal fluid

ideal drug therapy—safe, effective, timely, and cost-conscious medication use

immunity—the condition of being resistant to a particular disease (e.g., polio)

immunomodulators—agents that adjust the immune system to a desired level

incompatibility—a lack of compatibility; an undesirable effect when two or more substances are mixed together

incubation—the period between exposure to an infective disease process and the symptoms of infection

independent pharmacy—a retail pharmacy owned and operated by an individual pharmacist or group of individuals, as contrasted with chain drug stores

indirect-contact transmission—infection through contact with a contaminated object

individual prescription system—a system in which a multiple-day supply of each medication is dispensed for the patient upon receipt of prescriptions or medication orders

infection—the state or condition in which the body (or part of it) is invaded by an agent (microorganism or virus) that multiplies and produces an injurious effect (active infection)

infection control—the use of appropriate procedures and education to minimize the transfer of infections from one to another

infiltration—occurs when an intravenous solution is infused into the surrounding tissues instead of directly into the vein as intended

inflammation—a condition characterized by pain, heat, redness, and swelling

infusion—the introduction of a solution into a vein by gravity or by an infusion control device or pump

infusion pump—regulates the flow of an intravenous solution

infusion therapy—the introduction of fluid into the body, usually by intravenous routes

in-house pharmacy—a pharmacy located within the facility/hospital

injection—the introduction of a fluid substance into the body by means of a needle and syringe

inpatient—a patient who requires the use of a hospital bed and is registered in the hospital to receive medical or surgical care

input devices—keyboards, light pens, optical scanners, bar code readers, etc.

inscription—on a prescription, contains the name of the drug, the drug strength, and dosage form

institutional pharmacy—pharmacy services provided in hospitals, nursing homes, health maintenance organizations, prisons, mental retardation facilities, or other settings, wherein groups of patients are provided formal, structured pharmacy programs

intensive care unit (ICU)—a unit within a hospital where the patient receives constant and vigilant attention

intermittent infusion—the administration of an IV infusion over a period of time followed by a period of no administration. The same cycle usually is repeated at scheduled times, hence the name *intermittent*

intermittent injection—the administration of a drug over 15 minutes to 4 hours, after which there is a period of no drug administration, followed again by cycles of administration and periods of no administration

International System of Units (SI)—commonly known as the metric system for weights and measures

intoxication—a state of being poisoned by a drug or being inebriated with alcohol

intra-arterial—the injection of a sterile preparation into an artery

intra-articular—the injection of a sterile preparation in a joint, such as the elbow or knee

intracardia—the injection of a sterile preparation directly into the heart

intradermal (ID)—situated or applied within the skin

intramuscular (IM)—within the muscle

intraocular—within the eye

intraperitoneal—a sterile preparation is injected into the peritoneal or abdominal cavity

intrapleural—a sterile preparation is injected into the sac surrounding the lungs

intrasynovial (IS)—an injection directly into joint fluid

intrathecal—within the subdural space of the spinal cord

intravascular—injection into a blood vessel

intravenous (IV)—within a vein; administering drugs or fluids directly into the vein to obtain a rapid or complete effect from the drug

intraventricular—injection into a ventricle of the brain or heart

intravesicular—a preparation instilled into the urinary bladder

intravitrial—a sterile preparation is injected into the vitreous chamber of the eyeball behind the lens

inventory—a complete listing of the exact amounts of all the drugs in stock at a particular time

investigational drugs—drugs that have not received approval for marketing by the Food and Drug Administration

iontophoresis—use of an electric current to cause an ionized drug to pass through the skin into the system circulation

ISO Class 5 area—International Organization of Standardization (ISO) classification of particulate matter in room air, with no more than 3,520 particles per cubic meter of air 0.5 microns and larger

ISO Class 7 area—International Organization of Standardization (ISO) classification of particulate matter in room air, with no more than 352,000 particles per cubic meter of air 0.5 microns or larger

ISO Class 8 area—International Organization of Standardization (ISO) classification of particulate matter in room air, with no more than 3,520,000 particles per cubic meter of air 0.5 microns and larger

iso-osmotic—having the same tone

isotonic—having the osmotic pressure

IV admixture—intravenous solutions to which medications are added

IV push—the administration of a drug by directly pushing the barrel of the syringe to inject its contents directly into a vein; also known as *bolus*

jaundice—a yellow appearance of skin and mucous membranes, resulting from the deposition of bile pigment

job description—a guideline written by the employer for the employee outlining the requirements and limits of the job

Joint Commission—a not-for-profit organization whose standards are set to ensure effective quality services (e.g., optimal standards for the operation of hospitals)

just in time (JIT)—an inventory strategy to minimize inventory levels, thus minimizing tying up large sums of money

Kardex—a card for each patient kept in a folder, used as a reminder of what, when, and to whom to administer medication

Kefauver-Harris Amendment—an amendment to the Federal Food and Cosmetic Act that required all new drugs marketed in the United States to be proven safe and effective

laboratory—a hospital department where chemical or biological testing is performed for the purpose of aiding diagnosis

lacrimal fluids—tears

laminar flow hood—a sterile work area with positive pressure air flow that filters the air

leaching—the effect of removing a soluble substance from a solution

legend medication—a drug that is only available to a patient with a prescription from a licensed prescriber; also known as *prescription medication*

leukemia—a disease characterized by an extremely high white blood cell count

levigation—mixing of particles with a base vehicle, in which they are insoluble, to produce a smooth dispersion of the drug by rubbing with a spatula on a tile

lipophilic—"lipid loving"

liposome—a small membrane that entraps and later releases an active ingredient

liter—a basic unit of liquid measure in the metric system

local area networks (LAN)—permit different systems (mainframe, minicomputers, and microcomputers), as well as computers made by different manufacturers, to communicate and share data

long-term care—health care provided in an organized medical facility for patients requiring chronic or extended treatment

long-term care facility—for individuals who do not need hospital care but are in need of a wide range of medical, nursing, and related health and social services

lotions—liquid preparations intended for external application

lozenge—a small, medicated or flavored disc intended to be dissolved in the mouth

LSD—lysergic acid diethylamide, a hallucinogen; also known as *beast, black sunshine, the chief*

Maimonides—Rabbi Moses ben Maimon, a Spanish-born teacher and physician

mainframe—the largest, most powerful type of computer system; is able to service many users at once and process several programs simultaneously; has large primary and secondary storage capacities

malaria—an infectious, fever-producing disease, transmitted by infected mosquitoes

malignant—a type of tumor that invades healthy tissue and becomes progressively worse

malpractice—a deviation from the standard of care that arises out of a professional relationship; also called *professional negligence*

managed care—the provision of health care services in the most cost-effective way

MAO inhibitors—a class of drugs that act as antidepressants by inhibiting the enzyme monoamine oxidase

marijuana—a substance, made from hemp, that has an effect on mood, perception, and psychomotor coordination; also known as *sinse, weed, herb, grass, dope, reefer, maryjane*

mastectomy—the removal of the breast

materials management—the division of a hospital pharmacy responsible for the procurement, control, storage, and distribution of drugs and pharmaceutical products

materia medica—the branch of pharmacy that deals with drugs and their source, preparation, and use

matrix management—an organizational concept that emphasizes the interrelationship between departments and the common area of decision making

maximum allowable cost (MAC)—based on wholesaler acquisition costs

Medicaid—a state health care coverage program with some federal funding assistance for persons with low income, minimal assets, and no health care coverage as mandated by Title XIX of the Social Security Act. Medicaid may go by different names in different states; often known as *medical assistance programs.*

medical information system (MIS)—state-of-the-art clinical information that may include anything from drug information applications to video conferencing between other hospitals

medical records—the hospital department responsible for the maintenance and review of patients' medical charts

Medicare—a federal health care coverage program for those 65 years of age and over, certain disabled persons, and persons with end-stage renal disease as mandated by Title XVIII of the Social Security Act of 1965. Medicare includes Part A and Part B, which cover both hospital care and outpatient services.

medication administration record (MAR)—a record maintained by the nursing staff containing information about the patient's medication and its frequency of administration

medication administrator—a person who administers or gives medication to patients

medication order—orders for all medications and intravenous solutions written on an order sheet or via computerized physician order entry on a hospital-wide computer system

medication regimen review (MRR)—the process to provide appropriate drug therapy for patients as part of the health care team; i.e., a licensed pharmacist must review medication use every month for all residents in a skilled nursing facility

medication-related problems (MRPs)—undesirable events a patient experiences involving drug therapy that interfere with a desired patient outcome

medication therapy management (MTM)—pharmacists are reimbursed for non-drug services such as drug therapy management for diabetes, anticoagulation, anemia, hypertension, and renal failure

medium—a solvent used in dissolution testing

memory—the storage of both data and instructions internally in a computer

meninges—the membrane that surrounds the brain and spinal cord

meningitis—inflammation of the meninges

meniscus—the outer surface of a liquid having a concave or crescent shape, caused by surface tension

metabolism—the process by which an organism converts food to energy needed for anabolism

metabolite—a chemical synthesized within cells as part of a metabolic pathway

metastasis—the spread of disease from one organ to another

meter—a basic unit of length in the metric system

metric system—a system of weights based on the meter, the gram, and the liter

micronized drug particles—very small drug particles that have a diameter in the smallest size range

microorganism—a microscopic plant or animal

milliequivalent (mEq)—one-thousandth of an equivalent weight

milling—reducing the particle size

Millis Study Commission—published a report in 1975 titled "Pharmacist for the Future." Its main premise stated that pharmacy is a knowledge profession.

minicomputer, microcomputer, or personal computer systems—systems used for well-defined and specialized applications

miotic—a drug that causes constriction of the pupil

mnemonic codes—short, easy-to-remember entries that represent a longer instruction; used to assist in the entry of data

mode of transmission—the way in which the susceptible host is moved between the portal of exit and the portal of entry

moiety—a part of a molecule that exhibits a particular set of chemical and pharmacologic characteristics

molecular form—the drug form that elicits biological responses regardless of dosage form

monastery—the dwelling place for persons under religious vows who live in ascetic simplicity

morgue—a place where a corpse is kept until released for burial

Moses Maimonides—a Hebrew physician, pharmacist and rabbi (1135–1208). A physician to the Sultan Saladin, author of a health book (*Book of Counsels*) and a handbook on poisons

mucolytic—a substance that liquefies, dissolves, or digests mucus

multidrug-resistant organism (MDRO)—microorganisms, predominantly bacteria, that are resistant to one or more classes of antimicrobial agents (antibiotics)

multiple sclerosis—a degenerative disease of the central nervous system

mydriatic—an agent that dilates the pupil of the eye

myocardial infarction (MI)—injury to the heart muscle (myocardium) due to inadequate oxygen supply caused by the occlusion of a coronary artery

narcotic—a pain-relieving drug that is habit forming and addictive

narcotic antagonists—agents that oppose or overcome the effects of a narcotic

National Association of Boards of Pharmacy (NABP)—formed in 1904 to assist member boards in developing pharmacy standards to protect the public health

National Association of Chain Drug Stores (NACDS)—an association of corporations represented by chief executive officers, many of whom are not pharmacists, and includes chain pharmacies, grocery store pharmacies, department store pharmacies, and discount outlets

National Community Pharmacists Association (NCPA)—formerly the National Association of Retail Druggists, formed in 1898; represents the interests of independent pharmacy owners

National Formulary—a database of drugs of established usefulness not found in the U.S. Pharmacopoeia

National Pharmacy Technician Association (NPTA)—the world's largest professional organization for pharmacy technicians in practice sites including community practice, hospitals, home care, long-term care, military institutions, and prison facilities, as well as management, education, and drug sales

nephritis—inflammation of the nephron

nephron—a functional unit of the kidney

neurosonology—the laboratory section of the neurology department, specifically referring to EEG, EMG, carotid Doppler, brain mapping, etc.

NKA—"no known allergies"

nomogram—a chart that determines body surface area from height and weight

non-adherence—forgetting or purposefully not taking medications as prescribed

nonmaleficence—the principle that pharmacists are obliged to "do no harm" to others in the practice of health care and/or pharmacy

nonprescription medications—also known as over-the-counter medications (OTCs), available for patients suffering from conditions that are considered self-treatable

nosocomial infections—an infection or illness that occurs as a result of the patient's stay in the hospital or health facility

not-for-profit—institutions that are not run for profit; these facilities are obliged to reinvest the excess revenue back into programs or building improvements for the benefit of the serviced population; these facilities are not obligated to pay taxes and have the ability to raise funds for charitable purposes

nursing home—provides long-term care to individuals needing extensive medical care as well as personal care around the clock

objective—the purpose or goal toward which effort is directed

obstructive jaundice—jaundice that results from an impediment to the flow of bile from the liver to the duodenum

occlusion—blockage of a blood vessel

Occupational and Safety Act of 1970—a federal law that assures every working man and woman in the nation safe and healthy working conditions; established the Occupational Safety and Health Administration (OSHA)

ointment—an oil-based, semisolid, external dosage form, usually containing a medicinal substance

oleaginous—resembling or having the properties of oil

Omnibus Budget Reconciliation Act (OBRA)—mandated some provisions that affect the profession of pharmacy: drug manufacturers are required to provide their lowest prices to Medicaid patients, and pharmacists are to provide drug use review and patient counseling

one-compartment model—the simplest case in pharmacokinetics, in which the body is thought to behave as a single homogeneous compartment

operating room—a unit in the hospital where major surgical procedures are performed

operational manual—lists those policies and procedures that affect the internal workings of the pharmacy department

orphan drugs—drugs used for diseases and conditions considered rare in the United States, for which adequate drugs have not yet been developed and do not generate incentives for drug manufacturers to research and develop

osteoporosis—a disorder characterized by abnormal porosity of bone, usually in older women

ostomy—an artificial opening into the gastrointestinal tract

outcome competency—the measurable, desired ability, knowledge, and skill achieved upon the completion of a program

outpatient department—an area of the hospital where various medical services are provided to patients who do not require a hospital bed (outpatients)

output devices—video display terminal (VDT), cathode ray tubes (CRT), printers, and plotters

over-the-counter medications (OTCs)—a drug that can be sold without a prescription

oxytocic—an agent that causes uterine contractions

palliative—a treatment that provides relief, but no cure for a condition

pandemic—a global epidemic disease

parenteral—a sterile, injectable medication; introduction of a drug or nutrient into a vein, muscle, subcutaneous tissue, artery, or spinal column; often refers to intravenous infusions of nutritional solutions; *see also* **total parenteral nutrition**

parenteral solution—sterile solutions intended for subcutaneous, intramuscular, or intravenous injection

passive diffusion—the movement of drug molecules from an area of high concentration to one of a lower concentration

pathogen—any virus, microorganism, or other substance causing disease

pathology—the study of the characteristics, causes, and effects of disease

patient accounting system—a component of the hospital information system; allows the hospital to bill and collect for its services

patient controlled analgesia (PCA) pump—a device used to administer continuous infusion, but that also allows the patient to provide boluses of pain medication as the need arises

patient medication profile—a record kept in the pharmacy of patient data and current drug therapy. It contains such information as initiation and discontinuation of medication orders and dosage form and strength. It also indicates any allergies, diagnosis, or other information pertinent to drug therapy

patient package insert (PPI)—an informational leaflet written for the lay public describing the benefits and risks of medications

patient profile—a document used to incorporate patient information, allergies, sensitivities, and all medications the patient is receiving, both active and discontinued

Patient's Bill of Rights—a declaration ensuring that all patients, inpatients, outpatients, and emergency service patients are afforded their rights in a health care institution

PC—personal computer

PCA—patient controlled analgesia

PCP—phencyclidine, a hallucinogen; also known as *busy bee, buzz, zombie*

peptic ulcer disease (PUD)—the ulceration of the stomach or duodenal lining

peptides—a compound of two or more amino acids

percentage—a percent number representing amount per hundred (e.g., 5 percent represents 5 parts per 100)

percutaneous—through the skin

per diem **reimbursement**—payment on a preset daily rate

peripheral devices—sent to a computer for processing; receive information from the central processing unit once the data have been processed

peripheral parenteral nutrition (PPN)—a short-term therapy used to provide nutrients directly into the peripheral veins; these solutions are lower in concentration of dextrose than TPN to prevent pain, irritation, and tissue damage

personal care and support services—the provision of nonprofessional services for patients in their place of residence

personal protective equipment (PPE)—protective gear worn by health care workers, made up of barriers used to prevent skin and mucous membrane exposure when contact with blood or other potentially infectious material is anticipated

pertussis—whooping cough; an acute infectious disease of the respiratory tract

pH—a measurement of acidity or alkalinity

pharmaceutical alternates—drug products that contain the same therapeutic moiety and strength but differ in the salt, ester, or dosage form

pharmaceutical care—the direct, responsible provision of medication-related care for the purpose of achieving definite outcomes that improve a patient's quality of life

pharmaceutical services—focus on rational drug therapy and include the essential administrative, clinical, distributive, and technical functions to meet this goal

pharmaceutics—the area of the pharmaceutical sciences that deals with the chemical, physical, and physiological properties of drugs and dosage forms and drug-delivery systems

pharmacist—a person who has (1) completed five, six, seven, or more years of formal education in a pharmacy school, and (2) is licensed to prepare and distribute drugs and counsel on the use of medication in the state in which he or she practices

pharmacogenetic polymorphism—genetic variations accounting for changes in severely decreased drug metabolism, or when a normal dose is given, toxic concentrations can result

pharmacogenetics—the study of the relationship between heredity and response to drugs

pharmacognosy—the study of therapeutic agents derived from natural sources (e.g., plants)

pharmacokinetics—the branch of pharmaceutics that deals with a mathematical description of drug absorption, distribution, metabolism, and excretion and their relationship to the dosage form

pharmacology—the science that deals with the origin, nature, chemistry, effects, and uses of drugs

pharmacopoeia—an authoritative treatise on drugs and their purity, preparation, and standards

pharmacotherapeutics—pertaining to the use of drugs in the prevention or treatment of disease

pharmacotherapy—the treatment of disease with medications

pharmacy—the professional practice of preparing, dispensing, monitoring, and educating about drugs

Pharmacy and Therapeutics Committee—the liaison between the department of pharmacy and the medical staff, consisting of physicians who represent the various clinical aspects; this committee selects the drugs to be used in the hospital. The pharmacy director is the secretary and a voting member of this committee

Pharmacy Code of Ethics—rules established for the profession by pharmacists that guide proper conduct for pharmacists

pharmacy, contemporary—a health service concerning itself with the knowledge of drugs and their effects on the body.

pharmacy intern—a person obtaining practical experience and training in a pharmacy to meet the requirements of the state board of pharmacy for licensure as a pharmacist

pharmacy mission—to help people make the best use of medication

pharmacy resident—a graduate from an accredited pharmacy school enrolled in a program designed to develop expert and/or specialized skills in pharmacy practice

pharmacy service—(1) the procurement, distribution, and control of all pharmaceuticals used within the facility; (2) the evaluation and dissemination of comprehensive information about drugs and their use; and (3) the monitoring, evaluation, and assurance of the quality of drug use

pharmacy technician—a person skilled in various pharmacy service activities not requiring the professional judgment of the pharmacist; has received formal or informal skill training to participate in numerous pharmacy activities in concert with and under the supervision of a registered pharmacist

Pharmacy Technician Certification Board (PTCB)—established in 1995 to provide a voluntary mechanism for a national certification program for pharmacy technicians

Pharmacy Technician Educators Council (PTEC)—a council with the mission to assist the profession of pharmacy to prepare high-quality, well-trained technical personnel through education and practical training programs

pharmacy, traditional—the art and science of compounding and dispensing medications

PharmD degree—the doctor of pharmacy degree earned after a six-year course of study; emphasizes clinical (patient-oriented) professional skills

phlebitis—inflammation of the veins

phlegm—viscous mucus secreted orally

603

physical therapy (PT)—physical manipulation for the purpose of rehabilitation

physician—an authorized practitioner of medicine

physician assistant—an authorized practitioner of medicine who works under the responsible supervision of a licensed physician

physician order entry system—direct entry of the physician's order by the physician into the computer, which can then be accessed by pharmacy and other health care disciplines

phytochemist—a person who studies plant chemistry and applies these chemicals to science

PICC—peripherally inserted central catheter

piggyback—refers to a small-volume IV solution (25–250 mL) that is run into an existing IV line over a brief period of time (e.g., 50 mL over 15 minutes)

pill—a small globular or oval medicated mass intended for oral administration

plasma—the fluid portion of the blood in which the blood cells are suspended

polymer—a high-molecular-weight substance made up of identical base units

polyurethanes—substances sometimes used for linkage in elastomers

pneumatic tube system—a method of sending medication orders through the hospital by placing it in a "tube" and sending it to a dispatcher, who then forwards it to the specific location

pneumonia—inflammation of the lungs, usually due to infection

Poison Prevention Packaging Act—a federal law mandating special packaging requirements that make it difficult for children under the age of five to open the package or container

policy—a defined course to guide and determine present and future decisions; established by an organization or employer who guides the employee to act in a manner consistent with management philosophy

polymorphism—a condition in which a substance occurs in more than one crystalline form

portal of entry—the route by which the agent enters the host; may be through breaks in the skin, inhalation of contaminants, or through insect bites

portal of exit—the route by which an agent moves from the reservoir to the susceptible host; may be through body secretions such as saliva, blood, and urine

PPN—peripheral parenteral nutrition

practice plan—an agreed-upon guide, written by pharmacists, on how pharmacy will be practiced in a particular setting

preferred drug provided (PDP)—a gatekeeper between individual and government payors under Medicare Part D

preferred provider organization (PPO)—an insurance plan that provides comprehensive health care through contracted providers

preferred vendor—the drug firm selected as the wholesaler

prefix—a word element attached to the beginning of a word to modify its meaning

prescriber—a person in health care who is permitted by law to order drugs that legally require a prescription; includes physicians, physician assistants, podiatrists, dentists, and nurse practitioners

prescription—permission, granted orally or in writing, from a physician for a patient to receive a certain medication on an outpatient basis that will help relieve or eliminate the patient's problem

prescription medication—a drug that is only available to a patient with a prescription from a licensed prescriber; also known as *legend medication*

preservatives—substances used to prevent the growth of microorganisms

primary engineering control (PEC)—a device such as a laminar flow workbench, biological safety cabinet, or compounding aseptic isolator, that provides an ISO Class 5 environment necessaryfor compounding sterile preparations

primary resources—original research articles published in journals such as the *American Journal of Hospital Pharmacy* and the *Journal of the American Medical Association*

prime vendor—a drug wholesaler who contracts directly with hospital pharmacies for the purpose of their high volume pharmaceuticals

prior approval—the prescriber must demonstrate evidence for an individual patient's need for a medication outside the approved formulary for it to be reimbursed

prn (pro re nata) order—drugs to be given as needed when a clinical situation arises

procedures—guidelines on the preferred way to perform a certain function; particular actions to be taken to carry out a policy

prodrug—a class of drugs, the pharmacological action of which results from their biotransformation in the body

product line management—an organizational concept that emphasizes the end product or category of services being delivered

prognosis—the expected outcome of the course of the disease

programs—instructions for a computer

propellant—a substance used to help expel the contents of a pressurized container

prophylaxis—prevention of or protection against disease

proportion—a proportion is formed using two ratios that are equal (e.g., $1/2 = 5/10$)

proprietary—facilities owned by one person, a family, a partnership, or a corporation; they are run like a corporate business and should make a profit for their investors

prospective drug review—a review of the patient's medication profile by a pharmacist to screen for any drug problems prior to the drug being dispensed

prospective payment system (PPS)—a method of third-party reimbursement with predetermined reimbursement rates; *see also* **diagnosis-related group (DRG)**

protected health information (PHI)—includes any individually identifiable health information, with the exclusion of employment records

proteins—macromolecules consisting of amino acids

protocol—a written description of how an activity, procedure, or function is to be accomplished

protozoa—single-celled parasitic organisms with the ability to move

psychiatric—relating to the medical treatment of mental disorders

psychotropic—a drug used to treat mental and emotional disorders

pulmonary—pertaining to the lungs

Pure Food and Drug Act of 1906—this law was passed by Congress because of concern of the risks to public health and safety associated with unsanitary and poorly labeled foods and drugs

purified protein derivative (PPD)—a product used as a skin test for tuberculosis antibodies

pyrogen—an agent that causes a rise in temperature; produced by bacteria, molds, viruses and yeasts

quality assurance—a method of monitoring actual versus desired results in an effort to ensure a certain level of quality that meets predetermined criteria

quality assurance program—a format that elaborates special basic quality assurance steps

quality standards—the minimum standards and results needed to achieve a desired level of quality

quasi-legal standards—recognized standards that are similar to laws

radiation—the use of X-rays, ultraviolet rays, or short radio waves for treatment or diagnosis

radiation therapy—the use of X-rays in the treatment of a disease

radiology (X-ray) department—an area of the hospital where diagnosis and treatment are performed using X-rays, radioisotopes, and other similar methods

radio-opaque—having the property of absorbing X-rays

radiopharmacy—a branch of pharmacy dealing with radioactive diagnostics

ratio—the relationship of two quantities (e.g., 1:10 is read as one part in 10 parts)

receptor—a cell component that combines with a drug or hormone to alter the function of the cell

recertification—a renewal of person's certification

reciprocity—the mutual exchange or interchange between two parties

reconstitute—to add a sterile solvent to a sterile active ingredient for injectable purposes

recovery room (RR)—an area in the hospital where patients are monitored and treated immediately after leaving the operating room

refractory—resistant to treatment or a stimulus

regulation—an authoritative rule dealing with details of procedure

regulatory law—the area of law that deals with governmental agencies and how they enforce the intent of the statutes under which they operate

rehabilitation facility—institutions that provide services to patients recovering from acute or traumatic events on a short-term basis

renal—pertaining to the kidney

reservoir—a place where an agent can survive

residents' rights—refers to those rights that residents have within a long-term care facility, such as confidentiality and maintenance of dignity

respiration—the breathing process

retailer—the company responsible for delivering product to patients

ribonucleic acid (RNA)—a single-stranded structure that is the molecular basis for protein synthesis

rickettsia—intercellular parasites that need to be in living cells to reproduce

robotics—technology based on a mechanical device, programmed by remote control to accomplish manual activities, such as picking medications according to a patient's computerized profile

rubella—German measles

rule of three—the process of pharmacy personnel checking a medication being prepared and dispensed three times before it is dispensed and administered to the patient

rules and regulations—standards promulgated by government agencies at the local, state, and federal levels

sanatorium—an institution for the treatment of chronic disease such as tuberculosis or nervous disorders

satellite pharmacy—a decentralized pharmacy staffed by at least a pharmacist and technician. The satellite usually handles all the needs of the units for which they are responsible.

scanners—optical recognition devices that can read preprinted characters or codes

Schedule I—a controlled substance with a high potential for abuse that currently has no approved medical use

Schedule II—drugs with high potential for abuse with severe psychological and/or physical dependence liability

Schedule III—controlled substance whose abuse may lead to moderate or low physical dependence or high psychological dependence

Schedule IV—controlled substance with less abuse potential and limited physical and psychological dependence

Schedule V—drugs and preparations with limited quantities of certain narcotic drugs

script—an abbreviated form of "prescription"

secondary plant metabolite—derived from primary plant metabolites

secondary resources—indexing and abstracting services used as part of a research strategy

secondary storage—data and programs maintained on tapes or discs

sedative—a drug used to allay anxiety and excitement; often used to help a patient sleep

sepsis—the presence of pathogenic organisms in the blood

serum—the clear fluid of the blood separated from solid parts

side effects—the known effects of a drug experienced by most people taking the drug; these are usually minor

sig—an abbreviation for *signa or* signatura; includes directions that should be given to the patient

signa—an abbreviation for *signatura* (*see* **signatura**)

signatura—directions given to the patient: how much medication to take, how often to take it, and when to take it

signs—objective bodily evidence of distress found by physical examination

site survey—the visit by representatives of the American Society of Health-System Pharmacists to review training programs to ascertain compliance with standards

skilled nursing facility (SNF)—*See* **nursing homes**

soft copy—visual display units

software—the actual programs for the computer system

solution—a homogeneous mixture of one or more substances dispersed in a dissolving solvent; a clear liquid with all components completely dissolved

solution balance—a single unequal arm balance used for weighing large amounts

solvation—the process by which a solute is incorporated into the solvent

solvent—a substance used to dissolve another substance

stability—a condition that resists change; for example, a drug maintains potency

standard—a reference to be used in evaluating institutional programs and services

standard of care—the acceptable level of professional practice by which the actions of a professional are judged

standard precautions—universal precautions developed by the Occupational Safety and Health Administration (OSHA) for infection control safety measures, designed to protect health care workers and patients from infections

standards of practice—rules that pharmacists establish for the profession that represent the preferred way to practice

staphylococcus (plural, staphylococci)—microorganism of the family *Micrococcaceae* that is the most common cause of localized suppurative infections

state board of pharmacy—a body established to ensure that the public is well served professionally by pharmacists

STAT order—*statim*; "to be given immediately"

sterile—free from microorganisms

sterilization—the act or process of rendering sterile; the complete destruction of microorganisms by heat or bactericidal compound

sterilizing filter—filters used to sieve, absorb, and entrap foreign particles to achieve sterilization

stop order—an instruction to stop medication. An automatic stop order requires a physician's renewal order for the medication or the medication will be discontinued

structure criteria—specifying necessary resources (e.g., equipment)

styptic—an agent that stops or slows bleeding by contracting blood vessels when applied locally

subcutaneous—under the skin

subcutaneously—under the skin; introduced beneath the skin (e.g., subcutaneous injections)

sublingual—under the tongue

subscription—an indication on a prescriber's prescription to the pharmacist of the amount of medication to be dispensed

sudorific—a substance that causes sweating; also called a *diaphoretic*

suffix—a word element attached to the end of a word to create a new word with a specific meaning

superscription—the "Rx" symbol on the prescription

supportive pharmacy personnel—another term for pharmacy technician

suppository—solid dosage forms for insertion into body cavities (e.g., rectum, vagina, urethra) where they melt at body temperature

surface active agents—substances that lower the surface tension of liquids

surfactants—surface active agents, commonly known as *wetting agents*

susceptible host—must be present for the agent to be transferred; the host is usually vulnerable to disease due to lack of resistance

suspending agents—chemical additives used in suspensions to "thicken" the liquid and slow the settling of particles

suspension—a liquid containing finely divided drug particles uniformly distributed

symptom—subjective evidence of a disease; evidence of disease as perceived by the patient

syncope—fainting; a transient loss of consciousness due to inadequate blood flow to the brain

syndrome—a group of signs and symptoms that characterize a particular abnormality

synergies—groups working together in cooperation

synergism—a joint action of agents in which the total effect of the combination is greater than the sum of their individual independent effects

synthesize—to produce by bringing elements together to form a chemical compound

syrup—a concentrated sugar solution that may have an added medicinal agent

systemic—relating to the body as a whole, rather than individual parts or organs

systemic action—affects the body as a whole

systemic side effect—an effect on the whole body, but secondary to the intended effect

system software—contains the operating system that includes master programs for coordinating the activities of the hardware and software in a computer system

systolic—the force exerted by the blood when the ventricles are in a state of contraction

table of contents—an index for easy referral to the appropriate policies and procedures

tablet—a solid dosage form of varying weight, size, and shape that contains a medicinal substance

tachycardia—rapid heart rate

tare—a weight used to counterbalance the container holding the substance being weighed

taring—deduction from the gross weight of a substance and its container made in allowance for the weight of the container

tax-free alcohol—ethyl alcohol obtained with no federal tax under applicable federal regulations; to be used only for diagnostic and therapeutic purposes

telephone order—an order for a drug or other form of treatment that is given over the phone to an authorized receiver by an authorized prescriber

teratogenic—a substance that interferes with normal prenatal development

tertiary resources—very general resources to use in the beginning of a search

testosterone—a hormone that produces secondary sex characteristics in the male

Theophrastus—a Greek philosopher and botanist who classified plants by pharmaceutical actions

therapeutic—provision of treatment of a disease, infirmity, or symptom by various methods

therapeutic alternates—drug products that contain different therapeutic moieties but that are of the same pharmacologic or therapeutic class

therapeutic effect—a healing, curative, or ameliorating effect

therapeutic equivalent—a drug product that, when administered in the same amount, will provide the same therapeutic effect and pharmacokinetic characteristics as another drug to which it is compared

therapeutic substitution—the substitution of one drug product with another that differs in composition but is considered to have the same or very similar pharmacologic and therapeutic activity

therapy—the treatment of disease

thermal sterilization—heat; moist-heat or dry-heat are methods of thermal sterilization

thrombophlebitis—inflammation of a vein with a secondary blood clot formation

thrombosis—the development or presence of a blood clot

tincture—an alcoholic or hydro-alcoholic solution containing a medicinal substance

T_{max}—in biopharmaceutics, indicates how long it takes to reach maximum drug concentration in the body's circulation

TO—an abbreviation for "telephone order"; sometimes referred to as VO (verbal order)

tocolytic—a substance that delays or prolongs the birth process

topical—pertaining to the surface of a part of the body

total parenteral nutrition (TPN)—intravenous nutrition comprised of any or all of the following: amino acids, dextrose, lipids, vitamins, minerals, trace elements, electrolytes, and water in a prepared sterile solution that infuses into a large central venous blood vessel. TPN provides all of the essential nutrients needed for patients to survive if they are unable to ingest nutrients.

toxic—poisonous

toxicity—the degree to which something is poisonous

toxicology—the scientific study of poisons and their actions, detection, and treatment of conditions caused by the

toxin—a poison

toxin, bacterial—a noxious or poisonous product that causes the formation of antibodies called antitoxins

TPN—total parenteral nutrition

trachea—the windpipe

tracheotomy—an incision into the trachea

training program—the whole course of study (didactic, laboratory, and experiential) to prepare the student for a career

tranquilizer—a drug to relieve anxiety or agitation

transdermal—entering through the dermis or skin, as in administration of a drug applied to the skin in ointment or patch form

triturate—to reduce particle size and mix one powder with another

troche—a small tablet intended to dissolve in the mouth to deliver medication to the mouth or throat

tuberculin skin test (TST)—a test performed to identify exposure to the tuberculosis bacillus

turnover rate—the rate of drug inventory; calculated by dividing the total dollars spent to purchase drugs in one year by the actual pharmacy inventory dollars

unidirectional flow—air flow moving in a single direction in a robust and uniform manner to sweep particles away from the critical processing area related to laminar air flow

unit dose—a single-use package of a drug. In a unit-dose distribution system, a single dose of each medication is dispensed prior to the time of administration.

unit-dose distribution system—medication is distributed in single dose or unit-dose form from the pharmacy for use by the individual administering the drug

universal claim form (UCF)—a pharmacy prescription claim form utilized to serve as the basis for reimbursement of prescriptions dispensed

Universal-Standard Precautions—a set of standards mandated by the Occupational Safety and Health Administration, based on Centers for Disease Control and Prevention recommendations to reduce the risk of occupational exposure to disease

urticaria—eruption or rash associated with severe itching

USP—the United States Pharmacopoeia

utilization review—the work of a committee that determines how use of resources meets criteria and standards

vaccination—introduction of a vaccine into the body to produce immunity to a particular disease (e.g., smallpox inoculation)

vaccine—a suspension of attenuated or killed bacteria, viruses, or rickettsia administered for the prevention, amelioration, or treatment of infectious diseases (e.g., tetanus)

valence—electrons that are associated with bonds between elements

validation—a proof or confirmation of validity

vascular—related to or containing blood vessels

vasoconstriction—the narrowing of blood vessels

vasoconstrictor—a process, drug, or substance that causes constriction of blood vessels

vasodilation—the relaxation of smooth muscles of the vascular system that produces dilation of the blood vessel

vasodilator—an agent or drug that causes dilatation of the blood vessels; increases the caliber of the blood vessels

vector-borne transmission—infection through contact with infection-carrying insects or animals

vehicle transmission—infection through contact with contaminated food or water

ventricular fibrillation—the rapid, ineffectual action of the ventricle of the heart

verbal order—an order for a drug or other treatment that is given verbally to an authorized receiver by an authorized prescriber

verification—confirmation of the truth of a fact

verified—reviewed and approved as true and authentic

vertical health integration—a process that provides a continuum of care for the patient from hospital care to ambulatory care, to home care, to long-term care

vertical hood—a biological containment hood used to prepare anticancer drugs and other selective injectables

vertical laminar flow hood—a workstation that provides a vertical flow of filtered air to maintain a particulate-free environment

vertigo—a sensation the patient experiences that the external world is revolving around the patient; dizziness

video display terminal (VDT)—displays computer activities; sometimes referred to as *CRT* (cathode ray tube)

virus—a submicroscopic agent of infectious disease that is capable of reproduction

viscosity—an expression of the resistance of a fluid to flow

vitamin—a general term for a number of organic substances that occur in many foods in small amounts required for normal growth and maintenance of life

VO—a verbal order

volatile—evaporates at low temperature

volumetric check—an accuracy check for the rate of flow for an intravenous infusion

wetting agent—a surface active agent that allows materials to penetrate into a solid surface

wholesaler acquisition costs—includes contracts negotiated between the provider and the pharmaceutical industry

word elements—in medical terminology, made up of word roots, prefixes, and suffixes

word root—the primary building block of words; the core word used to identify fundamental anatomic and physiologic nomenclature

written order—an order for a drug or other form of treatment that is written on the appropriate form by an authorized prescriber

NOTE: Page references in *italics* refer to figures, illustrations, and tables.

IMPORTANT! READ CAREFULLY: This End User License Agreement ("Agreement") sets forth the conditions by which Cengage Learning will make electronic access to the Cengage Learning-owned licensed content and associated media, software, documentation, printed materials, and electronic documentation contained in this package and/or made available to you via this product (the "Licensed Content"), available to you (the "End User"). BY CLICKING THE "I ACCEPT" BUTTON AND/OR OPENING THIS PACKAGE, YOU ACKNOWLEDGE THAT YOU HAVE READ ALL OF THE TERMS AND CONDITIONS, AND THAT YOU AGREE TO BE BOUND BY ITS TERMS, CONDITIONS, AND ALL APPLICABLE LAWS AND REGULATIONS GOVERNING THE USE OF THE LICENSED CONTENT.

1.0 SCOPE OF LICENSE

1.1 <u>Licensed Content</u>. The Licensed Content may contain portions of modifiable content ("Modifiable Content") and content which may not be modified or otherwise altered by the End User ("Non-Modifiable Content"). For purposes of this Agreement, Modifiable Content and Non-Modifiable Content may be collectively referred to herein as the "Licensed Content." All Licensed Content shall be considered Non-Modifiable Content, unless such Licensed Content is presented to the End User in a modifiable format and it is clearly indicated that modification of the Licensed Content is permitted.

1.2 Subject to the End User's compliance with the terms and conditions of this Agreement, Cengage Learning hereby grants the End User, a nontransferable, nonexclusive, limited right to access and view a single copy of the Licensed Content on a single personal computer system for noncommercial, internal, personal use only. The End User shall not (i) reproduce, copy, modify (except in the case of Modifiable Content), distribute, display, transfer, sublicense, prepare derivative work(s) based on, sell, exchange, barter or transfer, rent, lease, loan, resell, or in any other manner exploit the Licensed Content; (ii) remove, obscure, or alter any notice of Cengage Learning's intellectual property rights present on or in the Licensed Content, including, but not limited to, copyright, trademark, and/or patent notices; or (iii) disassemble, decompile, translate, reverse engineer, or otherwise reduce the Licensed Content.

2.0 TERMINATION

2.1 Cengage Learning may at any time (without prejudice to its other rights or remedies) immediately terminate this Agreement and/or suspend access to some or all of the Licensed Content, in the event that the End User does not comply with any of the terms and conditions of this Agreement. In the event of such termination by Cengage Learning, the End User shall immediately return any and all copies of the Licensed Content to Cengage Learning.

3.0 PROPRIETARY RIGHTS

3.1 The End User acknowledges that Cengage Learning owns all rights, title and interest, including, but not limited to all copyright rights therein, in and to the Licensed Content, and that the End User shall not take any action inconsistent with such ownership. The Licensed Content is protected by U.S., Canadian and other applicable copyright laws and by international treaties, including the Berne Convention and the Universal Copyright Convention. Nothing contained in this Agreement shall be construed as granting the End User any ownership rights in or to the Licensed Content.

3.2 Cengage Learning reserves the right at any time to withdraw from the Licensed Content any item or part of an item for which it no longer retains the right to publish, or which it has reasonable grounds to believe infringes copyright or is defamatory, unlawful, or otherwise objectionable.

4.0 PROTECTION AND SECURITY

4.1 The End User shall use its best efforts and take all reasonable steps to safeguard its copy of the Licensed Content to ensure that no unauthorized reproduction, publication, disclosure, modification, or distribution of the Licensed Content, in whole or in part, is made. To the extent that the End User becomes aware of any such unauthorized use of the Licensed Content, the End User shall immediately notify Cengage Learning. Notification of such violations may be made by sending an e-mail to infringement@cengage.com.

5.0 MISUSE OF THE LICENSED PRODUCT

5.1 In the event that the End User uses the Licensed Content in violation of this Agreement, Cengage Learning shall have the option of electing liquidated damages, which shall include all profits generated by the End User's use of the Licensed Content plus interest computed at the maximum rate permitted by law and all legal fees and other expenses incurred by Cengage Learning in enforcing its rights, plus penalties.

6.0 FEDERAL GOVERNMENT CLIENTS

6.1 Except as expressly authorized by Cengage Learning, Federal Government clients obtain only the rights specified in this Agreement and no other rights. The Government acknowledges that (i) all software and related documentation incorporated in the Licensed Content is existing commercial computer software within the meaning of FAR 27.405(b)(2); and (2) all other data delivered in whatever form, is limited rights data within the meaning of FAR 27.401. The restrictions in this section are acceptable as consistent with the Government's need for software and other data under this Agreement.

7.0 DISCLAIMER OF WARRANTIES AND LIABILITIES

7.1 Although Cengage Learning believes the Licensed Content to be reliable, Cengage Learning does not guarantee or warrant (i) any information or materials contained in or produced by the Licensed Content, (ii) the accuracy, completeness or reliability of the Licensed Content, or (iii) that the Licensed Content is free from errors or other material defects. THE LICENSED PRODUCT IS PROVIDED "AS IS," WITHOUT ANY WARRANTY OF ANY KIND AND CENGAGE LEARNING DISCLAIMS ANY AND ALL WARRANTIES, EXPRESSED OR IMPLIED, INCLUDING, WITHOUT LIMITATION, WARRANTIES OF MERCHANTABILITY OR FITNESS FOR A PARTICULAR PURPOSE. IN NO EVENT SHALL CENGAGE LEARNING BE LIABLE FOR: INDIRECT, SPECIAL, PUNITIVE OR CONSEQUENTIAL DAMAGES INCLUDING FOR LOST PROFITS, LOST DATA, OR OTHERWISE. IN NO EVENT SHALL CENGAGE LEARNING'S AGGREGATE LIABILITY HEREUNDER, WHETHER ARISING IN CONTRACT, TORT, STRICT LIABILITY OR OTHERWISE, EXCEED THE AMOUNT OF FEES PAID BY THE END USER HEREUNDER FOR THE LICENSE OF THE LICENSED CONTENT.

8.0 GENERAL

8.1 <u>Entire Agreement</u>. This Agreement shall constitute the entire Agreement between the Parties and supersedes all prior Agreements and understandings oral or written relating to the subject matter hereof.

8.2 <u>Enhancements/Modifications of Licensed Content</u>. From time to time, and in Cengage Learning's sole discretion, Cengage Learning may advise the End User of updates, upgrades, enhancements and/or improvements to the Licensed Content, and may permit the End User to access and use, subject to the terms and conditions of this Agreement, such modifications, upon payment of prices as may be established by Cengage Learning.

8.3 <u>No Export</u>. The End User shall use the Licensed Content solely in the United States and shall not transfer or export, directly or indirectly, the Licensed Content outside the United States.

8.4 <u>Severability</u>. If any provision of this Agreement is invalid, illegal, or unenforceable under any applicable statute or rule of law, the provision shall be deemed omitted to the extent that it is invalid, illegal, or unenforceable. In such a case, the remainder of the Agreement shall be construed in a manner as to give greatest effect to the original intention of the parties hereto.

8.5 <u>Waiver</u>. The waiver of any right or failure of either party to exercise in any respect any right provided in this Agreement in any instance shall not be deemed to be a waiver of such right in the future or a waiver of any other right under this Agreement.

8.6 <u>Choice of Law/Venue</u>. This Agreement shall be interpreted, construed, and governed by and in accordance with the laws of the State of New York, applicable to contracts executed and to be wholly performed therein, without regard to its principles governing conflicts of law. Each party agrees that any proceeding arising out of or relating to this Agreement or the breach or threatened breach of this Agreement may be commenced and prosecuted in a court in the State and County of New York. Each party consents and submits to the nonexclusive personal jurisdiction of any court in the State and County of New York in respect of any such proceeding.

8.7 <u>Acknowledgment</u>. By opening this package and/or by accessing the Licensed Content on this Web site, THE END USER ACKNOWLEDGES THAT IT HAS READ THIS AGREEMENT, UNDERSTANDS IT, AND AGREES TO BE BOUND BY ITS TERMS AND CONDITIONS. IF YOU DO NOT ACCEPT THESE TERMS AND CONDITIONS, YOU MUST NOT ACCESS THE LICENSED CONTENT AND RETURN THE LICENSED PRODUCT TO CENGAGE LEARNING (WITHIN 30 CALENDAR DAYS OF THE END USER'S PURCHASE) WITH PROOF OF PAYMENT ACCEPTABLE TO CENGAGE LEARNING, FOR A CREDIT OR A REFUND. Should the End User have any questions/comments regarding this Agreement, please contact Cengage Learning at Delmar .help@cengage.com.

StudyWARE™ to Accompany *Pharmacy Practice for Technicians, Fourth Edition*

Minimum System Requirements

- Operating systems: Microsoft Windows 2000 w/SP 4, Windows XP w/SP 2, Windows Vista w/SP 1
- Processor: Minimum required by Operating System
- Memory: Minimum required by Operating System
- Hard Drive Space: 10 MB
- Screen resolution: 800 x 600 pixels
- CD-ROM drive
- Sound card and listening device required for audio features
- Flash Player 9. The Adobe Flash Player is free, and can be downloaded from http://www.adobe.com/products/flashplayer/.

Setup Instructions

1. Insert disc into CD-ROM drive. The StudyWARE™ installation program should start automatically. If it does not, go to step 2.
2. From My Computer, double-click the icon for the CD drive.
3. Double-click the *setup.exe* file to start the program.

Technical Support

Telephone: 1-800-648-7450
8:30 A.M.-6:30 P.M. Eastern Time
E-mail: delmar.help@cengage.com

the terrible sea. He lifted peats on to the fire and lit a lantern from the flames. Then he told Jannet about the night he had found Gioga in the rock pool among the skerries; how, when he lifted her out of the water, a fur skin slipped away from her, and how he let the skin drown.

'What does that mean?' she asked, hardly daring to look at him.

'You know as well as I what that means. Gioga is not one of us, but one of them. She's a child of the sea.'

'Will she ever go back to them?'

'Not without her skin. She can't. She has to stay with us. No matter how many times the seal people had come for her, she could never return with them. She was quite safe, you see. You had no need to do what you did.'

Wind slammed against the door, then dipped into silence. The beasts lowed in their straw.

'Why didn't you tell me about the seal skin?'

'Why didn't you tell me about Hill Marliner?' he asked.

The husband and wife stared at each other, aware of their own guilt and ashamed of it.

'What will happen now?' asked Jannet.

'We will see,' Munroe said. 'When dawn comes, I think we will see.'

ALSO AVAILABLE IN LAUREL-LEAF BOOKS:

SNAKE DREAMER, *Priscilla Galloway*

TRULY GRIM TALES, *Priscilla Galloway*

ANGELS ON THE ROOF, *Martha Moore*

UNDER THE MERMAID ANGEL, *Martha Moore*

KISSING DOORKNOBS, *Terry Spencer Hesser*

WHIRLIGIG, *Paul Fleischman*

RADIANCE DESCENDING, *Paula Fox*

THIN ICE, *Marsha Qualey*

THE WAR IN GEORGIA, *Jerrie Oughton*

THE SQUIRE'S TALE, *Gerald Morris*